Commissioning Editor: Serena Bureau
Project Development Manager: Kim Benson
Production Manager: Mark Sanderson
Project Manager: Hilary Hewitt
Design Direction: Barrie Carr

Percutaneous Central Venous and Arterial Catheterisation

THIRD EDITION

IAN PETER LATTO MB, BS, FRCA, DA
Clinical Teacher, University of Wales College of Medicine, Cardiff
Consultant Anaesthetist, University Hospital of Wales, Cardiff

W. SHANG NG MB, BCh, FRCA
Clinical Teacher, University of Wales College of Medicine,
Cardiff Consultant Anaesthetist, University Hospital of Wales, Cardiff

PETER L. JONES RD, MB, BCh, FRCA
Clinical Teacher, University of Wales College of Medicine, Cardiff
Consultant Anaesthetist and Clinical Physiologist, University
Hospital of Wales, Cardiff

BRIAN JENKINS MB, BS, FRCA
Senior Lecturer in Anaesthetics, University of Wales College of Medicine,
Cardiff

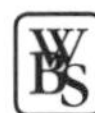 W.B. SAUNDERS

London • Edinburgh • New York • Philadelphia • St Louis • Sydney • Toronto 2000

WB SAUNDERS
An imprint of Harcourt Publishers Limited

First edition published in 1981
Second edition 1992

ISBN 0 7020 2509 7

Cataloguing in Publication Data:
Catalogue records for this book are available from the British Library and the US Library of Congress.

Note
Medical knowledge is constantly changing. As new information becomes available, changes in treatment, procedures, equipment and the use of drugs become necessary. The authors, contributors and the publishers have taken care to ensure that the information given in this text is accurate and up to date. However, readers are strongly advised to confirm that the information, especially with regard to drug usage, complies with the latest legislation and standards of practice.

Typeset by Kolam Information Services Pvt Ltd, Pondicherry, India

The publisher's policy is to use **paper manufactured from sustainable forests**

Printed in China

Contents

Authors and Contributors

Ian Peter Latto
MB BS FRCA DA
Clinical Teacher, University of Wales College of Medicine, Cardiff
Consultant Anaesthetist, University Hospital of Wales, Cardiff

W. Shang Ng
MB BCh FRCA
Clinical Teacher, University of Wales College of Medicine, Cardiff
Consultant Anaesthetist, University Hospital of Wales, Cardiff

Peter L. Jones
MB BCh FRCA
Clinical Teacher, University of Wales College of Medicine, Cardiff
Consultant Anaesthetist and Clinical Physiologist, University Hospital of Wales, Cardiff

Brian J. Jenkins
MB BS FRCA
Senior Lecturer in Anaesthetics, University of Wales College of Medicine, Cardiff

With contributions by

George P. Findlay
MB ChB FRCA
Consultant Intensivist, Critical Care Directorate, University Hospital of Wales, Cardiff
(Chapter 4)

I. Quiroga
LMC FRCS
Research Fellow in Transplantation, University Hospital of Wales, Cardiff
(Section 'Percutaneous Insertion of a Central Catheter for Haemodialysis' in Chapter 3)

With acknowledgement for assistance in producing the section on PICC lines

V. Aston
RGN
Chemotherapy Nurse Specialist
Velindre NHS Trust, Cardiff

Foreword

There are many situations in acute medicine and anaesthesia where catheterisation of the central veins is essential for the management of the seriously ill patient, and for repeated access to central veins. A large number of techniques have been developed to cannulate each vein, but their descriptions sometimes utilise unfamiliar anatomical terms. In the first edition in 1981, we standardised the terminology and offered detailed instructions. This approach proved to be of practical value and was extended into the second edition in 1992, adding a large section devoted to the paediatric patient.

The pace of change has increased so that my colleagues have, of necessity, decided to revise and update the text. Sections are added, directed to the intensive care unit, especially on avoiding infection and on arterial cannulation, which will also be useful to radiologists and others. I am pleased, and proud, that my colleagues continue to develop and improve the subject matter that is of great practical value. There are few practitioners in clinical practice who will not now find this book useful. It should reduce confusion and save lives.

Michael Rosen
CBE, Hon LID, FRCA, FRCOG, FRCS
Emeritus Professor of Anaesthetics
University of Wales College of Medicine, Cardiff
2000

Preface to the First Edition

Catheterisation of the great veins has become an important manoeuvre both for measuring the central venous pressure and for carrying out long-term intravenous alimentation. Furthermore, in an emergency – as after acute haemorrhage with peripheral vasoconstriction – it may be impossible to catheterise a peripheral vein percutaneously and only a central vein may be available for the rapid restoration of blood volume. Most hospital doctors will be faced with this situation at some time. Even clinicians who work regularly in the cardiovascular and neurosurgical fields, in which central venous catheterisation is frequently employed, may find their usual techniques unsuccessful. In such circumstances they have to perform an unfamiliar technique quickly yet safely perhaps without the benefit of previous experience. At that time it is often difficult to call to mind all the details of the numerous techniques available, which is our justification for bringing together the major methods of percutaneous central venous catheterisation in a practical handbook, using a systematic format and illustrating each technique by diagrams.

Our presentation of the major methods is not exhaustive and the basis of our selection is discussed in Chapter 1, 'Choosing the vein'. The principles governing the choice of equipment are described in Chapter 2, but, once again, it has proved impractical to discuss the whole range available.

In the remaining six chapters, we have made what we hope is the most useful selection from the different approaches to each vein, including a number of variations on some; for example, eleven techniques for cannulating the internal jugular vein are described, althought, even then, a number of minor variations have had to be excluded. The techniques chosen have not been selected on the results of controlled comparative trials; rather they reflect our opinions based on personal experience and a review of the literature. Since we have not tested each method personally, the original authors' escriptions of their techniques have been retained, although the anatomical terminology has, in some cases, been altered for the sake of uniformity. When it seemed helpful to clarify the description, we have done so in italics. The text also indicates when a technique was adopted by the original authors specifically for neonates or infants.

We hope this handbook will prove useful to those who work in the operating theatre, intensive therapy unit, casualty department, obsteric unit and all other units where central venous catheterisation may be required.

Michael Rosen
Ian Peter Latto
W. Shang Ng

Preface to the Third Edition

The usefulness of central venous access in a wide range of clinical applications remains as crucial as ever. An important and developing application is the percutaneous insertion of special catheters for haemodialysis. The shortcomings of repeated peripheral venepuncture have become more appreciated and nurse practitioners have eagerly taken up the use of peripherally inserted central catheters (PICC) in fields such as oncology, improving the quality of care that can be offered to patients.

There have been few major additions to the range of techniques suitable for central venous access. However, demand has stimulated improvements in catheter technology suitable for renal dialysis and PICC lines.

There is increasing interest in ultrasound devices designed to improve successful vascular access and to reduce complications. Whilst ultrasound guidance is useful in difficult cases and for teaching purposes, the majority of central venous cannulations will continue to be carried out using conventional anatomical landmarks.

Continuing reports of serious complications associated with central venous access suggest that training and supervision of operators could be improved. Those responsible for the care of patients who have central venous catheters in place must remain vigilant to the potential for many life-threatening complications.

Interventionist radiologists have claimed that they are the most appropriate specialists to insert central venous catheters for long-term use. They criticise the current technique of surgical cut-down as being unnecessarily invasive and more distressing for the patient. These procedures are often carried out under general anaesthesia with its additional risks. Furthermore, the cut-down technique may result in the vein being unsuitable for use again. Unquestionably, cut-down and 'blind' percutaneous techniques as practised by surgeons, anaesthetists and other clinicians are associated with a significant failure rate and incidence of complications. These twin problems should be reduced with improved training of operators and perhaps the increased use of ultrasound devices.

Radiologists claim that their ready access to venography and ultrasound devices must make their percutaneous insertion of central venous catheters more sure and less liable to complication. This sounds plausible but has not yet been subjected to detailed scrutiny. This reservation is reflected in studies in which – in spite of the apparent advantages offered by sophisticated aids – subclavian venepuncture and catheterisation by interventionist radiologists are still associated with significant complications such as pneumothorax and malpositioning. Other specialists have voiced their strong opposition to the concept of central venous lines being the sole preserve of radiologists.

What is certain is that central venous catheters will continue to be inserted by a variety of practitioners, including nurses, in a wide range of clinical settings. Interventionist radiologists have a role especially in the planned insertion of long-term catheters and possibly in 'problem' cases, particularly in paediatric practice. However, apart from other considerations, logistics alone will prevent them providing a universal central venous catheterisation service. It would seem sensible to review the pattern of work and requirements of any particular unit or hospital before investing in such a service.

The long-term care of patients with central venous catheters and the prevention of related infection is a specialised subject. A practitioner in intensive care medicine has contributed a new chapter devoted to this field.

A major addition to this new edition is a section dealing with the practical aspects of arterial cannulation. Practitioners who need central venous access for the care of their patients may also require arterial access for haemodynamic measurements as well as for sampling for biochemical analysis. It was thought that those who seek guidance for the one procedure would appreciate the availability of information concerning the other.

It is hoped that this one book brings together all the practical guidance necessary to achieve successful and complication-free vascular access.

The editors would like to record their appreciation of Professor Michael Rosen, who has now retired as one of the editors of this book. Professor Rosen conceived the idea for this book and remains the inspiration behind this work.

Ian Peter Latto
W. Shang Ng
Peter L. Jones
Brian J. Jenkins
2000

References

Adam A. Insertion of long-term central venous catheters: time for a new look (editorial). British Medical Journal 1995; **311**:341 (correspondence 1090–1).

Funaki B, Szymski GX, Hackworth *et al*. Radiologic placement of subcutaneous infusion chest ports for long-term central venous access. American Journal of Roentgenology 1997; **169**:1431.

Crowley JJ, Pereira JK, Harris LS, Becker CJ. Peripherally inserted central catheters: experience in 523 children. Radiology 1997; **204**:617.

Acknowledgements

We wish to thank members of the Department of Medical Illustration at the University Hospital of Wales for some of the artwork. We are indebted to various editors, publishers and manufacturers for permission to reproduce figures and tables.

Many thanks are due to the secretarial staff of the Department of Anaesthetics and Intensive Care Medicine at the University Hospital of Wales.

Special thanks go to Mrs Val Aston, RGN, Chemotherapy Nurse Specialist, Velindre NHS Trust, Cardiff, one of the leading exponents of this development in the United Kingdom, for her invaluable advice and information regarding PICC lines.

Part 1

Central Venous Catheterisation: General considerations and adult procedures

1 • Choosing the Vein

PETER LATTO

Before 1960 peripheral venous pressure was frequently used to judge the state of intravascular volume.[1] This technique was abandoned with the introduction of central venous pressure measurement. Surprisingly, though no longer used, peripheral venous pressure has been shown to reflect central venous pressure quite accurately under controlled circumstances.[1] The history of central venous catheters from the time of Stephen Hales in 1733 to the pioneering work of Bleichroder in 1905 and Forssmann in 1929 has been carefully reviewed by Kalso.[2]

The great majority of central venous catheters are used for measuring trends in central venous pressure or for infusing drugs or alimentation fluid into the central circulation. Small-diameter catheters are satisfactory for this purpose. In a few cases (probably less than 1%) a Seldinger technique with a vein dilator may be used to insert a large-diameter catheter into a central vein in order to facilitate rapid infusion of crystalloid or colloid solutions in shocked patients.

Clinical Trends

Cubital and femoral vein routes were reported to be most popular during the early years of central venous catheterisation.[2] Until the late 1970s in anaesthetic practice in the UK many clinicians appeared to use only the arm veins. In an unpublished survey in Cardiff in 1979 it was shown that 30 clinicians questioned used arm veins as their preferred route. Other routes were considered only if cannulation through arm veins was unsuccessful. If this was the case some anaesthetists attempted an alternative percutaneous route whilst others called for the assistance of a surgeon to perform a cut-down. Surgical cut-downs were certainly much more widely used before 1990 than they are today. However, with improved clinical skills and the availability of a wider range of equipment, it is now very rare in anaesthetic practice for an experienced clinician to fail with percutaneous techniques in adult patients. Since publication of the first edition of this book in 1981 one of the outstanding trends in central venous catheterisation practice has been the increasing use of the internal jugular vein. Indeed, this vein is now used routinely in most centres for cardiac anaesthesia. With the advent of the J wire, which facilitates successful cannulation, it can be confidently predicted that there will be a trend towards more frequent use of the external jugular vein. At the same time there appears to be a marked decrease in the use of the subclavian route in anaesthetic practice although this route is still widely used in the field of intensive care especially for the administration of parenteral nutrition.

The Cardiff anaesthetic records (approximately 20 000 patients per year between 1972 and 1977) show some trends in the overall use of central venous lines. In 1972 the incidence was 4.1% of all anaesthetics and in 1977 it was 6.7%. These figures have remained roughly constant, the rates between 1985 and 1988 (approximately 23 000 patients per year) being 6.8%, 6.8%, 6.9% and 7% respectively.

Local anaesthesia is usually adequate for cannulating superficial veins; whilst some clinicians cannulate deep veins under local anaesthesia, many wait until the patient has been anaesthetised. One report showed significant cardiovascular stimulation during percutaneous insertion of arterial and pulmonary artery catheters prior to induction of anaesthesia in patients with coronary artery disease,[3] although a later study did not substantiate this finding.[4] However, it was recommended that these patients should be sedated and treated with antianginal drugs if required. Clinicians carrying out such techniques in these patients should be adequately supervised if they have limited skill and experience.

The Learning Curve

Whilst experienced clinicians rarely fail in attempts to insert internal jugular vein catheters, many central venous catheters are inserted by inexperienced clinicians. In a 1982 study from Dallas, Texas, the success rate of medical house officers using jugular and subclavian veins was 363 out of 470 attempts (77%).[5] The success rate was improved if the attempt was made under elective circumstances and if the vein was initially located with a small seeker needle. Only 62% of attempts were successful when catheterisations were carried out during cardiopulmonary resuscitation. The authors recommended that no more than three attempts should be permitted with a large needle at the same site.

In another study involving intensive care patients the failure rate for subclavian and internal jugular routes was 19.4% for inexperienced and 10.1% for experienced clinicians.[6] The complication rate was 11% for inexperienced and 5.4% for experienced clinicians. Inexperienced clinicians caused fewer complications when attempts were carried out while patients were anaesthetised and mechanically ventilated than in conscious patients breathing spontaneously. The success rate for central venous cannulation is higher for experienced clinicians under elective circumstances in the operating theatre than when performed by inexperienced clinicians under emergency circumstances.

In yet a further study, house officers attempting to insert catheters in patients receiving intensive care had a success rate of only 74%.[7] A wide variety of insertion sites were used and both elective and emergency cases were studied. Their complication rate was 6.1%. Pleural complications were the most serious and insertion of chest drains was commonly needed. These authors recommended that the internal jugular vein should be used in preference to the external jugular or subclavian vein. Other authors have suggested that a medial antecubital vein should be used in emergency conditions to reduce the number of complications.[8] A Seldinger technique for arm veins with a vein dilator could be an added help. In seriously ill patients arm veins may be too small to successfully use a needle/cannula method. Manufacturers were urged to make suitable Seldinger guide wire equipment available.

Initial Training

How should the junior doctor acquire skills at central venous cannulation? It has been recommended that the trainee should practise initially on manikins or cadavers.[8] This advice does not, however, appear to be followed in many hospitals. In addition the trainee should be carefully supervised and possibly make his early attempts on aneasthetised rather than conscious patients. When learning a subclavian technique, the ideal clinical situation would be an anaesthetised or unconscious patient with a chest drain already *in situ*. It was stressed that clinicians should acquire expertise with both an internal jugular and a subclavian technique. Trainees should be taught to avoid if possible, but also to recognise, and treat any complications that might arise. The supericial veins of the arm and neck require less skill than the subclavian and internal jugular routes and the 'see one, do one, teach one' method of training is often used. Indeed techniques using these veins may even fit into the 'do one (under supervision), teach one' mould.

The Routes

A number of routes have been described for cannulating central veins, and for each of these routes a variety of techniques have been used. This wide choice often makes it difficult to determine the most suitable route and technique for a particular patient. In practice, decisions are commonly taken on empirical grounds, but a consideration of certain relevant factors would enable a more rational approach to be made. Such factors include the objectives of the cannulation, whether the patient is awake or unconscious, the expertise and experience of the operator, the success and complication rates of the technique, and the availability of suitable apparatus. The main indications for the different routes and techniques are shown in Table 1.1, and those factors to be considered when choosing a suitable route are detailed in Table 1.2.

Table 1.1 Indications for the various routes of cannulation.

Route	Indication
Arm	
Basilic vein	
Cephalic vein	For short-term use. Safe for the beginner
Forearm vein	
Axillary vein	
Proximal basilic vein	A rarely used alternative to distal arm veins
Cephalic vein in deltopectoral groove	
Chest	
Subclavian vein (supraclavicular infraclavicular)	Long-term access, e.g. parenteral nutrition, chemotherapy, haemodialysis
Neck	
External jugular vein	A safe alternative to arm veins
Internal jugular vein	For cardiac anaesthesia and major surgical procedures
Leg	
Femoral vein	Rarely used but a useful technique in paediatrics
Scalp	
Threaded through superficial veins	A technique used in neonates which avoids a cut-down

Table 1.2 Factors influencing the choice of method for central venous cannulation.

- Patient
  - Duration of time cannula likely to be required:
    - Long term
    - Intermediate
    - Short term
  - Suitability of vein for technique chosen
- Operator
  - Theoretical knowledge of the technique
  - Practical knowledge of the technique
  - Expertise in the technique
- Technique characteristics
  - Success rate for vein cannulation
  - Success rate for central placement
  - Complication rate
  - Applicability to different ages of patient
  - Ease of learning
  - Venepuncture of a visible and/or palpable vein or 'blind' venepuncture (especially important for the inexperienced clinician)
- Apparatus
  - Availability of suitable apparatus
  - Cost
  - Suitability of material for long-term cannulation
- Choice of cut-down or percutaneous technique
  - Cut-downs are now rarely required by experienced clinicians for adult patients (only used if percutaneous techniques fail)

Peripheral arm veins

The basilic, cephalic, or forearm veins may be the first choice for the inexperienced clinician since their use avoids the risk of the major complications associated with blind puncture of the internal jugular or subclavian veins. The peripheral approach is often indicated in patients undergoing short operative procedures under general anaesthesia. In a patient whose peripheral veins are constricted it may be helpful to await the vasodilation induced by anaesthesia. The basilic vein should be chosen in preference to the cephalic as central placement is more frequently successful in the former.[9] If the catheter is likely to be left in for a few days, the non-dominant arm should be chosen. Cannulation of superficial arm veins is specifically indicated in patients who are having anticoagulant therapy or who have a bleeding diathesis, as the development of a haematoma can be easily seen and compression applied.

Peripheral veins are, however, not always readily available, particularly in ill patients requiring long-term intravenous therapy. The veins may be thrombosed, inflamed, covered in plaster or dressings, or the preferred site may be burnt or infected. Sometimes veins are thrombosed as a result of previous surgical cut-down and ligation. In some patients, especially the obese, veins may be difficult to find. It may in some cases be useful to identify the vein either with a temperature-change strip or by a Doppler ultrasonic detector.

If percutaneous cannulation of arm veins is unsuccessful, an alternative route should be used.

Proximal arm veins

The proximal portion of the basilic vein and the distal portion of the axillary vein have been used successfully.[10,11] The cephalic vein, where it lies in the deltopectoral groove, has also been used for long-term catheterisation.[12]

The indications for selecting the proximal arm veins are the same as for the more distal veins, but there is the additional advantage of a larger vein. However, as these veins are usually not visible, venepuncture is more difficult than with distal arm veins. These sites are not commonly used, perhaps because of the paucity of references to the technique in the literature.

The external jugular vein

The external jugular vein is usually visible and easy to cannulate. It is, therefore, a useful superficial vein for the clinician unskilled in internal jugular techniques. Success appears to be related largely to the type of equipment used. Flexible catheters pass more easily around acute bends at the external jugular subclavian vein junction than do rigid catheters: rigid catheters are also more likely to penetrate the vein wall.[13] Blitt *et al.*[14] in 1974 used a modified Seldinger technique with a flexible J-shaped wire originally described by Judkins *et al.*[15] The J wire was threaded through the external jugular vein and manipulated into the superior vena cava, enabling the central venous catheter to be inserted into a central vein over the J wire. Successful central venous placement was reported in 96% of attempts. The experiences of other authors with J wires and other catheters are described in Chapter 8.

Stoelting[16] showed that the readings from a short (50 mm) catheter introduced into the external jugular vein reflected right atrial pressure in anaesthetised patients, both with controlled and spontaneous ventilation. A round-ended catheter that is placed just above the junction of the subclavian and external jugular vein will give accurate central venous pressure readings.[17] These are unaffected by head movement.

There are no specific contraindications, apart from local infection, to the use of the external jugular vein.

The internal jugular vein

The internal jugular vein now appears to have become the accepted route of choice for major surgical cases. However, the long-term nursing management of neck catheters can be difficult, particularly if the patient needs to be turned regularly. Contraindications include aneurysm of the carotid artery and local sepsis.

Internal jugular techniques can be arbitrarily divided into high and low approaches, according to their position in relation to the apex of the lung. A high approach should avoid the risk of pneumothorax. In the low approaches of English *et al.*[18] and Rao *et al.*[19] the reported incidences of pneumothorax were 0.2% and 0.3% respectively. Although some deaths have been associated with cannulation of the internal jugular vein,[20,21] many more have been reported following use of the subclavian vein route. In the young child the technique is more difficult to perform and the success rates may be reduced.[22] Ullman and Stoelting[23] suggest using a blood flow detector for localising the internal jugular vein. This could be especially helpful in young or obese patients, in whom anatomical landmarks may be difficult to locate. If failure occurs on one side the other can be used.

The subclavian vein

The subclavian vein has a wide calibre (1–2 cm diameter in adults) and is held open by surrounding tissue even in severe circulatory collapse. The vein is usually easily accessible to the anaesthetist during a surgical operation. In shocked patients there is a choice between the subclavian and the internal jugular vein because the latter can also be successfully cannulated using a guide-wire technique. The size of the vein allows for rapid infusion of fluid. The subclavian vein is the route most commonly adopted for long-term parenteral nutrition.

Use of the subclavian vein allows the catheter to be securely fixed on the chest wall with minimal subsequent movement, thus decreasing the risk of infection. Most authors report a high success rate for central placement, but serious complications occur much more frequently than with other routes. Pneumothorax is one of the most common problems, so the technique should be used with caution – if at all – in patients with severe lung disease. Attempts at cannulation on both sides are best avoided because of the risk of producing a bilateral pneumothorax. In patients in whom a thoracotomy is planned, ipsilateral cannulation is recommended as a chest drain will be used postoperatively.

This route is unsuitable for the inexperienced operator unless he is adequately supervised.

Use of Ultrasound for Difficult Central Venous Access

Many studies show a reduced incidence of multiple stabs and decreased time to successful catheterisation when ultrasound is used to facilitate the chosen technique. Ultrasound is used routinely in neonates by some operators. Very few operators use the technique routinely in adults, however.

Ultrasound has been used prospectively in adults to assess venous anatomy in cases where difficulty with catheterisation was anticipated.[24] The criteria used to define anticipated difficulty included altered surface anatomy, abnormal vascular anatomy, previous multiple puncture or sites, coagulopathy and previous complications. Internal jugular, subclavian and femoral veins were scanned at the bedside. The authors attempted to determine the optimum site for access and reason for previous failures. The information obtained enabled the optimum site for the attempts at venepuncture to be determined. A high (83%) first-pass success rate was achieved using information gained by ultrasound. In two patients *in situ* lines were rewired as other sites were considered unsuitable. Portable ultrasonography was quick, simple and safe to perform. It was able to provide information on previous failures and complications.

Central Venous Catheterisation in Infants and Children

The report of the National Confidential Enquiry into Perioperative Deaths (CEPOD)[25] published in 1989 contained no comment on the minimal requirements of training and current practice in anaesthesia for children. The authors however recognised that there was a problem that needed to be addressed urgently.

A clinician should not feel obliged to anaesthetise a child of less than 5 years of age on an occasional basis. Such young children should ideally be anaesthetised by clinicians regularly involved in paediatric anaesthesia. Similarly it is inappropriate for a clinician to be involved in inserting central venous catheters in such children on an occasional basis. These catheters should ideally be inserted by the designated paediatric anaesthetist. Some paediatric patients are, however, still anaesthetised by clinicians on an occasional basis. These patients are generally not high-risk cases and are very unlikely to need a central venous catheter. It is almost unheard-of for clinicians to fail with percutaneous techniques on the jugular or arm veins in adults; unfortunately, this is not the case with children. Under these circumstances some clinicians

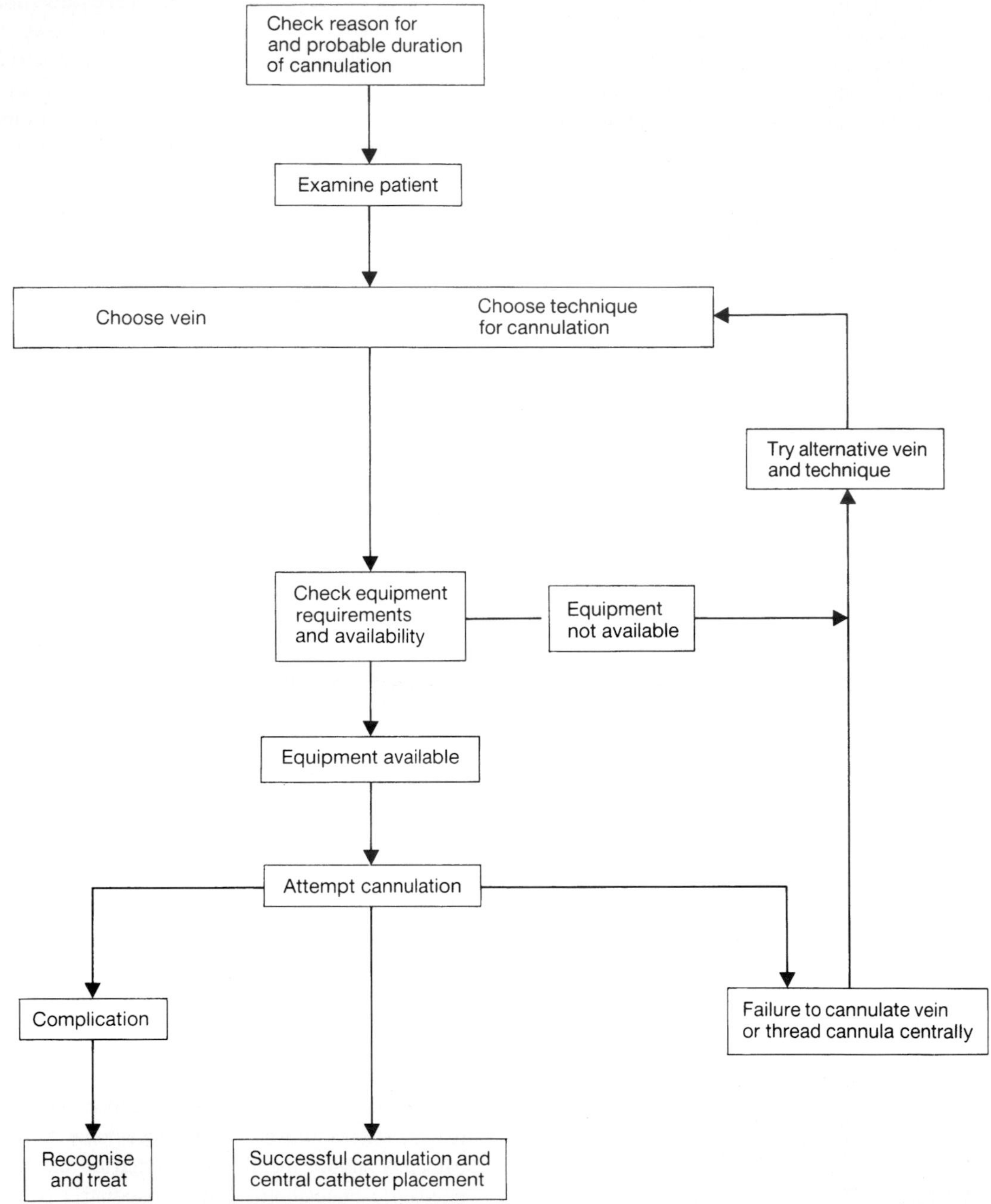

Figure 1.1 Central venous cannulation when operator is familiar with technique chosen.

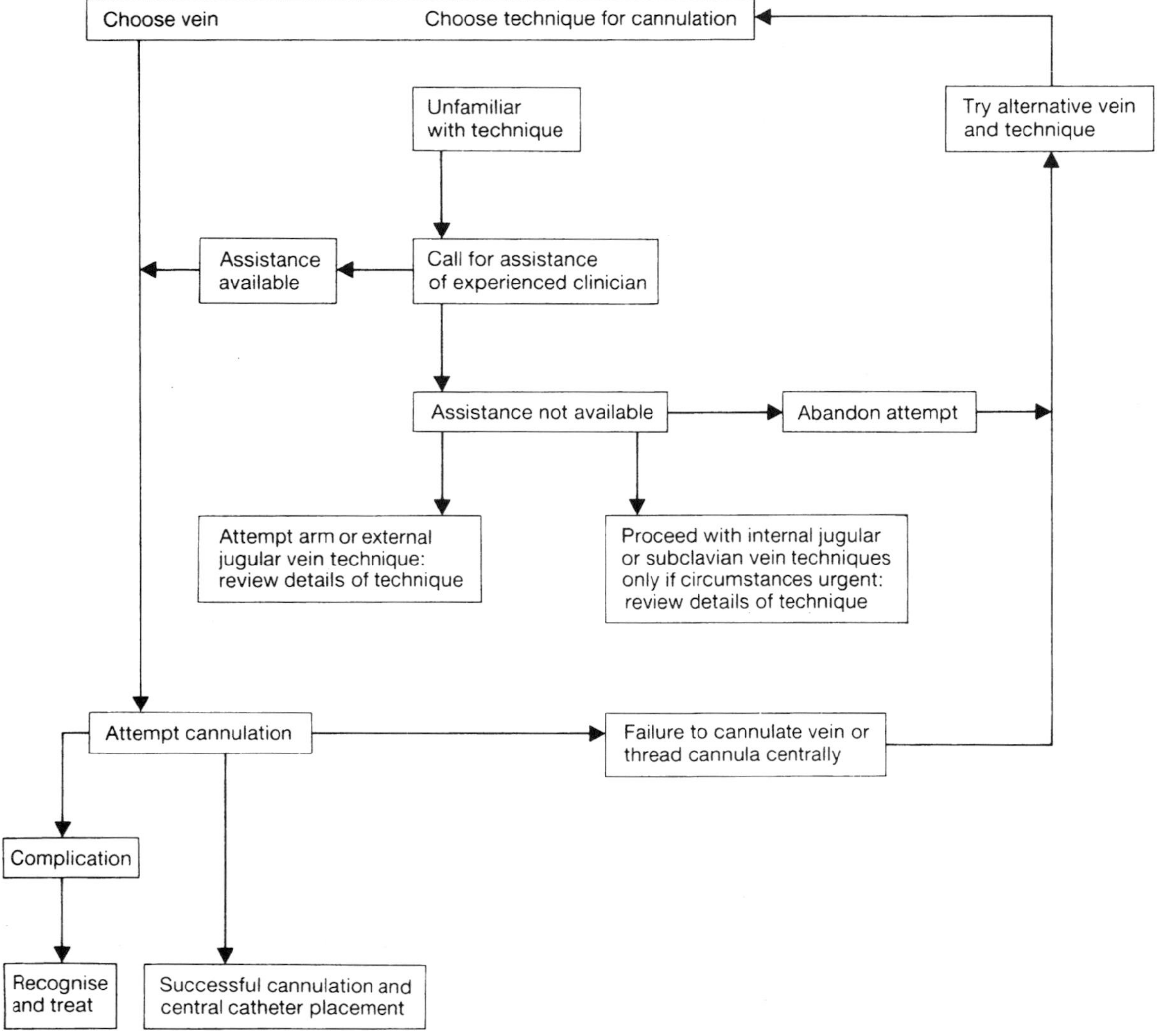

Figure 1.2 Central venous cannulation when operator is not familiar with technique chosen.

Table 1.3 Features of the different routes of central venous cannulation.

Feature	Arm veins	External jugular vein	Internal jugular vein	Subclavian vein
Ease of venepuncture for the inexperienced clinician	+++	+++	+	+
Complications relating to insertion of catheter	0	0	+	+++
Central placement success rate (%)	50–98 (normally approximately 80)	50–98 (depends on use of J wire)	90–100 (does *not* depend on type of catheter used)	90–98
Suitability for long-term parenteral nutrition	+	+	++	+++

attempt cannulation of the subclavian veins, others ask for a surgical cut-down.

Inserting a central venous catheter into a small peripheral arm vein in a child is technically more difficult than in an adult. Suitable guide-wire equipment is not usually available, therefore it is usual to attempt to cannulate other veins. The external jugular vein can be cannulated with minimal risk. Experience with internal jugular vein techniques should, however, first be obtained in adults. Prince *et al.*[26] compared their results of internal jugular vein cannulation in children with those of subclavian vein cannulation by Groff and Ahmed[27] in children less than 2 years old, and concluded that the use of the subclavian vein in patients of that age should be condemned. Our practice is to use a subclavian vein only as a last resort when attempts at internal and external jugular veins have failed. Alternatively a surgical cut-down may be used. In small infants, scalp veins have been used and catheters threaded through a needle into the superior vena cava.[28,29]

The Operator

No individual can be equally familiar with all the techniques described. Most anaesthetists have considerable experience with arm and jugular veins. The inexperienced clinician should select a technique that is intrinsically safe although possibly yielding a lower success rate. If a particular route is strongly indicated, the assistance of someone experienced in that technique should be sought unless circumstances are urgent. All trainee physicians should initially be supervised in the practical aspects of performing a technique until sufficient expertise is acquired.

It is an important ethical issue whether a technique with a known incidence of major complications should be employed solely to gain experience when alternative and less dangerous methods would suffice. This is justifiable only if the inexperienced operator is carefully supervised and facilities are readily available to institute effective treatment of complications.

The operator's choice of routes is ultimately limited by the equipment available. This may be a particular problem in the management of children. Flow diagrams showing the steps in central venous cannulation when the operator is experienced or inexperienced in the chosen technique are shown in Figures 1.1 and 1.2. Important features of the different routes are shown in Table 1.3.

Experience in Developing Countries

The 'Anaesthesia for Developing Countries' courses held annually in Oxford and Bristol are invaluable for any UK-trained anaesthetist who is contemplating working in such a country.[30] Equipment that is routinely available in the UK is frequently not available in less affluent countries. Pullman showed that a small amount of time spent in teaching both the insertion of central catheters and the use of adrenaline produced improvement in patient outcomes.[30] He noted that on his arrival in Fiji there was no regular supply of catheter kits. Fairly regular supplies were eventually obtained as his logistical skills improved.

KEY POINTS

- When the first edition of this book was published in 1981 anaesthetists in the UK used arm veins almost exclusively for placement of central venous catheters.
- The internal jugular vein is now probably the vein most frequently chosen by anaesthetists in the UK for central venous catheter placement.
- It is important therefore that an appropriate technique for internal jugular catheterisation is taught and that trainees are also instructed how best to avoid complications.
- The subclavian vein is now rarely used during anaesthesia, and rightly so. This vein is, however, used more widely in the intensive care unit.
- The external jugular vein deserves to be more widely used, particularly if difficulty is experienced in inserting internal jugular vein catheters.

- Particular expertise is required for placement of central venous catheters in neonates.
- In cases of difficulty (particularly in neonates) the use of ultrasound can be invaluable.
- Morbidity and mortality can be confidently anticipated when unsupervised, inexperienced staff persist in foolish attempts at subclavian catheterisation.

Under these circumstances, with no proper kits, the use of a short cannula in the external jugular vein[16,17] and a simple T piece for measuring pressure will be indicated. It is clear that there will not be enough money for disposable transducers and other expensive disposable apparatus in these countries.

References

1. Joseph DM, Phillip BK, Phillip JH. Peripheral venous pressure can be an accurate estimate of central venous pressure. Anesthesiology 1985; **65**:A166.
2. Kalso E. A short history of central venous catheterization. Acta Anaesthesiologica Scandinavica 1985; **81**:7.
3. Lunn JK, Stanley TH, Webster LR, Bidwai AV. Arterial blood-pressure and pulse-rate responses to pulmonary and radial arterial catheterization prior to cardiac and major vascular operations. Anesthesiology 1979; **51**:265.
4. Waller JL, Zaidan JR, Kaplan JA, Bauman DI. Hemodynamic responses to preoperative vascular cannulation in patients with coronary artery disease. Anesthesiology 1982; **56**:219.
5. Bo-Linn GW, Anderson DJ, Anderson KC, McGoon MD. Percutaneous central venous catheterization performed by medical house officers: a prospective study. Catheterization and Cardiovascular Diagnosis 1982; **8**:23.
6. Sznajder JI, Zveibil FR, Bitterman H, Weiner P, Bursztein S. Central vein catheterization. Failure and complication rates by three percutaneous approaches. Archives of Internal Medicine 1986; **146**:259.
7. Sessler CN, Glauser FL. Central venous cannulation done by house officers in the intensive care unit: a prospective study. Southern Medical Journal 1987; **80**:1239.
8. Editorial. Central vein catheterisation. Lancet 1986; **2**:669.
9. Webre DR, Arens JF. Use of cephalic and basilic veins for introduction of central venous catheters. Anesthesiology 1973; **38**:389.
10. Spracklen FHN, Niesche F, Lord PW, Besterman EMM. Percutaneous catheterisation of the axillary vein. Cardiovascular Research 1967; **1**:297.
11. Ayim EN. Percutaneous catheterisation of the axillary vein and proximal basilic vein. Anaesthesia 1977; **32**:753.
12. Jacobs P, Jacobson J. Placement of central feeding catheters. British Medical Journal 1978; **2**:1789.
13. Guest J, Leiberman DP. Late complications of catheterisation for intravenous nutrition. Lancet 1976; **2**:805.
14. Blitt CD, Wright WA, Petty WC, Webster TA. Central venous catheterization via the external jugular vein. A technique employing the J-wire. Journal of the American Medical Association 1974; **229**:817.
15. Judkins MP, Kidd HJ, Frische LH, Dotter CT. Lumen-following safety J-guide for catheterization of tortuous vessels. Radiology 1967; **88**:1127.
16. Stoelting RK. Evaluation of external jugular pressure as a reflection of right atrial pressure. Anesthesiology 1973; **38**:291.
17. Shah MV, Swai EA, Latto IP. Comparison between pressures measured from the proximal external jugular vein and a central vein. British Journal of Anaesthesia 1986; **58**:1384.
18. English ICW, Frew RM, Pigott JF, Zaki M. Percutaneous catheterisation of the internal jugular vein. Anaesthesia 1969; **24**:521.
19. Rao TLK, Wong AY, Salem MR. A new approach to percutaneous catheterization of the internal jugular vein. Anesthesiology 1977; **46**:362.
20. Ayalon A, Anner H, Berlatzky Y, Schiller M. A life threatening complication of the infusion pump. Lancet 1978; **i**:853.
21. Wisheart JD, Hassan MA, Jackson JW. A complication of percutaneous cannulation of the internal jugular vein. Thorax 1972; **27**:496.
22. Vaughan RW, Weygandt GR. Reliable percutaneous central venous pressure measurement. Anesthesia and Analgesia 1973; **52**:709.
23. Ullman JI, Stoelting RK. Internal jugular vein location with the ultrasound Doppler blood flow detector. Anesthesia and Analgesia 1978; **57**:118.
24. Hatfield A, Bodenham A. Portable ultrasound for difficult central venous access. British Journal of Anaesthesia 1998; **81**:821P.
25. Campling EA, Devlin HB, Lunn JN. (1989). The report of the National Confidential Enquiry into Perioperative Deaths.
26. Prince SR, Sullivan RL, Hackel A. Percutaneous catheterization of the internal jugular vein in infants and children. Anesthesiology 1976; **44**:170.
27. Groff BD, Ahmed NO. Subclavian vein catheterization in the infant. Journal of Pediatric Surgery 1974; **9**:171.
28. Shaw JCL. Parenteral nutrition in the management of sick low birth weight infants. Pediatric Clinics of North America 1973; **20**:333.
29. Cockington RA. Silicone elastomer for nasojejunal intubation and central venous cannulation in neonates. Anaesthesia and Intensive Care 1979; **7**:248.
30. Pullman M. S_pRs: Don't forget developing countries. The ultimate management experience? Today's Anaesthetist 1998; **13**:126.

2 • Choosing the Equipment

SHANG NG

Introduction

The basic equipment required for catheterisation is a needle and a catheter of sufficient length to reach a central vein. The catheter can be introduced either through or over the introducing needle (Table 2.1). In a development of the technique, a cannula is first inserted into the vein over a needle; then, after removal of the needle, the catheter is threaded through the cannula. The guide-wire or Seldinger[1] technique also starts with a needle being introduced into the vein; a matching guide-wire is then passed through the needle, and, after removal of the needle, the catheter is introduced into the vein over the guide-wire. A modification of this technique makes use of a tapered vein dilator with a wide-bore cannula, through which a large catheter (e.g. a Swan–Ganz catheter) can be inserted into a small vein. The terms 'cannula' and 'catheter' are not clearly defined in the medical literature. Shorter lengths, such as are commonly used for peripheral intravenous infusions, are usually, but not always, referred to as cannulae. Longer lengths (usually over long needles), intended for cannulation of subclavian or internal jugular veins, are sometimes referred to as cannulae and sometimes as catheters according to the manufacturer. Very long tubing is always referred to as a catheter. Since there is no agreement on definitions, the terms for the shorter lengths of tubing are used interchangeably in this book.

Table 2.1 Types of equipment.

1. Catheter-through-needle
2. Catheter-over-needle
3. Catheter-through-cannula
4. Catheter-over-wire

Basic Types of Equipment

Catheter-through-needle devices

The catheter-through-needle equipment was the first to become widely available for introducing a long venous catheter, although rarely used now. The device is easy to use because, once the needle tip is successfully inserted into the lumen of the vein, the catheter can be advanced through the needle tip without difficulty. It is also easy to see 'flashback' of blood into the hub of the needle immediately the vein is entered. Since the catheter lies inside the introducing needle it does not have to be pushed through the skin and deeper tissues; consequently the catheter can be constructed of a soft, pliant material and the tip need not be sharp.The long catheters of this type are usually protected by a transparent sleeve, so facilitating a 'no touch' technique during insertion of the catheter.

A drawback with this technique is that there may be leakage of blood, because the catheter is smaller than the hole made by the needle. The main disadvantage, however, is that the catheter may shear if attempts are made to withdraw it while the needle tip is still in the vein. Reports of sheared catheters nearly always relate to the use of catheter-through-needle devices.[2,3] Since the needle cannot usually be removed from the catheter because there is a fixed hub on the catheter, a protective sheath is supplied to prevent thesharp needle tip from damaging or cutting the catheter. The catheter may still be sheared through, however, if the protective sheath is incorrectly applied or becomes dislodged. A solution to this problem is to deliberately cut off the fixed hub from the catheter and so enable the needle to be removed. A suitable adaptor, such as a Tuohy connector, is then attached to the cut end of the catheter.

Technique

The technique is shown in Figure 2.1.

(a) A percutaneous venepuncture is performed.
(b) The catheter is threaded through the needle and advanced along the vein. If the passage of the catheter is obstructed, both catheter and needle should be withdrawn from the vein and catheterisation attempted again. The catheter should on no account be pulled back through the needle.
(c) The needle is withdrawn over the catheter, and the protective device to prevent the needle cutting the catheter is attached.

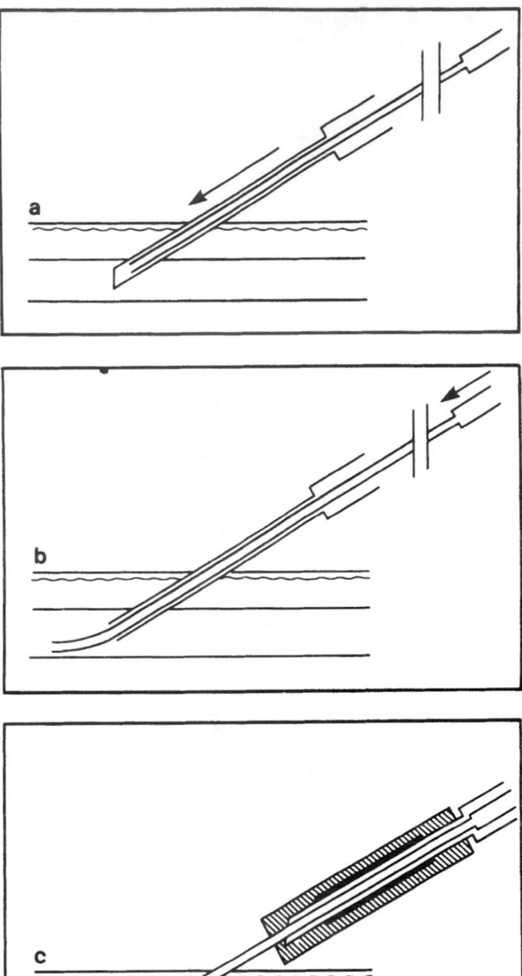

Figure 2.1 Catheter-through-needle devices: technique of use.

This type of device has been universally condemned[4,5] and is no longer produced by leading suppliers.

Catheter-over-needle devices

The catheter-over-needle device was developed to eliminate the risk of the needle cutting through the catheter. The needle is inside the catheter and both are inserted together when the vein is punctured. The needle is then withdrawn and the catheter advanced along the vein. Long and short versions of the catheter-over-needle device are available (Figure 2.2). In the long catheter, such as is used for catheterisation through arm veins, a syringe cannot be attached to aspirate blood and accelerated 'flashback' is the only reliable indication of entry into the vein. Furthermore, the needle tip protrudes beyond the catheter and so, although blood in the catheter may indicate that the needle tip is in the vein, it does not guarantee that the catheter tip is also in the vein.

The shorter catheter is simply an extra-long cannula (Figure 2.2a) intended for cannulation of the subclavian or internal jugular vein. A syringe can be attached to the needle so that blood can be aspirated to indicate successful venepuncture. Again, this does not guarantee that the cannula tip is also inside the vein.

(a)

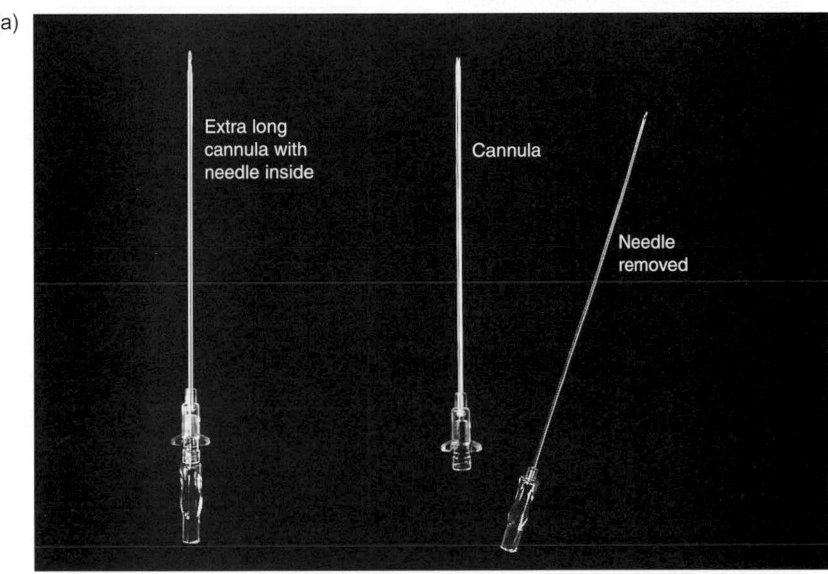

(b)

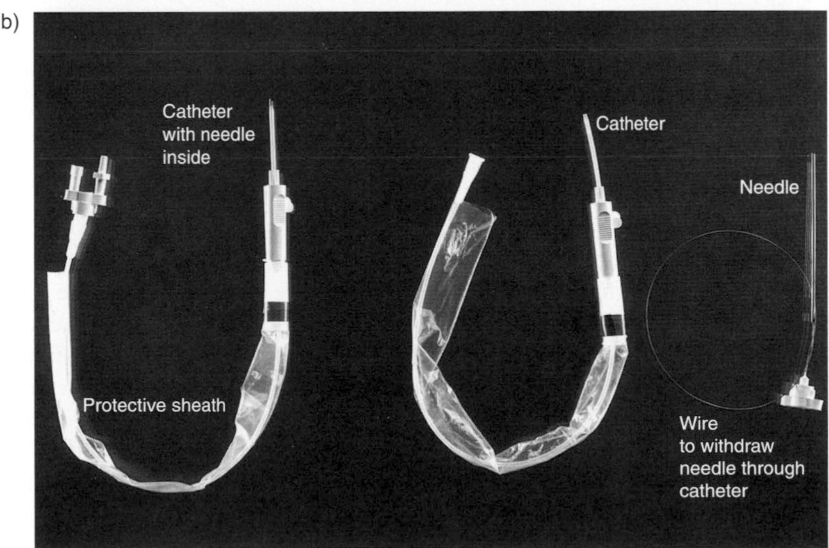

Figure 2.2 Catheter-over-needle devices.

In both long and short types the catheter tip has to be fairly sharp and rigid since it must be pushed through the skin. It can therefore injure the vein as it is advanced or later, when in position. One advantage is that the hole made in the vein by the needle is smaller than the size of the catheter, so leakage of blood is less likely than with catheter-through-needle devices. Because the long cannula with long needle device is flexible, the operator may have to grasp the cannula near its distal end in order to push it through the skin and deeper tissues.

Because of its length, the long cannula on long needle has, not unexpectedly, been associated with inadvertent injury to most superior mediastinal structures.

Technique

The technique is shown in Figure 2.3.

(a) A percutaneous venepuncture is made with the needle and closely fitting catheter. The needle tip is advanced a further short distance (3–4 mm) to ensure that the catheter tip is also in the vein.
(b) The needle is withdrawn into the catheter, which is advanced into the vein.
(c) The needle is then completely removed and discarded.

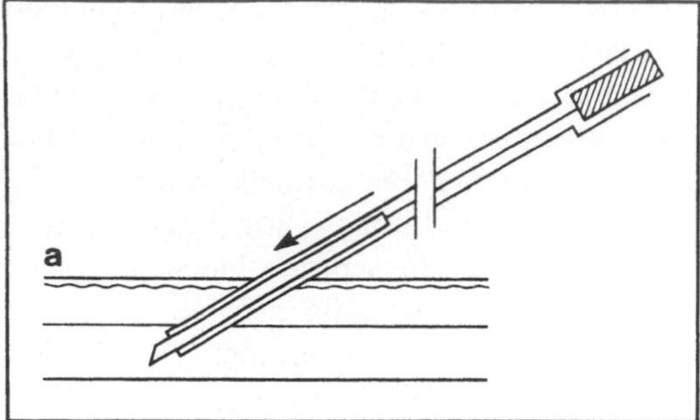

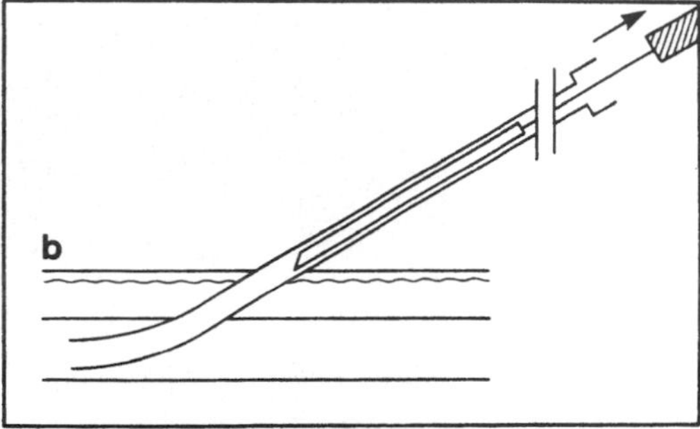

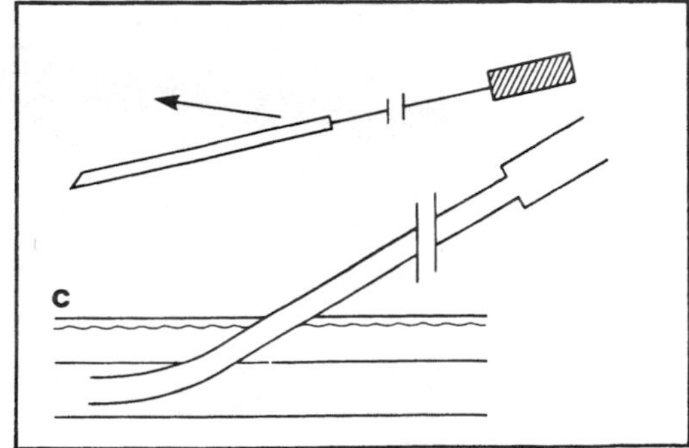

Figure 2.3 Catheter-over-needle devices: technique of use.

Catheter-through-cannula devices

The catheter-through-cannula device (Figure 2.4) was devised to preserve the advantages of both the catheter-through-needle and catheter-over-needle devices whilst overcoming their drawbacks.

Venepuncture is performed with a short cannula with the needle inside. A syringe can therefore be attached to the needle and successful venepuncture easily detected. The cannula tip must still be fairly sharp and rigid since it has to be pushed through the skin and wall of the vein, but the catheter tip that is subsequently inserted through the cannula can be of a much safer material and design. The needle is removed before the catheter is inserted to eliminate the risk of damaging the catheter.

Certain disadvantages remain. It is still possible that the cannula tip does not lie within the lumen of the vein with the needle tip. Furthermore, the catheter is smaller than the hole in the vein so blood may leak around the catheter. The syringe must usually be detached from the cannula to insert the catheter, and at this point there is a risk of air embolism and bacterial contamination (Figure 2.4).

In all these types, if the introducing cannula is left in the lumen of the vein and the proximal end is open to the atmosphere, there is a danger of serious air embolism.[6] The cannula tip should always be withdrawn from the vein, even if only to lie subcutaneously, where it can protect the catheter from kinking.

(a)

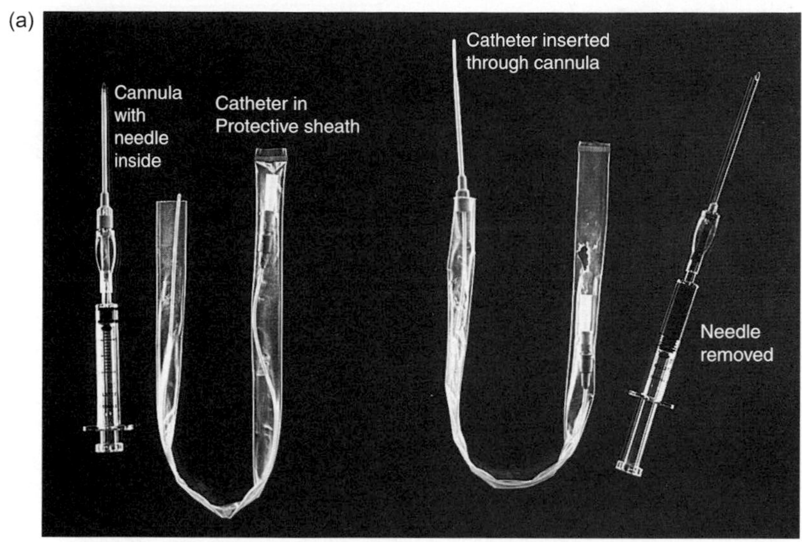

(b)

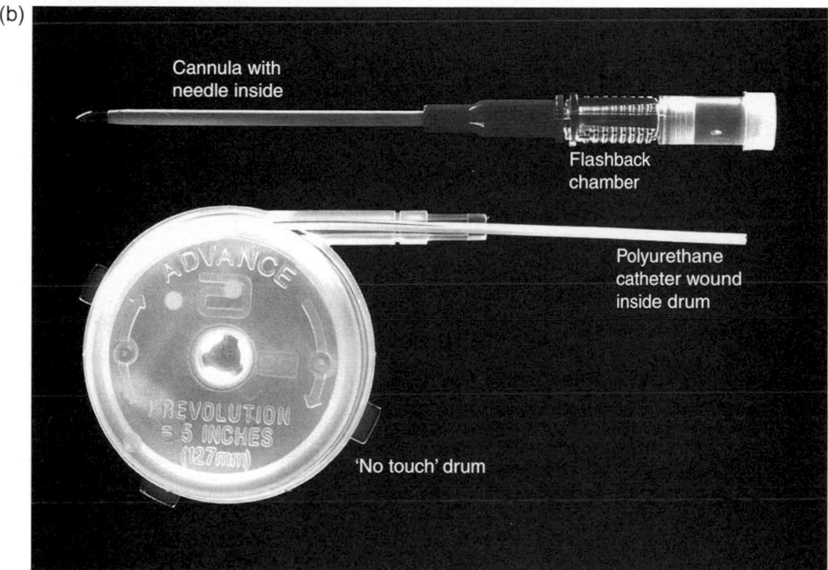

Figure 2.4 Catheter-through-cannula devices.

The catheter-through-cannula device is recommended for general use in catheterisation of veins at any site.

Technique

The insertion of a catheter-through-cannula device is shown in Figure 2.5.

(a) A percutaneous venepuncture is made with the short needle and introducing cannula.
(b) The needle is withdrawn completely and the catheter inserted through the cannula into the vein.
(c) The cannula should be withdrawn from the vein to be outside the skin *or* at least withdrawn from the vein but left subcutaneously.

Catheter-over-wire devices

The catheter-over-wire technique, originally described for arterial cannulation,[1] can also be used for central venous catheterisation of any route, but is particularly indicated for subclavian or jugular vein techniques. The catheter is inserted into the vein over a guide-wire. The guide-wire is flexible and has an even more flexible leading end with a rounded tip. A kinked or otherwise damaged wire should not be used. The main advantage of this technique is that the initial 'blind' needling of the vein can be performed with a smaller-gauge needle (just wide enough to admit the appropriate guide-wire). Trauma to important structures, including inadvertent arterial puncture with haematoma formation, is thus minimised. The guide-wire technique is especially suited to catheterisation of the small deep veins of infants and children. Although this is a through-the-needle technique, there is no risk of damage to the catheter since the needle is completely removed before the catheter is introduced.

Inserting a long guide-wire with its accompanying catheter from a peripheral arm vein is often difficult because of obstruction by valves or branching of veins. Therefore the guide-wire method is indicated only rarely when a peripheral arm vein is used, being more suited to cannulation of the subclavian, internal jugular, or femoral vein. Nevertheless, the guide-wire technique may be used with advantage.[7] Since the catheter has to be pushed through the skin, it must be fairly rigid, sharp and tapered and is thus likely to damage the wall of the vein as it is advanced and subsequently when it lies in the vein. A useful development is first to insert a short, tapered cannula (vein dilator) over the guide-wire; this vein dilator carries a shorter, wide-bore cannula. The taper dilates the vein and so allows the large cannula to be inserted. After removal of the vein dilator (and guide-wire) a catheter with a soft tip can easily be advanced through the wide-bore cannula.

In the basic guide-wire technique the hole made by the needle is smaller than the catheter so leakage of blood is unlikely. This advantage is absent when an introducing cannula is used. Full aseptic precautions including adequate towelling of the

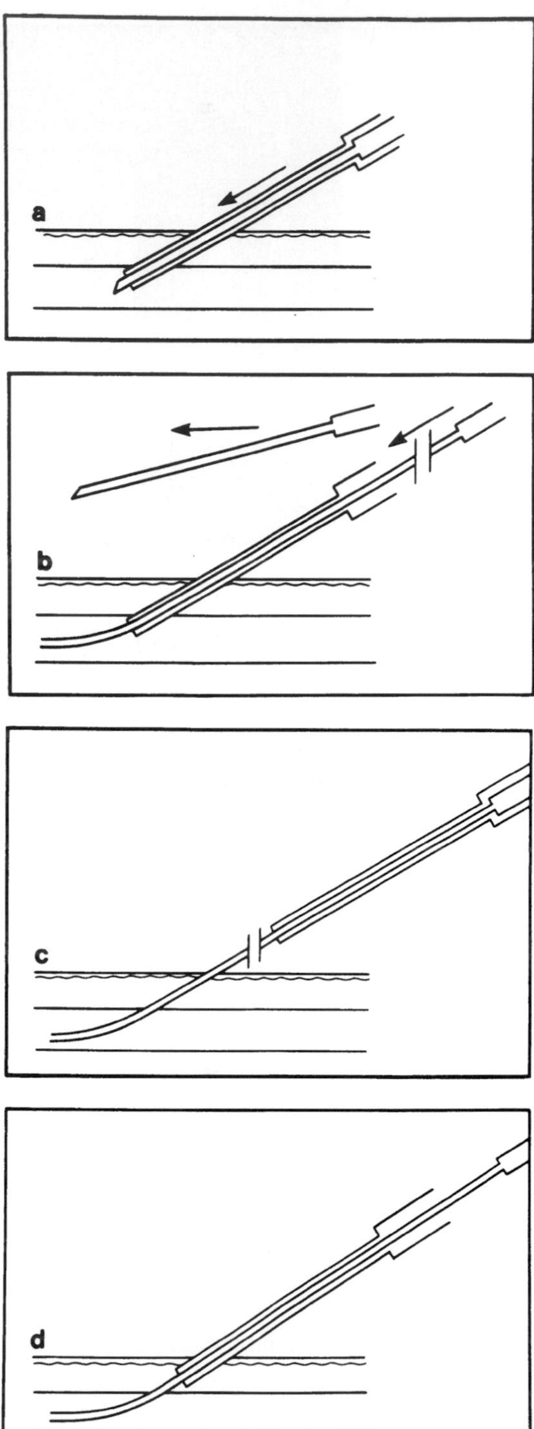

Figure 2.5 Catheter-through-cannula devices: technique of use.

area are essential, because a 'no touch' technique cannot be applied.

This technique can be used to insert single and multilumen catheters and is the method advocated for inserting a Swan–Ganz catheter. The technique is not only potentially safer, but can also increase the success rate.[8] It is safer for two reasons: first, there is less risk of harm to deep structures; and second, the method eliminates the danger of air embolisation, which is an inherent hazard of through-cannula devices when an open-ended introducer is inadvertently allowed to communicate with the vein.[9,10]

Some clinicians may be deterred from using a guide-wire method because of its apparent expense. However, the cost of the equipment is outweighed by the advantage of successful and safer catheterisation.

Technique without a vein dilator

The technique is illustrated in Figure 2.6.

(a) The guide-wire must be smooth (unkinked) and able to pass through the needle. The more flexible end is identified by palpation. The catheter must fit closely over the wire without too much free movement. The guide-wire must be at least 100 mm longer than the catheter. A percutaneous venepuncture is made with the needle attached to a syringe. The syringe is removed and steps taken to avoid air embolism.
(b) The flexible guide-wire (lubricated with a heparinised saline solution to prevent clotting) is inserted through the needle with the more flexible end leading, a short distance (4–5 cm) into the vein.
(c) The needle is removed over the wire and discarded.
(d) The catheter is inserted over the wire, which is again lubricated, until the wire protrudes through the outside end. Both catheter and wire are pushed through the skin. A small incision made with a scalpel assists the passage of the catheter through the skin.
(e) The catheter and wire together are passed into the vein for a sufficient distance to ensure that the catheter tip lies in the desired position.
(f) The guide-wire is removed carefully, retaining the catheter in position.

A useful 'extra' gained from the guide-wire technique is the correlation between guide-wire distortion and misplacement of the catheter tip when introduced through the infraclavicular subclavian vein route. If the wire is seen to be deviated cranially when it is withdrawn, then the inference is that the catheter has been misplaced into a neck vein.[11]

Technique with a vein dilator

This technique begins as described above; subsequent steps are shown in Figure 2.7.

(a,b) As above (see also Figure 2.6).
(c) The needle is removed over the guide-wire and discarded. A tapered vein dilator carrying a cannula is inserted over the wire, which is again lubricated with heparinised saline. The wire and vein dilator are pushed through the skin into the lumen of the vein.
(d) The wide-bore outer cannula is pushed over the vein dilator, through the skin and into the lumen of the vein.
(e) The guide-wire and vein dilator are removed, allowing a catheter (e.g. a Swan–Ganz) to pass readily through the wide-bore cannula.
(f) The tip of the large cannula is withdrawn outside the vein to act as a protective sheath, or is withdrawn completely outside the skin.

In a simpler progression the vein dilator is removed and the catheter inserted over the guide-wire, along the dilated passage, into the vein.

A combined guide-wire and vein dilator can increase the success rate of central venous catheterisation through antecubital fossa veins.[12] Catheters inserted through tributaries of the basilic vein have a far better chance of reaching a satisfactory central position than those inserted through the cephalic vein. However, an operator may be deterred from using a very small basilic vein to insert a large (13 gauge) cannula and opt for a larger cephalic vein which results in a poorer chance of successful central positioning. With the wire/dilator technique a small-gauge needle (18 gauge) is used to puncture the vein and to introduce a wire. Over

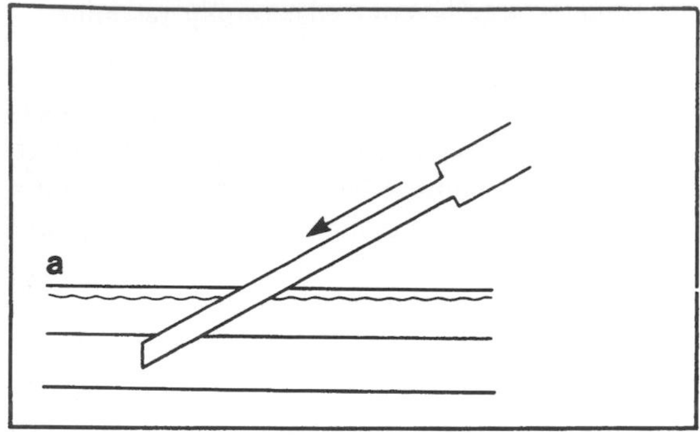

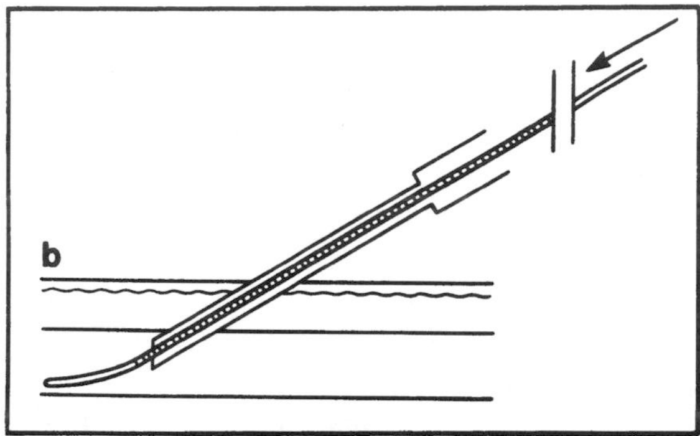

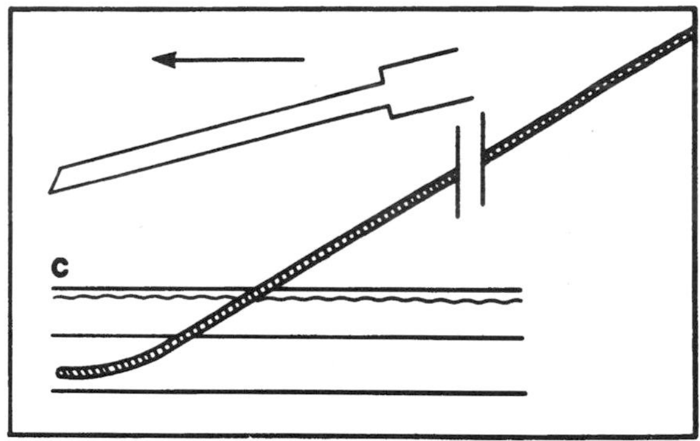

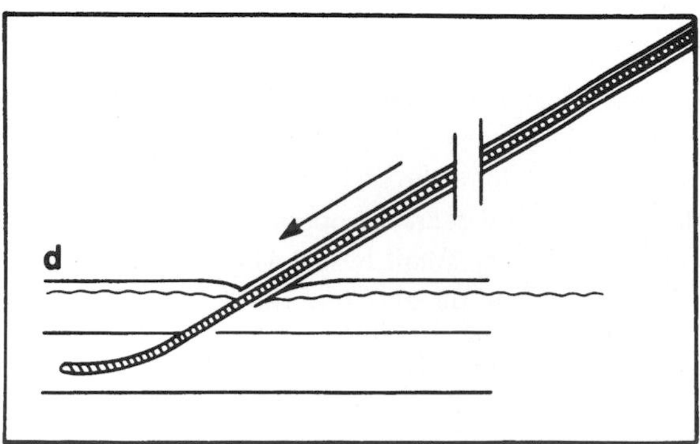

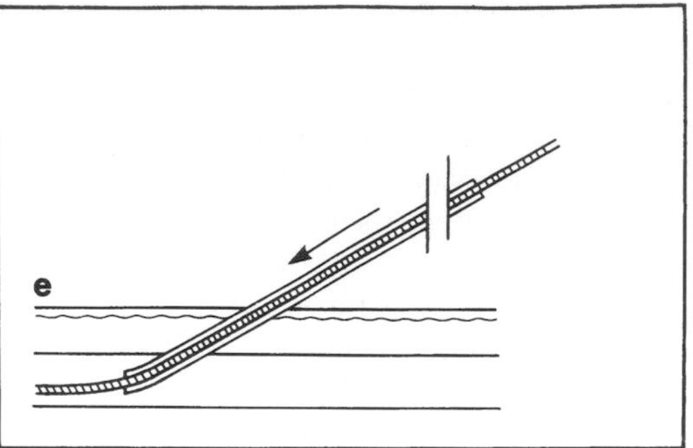

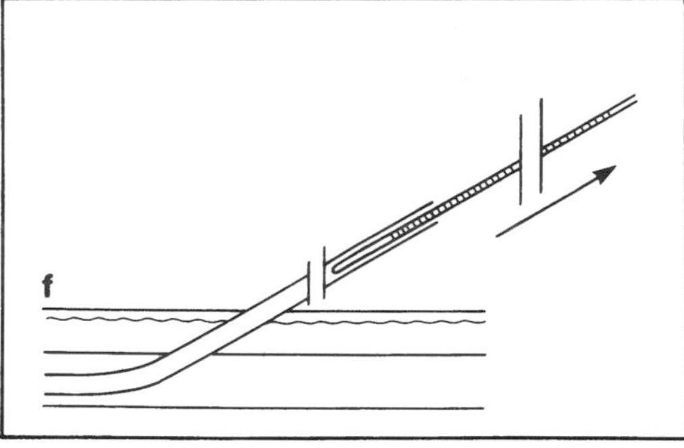

Figure 2.6 Catheter-over-wire devices: technique of use without a vein dilator.

this wire a vein dilator is then inserted progressing to the introduction of a large introducer allowing the long catheter to be advanced centrally. This technique then permits successful catheterisation through a basilic vein even if it is quite small.

Guide-wires

Flexible but straight guide-wires were originally used to facilitate percutaneous vascular catheterisation[1] and are still used extensively in angiographic techniques (Figure 2.8). The J-tipped guide-wire was developed to overcome the difficulties encountered with the straight wire in negotiating tortuous or atheromatous arteries.[13,14] At the same time less damage to endothelial structures seemed likely. The smooth convexity of the J facilitates smooth advancement and enables the wires to 'turn corners' where a straight wire would be stopped by engagement of the tip in the wall of the vessel (Figure 2.9).

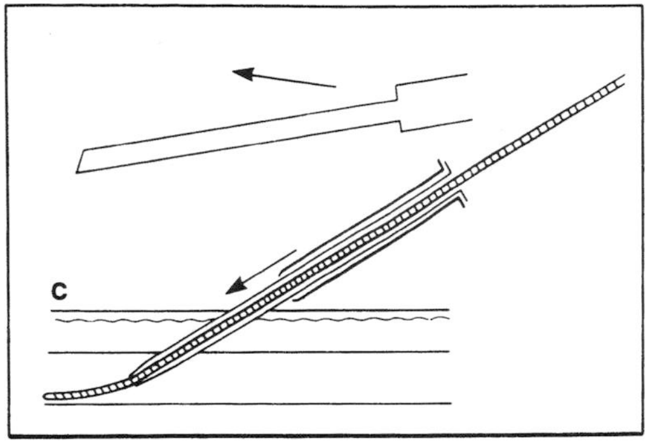

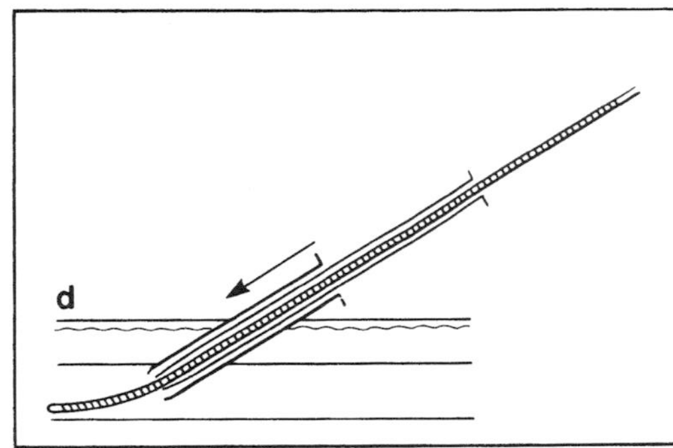

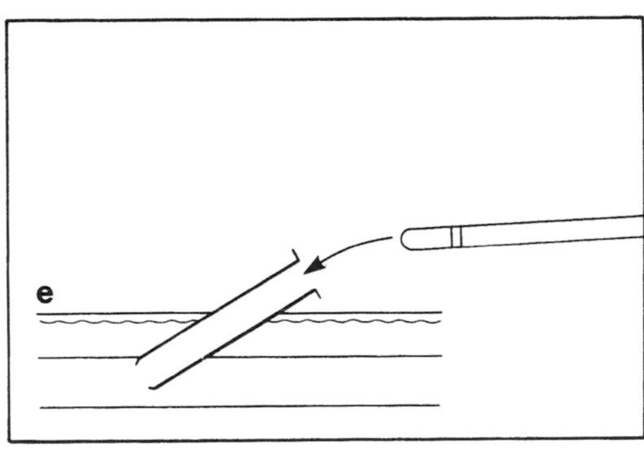

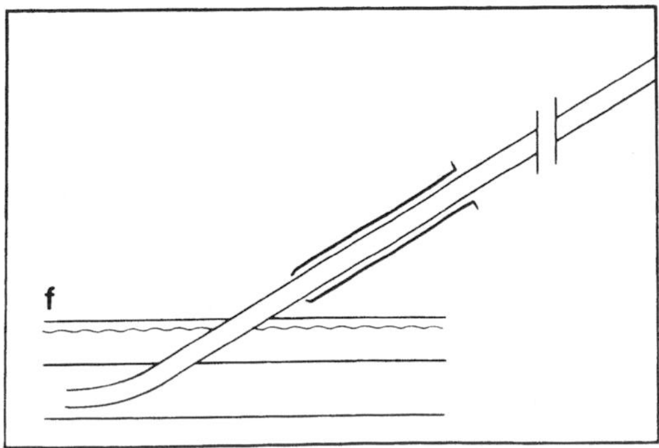

Figure 2.7 Catheter-over-wire devices: technique of use with a vein dilator.

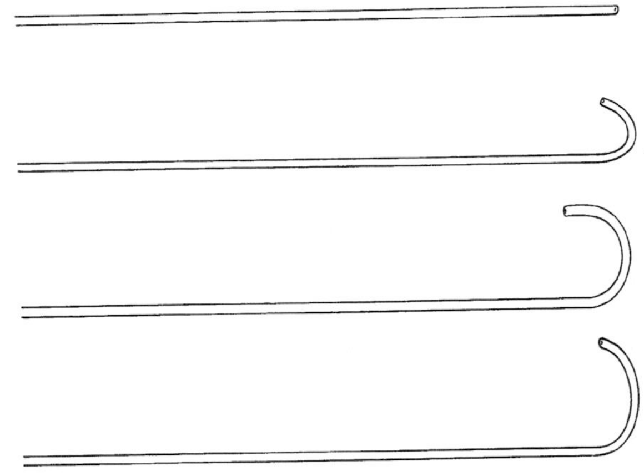

Figure 2.8 Flexible wire catheter guides. Straight and a variety of J-tipped wires. Reproduced with kind permission of Blitt *et al.* (1982).[18]

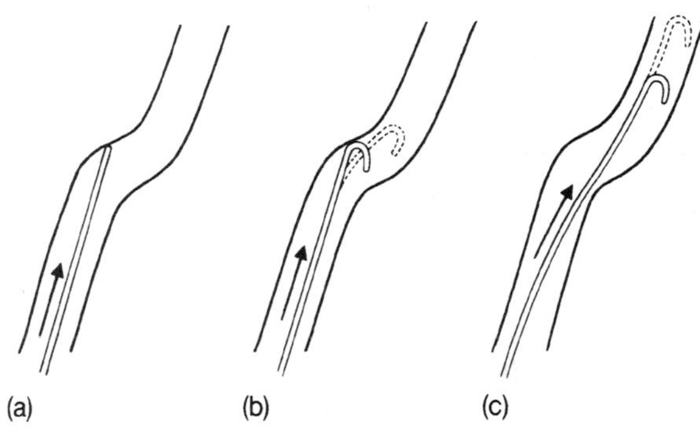

Figure 2.9 Schematic representation of obstruction to guide-wire tip and advantage of J-tipped (b and c) over the straight tip (a).

Blitt pioneered the use of the J-tipped wire in venous cannulation in 1974[15] when he described its advantage in obtaining virtually complete success in external jugular vein catheterisation. With conventional catheter devices, experience with this route is often disappointing, failure usually being attributed to tortuosity and acute angulation of the course of this vein together with the obstruction presented by venous valves. Similar success with the J wire has not always been found by others[16,17] but many workers have found the J-tipped wire advantageous and Blitt's further studies reinforce its value.[18]

The J wire has also been used to significantly increase successful venous catheter positioning when antecubital fossa veins are used. When the wire could be introduced into the basilic vein, all catheters reached a satisfactory position; 78% success was gained through the cephalic vein.[7]

Guide-wires are not without their own hazards. Straight wires have been implicated in perforation of central vessel walls leading to pericardial tamponade.[17] Other complications have been reported.[19]

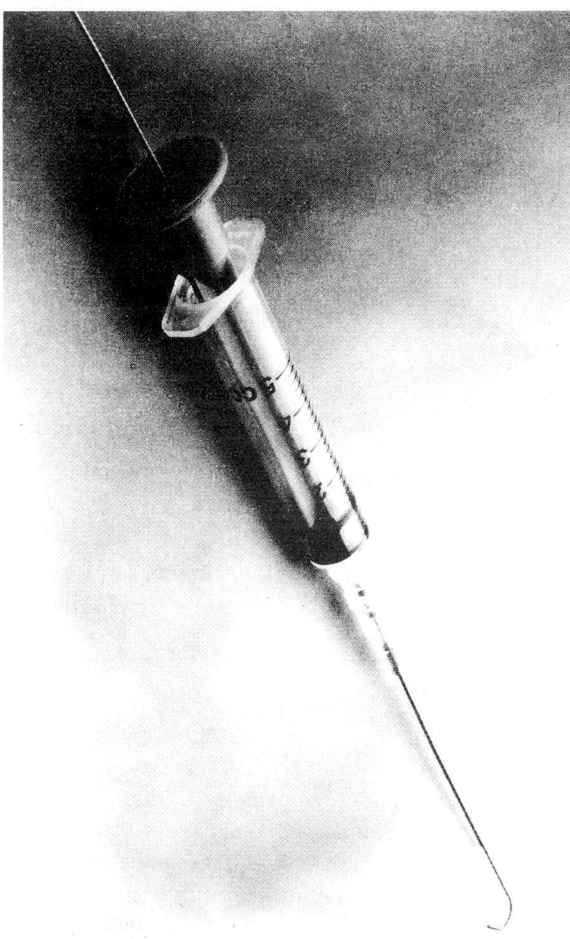

Figure 2.10 Arrow® Raulerson Syringe with the guide-wire passing through the syringe. Reproduced with kind permission of Arrow International Inc.

One of the causes of failure with the guide-wire technique is displacement of the introducing needle tip out of the lumen of the vessel due to movement when a firmly fitted syringe is disconnected from the needle hub. In addition air embolism is a danger with the needle hub open to the atmosphere. These dangers have been eliminated by an ingenious device (Figure 2.10) now commercially available, the Safety Syringe (Arrow International Inc., Reading, Pa, USA). The J wire is introduced into the vein through a channel in the specially constructed syringe plunger without the need to disconnect the syringe.

Precautions when using guide-wires

A straight guide-wire may be selected for vessels having a linear configuration. A J-tipped wire is indicated for veins that have a tortuous course such as the external jugular vein. Some authorities advise the routine use of J-tipped wires to minimise endothelial damage.[20] This would seem to be sound advice.

Technical complications which can occur with the wire include knotting of the most flexible portion of the straight wire, separation of the helical portion of a straight wire and displacement of the rounded tip of a J wire. Complications can be avoided if the following precautions are taken:

(a) Inspect the wire for defects before insertion.
(b) Consider a guide-wire to be a delicate and fragile instrument.
(c) When resistance to insertion is met, remove and inspect the wire for damage; reposition the introducer so that no resistance to its passage is felt.
(d) Enlarge the skin puncture with a pointed scalpel blade to enable smooth, one-step passage of the catheter insertion over the wire.
(e) If multiple manipulations are needed, reinspect the wire and replace if necessary.
(f) Always inspect the wire for complete removal at the end of the procedure.
(g) Do not reuse disposable guide-wires.

Multiple-Lumen Catheters

A multiple-lumen catheter is a central venous catheter with more than one completely separate channel. It may be double- or triple-lumen, the latter appearing to be most popular (Figure 2.11). Four- and five-lumen catheters are now widely available. Only double-lumen catheters are available for paediatric use. They are necessarily large catheters with external diameters of 2.3 mm or more, compared with single-lumen catheters which are not usually more than 2 mm (14 gauge) across. A typical arrangement of the channels in a triple-lumen catheter as seen longitudinally is shown in Figure 2.12.[21] The distal ports of the three channels are staggered along a short length of catheter to minimise mixing of infusates as they exit.

Manufacturers produce a variety of designs with different cross-sectional arrangements of the separate lumina (Figure 2.13). A typical arrangement for double-lumen catheters is shown in Figure 2.13a. The most common arrangement in triple-lumen catheters is one large lumen (16 gauge) and two smaller (18 gauge) ones (Figure 2.13c,d). The lumen diameter determines the flow rate through the channel. The wall thickness determines to some extent the catheter's strength. Any particular configuration of lumen diameters therefore represents a compromise.

Catheter lengths available are 15 cm and 20 cm for right-sided internal jugular and subclavian veinentry sites, whilst longer catheters (25 cm and

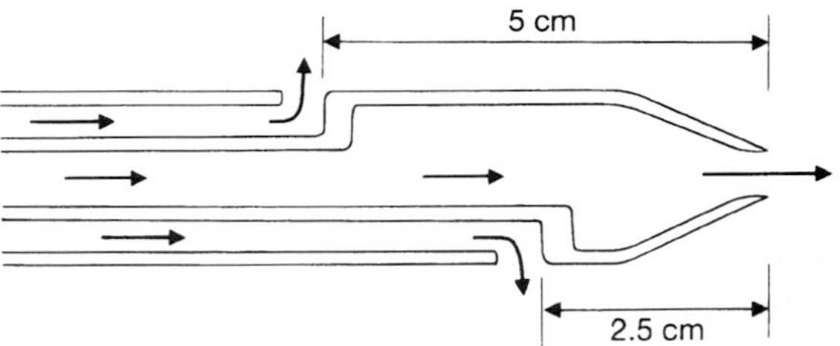

Figure 2.12 Longitudinal section of the distal end of a triple-lumen catheter. Reproduced by kind permission of Coe and Coates (1988).[21]

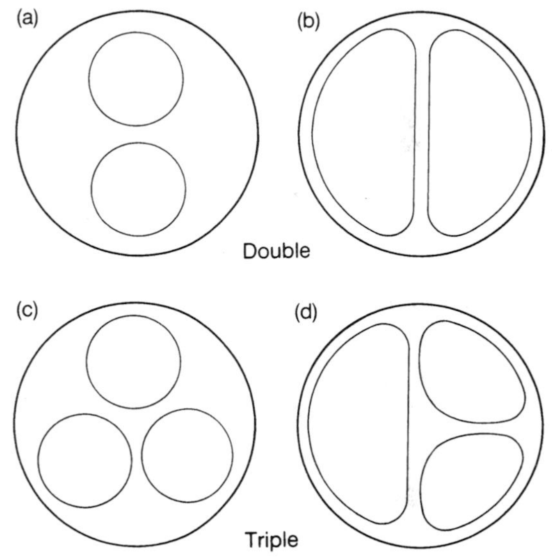

Figure 2.13 Cross-section of double-and triple-lumen catheters showing how lumen size can vary.

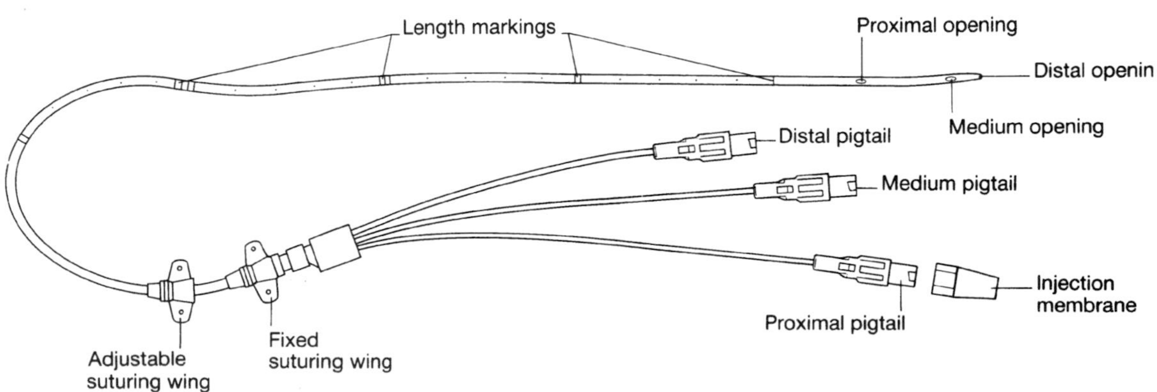

Figure 2.11 Features of a triple-lumen catheter.

30 cm) cater for left-sided attempts. Most catheters incorporate distance markings.

Paradoxically, the first of what was essentially a multilumen central venous catheter produced commercially was the most complex. This was the pulmonary artery flotation catheter which, although a single device, incorporated not only a thermistor and balloon-tipped pulmonary artery catheter but also a separate catheter with its own lumen opening into the right atrium for injecting an indicator solution for estimating cardiac output. The nature of its construction prevents the flotation catheter itself from being guided into the vein over a flexible wire, so the introduction of the flotation catheter spawned a number of introducer kits which facilitated insertion of the large-bore catheter. The introducer and vein dilator themselves necessitated a guide-wire for their insertion. There appears therefore to have developed from this available technology the production of the simpler multilumen catheter. The first double- and triple-lumen venous catheters were made available in 1982 (Arrow-Howes Multi-Lumen Central Venous Catheter, Arrow International Inc.). Similar designs are now widely available from all leading manufacturers.

Multilumen central venous catheters provide several benefits in situations where several routes of venous access are needed for the effective management of the patient. For example, in many patients undergoing intensive therapy, central venous access is needed for drug administration, blood sampling, pressure measurements and intravenous infusions of both crystalloids and parenteral nutrition fluids. If all these functions are being carried out through a single-lumen catheter there are obvious hazards resulting from the constant interruption of and surges in drug delivery and the mixing of infusates, apart from the practical inconvenience. In addition, the advantage of the multilumen catheter is very apparent in reducing the hazards inherent in making several separate venepunctures into deep neck veins to secure several individual venous channels.[22]

Additional lumina are useful in managing patients in critical care areas. When catheters with several exit orifices are used, great care is needed in inserting an adequate length of catheter into the vein. The exit lumina of the ports are disposed over a significant length of the distal end of the catheter. The most external port can be in danger of being extravascular even when an apparently adequate length of catheter has been inserted. Extravasation has been reported in one case involving a five-lumen Medex catheter (Medex Medical, Rossendale, UK) in which the most external lumen is 8.75 cm from the tip.[23]

The main disadvantages appear to be cost and the risk of interaction of the different infusates as they emerge from the exit ports, which must necessarily be close together. Catheter infection and catheter-related sepsis are well documented in relation to single-lumen catheters[24–27] and an increased incidence might have been expected with multiple-lumen catheters. Critical appraisal of such reports suggests that catheter-related sepsis is more likely to be expected in patients with multilumen catheters because they are more seriously ill and require more handling of their catheter and connections.[28] Breach of catheter management protocol is also an important contributing factor.[29] However, several careful prospective studies indicate that multilumen catheters may be safely used in severely ill patients requiring total parenteral nutrition provided that the care protocol is adhered to.[28,30–32] Prospective comparative studies with single-lumen catheters support the safety of multilumen catheters although the risk of catheter sepsis is no less.[33] With these conflicting reports in mind it is probably wise to use a channel of a triple-lumen catheter for parenteral nutrition only in the short term if such a catheter has been deemed necessary for the overall management of the patient. If intravenous feeding is likely to be long term, then at a later stage a dedicated tunnelled, single-lumen catheter can be inserted. A practical disadvantage of relying on venous access only through a multilumen catheter is that 'all one's eggs are in one basket'. If the multilumen catheter has to be removed, all venous access is lost in one move.

Insertion of multiple-lumen catheters

The recommended method of inserting these catheters is with the Seldinger guide-wire technique and vein dilator (see pp. 19–20 and 21). Before proceeding examine the catheter and identify each channel with its own proximal pigtail (usually colour coded). Irrigate each channel with heparinised saline.

1. Perform venepuncture of the chosen vein using the small-gauge wire introducer needle.
2. Insert the guide-wire to the superior vena cava and remove the needle. Allow a length of wire outside the skin sufficient to thread the whole length of the catheter plus an extra 2–3 cm to hold the wire as the catheter is slid into the vein over the wire.
3. Enlarge the puncture with a sharp-pointed scalpel blade.
4. Advance the vein dilator over the wire into the vein.
5. Remove the vein dilator.
6. Thread the catheter tip over the wire and insert it to its required length.
7. Remove the wire and confirm satisfactory positioning by easy aspiration of blood from each channel, flushing each lumen with heparinised saline.
8. Secure and apply a dressing to the puncture site.
9. Confirm position of catheter tip with a chest X-ray.

Some catheters are inserted using a catheter-through-cannula technique (see pp. 16–17 and 18). The introducer cannula can be peeled apart and removed, so eliminating any danger of air embolism which may exist with a through-the-cannula technique where the introducer cannula is left in the vein. This technique is probably only necessary for inserting the very soft silicone elastomer multilumen catheters.

Size of Needles, Catheters and Guide-wires

Table 2.2 gives some guidance in the selection of suitably sized equipment.

The introducing needle and cannula

Length

For puncturing visible superficial veins the introducing needle and cannula can be short (about 40 mm). When attempting puncture of deep veins the length must be adequate to reach the vein – something that may be difficult to estimate accurately in an obese patient. An introducer may need to be up to 70 mm long to gain entry to the subclavian vein, although a shorter length (40–60 mm) is adequate for puncture of the internal jugular vein.

In the case of the long cannula over the long needle, a sufficient length of cannula must be inserted into the vein for its tip to reach a satisfactory central venous position. This requirement determines the minimum length of the needle. Since the long needle is flexible it is difficult to control the tip accurately when attempting to puncture a vein. The risk of traumatic complications may thus be increased.

Diameter

Peripheral veins in particular can vary widely in size and may not even be visible or palpable in states of circulatory collapse, whereas the subclavian vein is always held open by its surrounding tissues. Veins can usually be distended by adopting aids such as a tourniquet or glyceryl trinitrate ointment in the case of peripheral arm veins or a head-down position in the case of internal jugular and subclavian veins. Generally, in adults, a 14 gauge or 16 gauge outside diameter (OD) introducing needle or introducing cannula is appropriate for central venous cannulation through large proximal veins. In the case of superficial veins the operator can make a decision only after inspecting the veins. Whenever the chosen vein is constricted or small, a guide-wire technique will allow the use of a smaller-gauge introducing needle and the subsequent insertion of a large-diameter catheter, using a vein dilator if necessary. Much smaller introducing needles or cannulae (18 gauge or smaller) have to be used in infants.

Cannulae and catheters

Length

The minimum length of a central venous cannula or catheter should equal the distance from the skin puncture to the desired central venous position

Table 2.2 Sizes of needles, catheters and guide-wires (adults).

Route of insertion	Introducer and long catheter			Long cannula with long needle	Introducer, guide-wire and catheter			
	Outside diameter of introducing needle or cannula gauge)	Minimum length of introucing needle or cannula (mm)	Minimum length of catheter* (mm)	Minimum length† (mm)	Outside diameter of introducing needle for guide-wire (G) (mm)	Outside diameter guide-wire (mm)	Minimum length of catheter (mm)	Length of guide-wire
Arm veins	14 or 16	short (40)	600	Not applicable	18(1.2)	0.77	600	
Internal jugular vein	14 or 16	short (40) Some techniques require 70	200	130	18(1.2)	0.77	200	Must exceed length of catheter by at least 100 mm
Subclavian vein	14 or 16	Mid-clavicular insertion 60 More lateral 70	200	130	18(1.2)	0.77	200	
External jugular vein	14 or 16	Short (40)	200	130	18(1.2)	0.77	200	
Femoral vein	14	Short (40)	600	Not applicable	18(1.2)	0.77	600	

* The catheter length allows for surplus catheter outside the skin for secure fixation.

† The design precludes excess length for fixation of catheter.

with sufficient length outside the skin to facilitate secure fixation. This distance should be estimated on the skin surface of the patient when selecting equipment.

Diameter

The outside diameter of the catheter in a through-needle or through-cannula device must be related to the type of introducer, as it must be smaller than the needle or introducing cannula in order to pass through it. If the catheter is to be inserted over the needle, the inside diameter of the catheter is also relevant. In most commercially available equipment the introducing needle and catheter are closely matched. In a guide-wire technique the wire must pass easily through the introducing needle; furthermore, the internal diameter of the catheter and the outside diameter of the wire must form a close fit.

Catheter Material

The ideal catheter material is chemically inert, non-thrombogenic, flexible, radio-opaque, and transparent (Table 2.3).

Most plastics contain various additives which may produce chemical phlebitis. These additives may comprise as much as 50% of the plastic material[34] and include plasticisers, stabilising agents, antioxidants, barium or tungsten salts for radio-opacity, and colouring material. The only way to determine whether these substances may leach out in the body is by subjecting the catheter material tobiological implant tests. Most British and American manufacturers use only tested materials. Silicone elastomer catheters have been generally considered to be the most biologically inert, but the validity of this has been questioned.[35]

Physical characteristics

Physical damage to the wall of the vein is related to the stiffness of the catheter. Stiff catheters generate thrombosis by pressure on the vein wall,[36] whilst flexible catheters that float in the bloodstream are less likely to produce injury.[37] Catheters made of polyethylene and polypropylene are relatively stiff and thrombogenic.[36–41] Fluorocarbons represent some improvement over the earlier materials, and fluoroethylene propylene (Teflon FEP) in

Table 2.3 Choice of material of catheter.

Type of material	Thrombogenic	Stiffness	Short-term use (48 h)	Long-term use
Polyethylene	++	++	Suitable	Unsuitable
PVC or nylon				
Polypropylene	++	+++	Suitable	Unsuitable
Fluorocarbons				
Teflon TFF	+	+	Suitable	Uncertain
Teflon FEP	+	+	Suitable	Uncertain
Polyurethane	+	0/+	Suitable	Suitable
Hydromer-coated polyurethane	0	0 (when wet)	Suitable	Alternative material of choice
Silicone elastomer	0	0 (pliable but difficult to insert, stylet needed)	Suitable	Material of choice based on long experience

particular has been shown to cause fewer venous complications than the older materials and tetrafluoroethylene (Teflon TFE).[42,43] Teflon FEP was widely used in the manufacture of cannulae. Most of these materials have now been dropped by manufacturers in favour of polyurethane. Polyurethane (PU) catheters have superior mechanical properties (tensile strength, wearing resistance many times that of silicone elastomer, ability to recover original shape after deformation). In addition PU is resistant to oils, oxidation hydrolysis and thermal degradation. In practice, these properties confer advantages in resisting kinking, bending and deformation compared with the plastics that were previously popular (Teflon, polyethylene and polyvinyl chloride). The softest and most flexible material is silicone elastomer, which is still generally regarded as the least thrombogenic and traumatic of currently available catheter materials. However, silicone elastomer catheters are so soft that they are difficult to insert into veins unless a stylet is employed. These catheters are much more fragile than PU catheters and are relatively easily ruptured when distended.[35]

Thrombogenicity

Whilst catheter stiffness has been implicated in the initiation of thrombus formation, making silicone elastomer (SE) with its soft characteristics preferable, it is possible that the chemical composition of the catheter is a more important factor in determining the incidence of clinical thrombophlebitis. Comparing equally soft PU and SE catheters, thrombophlebitis occurred significantly less often with the PU catheter.[35] Other experimental studies show a wide range of thrombogenicity between different materials. Comparing PU, Hydromer-coated PU, PVC and SE catheters, Hydromer-coated PU appeared the best, followed by SE. Plain PU was the worst.[44]

Hydromer is the commercial name for a polymer made from polyvinylpyrrolidone (PVP) and an isocyanate prepolymer. The Hydromer polymer so formed is a hydrophilic substance (i.e. it absorbs water) and forms a gel. When a Hydromer-coated catheter is wetted, water is absorbed onto the coating and the resulting gel acts as a barrier between the blood flowing past in the vessel and the catheter material (a foreign substance which would normally lead to platelet deposition). Thus any tendency for the initiation of thrombosis is inhibited. A practical advantage of a Hydromer-coated catheter is that when wetted by body fluids (including blood) the catheter becomes exceptionally slippery, which assists easy passage of the catheter and reduces trauma to the blood vessel.

Heparin coating and bonding have proved disappointing for protecting catheters against the risk of thrombogenesis in long-term catheterisation. Studies show no benefit compared with uncoated catheters.[45,46]

Catheters should be radio-opaque since it has been shown by many authors that an X-ray is the only reliable method of determining the position of the catheter tip. Radio-opaque catheters constructed of all the materials mentioned above are now commercially available. Catheters of transparent material allow air bubbles and particles to be easily seen. The older materials are transparent but some Teflon and silicone elastomer catheters are opaque.

Most catheter materials are suitable for short-term catheterisation (up to 48 hours) and selection is therefore determined by availability, ease of insertion and cost. For long-term use, non-thrombogenicity, flexibility and chemical inertnessare paramount and override the requirements for ease of insertion and radio-opacity. Silicone elastomer catheters are therefore recommended for longer-term catheterisation, especially for prolonged intravenous alimentation. Of the other materials, polyurethane and Hydromer-coated polyurethane catheters are to be preferred for long-term use.

Apparatus used in Long-term Central Venous Access

Long-term central venous access has become an integral requirement in the management of an increasingly wide spectrum of disease. The needs of patients in this category have led to the development of special devices to avoid the shortcomings of simpler catheter systems which include the frequent occurrence of catheter-related pain, phlebitis and infections.[47] With repeated treatments some patients have simply run out of accessible veins.

The components of these specialised systems comprise a suitable catheter which was formerly invariably made of silicone elastomer, although newer materials such as Hydromer-coated polyurethane have now been advocated for long-term catheters. Traditionally, the catheter was inserted into a suitable vein (usually the subclavian) using a surgical cut-down procedure. Catheters can, however, also be inserted satisfactorily with percutaneous techniques although it appears that surgical cut-down retains its popularity in these special cases. The catheter is then tunnelled subcutaneously to a distal site where it terminates in one of two possible ways (Table 2.4). In the first type, where the catheter is led through a skin exit site, a Dacron cuff surrounds the catheter before it emerges. The Dacron cuff is designed to encourage local fibrosis, which acts as a physical barrier to the entry of bacteria along the track of the catheter as well as anchoring the catheter securely. In the second type of device (Figures 2.14 and 2.15), the catheter ends in a reservoir (e.g. Port-a-Cath) which has been implanted subcutaneously. The reservoir has a self-sealing silicone diaphragm through which entry is made into the reservoir by percutaneous puncture. A needle with a special Huber point is available (Viggo Products, Swindon, UK). The tip of this needle is designed to displace rather than tear the fibres of the silicone diaphragm of the reservoir.[48] A Dacron cuff is again often incorporated in this system.

A recent innovation has been the introduction of a cuff made of biodegradable collagen to which silver ion has been chelated.[49] The cuff has been

Table 2.4 Long-term central venous catheter devices.

Catheter type	Description	Examples
Tunnelled silicone catheter	Silicone catheter tunnelled subcutaneously exiting the skin medial to the nipple. Dacron cuff around catheter at least 3 cm away from the skin entry site	Hickman – single or double lumen Broviac – smaller lumen Quinton – double lumen Groshong – single or double lumen special sealing valve at tip allowing saline instead of heparin to maintain patency
Subcutaneous infusion port	Silicone catheter tunnelled subcutaneously ending in a self-sealing silicone reservoir implanted beneath the skin	Mediport Infus-a-Port Port-a-Cath Vascuport

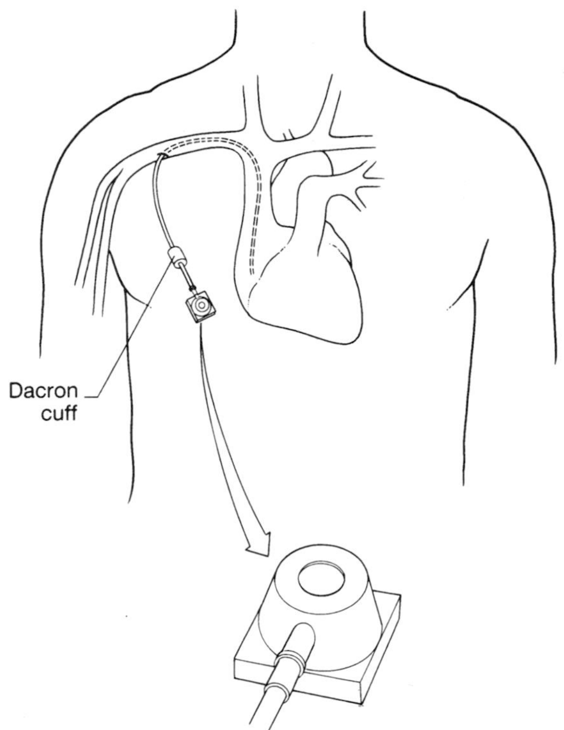

Figure 2.14 The long-term central venous catheter with a subcutaneously implanted reservoir (Port-a-Cath type). Note Dacron cuff. Reproduced with kind permission of Clarke and Raffin (1990).[52]

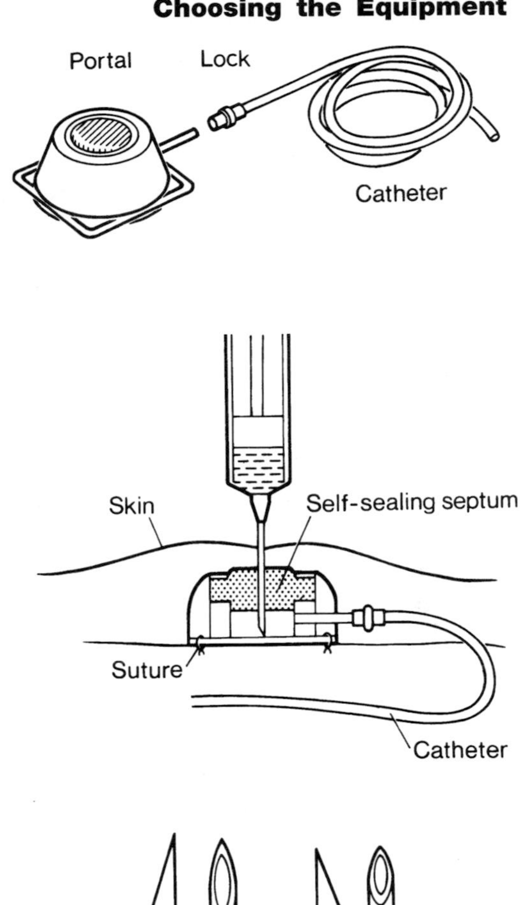

Figure 2.15 The Port-a-Cath system and diagram showing percutaneous access to the portal using the Huber point needle. Reproduced with kind permission of Soo *et al.* (1985).[53]

developed to be used with percutaneously inserted catheters. It is attached to the catheter prior to insertion into the vein. Subsequently, subcutaneous tissue grows into the collagen and as with the Dacron cuff, provides a barrier to bacteria and secures the catheter. In addition, the silver ion acts as a chemical barrier to the passage of organisms. Studies give encouraging results in the reduction of catheter-related sepsis and the enhanced life span of catheters.

Unfortunately, even these sophisticated techniques have not fully prevented a significant incidence of catheter-related problems, especially catheter infections. Nevertheless, experience over many years confirms the value of these specialised devices in long-term central venous catheter survival, but only if strict recommendations concerning their insertion and maintenance are adhered to (see Chapter 3).

Double-lumen Central Venous Haemodialysis Catheters

Double-lumen central venous haemodialysis catheters were introduced to provide permanent access for renal dialysis and to spare peripheral vessels for the creation of more durable arteriovenous fistulae. The method of insertion is identical to any guide-wire technique. It is crucial to place both distal orifices of the catheter in a large-diameter vein to obtain adequate flows for the dialysis machine. Full patency and adequate free flow of blood through both lumina of the catheter must be established before the catheter is fixed in position.

These catheters have integral clamping devices to prevent air embolism. When not in use the catheter is regularly flushed with heparinised saline. The majority of these catheters will function for up to 2 months. Replacement of the catheter can be performed over a guide-wire provided that the original catheter is not the source of sepsis and is not blocked by thrombus.[50,51]

PICC Lines

The peripherally inserted central venous catheter (PICC) has been developed to facilitate intravenous therapy over a medium to long-term period and so avoid the need to resort to more invasive techniques. These devices are essentially long catheters designed to be inserted through the veins around the antecubital fossa. Important elements of these catheters include the use of silicone elastomer and detailed design to permit insertion and facilitate nursing management. These catheters are described in more detail in Chapter 3.

References

1. Seldinger SI. Catheter replacement of needle in percutaneous arteriography: new technique. Acta Radiologica 1953; **39**:368.
2. Taylor FW, Rutherford CE. Accidental loss of plastic tube into venous system. Archives of Surgery 1963; **86**:177.
3. Bennett PJ. Use of intravenous plastic catheters. British Medical Journal 1963; **2**:1252.
4. John GE. Serious accidents involving intravenous catheters. DHSS DS (Supply) 6/72. DHSS Circular, 1972.
5. Farman JV. Which central venous catheter? British Journal of Clinical Equipment 1978; **32**:210.
6. Ross SM, Freedman PS, Farman JV. Air embolism after accidental removal of intravenous catheter. British Medical Journal 1979; **1**:987.
7. Smith SL, Albin MS, Ritter RR, Bunegin L. CVP catheter replacement from the antecubital veins using a J-wire catheter guide. Anesthesiology 1984; **60**:238.
8. Belani KG, Buckley JJ, Gordon JR, Castenda W. Percutaneous cervical central venous line placement: a comparison of the internal and external jugular vein routes. Anesthesia and Analgesia 1980; **59**:40.
9. Peters JL, Armstrong R. Air embolism occurring as a complication of central venous catheterization. Annals of Surgery 1978; **187**:375.
10. Editorial. Central venous catheterisation. Lancet 1986; **2**:669.
11. Miller JDB, Broom J. Early non-radiological recognition of misplacement of central venous catheter. British Medical Journal 1983; **287**:95.
12. Bowdle, TA. Improved technique for placement of Sorenson CVP catheter. Anesthesia and Analgesia 1984; **63**:1143.
13. Baum S, Abrams HL. A J-shaped catheter for retrograde catheterization of tortuous vessels. Radiology 1964; **83**:436.
14. Judkins MP, Kidd HJ, Frische LH, Dotter CT. Lumen-following J-guide for catheterization of tortuous vessels. Radiology 1967; **88**:1127.
15. Blitt CD, Wright WA, Petty CP, Webster TA. Central venous catheterization via the external jugular vein. A technique employing the J-wire. Journal of the American Medical Association 1974; **229**:817.
16. Blyth PL. Evaluation of the technique of central venous catheterisation via the external jugular vein using the J-wire. Anaesthesia and Intensive Care 1985; **13**:131.
17. Wilkie M, Hughes M. Complications of central venous cannulation. British Medical Journal 1988; **297**:1126.
18. Blitt CD, Carlson GL, Wright WA, Otto CW. J-wire versus straight wire for central venous system cannulation via the external jugular vein. Anesthesia and Analgesia 1982; **61**:536.
19. Schwartz AJ, Harrow JC, Jobes DR, Ellison N. Guide wires – a caution. Critical Care Medicine 1981; **9**:347.
20. Kaye CG, Smith DR. Complications of central venous cannulation. British Medical Journal 1988; **297**:572.
21. Coe AJ, Coates DP. Triple lumen catheters. British Journal of Hospital Medicine 1988; **39**:313.
22. Powell H. Safety first with triple lumen. Murmurs (Lilly Cardiac Care) 1988; **5**:27.
23. Walker C, Jackson D, Dolan S. The potential for extravasation using a new five lumen catheter [letter]. Anaesthesia 1997; **52**:716.
24. Mogenson JV, Frederiksen W, Jensen JK. Subclavian vein catheterization and infection: a bacteriological study of 130 catheterization insertions. Scandinavian Journal of Infectious Disease 1972; **4**:31.
25. Bernard RW, Stahl WM, Chase RM. Subclavian vein catheterization: a prospective study. II. Infectious complications. Annals of Surgery 1971; **173**:191.
26. Applefield JA, Carruthers TE, Reno DJ *et al.* Assessment of the sterility of long-term cardiac catheterization using the thermodilution Swan-Ganz catheter. Chest 1978; **74**:377.
27. Michel L, Marsh M, McMichan JC *et al.* Infection of pulmonary artery catheters in critically ill patients. Journal of the American Medical Association 1981; **245**:1032.

28. Payne-James JJ, Doherty J, Rees RG, Silk DBA. A prospective evaluation of a multi-lumen central venous catheter in patients requiring total parenteral nutrition. Intensive Therapy and Clinical Monitoring Aug/Sept 1989; **89**:213.
29. Clarke PJ, Ball MJ, Tunbridge A, Kettlewell MGW. The total parenteral nutrition service: an update. Annals of the Royal College of Surgeons 1988; **70**:296.
30. Kelly CS, Ligas JR, Smith CA, Madden GM, Ross KA, Becker DR. Sepsis due to triple lumen central venous catheters. Surgery, Gynecology and Obstetrics 1986; **163**:14.
31. Paterson-Brown S, Parry BR, Sim AJW. The role of double-lumen catheters in intravenous nutrition. Intensive Therapy and Clinical Monitoring 1987; **8**:54.
32. Kaufman JL, Rodriguez JL, McFadden JA, Brolin RE. Clinical experience with the multilumen central nervous catheter. Journal of Parenteral and Enteral Nutrition 1986; **10**:487.
33. Miller JJ, Venus B, Mathru M. Comparison of the sterility of long-term central venous catheterization using single lumen, triple lumen, and pulmonary artery catheters. Critical Care Medicine 1984; **12**:634.
34. Mitchell DC. Putting up a drip. Info No. 12. Queensborough, Kent: Abbott Laboratories. 1975.
35. Linder L, Curelaru I, Gustavsson B, Hansson H, Stenqvist O, Wojciechowski J. Material thrombogenicity in central venous catheterization: a comparison between soft, antebrachial catheters of silicone elastomer and polyurethane. Journal of Parenteral and Enteral Nutrition 1984; **8**:399.
36. Indar R. The danger of indwelling polyethylene cannulae in deep veins. Lancet 1959; **1**:284.
37. Hoshal VL, Ause RG, Hoskins PA. Fibrin sleeve formation on indwelling subclavian central venous catheters. Archives of Surgery 1971; **102**:353.
38. Wyatt R, Glaves I, Cooper DJ. Cannulation of the radial artery. Lancet 1974; **2**:156.
39. Frazer IH, Eke N, Laing MS. Is infusion phlebitis preventable? British Medical Journal 1977; **2**:232.
40. Pottecher T, Forrier M, Picardat R, Krause D. Central venous catheter thrombogenicity. European Journal of Anaesthesia 1984; **1**:361.
41. Stenqvist O, Curelaru I, Linder L, Gustavsson B. Stiffness of central venous catheters. Acta Anaesthesiologica Scandinavica 1983; **27**:153.
42. Dinley RJ. Venous reactions related to indwelling plastic cannulae: a prospective clinical trial. Current Medical Research and Opinion 1976; **3**:607.
43. Thomas FW, Evers W, Racz BG. Post infusion phlebitis. Anesthesia and Analgesia: Current Researches 1970; **49**:150.
44. Borow M, Crowley JG. Evaluation of central venous catheter thrombogenicity. Acta Anaesthesiologia Scandinavica 1985; **81**(suppl):59.
45. Bennegard L, Curelaru I, Gustavsson B, Linder LE, Zachrisson BF. Material thrombogenicity in central venous catheterization. I. A comparison between uncoated and heparin-coated, long, antebrachial polyethylene catheters. Acta Anaesthesiologica Scandinavica 1982; **26**:112.
46. Mollenholt P, Eriksson I, Andersson T. Thrombogenicity of pulmonary-artery catheters. Intensive Care Medicine 1987; **13**:57.
47. Peters JL, Belsham PA, Taylor BA, Watt-Smith S. Long -term venous access. British Journal of Hospital Medicine 1984; **32**:230.
48. Shanbhogue LKR, Bruce J, Bianchi A. Implantation of a central venous access device. Journal of the Royal College of Surgeons of Edinburgh 1990; **35**:252.
49. Maki DG, Cobb L, Garman JK, Shapiro JM. An attachable silver-impregnated cuff for prevention of infection with central venous catheters: a prospective randomized multicenter trial. American Journal of Medicine 1988; **85**:307.
50. Dunn Y, Nylander W, Richie R. Central venous dialysis access: experience with dual lumen silicone rubber catheters. Surgery 1987; **102**:784.
51. Schwab SJ, Buller GL, McCann RL *et al.* Prospective evaluation of a Dacron cuffed haemodialysis catheter for prolonged use. American Journal of Kidney Disease 1986; **11**:166.
52. Clarke DE, Raffin A. Infectious complications of indwelling long-term central venous catheters. Chest 1990; **97**:966.
53. Soo KC, Davidson TI, Selby P, Westbury G. Long-term venous access using a subcutaneous implantable drug delivery system. Annals of the Royal College of Surgeons of England, 1985; **67**:264.

3 • Practical Aspects of Technique

SHANG NG

Each technique of central venous catheterisation is described separately below, but there are a number of important practical procedures which can increase the likelihood of a successful and safe cannulation in all methods. Guidance in these procedures is presented in roughly the sequence in which an operator may need them during central venous catheterisation.

Identification of Anatomical Planes

In many of the techniques described in this book it is necessary to relate the direction in which the needle is advanced to conventional anatomical planes (Figure 3.1). This is important in order to avoid ambiguity in the descriptions.

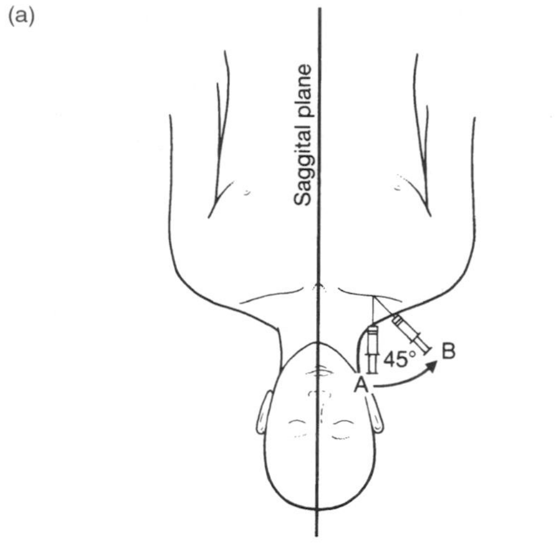

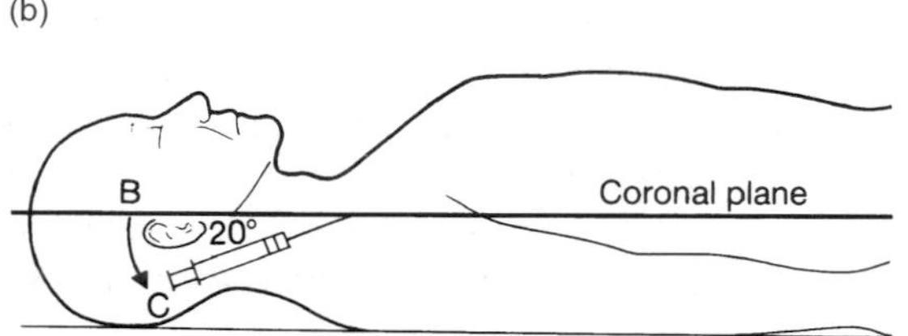

Figure 3.1 Identification of anatomical planes. (a) Needle and syringe moved 45° away from *sagittal* plane (A to B). (b) Needle and syringe depressed 20° below the *coronal* plane (B to C).

Prevention of Air Embolism

There is a risk of air embolism whenever a vein is cannulated and particularly when it is a large vessel such as the internal jugular or subclavian vein.[1] This complication can occur through a leak or a disconnection (deliberate or accidental) which opens the system to the atmosphere. It has been estimated that a fatal dose of air – 100 ml – can enter through a 14 gauge cannula in 1 second. Attention to the following points can greatly diminish the danger.

Position

If the venous pressure at the site of the venepuncture can be increased by correct positioning of the patient the risk of aspiration of air is diminished. For instance, in approaches to the subclavian and jugular veins a head-down tilt (10–30°) is necessary – besides distending the vein and facilitating successful venepuncture this also prevents air embolism. The same advantages follow the use of a tourniquet during puncture of the arm veins. It is important to remember, however, that when the tourniquet is released the open hub on the needle or catheter must be kept below the level of the patient's right atrium until it is closed by means of a stopcock or connected to an infusion system. These precautions also apply when catheterising the femoral vein.

Air leaks

Most techniques employ a syringe attached to a needle. It is essential to check that the joint between syringe and needle (or introducing cannula) is airtight. Some cannulae incorporate an on/off

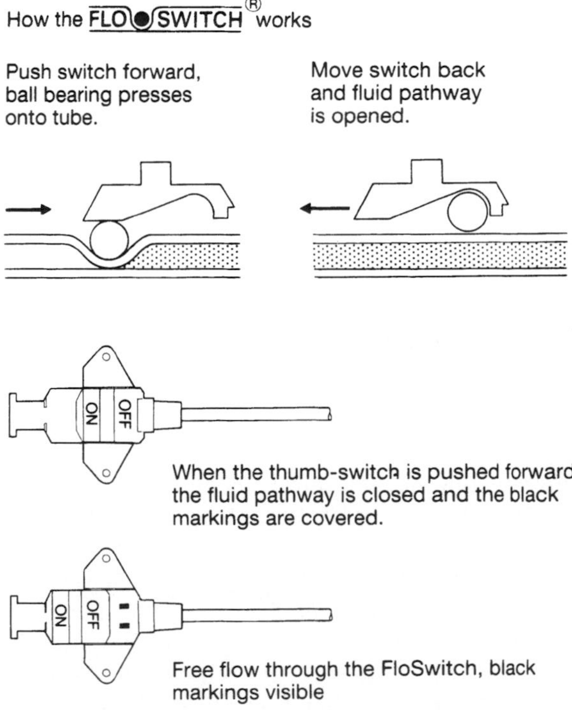

Figure 3.2 FloSwitch.

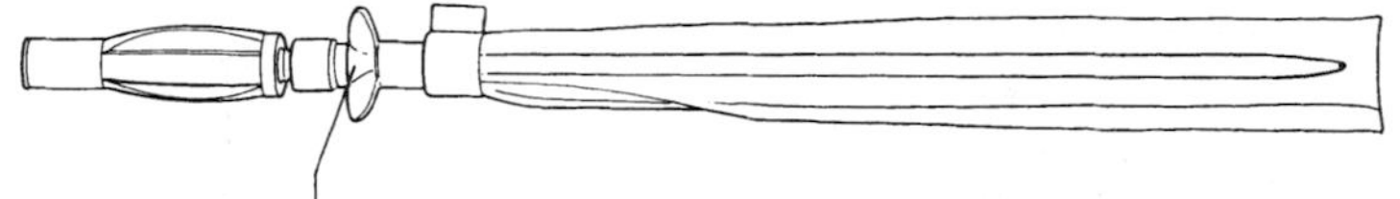

Figure 3.3 Flexihub.

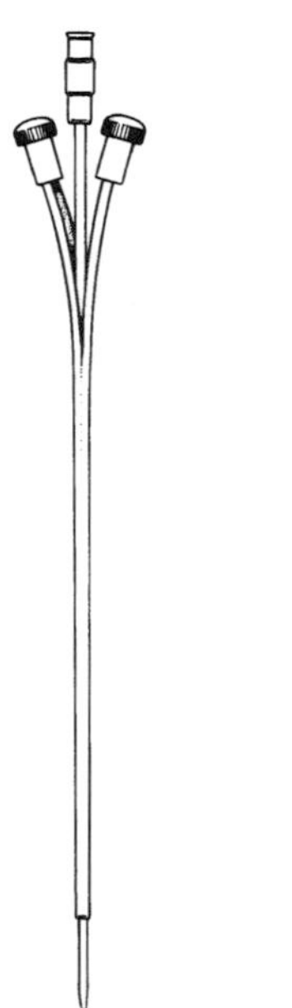

Figure 3.4 Split introducer. Reproduced with kind permission of Wood (1985).[70]

switch at the hub (FloSwitch, Viggo-Spectramed, Swindon, UK, Figure 3.2) or a flexible hub (Flexihub, H.G. Wallace Ltd, Colchester, UK, Figure 3.3) which can be compressed between the fingers. These types of device help to prevent the entry of air during cannulation and when connections are being made.

A less obvious danger of air embolism exists when a catheter is introduced into the vein through a wide-bore cannula which is left with its tip in the vein,[2] for air can pass through the space between the catheter and the wide-bore cannula. If the catheter is accidentally withdrawn, there is a very wide passage for air to reach the vein. It is therefore essential to withdraw the introducing cannula completely from the interior of the vein.

Split introducer cannulae, as their name suggests, can be peeled apart and removed entirely from the vein after successful insertion of a catheter with a fixed hub (Figure 3.4).

Patient's respiration

If the patient is inhaling deeply when the system is open to the air, the subatmospheric pressure within the thorax may suck air into the venous system. Therefore, a conscious patient should be instructed not to breathe deeply during the procedure. If an anaesthetised or unconscious patient is attached to a breathing circuit the venous pressure should be increased by holding the lungs briefly in inflation at any critical time.

Initial Location of the Vein with a Small-gauge Needle

The technique of using a small-gauge needle to locate the vein can be employed usefully in any approach in which venepuncture is 'blind'. Exploration with a small-gauge needle minimises injury and haematoma formation should an artery be inadvertently punctured.

This technique has been advocated for the internal jugular route,[3,4] and the subclavian route.[5]

Directional guide

A 21 gauge or 22 gauge outside diameter needle of suitable length is attached to a syringe. If local anaesthetic solution is being infiltrated subcutaneously, the same needle can be introduced more deeply to locate the vein.[6] A slight negative pressure is maintained on the syringe as the needle is advanced until a 'flashback' of blood indicates entry into the vein. The position of the vein is noted, the small needle removed (or left in position as a guide) and venepuncture with the larger needle attempted along a parallel track.

Guide-wire technique

If a guide-wire technique is used, the small-gauge wire introducer needle can serve also as the locating needle. However, in many commercially available kits, the introducer needle is sometimes, it seems, unnecessarily long and large (18 or 16 gauge). In these cases a small-gauge (21 or 22) short needle is recommended to find the vein first.

Fixation of the Catheter

The catheter must be securely fixed in position as soon as it has been successfully inserted. This is necessary for two reasons. First, the catheter will not be lost into the vein if it is inadvertently cut across outside the skin. This complication is usually associated with catheter-through-needle devices[7,8] but any catheter may fracture or be accidentally cut.[9,10] A 'lost' catheter must be removed because of the high risk of infection; if the fragment has entered the heart it can be removed either by a Dormia catheter device[11] passed into the heart or, if this is unsuccessful, by open heart surgery. Second, securing the catheter prevents any movement, which produces mechanical and chemical irritation of the intima of the vein encouraging local thrombophlebitis.[12] Furthermore, preventing movement reduces the chance of infection produced by the inward migration of bacteria proliferating at the site of skin puncture.

Adhesive tape can be used when the catheter is to be in position for a short time only (for example, during an operation). Tape soon loses its adhesiveness and skin reactions commonly occur. For anchoring the catheter for a long period a skin suture is especially recommended. In comparison with adhesive tape, it is likely to be more effective in reducing the risk of catheter embolism if the catheter is accidentally cut across.

Adhesive tape

Narrow (1 cm) adhesive tape is passed beneath the catheter, adhesive side facing upwards, crossed over above the catheter, ensuring that the catheter is gripped firmly, and attached to the skin. Tincture of benzoin applied to the skin before the tape is attached improves its adhesion and may also reduce damage to the underlying skin.

Skin suture

A 3–0 silk or fine wire stitch is inserted through the skin and subcutaneous tissue and tied loosely over the catheter. The two ends of the suture are then passed around the catheter and firmly tied. In this way the catheter is securely fastened without any direct pressure by the catheter on the skin.

Bio-occlusive dressing

The use of thin, transparent adhesive dressings has gained popularity following claims that they prevent contamination at the point of entry of the cannula and isolate the catheter from the surrounding area, while allowing frequent inspection without the need to remove the dressing.

Correct Positioning of the Catheter Tip

The tip of a central venous catheter inserted for the measurement of central venous pressure or for long-term parenteral nutrition should lie in a large intrathoracic vein. The preferred position[13] (Figure 3.5a) is in the upper part of the superior vena cava above the pericardial reflection, to avoid any danger of perforation or erosion of the lower portion of the superior vena cava, right atrium or right ventricle, which could lead to pericardial haemorrhage and cardiac tamponade.[14,15] In one study there was an 87% mortality rate among 16 patients who developed cardiac tamponade following the use of a central venous catheter.[13] An additional reason for ensuring that a catheter does not enter the heart is the risk of provoking dysrhythmias.[9] Even with the catheter tip positioned above the pericardial reflection, perforation of the subclavian or innominate veins can still give rise to the serious complications of hydromediastinum or hydrothorax.[16,17]

The danger of placing the catheter tip within the pericardial reflection has been well publicised. The practice of identifying the position of the catheter tip after insertion has been recommended by all authors in this field. Yet up to the time of writing a steady stream of reports of cardiac perforation and lethal or near-fatal consequences have continued to be published.[33]

Insertion of the catheter deep into the right atrium can be detected easily on a chest X-ray and failure to remedy this cannot be excused. However, even in carefully positioned catheters the tip may still be placed in a dangerous position because of the difficulty in recognising accurately the level of pericardial reflection on a supine portable anteroposterior (AP) chest X-ray. Bony landmarks which may be reliable in a posteroanterior chest film may vary in position considerably on an AP film because of parallax errors. Inserting the catheter to a predetermined length may also be unsatisfactory.

In an audit of catheters placed by the infraclavicular route to a standard depth of 15 cm, more than half the tips were in 'too far'.[33] The authors recommended a tailored technique in which the distance from skin to venepuncture was first determined. An additional length was added to this equal to the distance between the proximal port and the distal port plus a further 3 cm. This extra 3 cm would allow for any catheter migration towards the skin leading to a risk of extravasation from the proximal port in the event that this came to lie outside the lumen of the vein. When this technique was used only a small proportion of catheter tips were sited 'too far'.

These workers proposed that any recommendation of insertion into the subclavian and internaljugular veins further than 15 cm would be excessive.

There are occasional indications for deliberately placing a catheter in the right atrium – for instance, to aspirate air which may reach the heart from the site of operation in certain neurosurgical procedures.[18] If the catheter is inserted through the femoral vein, the tip should lie in the inferior vena cava below the diaphragm.

Numerous investigations have shown that if the catheter tip is placed blindly it may settle in an unsatisfactory site, irrespective of the route of insertion.[19–26] The position of the catheter tip is deemed unsatisfactory if it lies in a peripheral vein (Figure 3.5b), in an internal jugular vein (Figure 3.5c), or in the heart (Figure 3.5d).

Even when a sufficient length of catheter has been advanced into the vein, the tip may still not have reached a central position. The catheter may curl back on itself and pass retrogradely. A catheter inserted through an arm vein may traverse the intrathoracic veins and emerge in the other arm vein. A catheter can find its way into the internal jugular vein from any route of insertion (other than through the femoral vein), but this most frequently happens with catheters inserted through arm veins.[19,24,25,27,28] Inserting too great a length of catheter so that it enters the right atrium or right ventricle is a common occurrence. The catheter may even enter the pulmonary artery.[9] A catheter lying in the internal jugular vein may be satisfactorily repositioned by withdrawing an appropriate length, but the catheter should not be reinserted as the portion withdrawn is no longer sterile. Withdrawing the appropriate length of a catheter that has entered the heart results in a perfectly positioned catheter in the superior vena cava.

The following steps should be taken when any central venous catheter is inserted:

1. The catheter (kept in the sterile coverings) should be placed against the skin and the length from the intended skin puncture site to a satisfactory central position roughly estimated. This length can later be rechecked using the stylet (if provided) after inserting the catheter. In many commercially available kits, distance markings are printed on the catheter which enables the precise length inserted to be known.
2. When the catheter is in place it should be possible to aspirate and reinject blood freely without undue resistance.
3. When a manometer is connected, oscillations should be seen which are synchronous with respiration and pulse.

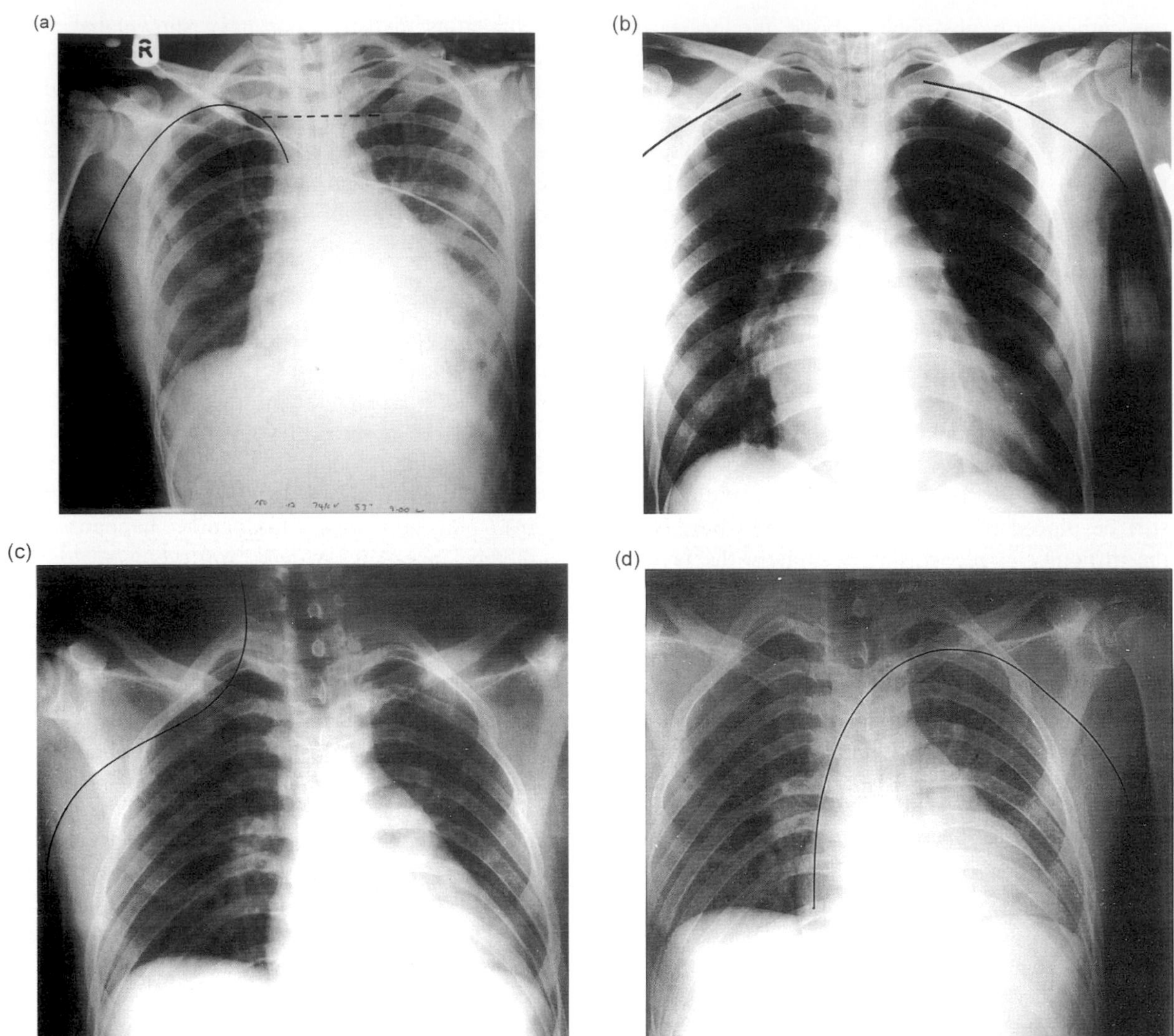

Figure 3.5 (a) Correct positioning of the catheter tip in the upper part of the superior vena cava. (b) Incorrect positioning of the catheter tip in a peripheral vein. (c) Incorrect positioning of the catheter tip in an internal jugular vein. (d) Incorrect positioning of the catheter tip in the heart.

4. A chest X-ray is the only certain method of identifying the position of the tip and should be taken as soon as possible. However, if the catheter is not made of radio-opaque material, it must be filled with a radio-opaque medium such as Urografin 60% (sodium diatrizoate injection). In adults the catheter tip should lie no more than 2 cm below a line joining the lower surfaces of the ends of the clavicle on a posteroanterior chest X-ray (Figure 3.6).[13] This line corresponds to the division of the superior vena cava into a portion well above and a portion below the pericardial reflection (see Figure 3.5a). If the catheter has been inserted into the inferior vena cava, its tip should lie below the level of the diaphragm.

Only after ascertaining the position of the catheter tip should the administration of intravenous fluid be started.

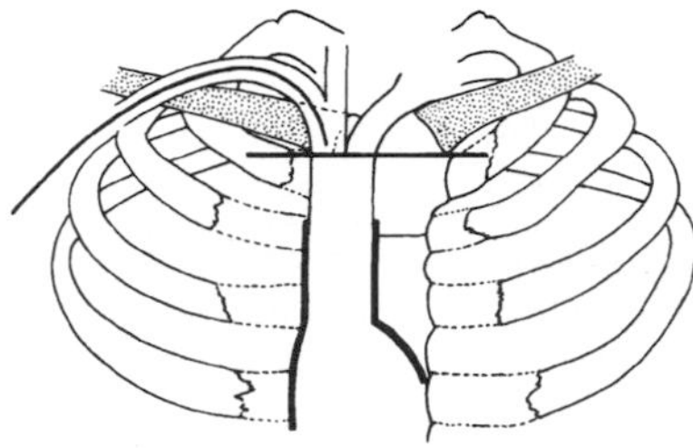

Figure 3.6 Outline diagram of central veins superimposed on skeletal appearance of posteroanterior chest radiograph. Line is drawn below lower surface of each clavicle (shaded), and we suggest that tip of catheter should lie no more than 2 cm below this. Heavy lines represent pericardial reflections around superior vena cava. Reproduced from Greenall *et al.* (1975) with kind permission of the BMJ Publishing Group.[13]

Ultrasound-aided central venous catheterisation

An ultrasound apparatus, if available, can facilitate and make the insertion of a central venous catheter safer under direct imaging. The method gives immediate and accurate confirmation of correct positioning of the catheter tip. Ultrasound techniques have been used in catheterisation through subclavian and internal jugular vein routes.[30–32]

Several suppliers now offer compact, portable ultrasound apparatus suitable for aiding central venous cannulation. One particular device has been specifically designed for central venous cannulation. The miniature ultrasound scanner is dedicated to internal jugular vein puncture (Site-Rite, Dymax Corporation, Pittsburgh, Pa, USA). The scanner incorporates a needle guide enabling accurate advancement of the needle tip into the vein as the operator watches a clear display (Figure 3.7).

Visualisation of the procedure in this way can reduce the number of attempts required to gain satisfactory entry into the vein and increase the rate of successful cannulation. This is accompanied by a convincing reduction in the incidence of complications.[34–36] One study involved over 1200 internal jugular vein cannulations. When venepuncture was guided by anatomical landmarks, there was a success rate of 88% after an average of 2.5 attempts. With visual display from the ultrasound probe (Site-Rite, Dymax) a 100% success

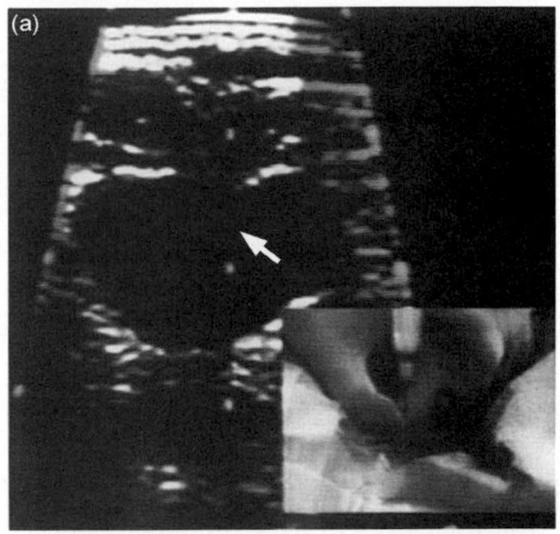

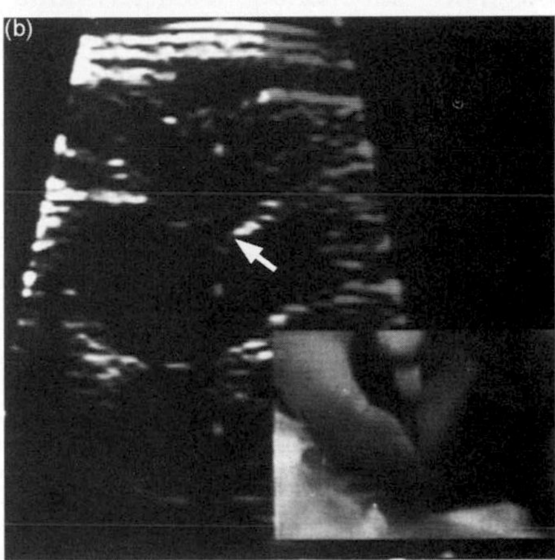

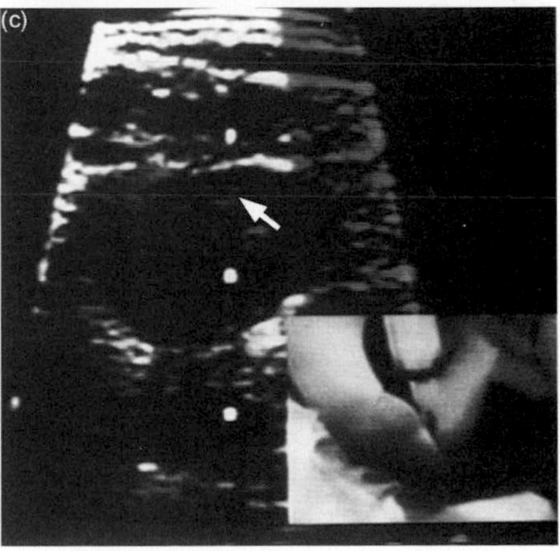

Figure 3.7 Ultrasound display of venepuncture of internal jugular vein using the Site-Rite scanner. (a) Arrow shows the vein wall being invaginated as the needle approaches the vein. (b, c) Vein wall springs back as the needle penetrates and is advanced into the lumen.

rate was achieved with 1.3 attempts with significantly less complications.[34] Similar results were found in a study involving 95 infants. When anatomical landmarks were used, there was a success rate of 76% after an average of 3.3 attempts in 14 minutes with complications of 36% (mainly carotid artery puncture). With visual display of ultrasound guidance (Site-Rite, Dymax) a 100% success rate was achieved with 1.3 attempts in 4 minutes with no complications at all.[35]

Ultrasound-guided cannulation devices would thus seem to promise easy and risk-free cannulation of deep veins. Many studies have supported this promise.[36] However, in a large study where infraclavicular subclavian catheterisation was attempted under controlled non-emergency conditions, ultrasound guidance had no effect on the rate of complications or failures. However, in this series, ultrasound was only used to identify the subclavian vein and mark its position on the skin. Real-time ultrasound guidance was not used for actual placement of the catheter.[37] In contrast, in another study of less experienced operators (fewer than 30 successful attempts previously) the ultrasound-assisted technique showed a clear advantage in terms of success and enabled salvage of a number of instances in which the use of landmarks alone had failed. The ultrasound device used in this study (Sife-Rite, Dymax) gives a real-time image.[38]

A direct comparison of internal jugular vein catheterisation using conventional landmarks compared with ultrasound guidance with an audible (but not a visual) signal again showed no advantage gained with the ultrasound device in 'easy' patients. However, the ultrasound machine did enable avoidance of carotid artery puncture by correctly distinguishing artery from vein.

The particular device used seems to dictate the differing experiences that have been reported. Clearly, a distinction should be made between devices that give visual guidance (e.g. Site-Rite, Dymax) and those that give only an auditory signal (e.g. SMART Needle[39]). The author's experience is that the Site-Rite instrument with its real-time visual display enhances successful cannulation. With experienced operators, the particular advantage of ultrasound guidance is really only apparent in difficult cases where there is distortion of normal anatomy. This may be a feature in patients who have undergone previous catheterisation, surgery or radiotherapy in the clavicular region. Ultrasound guidance techniques are certainly worthwhile adjuncts in training programmes.[71]

ECG guided placement of central venous catheters

Electrocardiographic (ECG) guidance was first used in helping position the tip of a ventriculoatrial catheter being inserted for the treatment of hydrocephalus.[40] Precise positioning in the right atrium-was crucial to the proper functioning of the catheter. The method eliminated the need for a confirmatory X-ray during the operation. In neurosurgery, the technique has also been used to accurately position a central venous catheter tip to aspirate air embolus[18] as well as for venous pressure measurement.[41]

The key to the technique is recognition of the large negative or biphasic P wave of the ECG trace as the fluid-filled catheter acting as an exploring electrode is advanced into the right atrium (Figure 3.8).

A good success rate of 81% has been achieved using a catheter filled with electrolyte connected through a metal stopcock and wire to the V_5 lead of the ECG monitor. The conducting fluids used were 8.4% sodium bicarbonate (readily available) and 4% saline (made up). The time taken was 5–15 minutes.[42]

Other authors have made useful recommendations.[43] Their usual ECG configuration consisted of:

right arm lead to the right shoulder
left arm lead to the left shoulder
left leg lead to the upper half of the sternum.

When ECG-guided central venous catheterisation was needed, the following adjustments were made:

right arm as above
left leg lead to the left shoulder
left arm lead was clipped to the distal end of the guide-wire inside the catheter.

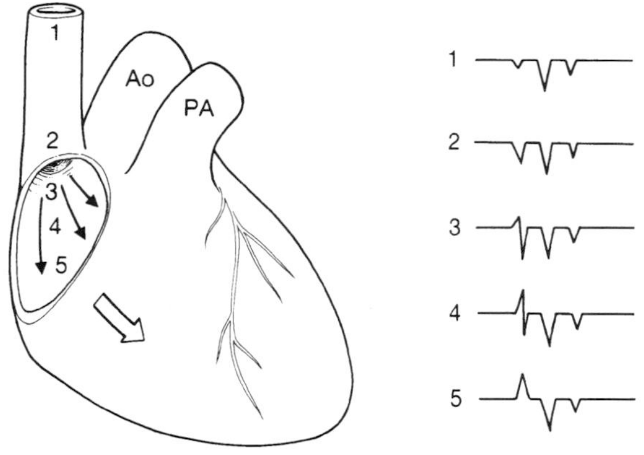

Figure 3.8 The P wave which is negative at first becomes progressively more negative as it approaches the sinoatrial (SA) node in the atrium. When the tip of the catheter enters the atrium and lies near the SA node, the P wave becomes large and biphasic. As the tip is advanced further into the atrium the wave becomes positive. Ao, aorta; PA, pulmonary artery. Reproduced with kind permission of Cucchiara *et al.* (1980).[42]

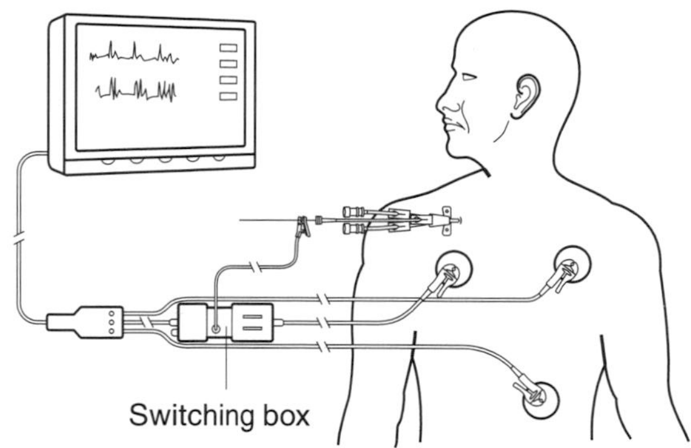

Figure 3.9 TThe Certodyn universal adaptor facilitates switching from intra-vascular to standard ECG.

Alternatively, if the catheter had no metal stylet or wire, the catheter was filled with saline and attached to a saline drip. The left arm lead was then clipped to a metal needle inserted into the drip tubing.

A purpose-made device is commercially available.[44] The Arrow-Johans RAECG Adapter is a disposable 20 mm long plastic Luer-Lok adaptor which has a steel nipple pressed through its wall so permitting contact with the intravascular conductive electrolyte fluid path.

There appear to be few complications associated with this technique so its lack of popularity probably results from uncertainty about the methodology. Its value in paediatric work has been described in a series of 807 catheters placed in children over a period of 10 years. The authors have found it a highly reliable technique and one that avoids the need for radiological control to ensure correct placement of the catheter tip.[45]

Difficulties with assembling the correct apparatus have been eliminated by the easy-to-use Cavafix-Certodyn SD system (Braun Melsungen AG, Germany). This comprehensive kit is designed to ensure reliable placement of the central venous catheter using the Seldinger guide-wire technique and an intra-atrial ECG lead option. The advantage of the Cavafix-Certodyn SD system is the incorporation of a conducting intraluminal wire instead of an electrolyte solution which can lead to better conductance and a less distorted signal.[46]

The intraluminal guide-wire is connected by a switching box (Certodyn Cab) to the extremity electrodes and the ECG monitor. This enables a change from normal two-limb lead ECG to a bipolar intravascular ECG (Figure 3.9).

Catheter tip location in the right atrium is indicated by a significantly elevated P wave. ECG guidance is then used to withdraw from the atrium into the superior vena cava. The catheter is withdrawn by 3 cm or until a normal-size superior vena cava P wave is seen (Figure 3.10).

The atrial ECG guidance technique has a success rate of between 81% and 100%. Failures can be accounted for by existing myocardial pathology, catheter looping, catheter being too short to reach the right atrium from the site of venepuncture, and catheter malpositioning in arm or neck veins (Salmela 1993).

Avoiding Inadvertent Arterial Cannulation

Arterial puncture is probably the most frequent complication associated with central venous cannulation and is potentially fatal. The incidence

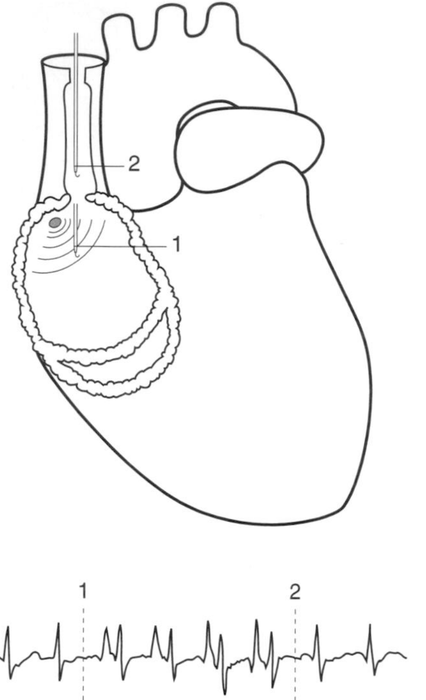

Figure 3.10 Catheter tip location in the right atrium is shown by P wave changes. (1) Catheter tip is in right atrium, indicated by an elevated P wave. (2) The catheter tip has been removed from the right atrium and the P wave has normalized. The cathetor is withdrawn a further 2–3 cm to reach its final position.

in one series of over 1000 attempts to cannulate the internal jugular, subclavian or femoral veins was 3% (14.1% in those with congenital heart disease).[48]

Detection of arterial puncture can sometimes be problematical especially in patients with desaturated arterial blood (e.g. cyanotic heart disease). If the operator is unaware that the device is in an artery and proceeds with the use of a vein dilator and large cannula, there is a potential for a major catastrophe.

Ultrasound devices if available can reduce the risk. Another technique to detect arterial puncture reliably is to connect the needle to a continuous display of pressure detected by the advancing needle. In this way cannulation of the artery can be avoided.[48]

Moving the Site of Entry of a Central Venous Catheter

Normally, the sites where the skin and the vein are punctured lie close to each other. In consequence the track can easily become infected, especially in longer-term catheterisation. This risk can be reduced by widely separating the two puncture sites by means of a subcutaneous tunnel. The technique has been used with catheters inserted for intravenous alimentation through the subclavian vein[49,50] as well as through the internal and external jugular vein[51] routes in both adults and children. Particularly strong indications for using a subcutaneous tunnel are the presence of skin infection, burns or a tracheostomy wound near the point where the catheter enters the skin.[51] Moving the entry point of the catheter could be especially advantageous in the case of catheters inserted into the subclavian vein by the supraclavicular route. The supraclavicular fossa tends to collect secretions and perspiration and is difficult to keep dry; furthermore, because of the irregular contour, it is not easy to secure the catheter with adhesive tape or to hold a dressing in place. For similar reasons, the use of the technique in femoral vein catheterisation could reduce the high rate of infection associated with the route. However, contradictory reports have questioned the value of tunnelling in the reduction of catheter-related sepsis.[52] Nevertheless, the technique remains widely practised.

There are now many commercially available composite long-term catheter tunnelling kits which are both convenient and effective. Hickman–Broviac catheters are widely used for longer-term central venous catheterisation. They are universally tunnelled and have the advantage of a Dacron cuff around the catheter as it lies subcutaneously. Over a period of several weeks, fibrous tissue grows into and around the Dacron cuff anchoring it and acting as a barrier to the spread of infection from the skin entry site. These long-term catheters have customarily been inserted by surgical cut-down procedures, but apparatus for percutaneous insertion is now available from leading manufacturers (see Chapter 2).

Percutaneous Insertion of Long-term Central Venous Catheter with Tunnelling Procedure

Insertion of guide-wire

Perform the procedure under aseptic conditions.

1. Locate the central vein with a small-gauge needle (22 gauge).
2. Enlarge the skin puncture site with a scalpel blade.
3. Perform venepuncture with the introducer needle and cannula or needle alone guided by the locator needle.
4. Insert guide-wire through the introducer and advance it to a satisfactory central position confirmed by fluoroscopy if available (Figure 3.11). Hold guide-wire firmly in place.

Forming a subcutaneous tunnel

1. Infiltrate local anaesthetic solution just below and medial to the nipple and make the incision for the tunnel.
2. Insert the tunnelling needle with its dilator into this skin incision and advance the assembly, so creating a subcutaneous tunnel, until the tip protrudes through the upper incision. Remove the tunnel needle leaving the tunnel dilator in place (Figure 3.12).
3. Insert the guide-wire into the tip of the tunnel dilator and push it through until it emerges at the lower end. Grasp the wire and pull it through the dilator leaving a 5 cm loop of wire at the upper incision. Grasping this loop firmly, remove the dilator.
4. Thread the tip of the central venous catheter over the guide-wire and advance it upwards through the tunnel until it emerges in the upper incision. Guide it over the wire loop, while maintaining the loop, into the vein until the correct length has been inserted into the superior vena cava (Figures 3.13 and 3.14). Traction on the lower end of the catheter will now straighten out the redundant loop by pulling it into the tunnel.

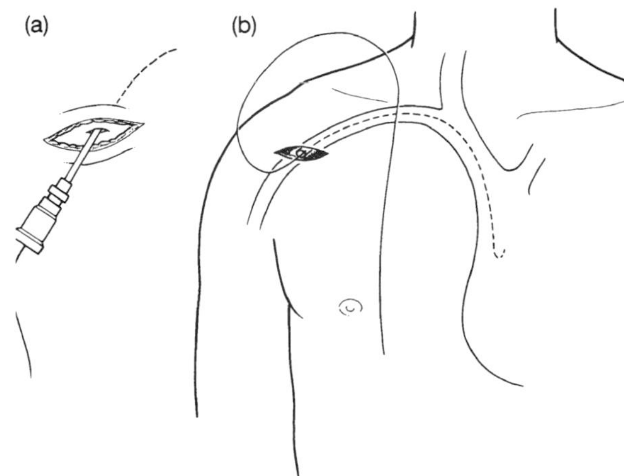

Figure 3.11 (a) Introduction of spring wire guide. (b) Final position of wire guide after removal of introducer.

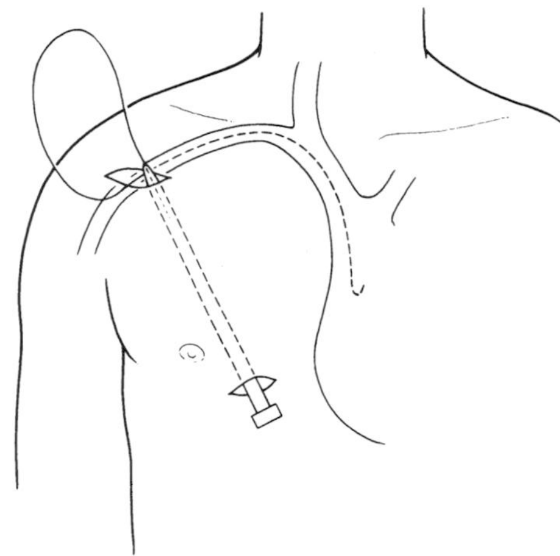
Figure 3.12 Insertion of wire guide through tunnel dilator.

Placing a Dacron cuff around the catheter

1. Dilate the lower incision by blunt dissection with an artery forceps to about 3 cm into the tunnel.
2. Position the Dacron cuff by pushing the silicone sleeve on which it is mounted along the catheter so that it lies no less than 3 cm inside the tunnel (Figure 3.15). Tie the cuff firmly to the catheter by means of a suture around the silicone sleeve. Remove the guide-wire.

3. Secure the catheter with the temporary catheter clamp provided (Figure 3.16) until fibrosis into the Dacron cuff fixes the catheter (about 10–14 days).
4. Close the two incisions with sutures and apply suitable dressings.

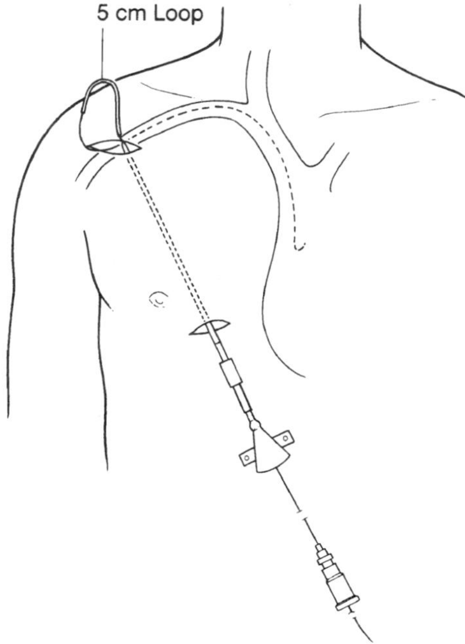

Figure 3.13 Threading catheter over spring wire guide in subcutaneous tunnel.

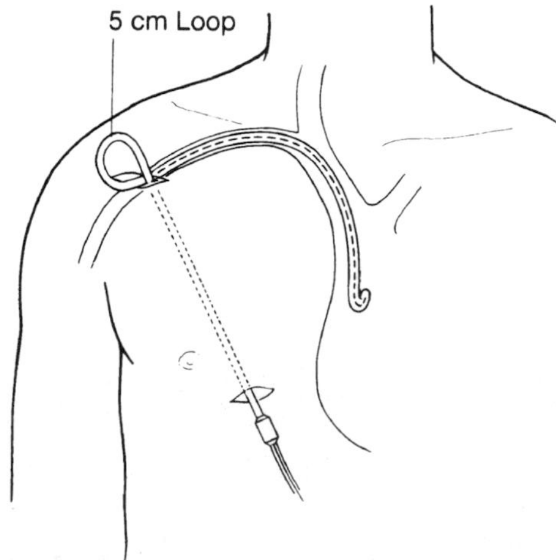

Figure 3.14 Maintaining 5 cm loop during introduction of the catheter into the superior vena cava.

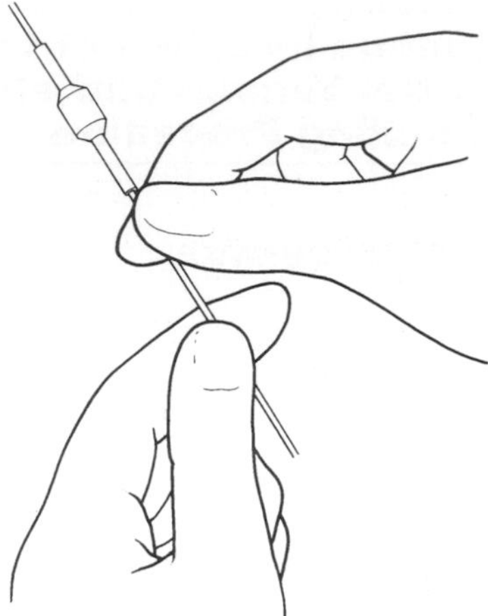

Figure 3.15 The Dacron cuff over silicone sleeve can be repositioned along the catheter by firmly grasping the catheter and pushing on the proximal end of the silicone sleeve (not cuff).

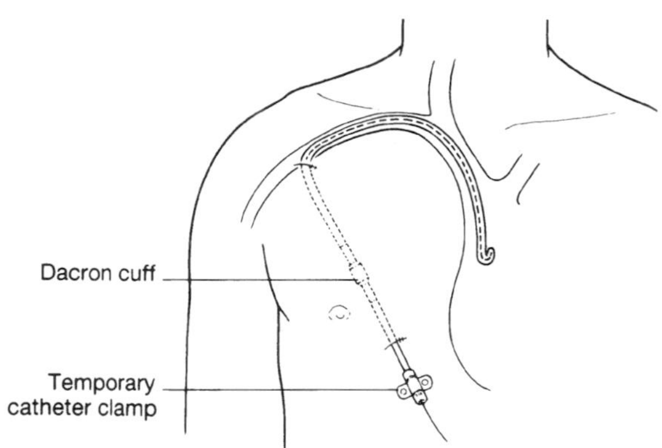

Figure 3.16 Completed procedure showing position of Dacron cuff and temporary catheter clamp.

Percutaneous Insertion of a Central Catheter for Haemodialysis

Percutaneous insertion of central catheters for haemodialysis is now commonly practised. Furthermore, the setting in which the procedure is carried out is diversifying to include general wards, intensive care units and operating theatres. Correct placement of the catheter is a prerequisite for efficient dialysis and a low morbidity rate.

Patient category

The technique is suitable for:

temporary access to the venous circulation for haemodialysis or haemofiltration in acute potentially reversible failure

temporary or medium-term access to the venous circulation in patients with the need for acute haemodialysis where early recovery of renal function is not expected.

Preferred sites

The right internal jugular vein is the preferred site for insertion as the rigidity and large size of these catheters favours a straight line of insertion into the superior vena cava. The length of time the catheter may be *in situ* is prolonged in comparison with temporary central monitoring catheters. Internal jugular catheters may be unpopular with patients because they are obtrusive and uncomfortable. Catheters are available with a 180° preformed bend at the skin level to bring the connecting hubs down towards the anterior chest wall.

Insertion into the subclavian vein is to be avoided. Subclavian vein stenosis is common, possibly due to the relatively rigid catheter having to conform to the curvature of the subclavian to superior vena cava route. Importantly, this may lead to clinically evident subclavian vein occlusion or occult stenosis. Either of these situations will exclude the use of this arm for an arteriovenous fistula for future permanent haemodialysis access as venous hypertension and swelling of the arm are inevitable. Lack of sites for permanent vascular access may severely compromise the long-term survival of the patient.

Early consideration should be given to the insertion of semi-permanent dialysis catheters, rather than the traditional temporary catheters, to reduce morbidity.

A femoral approach can be useful when the patient has acute fluid overload and is in urgent need of dialysis but cannot lie flat.

Equipment used

Temporary catheter (e.g. Vascath or DuoFlow)
Semi-permanent catheter (e.g. Permacath)

Technique

Temporary venous dialysis access (Figure 3.17)

The catheter is a tapered double lumen tube. The 'arterial' limb is used to extract the blood from the central venous system to the dialysis or haemofiltration circuit and the 'venous' limb is used to return the blood to the central venous system.

Meticulous sterile technique with or without prophylactic antibiotic is required, as the catheter may need to stay in for several weeks.

A high approach to the right internal jugular vein using a Seldinger technique, as described elsewhere is this book, is the preferred technique. Large dilators passed over the wire are used, therefore controlled venous puncture is important. Radiological

Figure 3.17 Catheter for short-term dialysis access.

screening of the position of the wire is not essential particularly when the right internal jugular approach is used. However, screening of the position of the wire is helpful if the wire will not pass easily and with left-sided approaches. Sometimes the wire can pass easily but not into the superior vena cava. If as a result, the catheter tip is not in the superior vena cava or right atrium the high volume flow on the extracting limb will cause collapse of the vein and inadequate dialysis.

Once the wire is in position a cut is made alongside the wire so that the dilators and catheter can pass easily over the wire. The track is dilated over the wire. The catheter is passed over the wire so that the tip lies at the superior vena cava/right atrial junction. The catheter is secured into position with a non-absorbable suture. Patency of the limbs of the catheter can be preserved with 1 ml of 1,000 units per ml heparin when not in use.

Semipermanent venous dialysis access

Semipermanent catheters are large-bore, cuffed, and softer than the temporary catheters (Figure 3.18). The cuff allows tissue ingrowth after a few weeks. This ingrowth stabilises the position of the catheter so that securing sutures can be removed and bacterial translocation along the outside of the catheter to the circulation is restricted. The softness of the catheter increases comfort and reduces venous stenosis by comforming better to the venous anatomy. For these reasons, insertion of these catheters is preferable when dialysis access is required for more than a few days. However, the softness of the catheter means that it cannot be forced through the tissues to make its own track to the central vein. Developments in catheter technology now allow this type of catheter to be inserted percutaneously under local anaesthesia where insertion was previously an open surgical procedure. The right internal jugular approach should be used and considerations regarding the use of the Seldinger wire technique as above should be followed.

The wire is screened into the right atrium.

Select a catheter entry point in the skin on the anterior chest wall allowing a subcutaneous tunnel of approximately 10 cm to the point of insertion of the wire into the neck. Anaesthetise this track by local infiltration.

Make a cut in the skin at the catheter insertion point large enough to allow entry of the catheter and its cuff.

Make a cut in the neck where the wire enters the neck and the catheter is brought along the subcutaneous tunnel and out in the neck alongside the wire. The cuff is brought midway into the tunnel.

Pass a large dilator over the wire into the central vein. Place a 'peelable' sheath over the dilator and insert both together into the central vein. Remove the wire and dilator.

Pass the catheter down the inside of the sheath into the central vein. Pull away the sheath by splitting it into two halves by opposing traction. Remove the sheath. The catheter is now in place.

Screening should be used to ensure the tip lies at the superior vena cava/right atrial junction. The amount of catheter inserted can be adjusted by altering the position of the cuff within the subcutanous tunnel. Kinking at the neck incision where the catheter turns deeply can be avoided by making a small subcutaneous pocket by blunt dissection.

Patency of the lumina of the catheter can be preserved by filling them with 1 ml of 1000 U/ml heparin when not in use.

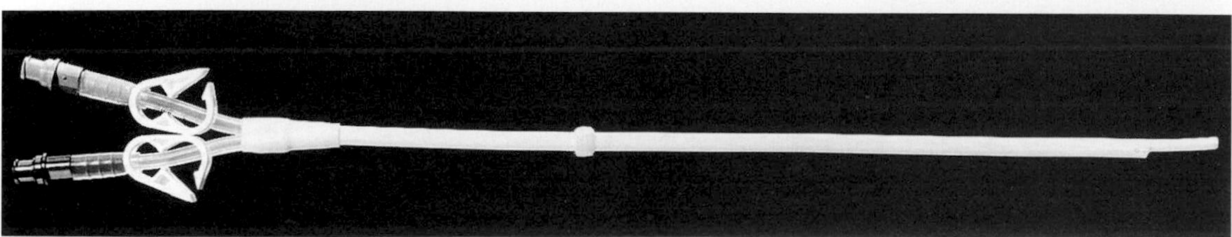

Figure 3.18 Semipermanent catheter.

Possible complications

Complications are as described for any percutaneous approach to a central vein (Table 3.1).

Table 3.1 Complications of insertion of long-term central venous catheters.

Subclavian	Stenosis or occlusion, pneumothorax, mediastinal haemorrhage, brachial plexus injury, sepsis
Internal jugular	Carotid artery and cranial nerve injury, pneumothorax, sepsis
Femoral	Stenosis, deep vein thrombosis, femoral artery damage, high incidence of sepsis

Insertion of a Flotation (Swan–Ganz) Catheter

The balloon-tipped flotation catheter introduced into clinical practice in 1970 by Swan and Ganz[54] enabled the pulmonary artery to be catheterised for the measurement of pressures without calling on the manipulative skill and radiological control demanded by other methods of cardiac catheterisation. The Swan–Ganz catheter has been further developed for measuring cardiac output by the thermodilution technique,[55] for cardiac pacing,[56] for electrocardiography,[57,58] for pulmonary angiography[59] and for fibreoptic mixed venous blood oximetry,[60] and is now used in a wide variety of clinical situations.[61]

The common indications for the insertion of a Swan–Ganz catheter include the management of post-traumatic, surgical and septic shock in order to optimise tissue oxygen transport; in cardiogenic shock to correct pulmonary wedge pressure and to improve cardiac index; in profound hypoxaemia to improve oxygen delivery and oxygen consumption; in cardiac surgery for coronary artery disease to aid early detection of myocardial ischaemia, and to manipulate preload and afterload.[62] The main contraindications (Table 3.2) are pathological conditions or prostheses of the valves of the right heart, presence of an endocardial pacemaker and severe bleeding disorders.

Table 3.2 Contraindications to insertion of a Swan–Ganz catheter and complications associated with Swan–Ganz catheterisation.

Contraindications
Prosthetic tricuspid or pulmonary valve
Tricuspid and pulmonary valve disease
Cardiac septal defects
Left bundle branch block
Endocardial pacemaker *in situ*
Untreated severe coagulopathy and thrombocytopenia
Complications
Arrhythmias
Arterial punctures and pneumothorax
Pulmonary artery rupture
Pulmonary infarction and thrombosis
Catheter-related sepsis
Damage to tricuspid valve and pulmonary valve by the catheter
Endocarditis
Balloon rupture

Choice of vein and technique of cannulation

A Swan–Ganz catheter may be inserted into any vein used for central venous catheterisation. Surgical cut-down on an antecubital fossa vein may be used and cut-down on the proximal basilic vein has also been advocated[63] but percutaneous insertion is easier and is possible in most cases.[64]

Percutaneous cannulation of a vein in the antecubital fossa is most comfortable for the conscious patient[65] but the vein may be too small to admit the larger size Swan–Ganz catheter and it may be difficult to advance the catheter in the shoulder region.[66] Operators with the appropriate skill may prefer the external jugular, subclavian or femoral vein routes, but percutaneous insertion through the right internal jugular vein is the most favoured because of its short, direct path to the right atrium.[66,67] The route of insertion selected will depend upon the experience of the operator, the accessibility of the vein and the equipment available.

A cannula of adequate size has to be inserted into the chosen vein to admit the Swan–Ganz catheter. The cannula can be inserted directly into the vein, although to use a modified Seldinger (guide-wire) and vein dilator technique (see pp 19–20 and 21) is preferable and safer, especially in deep vessels such as the internal jugular or subclavian veins.[64,67,68] Because of its construction, the Swan–Ganz catheter cannot be inserted by the conventional guide-wire technique.

Equipment

Flotation catheter

For adults a 6F (1.8mm OD) or 7F (2.1mm OD) flotation catheter is suitable. For children the catheter should be 5F (1.5mm OD).

Introducing cannula

The introducing cannula may have to be one size larger than the Swan–Ganz catheter in order to accommodate the deflated balloon.

Catheter-through-cannula device

Cannula diameter 12 gauge (OD) to pass a 7F Swan–Ganz catheter. Cannula length is appropriate for the chosen vein.

Modified guide-wire (Seldinger) technique using a vein dilator

Diameter of the final wide-bore cannula is 8F to admit a 7F Swan–Ganz catheter, and 6F to admit a 5F Swan–Ganz catheter. (Sets containing matching guide-wire, vein dilator and wide-bore cannula are now commercially available from several manufacturers.)

Flushing solution

Sodium chloride 0.9% (500ml with heparin 500 IU added).

General

Trolley equipped for central venous catheterisation using aseptic technique; two 20ml syringes containing heparinised saline; scalpel to incise skin if a guide-wire technique is used; pressure recording system; electrocardiograph; defibrillator; cardiac arrest trolley.

Precautions

Do not use a resterilised Swan–Ganz catheter. Use aseptic technique to insert the catheter. Identify the balloon inflating stopcock.

Procedure

1. Check that the balloon is intact by inflating to the recommended volume. Do not inject fluid into this lumen.
2. Fill the lumen of the monitoring catheter with heparinised saline.
3. Cannulate the chosen vein. Insert guide-wire and vein dilator. Finally, insert the introducer.
4. Insert the Swan–Ganz catheter into the vein and connect the pressure-monitoring lumen to the recording apparatus.
5. Advance the catheter into the thorax. Its arrival can be recognised by an increased fluctuation in pressure with respiration. When the patient is asked to cough, the pressure rises sharply to about 40 mmHg.
6. Advance the catheter further (into the lower part of the superior vena cava close to the right atrium). The length of the catheter inserted will depend on the site of insertion. For an average-sized adult it will be:
   right antecubital fossa vein 35–40cm
   left antecubital fossa vein 45–50cm
   internal jugular vein 10–15cm
   subclavian vein 10cm
   femoral vein 35–45cm
7. Inflate the balloon with the recommended volume and advance the catheter slowly to allow it to be carried along in the main blood flow. Watch the pressure trace and observe the following characteristic changes as the catheter traverses the chambers of the heart (Figure 3.19):

   Right ventricle: the atrial trace alters to the large ventricular trace (often accompanied by premature ventricular contractions).

   Pulmonary artery: the trace alters – the systolic pressure remains the same but the diastolic pressure rises.

   Pulmonary artery wedged position: the trace alters and shows a pressure approximately equal

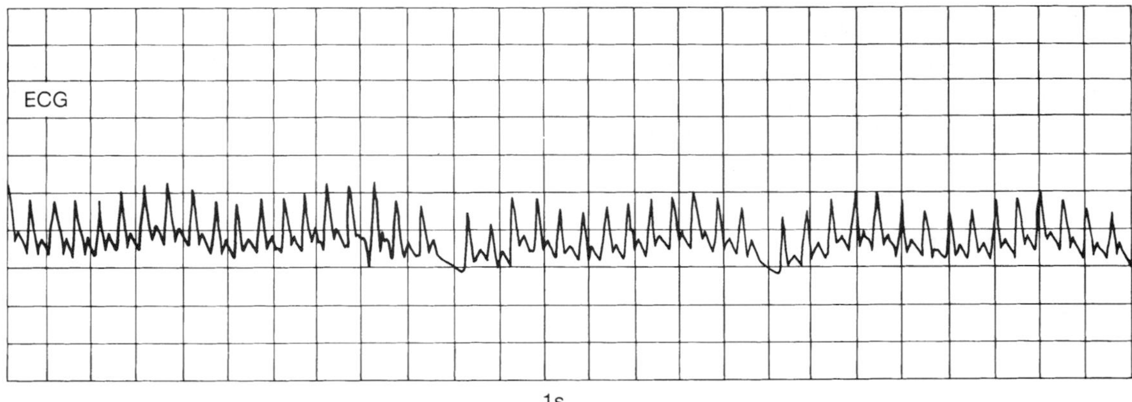

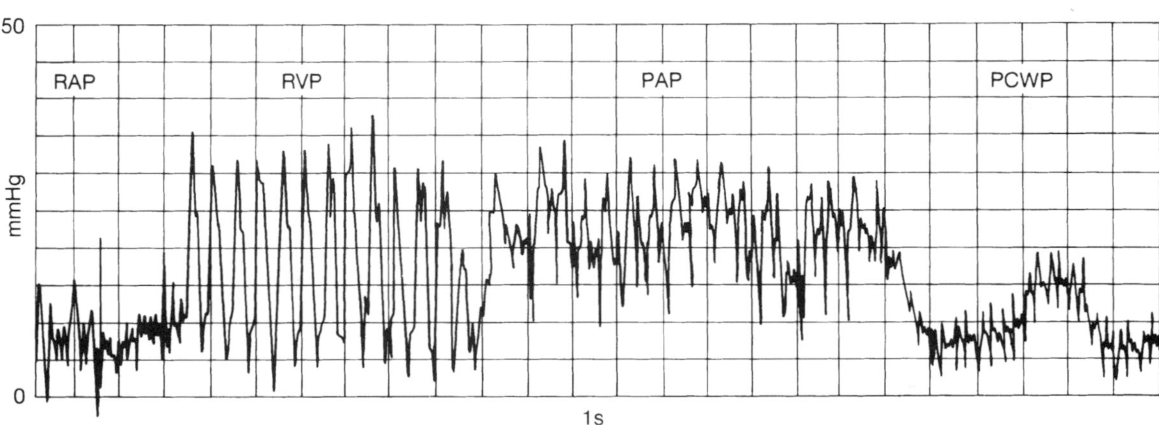

Figure 3.19 Inserting a pulmonary artery flotation catheter: the characteristic pressure trace as the catheter traverses the right atrium (RAP), the right ventricle (RVP) and enters the pulmonary artery (PAP), PCWP, pulmonary capillary wedge pressure. Rreproduced with kind permission of George and Banks (1983).[69]

to the pulmonary artery diastolic pressure.

8. As soon as the catheter shows the pulmonary artery wedge pressure (PAWP), stop advancing the catheter. Deflate the balloon and confirm that the trace returns to that of the normal phasic pulmonary artery pressure. From now on, the balloon should be reinflated intermittently and for short periods only in order to measure PAWP.

   If the catheter has not reached the pulmonary artery when about 60 cm of catheter has been inserted, withdraw the catheter to the right atrium and attempt again. The catheter must never be withdrawn while the balloon is inflated; serious damage to the heart valves or vessels can occur.
9. Protect the length of catheter outside the puncture site with a sterile dressing and secure it temporarily with adhesive tape.
10. Check the position of the catheter with a chest radiograph. The catheter tip is in an ideal position when it lies in one of the main branches of the pulmonary artery (Figure 3.20). If intermittent right ventricular complexes appear, the catheter tip has probably 'recoiled' into the right ventricle. The catheter should be advanced 1–2 cm before it is secured.
11. After recording the end-expiratory pulmonary capillary wedge pressure, deflate the balloon. The pressure measured can only be regarded as valid if the pressure trace then returns to a pulmonary artery pressure waveform. When satisfactory wedging has been obtained, extend the protective sheath (if supplied) to cover the

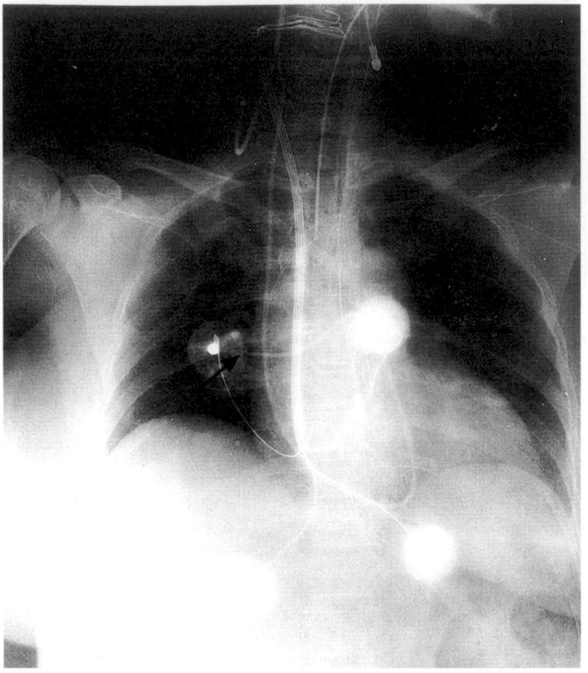

Figure 3.20 Chest radiograph showing the correct position for a monitoring flotation catheter.

full length of the catheter outside the skin so that manipulations of the catheter can be made later in a 'no touch' manner. Secure the collar onto the introducer cannula. Fix the catheter with skin sutures and cover with a bio-occlusive dressing.

Problems

Failure to enter the right atrium: the catheter has inadvertently entered the internal jugular vein or contralateral subclavian vein or even coiled up in the superior vena cava. Prevention is probably helped by inserting the catheter through the right internal jugular vein and by pointing the catheter tip in the right direction. Withdraw and reinsert. If persistently unsuccessful it may be necessary to resort to the aid of an image intensifier to guide the catheter along the correct path.

Failure to pass through the tricuspid or pulmonary valve: reduce the size of the balloon or deflate it completely before advancing further.

Failure to enter the pulmonary artery: if the ventricular trace persists or reappears after advancing the catheter 10–20 cm after its first appearance, the catheter is coiling up on itself and there is a danger of knotting. Deflate the balloon and pull it back into the atrium, then readvance. Several attempts may be made before resorting to the image intensifier.

Catheter obstruction: if the catheter tip appears to be stuck against the wall or at the bifurcation of branches of the pulmonary artery the pressure trace will steadily rise above the expected value. Deflate the balloon and draw it back. Wedge again with a smaller volume of air in the balloon.

It is essential that the catheter is free of blood and air and well flushed with heparinised saline before it is connected to a pressure transducer. Omitting these measures can result in a poor trace and inaccurate measurements. Many of the complications of pulmonary artery catheters can be avoided if the catheter is not left *in situ* for more than 48–72 hours. Table 3.2 shows the complications most commonly encountered.

Maintenance of the Swan–Ganz catheter

1. The pulmonary artery pressure trace should be continuously displayed so that 'spontaneous wedging' may be promptly diagnosed. This occurs if the catheter material softens, when the tip migrates into the smaller branches of the pulmonary artery and into a wedged position. If flushing does not remove a wedged trace, withdraw the catheter 1–2 cm.
2. Take careful precautions on reinflating the balloon to measure PAWP. It is possible that the catheter tip may migrate into a more distal branch of the pulmonary artery and inflating the balloon to its full volume may cause local damage. Therefore always reinflate slowly and with increments of 0.1–0.2 ml until the PAWP trace is obtained. If a much smaller volume is required to elicit PAWP, withdraw the catheter 1–2 cm until the full volume is needed to obtain a wedged pressure. Always deflate the balloon prior to moving the catheter.
3. Continously flush the catheter with heparinised saline, with a 'fast flush' at hourly intervals. If a

continuous flush is not available, flush every 10 minutes.

4. Use an aseptic technique during any manipulation or inspection of the catheter.
5. Radiograph the chest at least once a day.

Insertion of a PICC

The peripherally inserted central venous catheter (PICC) is specifically designed to facilitate intravenous therapy over a medium to long-term period (Table 3.3). It is inserted through a suitable vein in the arm. A conventional short cannula inserted into a peripheral vein rarely remains satisfactory for more than 48–72 hours and especially if irritant substances are infused through it. A PICC reduces the need for repeated venepunctures and attendance at hospital or clinic.

These catheters are inserted by suitably trained nurses. Maintenance of the PICC in the home environment can be taught to patients' carers. Indeed, PICC lines have been shown to be a realistic alternative to the conventional but more invasive Hickman line. These advantages can mean a great deal in comfort and convenience to patients undergoing lengthy and unpleasant treatments such as chemotherapy.

Central venous catheters introduced through the arm veins are not new but the success of the PICC can probably be attributed in great part to the careful training of nursing personnel in the insertion and management of central catheters. Also of major importance has been the commercial availability of well-designed kits and the selection of silicone elastomer catheters. Silicone rubber catheters cause the least phlebitis.

Table 3.3 Some indications and contraindications for inserting a PICC.

Extended intravenous therapy for:
Antibiotics
Fluids
Pain control
Chemotherapy
Parenteral nutrition
Intravenous therapy in the patient's home
Blood sampling (difficult with small-lumen silicone catheters and probably unwise as occlusion of the catheter with blood clot is likely)
Contraindications for a PICC
No suitable veins in the antecubital fossa of both arms
Local infection
Significant bleeding disorder

The catheters used may be single or multilumen (Figure 3.21). The portion outside the skin ends in a hub which is covered by an injection cap. Each catheter has an occluding clamp for use when required. Alternatively, the catheter is capped by a non-return valve to prevent back-flow, eliminating the need for a clamp.

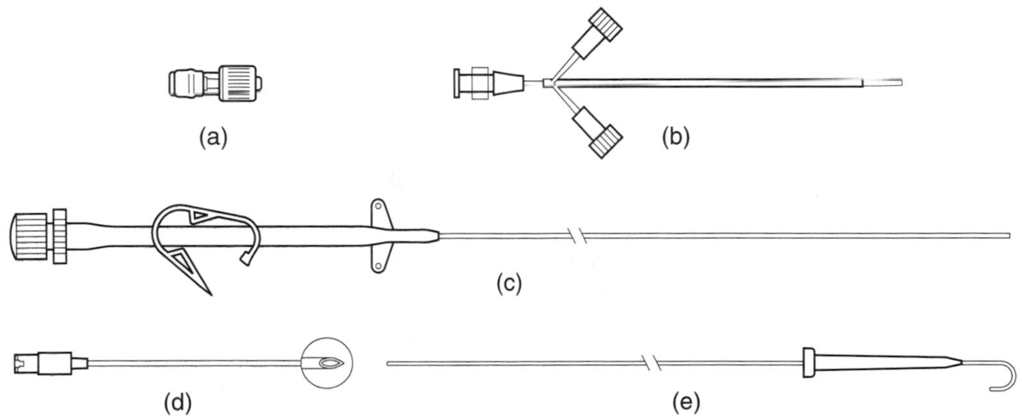

Figure 3.21 Main components of a PICC Tray. (a) Medicinal rubber cap. (b) Sheath introducer with 'peel-away' walls. (c) Central venous catheter (50–60 cm long) with wire guide obturator inside. Usually contructed of silicone rubber. May be multilumen (d) Venepuncture needle. (e) Guide wire for inserting sheath introducer..

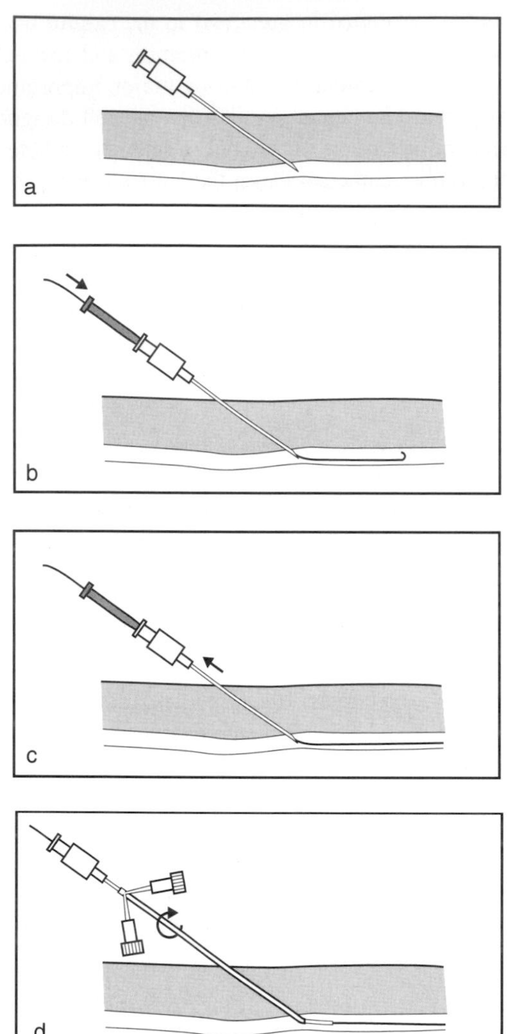

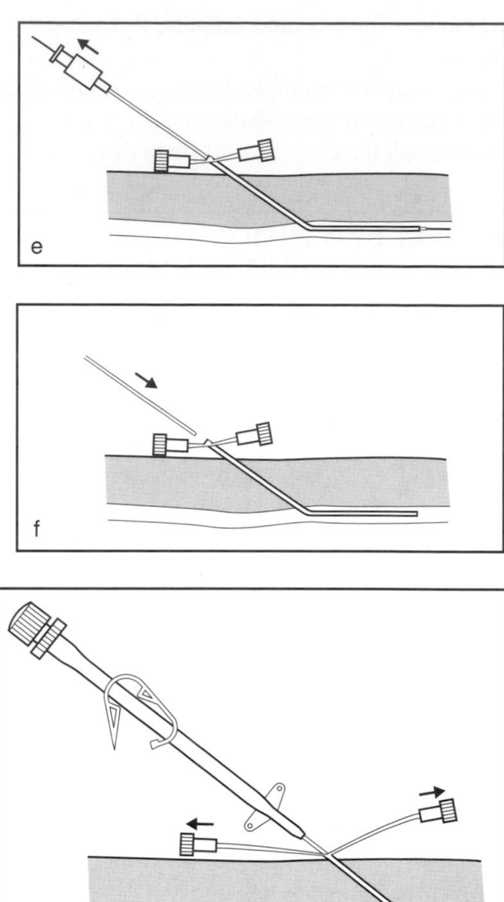

Figure 3.22 Inserting a PICC. (a-g) Steps illustrating the use of a guide wire technique are included for completeness, although this method is not always used.

The catheter can be inserted into the vein through an introducer which is inserted into the vein as a first step. The introducer can be made as a 'peel-away' device which enables the whole introducer to be removed from around the catheter.

A more elaborate method which may be applicable when the chosen vein is small, is the Seldinger (guide-wire) technique (Figures 3.22). The guide-wire method enables a large-gauge catheter to be inserted eventually with ease into a relatively small vein since the vein is first accessed by a small introducer needle.

Veins in the antecubital fossa are the most suitable. Successful entry of the catheter into the central veins is more likely through veins on the medial side (basilic vein) compared with those running up the lateral side (cephalic vein) of the arm. Venepuncture just below or just above the elbow flexure improves patient comfort and reduces kinking. In practice the choice of veins may be limited because of previous venepunctures, obesity or anatomical variation.

Cannulation can be carried out in any location (including at the bedside) provided suitable equipment and lighting are available.

Equipment

Commercially available PICC trays contain all items necessary: these comprise a small-gauge needle (25 gauge), larger needle (22 gauge), local anaesthetic solution (lignocaine 1% or 2%), iodine solution, sponges, fenestrated drape, syringe, scalpel blade, suture with needle, 36 in (90 cm) measuring tape. Central venous catheter (50–60 cm length) with its wire guide obturator inside.

A topical anaesthetic gel such as Ametop (Smith & Nephew Healthcare Ltd, Hull, UK) may be applied about 45 minutes prior to cannulation instead of local anaesthetic injection.

Position of the patient

Semi-reclining. A small rolled towel under the elbow to extend the arm slightly helps to throw the antecubital veins into prominence.

Procedure

Wash hands. Assemble all necessary equipment. Take the cover off the PICC tray.

Estimate the length of catheter that will be needed by measuring the distance from 1 cm outside the planned site of venepuncture to three fingers'-width above the suprasternal notch. If left-sided insertion is planned, an additional 2–3 cm of catheter will be needed.

If necessary, trim the catheter using sterile scissors. To do this, firstly withdraw the stylet in the catheter backwards from the portion of the catheter that is to be trimmed. Make a sharp 90° cut leaving no ragged edges.

Apply a tourniquet to distend the vein.

Use aseptic technique for insertion of the line. Prepare the skin over the proposed venepuncture site with antiseptic solution. Position sterile towelling over a wide area to ensure an aseptic environment.

Infiltrate the skin and subcutaneous tissue with 0.5–1 ml lignocaine 1% if topical anaesthetic gel has not been used.

Attach a syringe to the introducer needle.

1. Perform venepuncture with the introducer needle. Release tourniquet (Fig. 3.22a).

   The following description applies to the use of a guide-wire insertion technique. If this is not applicable as in the case of systems which allow the catheter to be advanced directly through a cannula then steps 1–4 are not relevantand the description should be taken up at point 5.
2. Insert the straight end of the guide-wire into the hub of the introducer and advance it 5–10 cm. Remove the introducer needle (Fig. 3.22b,c).
3. Enlarge the skin puncture a little with the tip of the scalpel provided in the tray.
4. Advance the sheath introducer assembly over the guide-wire onwards into the vein, ensuring that the wire protrudes 1–2 cm from the open end of the introducer (Fig. 3.22d).
5. Remove the introducer and J wire from the peel-away sheath introducer, applying a finger over the open end of the sheath to prevent air entering the vein (Fig. 3.22e).
6. Insert the catheter with its obturator stylet through the introducer and steadily insert the whole length of the catheter. Flush the catheter with isotonic saline approximately every 10 cm to assist passage of the vein and reduce damage to the vein wall (Fig. 3.22f).

   Turning the patient's head to the side of insertion and dropping the chin downwards may help prevent the catheter tip from going upwards into the internal jugular vein.
7. When the catheter is fully in place, if a peel-away sheath has been used, grasp the two knobs on the peel-away sheath, pull upwards and outwards at the same time to remove the sheath. If a simple cannula has been used as a catheter introducer, slowly withdraw it from the skin puncture site (Fig. 3.22g).

Prime the extension tube with its medicinal rubber cap, with isotonic saline. Attach this to the catheter after withdrawing its metal obturator stylet. Alternatively, if the extension tubing is integral with the catheter, attach a suitable connector.

Aspirate with the syringe containing isotonic saline to confirm withdrawal of blood, then flush the catheter with saline. Flush the line with heparinised saline. Clean and dry the skin around the puncture site. Place a sterile swab over the puncture site to prevent undue bleeding. Form a loop with the extension tubing and apply appropriate fixing tapes.

Apply a transparent occlusive dressing to the assembly, making sure that the clamp (if used) is outside the dressing. Apply any other securing tapes as necessary. Suitably label the PICC line including the date of insertion. Take a chest X-ray to confirm correct positioning of the catheter tip. If the position is unsatisfactory, manipulation (partial withdrawal or reinsertion) must be carried out with aseptic technique.

Nursing management of PICC

Remove the swab no later then 4 days after insertion so that the puncture site can be observed. Change the transparent dressing using aseptic technique, every 7 days as long as it is dry and occlusive. Observe the venepuncture site daily for signs of drainage, swelling or tenderness. If redness and tenderness develop, apply a heating pad to the area for 2–3 days. This effectively deals with the usual mechanical phlebitis. Onset of redness and pain after 7 days is more likely to be due to infection.

If the catheter is heparin locked, change the rubber medicinal cap every 7 days and flush the catheter every 12 hours with 2.5 ml of heparinised saline. Proprietary needleless connectors should be changed and flushed according to manufacturer's instructions or local policy.

Catheters should be flushed once weekly. Isotonic saline should be injected to produce turbulent flushing to clean the line. In order to avoid excessive pressures with the risk of rupturing the line, the syringe must be of 10 ml or larger type.

References

1. Flanagan JP, Gradisar IA, Gross RJ, Kelly TR. Air embolus – a lethal complication of subclavian venepuncture. New England Journal of Medicine 1969; **281**:488.
2. Ross SM, Freedman PS, Farman JV. Air embolism after accidental removal of intravenous catheter. British Medical Journal 1979; **1**:987.
3. Daily PO, Griepp RB, Shumway NE. Percutaneous internal jugular vein cannulation. Archives of Surgery 1970; **101**:534.
4. Prince SR, Sullivan RL, Hackel A. Percutaneous catheterization of the internal jugular vein in infants and children. Anesthesiology 1976; **44**:170.
5. Haapaniemi L, Slatis P. Supraclavicular catheterisation of the superior vena cava. Acta Anaesthesiologica Scandinavica 1974; **18**:12.
6. Ryan JA. Complications of total parenteral nutrition. In: Fischer JE, ed. Total Parenteral Nutrition. Boston: Little, Brown, 1976, p. 55.
7. Bennett PJ. Use of intravenous plastic catheters. British Medical Journal 1963; **2**:1252.
8. Taylor FW, Rutherford CE. Accidental loss of plastic tube into venous system. Archives of Surgery 1963; **86**:177.
9. Farman JV. Which central venous catheter? British Journal of Clinical Equipment 1978; **32**:210.
10. Parulkar DS, Grundy EM, Bennett EJ. Fracture of a float catheter. British Journal of Anaesthesia 1978; **50**:201.
11. Zwiauer K, Grabenwoger F, Lachmann D *et al.* Non-surgical removal of iatrogenic intracardiac foreign bodies. A study in a 5 month old infant. Monatsschrift Kinderheilkunde 1987; **135**:784.
12. Ryan JA, Abel RM, Abbott WM *et al.* Catheter complications in total parenteral nutrition. A prospective study of 200 consecutive patients. New England Journal of Medicine 1974; **290**:757.
13. Greenall MJ, Blewitt RW, McMahon MJ. Cardiac tamponade and central venous catheters. British Medical Journal 1975; **2**:595.
14. Csanky Treels JC. Hazards of central venous pressure monitoring. Anaesthesia 1978; **33**:172.
15. James OF, Tredarea CR. Cardiac tamponade caused by caval catheter – a radiological demonstration of an unusual complication. Anaesthesia and Intensive Care 1979; **7**:174.
16. Adar R, Mozes M. Fatal complications of central venous catheters. British Medical Journal 1971; **3**:746.
17. Rudge CJ, Bewick M, McColl I. Hydrothorax after central venous catheterization. British Medical Journal 1973; **3**:23.
18. Michenfelder JD, Terry HR, Dow EF, Miller RH. Air embolism during neurosurgery: a new method of treatment. Anesthesia and Analgesia: Current Researches 1966; **45**:390.
19. Deitel M, McIntyre JA. Radiographic confirmation of site of central venous pressure catheters. Canadian Journal of Surgery 1971; **14**:42.
20. Gilday DL, Downs AR. The value of chest radiography in the localization of central venous pressure catheters. Canadian Medical Association Journal 1969; **101**:363.
21. Johnston AOB, Clark RG. Malpositioning of central venous catheters. Lancet 1972; **2**:1395.
22. Kellner GA, Smart JF. Percutaneous placement of catheter to monitor 'central venous pressure'. Anesthesiology 1972; **36**:515.
23. Kuramoto T, Sakabe T. Comparison of success in jugular versus basilic vein techniques for central venous pressure catheter positioning. Anesthesia and Analgesia: Current Researches 1975; **54**:696.
24. Langston CS. The aberrant central venous catheter and its complications. Radiology 1971; **100**:55.
25. Ng WS, Rosen M. Positioning central venous catheters through the basilic vein. A comparison of catheters. British Journal of Anaesthesia 1973; **45**:1211.
26. Sorensen TIA, Sonne-Holm S. Central venous catheterization through the basilic vein or by infraclavicular

puncture?: a controlled trial. Acta Chirurgica Scandinavica 1975; **141**:322.

27. Bridges BB, Carden E, Takacs FA. Introduction of central venous pressure catheters through arm veins with a high success rate. Canadian Anesthetists Society Journal 1979; **26**:128.
28. Burgess GE, Marino RJ, Peuler MJ. Effect of head position on the location of venous catheters inserted via basilic veins. Anesthesiology 1977; **46**:212.
29. Williamson J. Prevention and early recognition of complications of central venous catheterization. American Heart Journal 1976; **92**:667.
30. Sukigara M, Yamazaki T. Ultrasonic real time guidance for subclavian venepuncture. Surgery, Gynecology and Obstetrics 1988; **167**:239.
31. Schering A, Klein A, Jantzen JP. Catheterization of the internal jugular vein using sonography. Anasthesie Intensivtherapie Notfallmedizin 1987; **22**:229.
32. Switzer DF, Nanda NC, Harris P, Bren W. The use of two dimensional Doppler technique in facilitating percutaneous catheterization of the subclavian vein. Pacing and Clinical Electrophysiology 1988; **11**:13.
33. Chalkiadis GA, Goucke CR. Depth of central venous catheter insertion in adults: an audit and assessment of a technique to improve tip position. Anaesthesia and Intensive Care 1998; **26**:66.
34. Denys BG, Uretsky BF, Reddy PS. Ultrasound-assisted cannulation of the internal jugular vein. A prospective comparison to the external landmark-guided technique. Circulation 1993; **87**:1557.
35. Verghese S, McGill WA, Patel R *et al.* Internal jugular vein cannulation in infants: palpation vs. imaging. Anesthesiology 1996; **85**(3A):1078.
36. Branger B, Dauzat M, Zabadani B, Vecina F, Lefranc JY. Pulsed Doppler sonography for the guidance of vein puncture; a prospective study. Artificial Organs 1995; **19**:933.
37. Mansfield PF, Hann DC, Fornage BD, Ota DM. Complications and failures of subclavian vein catheterization. New England Journal of Medicine 1994; **331**:1735.
38. Gualtieri E, Deppe SA, Sipperly ME, Thompson DR. Subclavian venous catheterization: greater success rate for less experienced operators using ultrasound guidance. Critical Care Medicine 1995; **23**:692.
39. Vucevic M, Tehan B, Gamlin F *et al.* The SMART needle. A new Doppler ultrasound-guided vascular access needle. Anaesthesia 1994; **49**:889.
40. Robertson JT, Schick RW, Morgan F, Matson D. Accurate placement of ventriculo-atrial shunt for hydrocephalus under electrocardiographic control. Journal of Neurosurgery 1961; **18**:225.
41. Colley PS, Artru AA. EKG guided placement of CVP catheters via arm veins: success rate, placement time and optimal conductive solutions. Anesthesia and Analgesia 1984; **63**:175 [abstracts p. 200].
42. Cucchiara RF, Messick JM, Gronert GG, Michenfelder JD. Time required and success rate of percutaneous right atrial catheterization: description of a technique. Canadian Anaesthetists Society Journal 1980; **27**:572.
43. Farag H, Gyamfi YA, Naguib M. Non-radiological recognition of misplacement of central venous catheter. British Medical Journal 1983; **287**:761.
44. On Target (Arrow International Inc.) Vol. 1, No. 1.
45. Parigi GB. Accurate placement of central venous catheters in pediatric patients using endocavity electrocardiography: reassessment of a personal technique. Journal of Pediatric Surgery 1997; **32**:1226.
46. Corsten SA, Boudewijn van D, Bakker NC, de Lange JJ, Scheffer GJ. Central venous catheter placement using the ECG-guided Cavafix-Certodyn SD catheter. Journal of Clinical Anesthesia 1994; **6**:469.
47. Salmela L, Aromaa U. Verification of the position of a central venous catheter by intra-atrial ECG. When does this method fail? Acta Anaesthesiologica Scandinavica 1993; **37**:26.
48. Oliver WC, Nuttall GA, Beynen FM, Raimundo HS, Abenstein JP, Arnold JJ. The incidence of artery puncture with central venous cannulation using a modified technique for detection and prevention of arterial cannulation. Journal of Cardiothoracic and Vascular Anesthesia 1997; **11**:851.
49. Broviac JW, Cole JJ, Scribner BH. A silicone rubber atrial catheter for prolonged parenteral alimentation. Surgery, Gynecology and Obstetrics 1973; **136**:602.
50. Powell-Tuck J, Nielsen T, Farwell JA, Lennard-Jones JE. Team approach to long-term intravenous feeding in patients with gastro-intestinal disorders. Lancet 1978; **2**:825.
51. Parsa MH, Habit DV, Ferrer JM. Techniques for placement of long-term indwelling superior vena cava catheters. Monograph and film presented at the Fifty-sixth Annual Clinical Congress of the American College of Surgeons, Chicago, October, 1970.
52. Moran KT, McEntee G, Jones B *et al.* To tunnel or not to tunnel catheters for parenteral nutrition. Annals of the Royal College of Surgeons of England 1987; **69**:235.
53. Alfieris GM, Wing CW, Hoy GR. Securing Broviac catheters in children. Journal of Pediatric Surgery 1987; **9**:825.
54. Swan HJC, Ganz W, Forrester J, Marcus H, Diamond G, Chonette D. Catheterisation of the heart in man with use of a flow directed balloon-tipped catheter. New England Journal of Medicine 1970; **283**:447.
55. Forrester JS, Ganz W, Diamond G, McHugh T, Chonette DW, Swan HJC. Thermodilution cardiac output determination with a single flowdirected catheter. American Heart Journal 1972; **83**:306.
56. Meister SG, Banka VS, Helfant RH. Transfemoral pacing with balloon-tipped catheters. Journal of the American Medical Association 1973; **225**:712.
57. Meister SG, Banka VS, Chadda KD, Helfant RH. A balloon tipped catheter for obtaining His bundle electrograms without fluoroscopy. Circulation 1974; **49**:42.
58. Chatterjee K, Swan HJC, Ganz W, Gray R, Loebel H, Forrester JS, Chonette D. Use of a balloon-tipped flotation

electrode catheter for cardiac monitoring. American Journal of Cardiology 1975; **36**:56.

59. Wilson JE, Bynum LJ. An improved pulmonary angiographic technique using a balloon-tipped catheter. American Review of Respiratory Diseases 1976; **114**:1137.
60. Woodcock TC, Murray S, Ledingham I. Mixed venous oxygen saturation changes during tension pneumothorax and its treatment. Anaesthesia 1984; **39**:1004.
61. Pace NL. A critique of flow-directed pulmonary arterial catheterisation. Anesthesiology 1977; **47**:455.
62. Pierce T, Woodcock T. How to insert a pulmonary arterial flotation catheter. British Journal of Hospital Medicine 1989; **42**:484.
63. Mandel S, Barash P. The proximal basilic vein: a new approach for introduction of a flow-guided catheter into the pulmonary artery. Journal of Thoracic and Cardiovascular Surgery 1976; **71**:376.
64. Swan HJC, Ganz W. Use of balloon flotation catheters in critically ill patients. Surgical Clinics of North America 1975; **55**:501.
65. George RJD. How to insert a flotation catheter. British Journal of Hospital Medicine 1980; **23**:296.
66. Civetta JM, Gabel JC. Flow directed-pulmonary artery catheterization in surgical patients: indications and modifications of technic. Annals of Surgery 1972; **176**:753.
67. Kaplan JA, Miller ED. Insertion of the Swan–Ganz catheter. Anesthesiology Review 1976; **1**:22.
68. Ellertson DG, McGough EC, Rasmussen B, Sutton RB, Hughes RK. Pulmonary artery monitoring in critically ill surgical patients. American Journal of Surgery 1974; **128**:791.
69. George RJD, Banks RA. Bedside measurement of pulmonary capillary wedge pressure. British Journal of Hospital Medicine 1983; **29**:286.
70. Wood SR. Placement of a tunnelled catheter with a fixed hub using a split introducer. British Journal of Parenteral Therapy 1985; **6**:96.
71. Troianos CA, Jobes DR, Ellison N. Ultrasound-guided cannulation of the internal jugular vein. A prospective, randomized study. Anesthesia and Analgesia 1991; **72**:823.

4 • Central Venous Catheter-associated Infections

GEORGE FINDLAY

Introduction

Central venous catheters (CVCs) are integral to the management of critically ill patients in modern intensive care. They allow delivery of life-saving fluids, such as vasoactive drugs, parenteral nutrition, antimicrobial agents, and blood or blood products. They also enable the haemodynamic status of critically ill patients to be monitored and guide treatment of such patients. It is estimated that in the USA up to 5 million CVCs are used annually,[1] whilst in the UK a figure of 200 000 CVCs is quoted.[2] There are recognised mechanical risks associated with the placement of CVCs;[3] however, a worrying trend is the explosive rise in the rate of intravascular line infection and bacteraemia.[4] In the USA it is estimated that more than 50 000 cases of CVC-related bacteraemia occur annually with an attributable mortality of 10–20%.[5,6] Indeed, 90% of all nosocomial bacteraemias are secondary to the use of CVCs.[1] The prevention, diagnosis and appropriate management of CVC-related infection is obviously of great importance.

Definitions

There is a huge body of literature covering aspects of CVC-related infections and a source of confusion is the differing terminology used by investigators and reviewers. The term 'catheter-related sepsis' is often used: in this context 'sepsis' usually denotes 'bacteraemia' and not the clinical syndrome of sepsis. It would be more informative to use the term 'catheter-related bacteraemia' (CRB) and reserve 'sepsis' for bacteraemia associated with the clinical syndrome of sepsis. Table 4.1 sets out the most commonly used definitions.[7] The most widely used method of semiquantitative culture was described by Maki and involves rolling the catheter segment on agar plates, thus sampling

Table 4.1 Definitions of CVC-related infections.

Site infection	Pus or ≥15 colonies on semiquantitative culture or ≥ 10^3 colonies on quantitative culture of the intracutaneous (proximal) catheter segment
Site colonisation	< 15 colonies on semiquantitative culture or <10^3 colonies on quantitative culture of the intracutaneous (proximal) catheter segment
Catheter infection	≥15 colonies on semiquantitative culture or ≥10^3 colonies on quantitative culture of the intravascular (distal) catheter segment
Catheter colonisation	<15 colonies on semiquantitative culture or <10^3 colonies on quantitative culture of the intravascular (distal) catheter segment
Catheter-related bacteraemia	Positive blood and catheter segment culture for the same organism

only the extraluminal surface, and counting the colonies of pathogens after culture.[8] The quantitative culture, described by Cleri, involves submerging the catheter segment in broth, thus including both extraluminal and intraluminal organisms.[9]

Routes of infection

There are five principal routes by which microorganisms can gain access to intravascular catheters. These are extraluminal; intraluminal; contaminated infusates; haematogenous seeding; and impaction of organisms at the time of insertion (Figure 4.1). The two most important routes of infection are thought to be extraluminal contamination, where organisms on the patient's skin migrate from the insertion site down the intracutaneous tract on the external catheter surface,[10] and intraluminal passage via the internal lumen of the catheter, primarily due to catheter hub and Luer connector colonisation.[11,12] More recently it has been shown that impaction of organisms at the time of catheter insertion occurs despite seemingly adequate skin preparation. In a study of 30 patients undergoing open heart surgery the distal tip of the CVC was sampled *in situ*

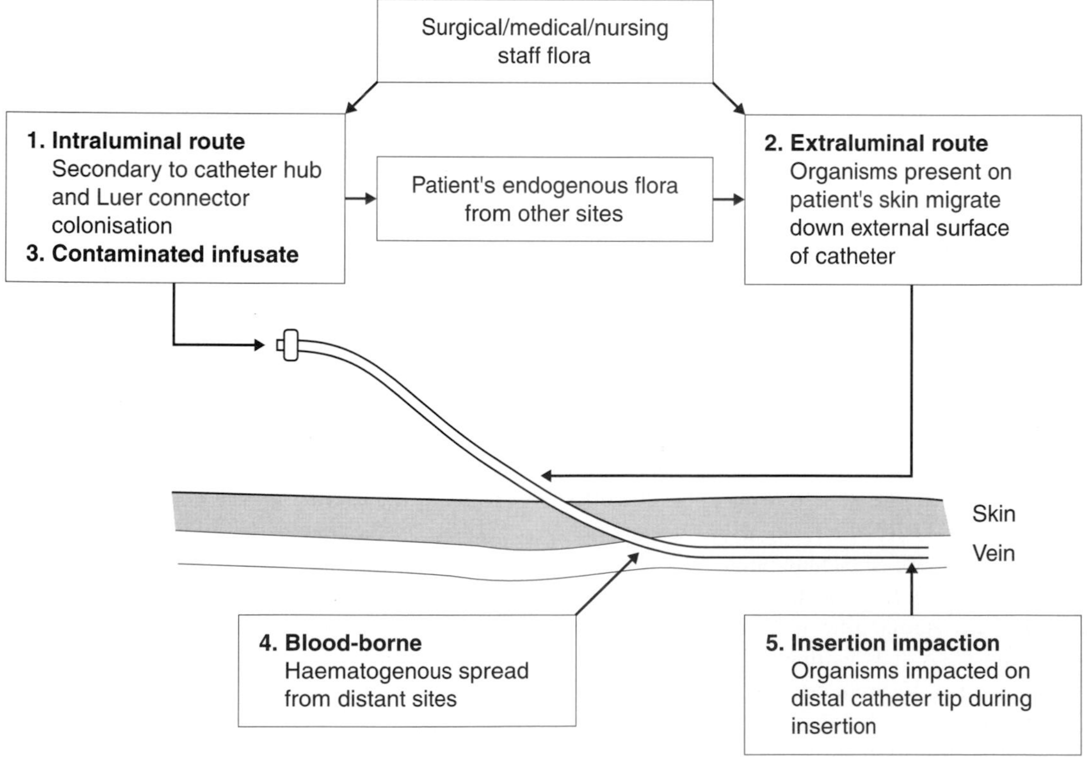

Figure 4.1 The five principal routes of microbial contamination of CVCs.

90 minutes after insertion under aseptic conditions, including the application of alcoholic chlorhexidine for more than 2 minutes.[13] The finding that 16% of CVC tips were contaminated suggested the hypothesis that organisms had been impacted onto the CVC tip during insertion. Bacteria were isolated from skin insertion sites (66%), and from the introducer needle and guide-wires (50%), giving weight to this theory.

Recognition

The diagnosis of catheter-related infection can be made on the basis of either clinical criteria or laboratory investigations.

Clinical diagnosis

The clinical diagnosis may be of localised infection at the catheter insertion site or catheter infection/bacteraemia. Localised infection is normally obvious and includes the presence of erythema and exudate at the catheter insertion site. Patients with catheter infection/bacteraemia may present with one or more of the following:

- low-grade pyrexia with no obvious source
- intermittent pyrexia following flushing of the catheter
- persistence of signs of infection despite broad-spectrum antibiotic therapy
- no clinical signs.

Both localised infection and systemic infection may be present concurrently.

Microbiological diagnosis

Insertion site infection

The diagnosis of localised infection is supported by the isolation of organisms from swabs of insertion site exudate, particularly if a single organism is isolated which is a recognised pathogen.

Catheter infection/bacteraemia

The diagnosis of catheter infection/bacteraemia relies on blood cultures and catheter tip cultures. Culture of the catheter tip requires removal of the catheter, which may be unwarranted. The isolation of the same micro-organism from the catheter tip and from blood cultures, or the isolation of the same micro-organism from peripheral blood cultures and catheter blood cultures, with more organisms being isolated from the latter, are highly suggestive of catheter-related bacteraemia. Significant improvements in the yield of organisms can be made by increasing the sampling volume, and therefore at least 20–30 ml of blood should be taken.

Insertion site/catheter hub swabs

Much has been written about the use of swabs of catheter insertion sites or hubs as a predictor of catheter-related infection. However, insertion site swabs, in the absence of obvious signs of infection, may represent commensals only and may lead to confusion. Similarly, hub swabs may provide information that is easily misinterpreted.

Non-specific clinical signs are common in the critically ill and the diagnosis of catheter-related infection must often be considered. Owing to the severity of the illness it may not be possible to await microbiological confirmation or refutation of this differential diagnosis and it is thus important to formulate guidelines for the management of suspected catheter-related infection. In the absence of guidelines the risks are either excessive rates of catheter removal and insertion of a new CVC, with all the associated procedural risks, or inappropriate non-removal of catheters with the associated risks of sepsis.

Risk Factors and Possible Interventions

There are many variables in infectious complications of CVCs, each one offering a potential therapeutic option (Table 4.2).

Table 4.2 Variables in infectious complications of central venous access.

Catheter manufacture and design
Surface characteristics
Composition
Single or triple lumen
Antibiotic or antiseptic bonded
Choice of insertion site
Catheter insertion
Preparation of the site
Difficulty of insertion
Insertion technique
Care of insertion site
Dressing type
Local application of ointments
Frequency of dressing changes
Infusate and apparatus
Administration set
Filters
Apparatus manipulation
Patient characteristics
Underlying illness
Immune compromise
Antibiotic administration
Duration of catheterisation

Catheter Manufacture and Design

Catheters vary in composition and design. Newer types have a reduced risk of colonisation. Catheters with a smooth topography are less likely to be colonised.[14] Coating catheter surfaces with compounds such as polytetrafluoroethylene (Teflon) or Hydromer has also been shown to reduce microbial colonisation.[15] Percutaneous catheters with a silver-impregnated collagen cuff have been developed, but a prospective study has shown no benefit[16] and indeed some studies have shown a worrying increase in fungaemia in association with this cuff.[17,18] A recent approach is the chemical bonding of antimicrobial agents (antibiotics or antiseptics) to the catheter surface. Several studies have demonstrated that the use of benzalkonium chloride,[19] silver sulphadiazine and chlorhexidine,[20,21] cefazolin[22] and vancomycin[23] are all associated with lower rates of microbial colonisation and catheter-related bacteraemia. Two prospective, randomised double-blind trials have compared catheters bonded with minocycline–rifampicin[24] and chlorhexidine–silver sulfadiazine.[25] Both of these large, well-conducted studies demonstrated a significant reduction in catheter colonisation and catheter-related bacteraemia. Further investigation of these bonded catheters is warranted. Of concern, however, is the potential for misuse of such antibiotic-bonded catheters and the possibility of the emergence of resistant micro-organisms. There is debate over whether multiple-lumen CVCs pose a greater infection risk than single-lumen CVCs, owing to the increased potential for intraluminal infection via multiple routes of access. The evidence is contradictory but is mostly derived from non-randomised studies. In two prospective randomised studies comparing triple-lumen CVCs with single-lumen CVCs there was no statistically significant difference in infection rates.[26,27]

Site of insertion

The site of insertion is associated with different rates of infection. Although no study has shown that choice of site reduces catheter-related bacteraemia, there is good evidence to suggest that insertion site infection correlates with subsequent CRB.[28] The subclavian vein has lower rates of insertion site infection than the internal jugular vein, which has lower rates of insertion site infection than the femoral vein.[29,30] The difference in infection rates may be due to different skin colonisation rates. It therefore seems that the subclavian vein should be the preferred site, from the point of view of a reduction in infection, if no contraindication exists. This is more relevant for long-term catheters used in intensive care than for short-term perioperative use, when internal jugular cannulation may be more appropriate.

Catheter insertion

The ease of insertion and the level of experience of the operator have been claimed to influence infection rates. However, this factor is likely to be small compared with appropriate insertion site skin preparation and aseptic techniques. The patients' skin microflora is probably a major source of catheter infection and thorough skin preparation is thus essential. It has been shown that preparation with chlorhexidine was associated with lower incidence of catheter-related infections and bacteraemia compared with the use of povidone–iodine or alcohol.[31] However, in a study by Elliott *et al.*, despite preparation with 2% aqueous chlorhexidine for 2 minutes, 16% of CVC tips, sampled *in situ* 90 minutes after insertion, were contaminated.[13] Bacteria were also isolated from skin insertion sites (66%), the introducer needle and guide-wires (50%), demonstrating that skin preparation may not be adequate.

Care of the insertion site

Dressing

It is not clear whether a transparent semipermeable dressing, which is designed to exclude organisms but allow the passage of air to the skin and inspection of the insertion site, is superior to sterile gauze. Some studies have found no difference in site colonisation rate,[32,33] whilst others have found an increase in site colonisation, catheter infection and CRB with transparent dressings.[34] A meta-analysis on this topic concluded that transparent dressings increased the risk of catheter-related infection.[35] Since this analysis there have been significant advances in transparent dressings, with increased moisture vapour transmission rates. However, it appears that dry gauze dressings should be used preferentially as they are at least equivalent, and may be superior, to transparent dressings. Whatever dressing is used it should stabilise the catheter effectively, thus preventing the pump action of the catheter moving in and out of the skin, which can introduce micro-organisms subcutaneously.[36]

Frequency of dressing change

The frequency with which dressings are changed may influence the risk of infection. Practices differ from institution to institution, but it appears that the optimum interval for dressing changes is 72 hours, with no benefit being gained by more frequent changes.[37,38] With each dressing change the site should be inspected for the presence of signs of infection and should be cleaned with an antiseptic solution prior to re-dressing.

Antiseptic ointment

The use of antiseptic ointment at the insertion site has been investigated by some workers. Mupirocin, bacitracin and neomycin ointment have all been used with little or no impact on CRB.[39,40] As this strategy may encourage the emergence of resistant organisms it cannot be recommended.

Apparatus

Changing the infusate apparatus

The infusate apparatus can be a source of infection and routine changing of this apparatus is recommended.[41,42] The optimum replacement interval is 48–72 hours, as a further shortening of that time does not appear to improve the overall infection rate.[43] Additionally it would seem wise to change infusate apparatus at the time of any guide-wire change of CVC.

Care of injection ports

Manipulation of catheter hubs and injection ports may result in internal microbial contamination followed by intraluminal infection. In one study 23% of catheter hubs were colonised after only 4 days of catheterisation,[12] emphasising the importance of this route. Strategies need to be developed to eliminate this potential source of infection. One possible strategy is the use of closed ports, thus avoiding the problems of an open system, in particular the use of hub caps. The principle behind this system is shown in Figures 4.2 and 4.3. A recent development which may hold promise is the construction of catheter hubs containing reservoirs of antiseptics which may reduce infection via this route.[44] More pragmatically, the use of CVCs with the addition of extra access ports only if absolutely necessary, the minimal use of these access ports, and aseptic handling when using theseaccess ports, should be standard.

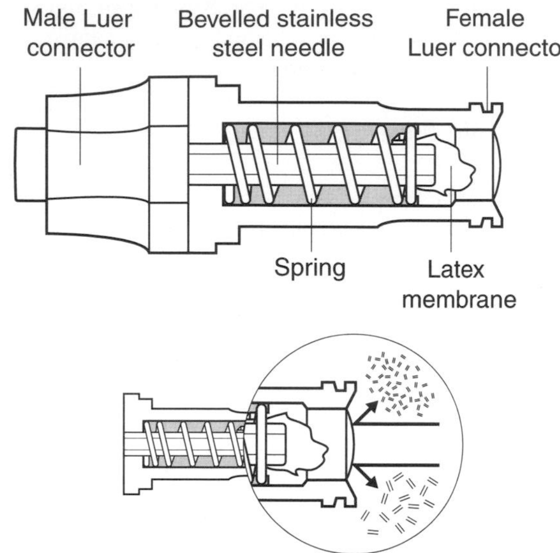

Figure 4.2 Example of a needleless closed system hub for use with CVCs (Bionector, Vygon, Cirencester, UK). The latex membrane provides a closed and cleanable surface which may reduce hub colonisation.

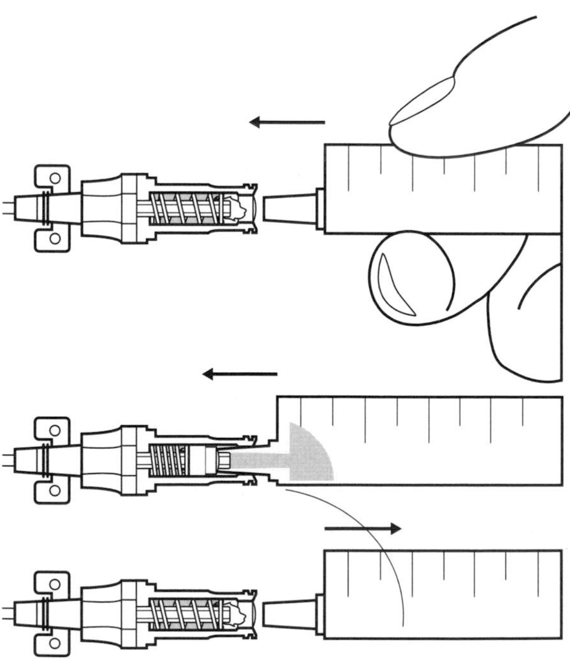

Figure 4.3 The Bionector in use illustrating the closed and cleanable system which is compatible with standard equipment.

Bacterial filters

The use of in-line filters has been shown not to decrease the infection rate in peripheral catheters but does not seem to have been evaluated in CVCs.[45]

Duration of catheterisation

The routine changing of CVCs in the absence of signs of infection is based on the evidence that a positive correlation exists between the duration of catheterisation and infection risk.[46] However, the evidence is that routine guide-wire exchanges every 3 days do not reduce the incidence of infectious complications and may increase mechanical complications.[47,48] Indeed, infection rates are similar for catheters routinely changed at 3 days or 7 days,[49] and a prospective randomised trial comparing three methods of catheter maintenance could not demonstrate a reduction in infection by routine exchange or replacement at 7 days compared with no routine changes.[50] In the absence of benefit, and in the presence of procedural risks, the routine changing of CVCs cannot be supported. Preferably, a CVC should be left *in situ* for as long as clinically indicated provided there is no evidence of catheter-related infection.

Management of Suspected Infection

The signs of CVC-related infection are non-specific and may have many other causes. It is therefore important to formulate clear guidelines for the management of suspected infection. In the absence of such guidelines removal and *de novo* insertion of CVCs (with associated procedural risks) or under-removal of CVCs (with increased risks of sepsis-related complications) may occur. The possible options for management of suspected CVC-related infection are outlined in Table 4.3 and guidelines for management are given in Figures 4.4 and 4.5.

Table 4.3 Approaches to managing suspected CVC related infection

Method	Advantages	Disadvantages
Systemic antibiotics	Removal of line not required	High failure rate
Antibiotic lock	Removal of line not required	Intermediate success rate
Removal of CVC and *de novo* replacement at new site	Removal of possible source of infection Possible to culture CVC	Removal of CVC may be inappropriate Risks of new CVC insertion
Guide-wire exchange of CVC	Removal of possible source of infection Possible to culture CVC Minimal risks of new CVC insertion	Colonisation of new CVC may occur
Endoluminal brush	Removal of line not required	Unproven technique May cause bacteraemia

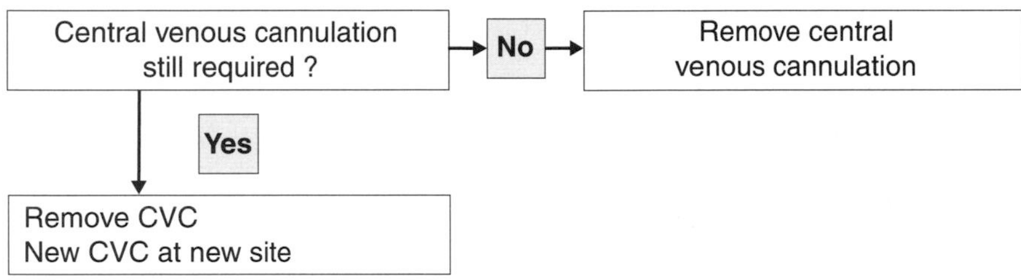

Figure 4.4 Guidelines for the management of suspected CVC-associated infection.

Obvious site infection

If there are obvious signs of site infection the CVC must be removed and inserted *de novo* at a distant site if still required (Figure 4.4). The use of broad-spectrum antibiotics while an infected line is in place is unlikely to be successful. Soon after catheter insertion a biofilm develops on the surface. This biofilm includes deposits of fibronectin, which can act as a specific binding site for micro-organisms. Many organisms, particularly *Staphylococcus epidermidis*, produce a glycocalyx slime which protects the organism from phagocytosis and antibiotic exposure. This is demonstrated by the ability of micro-organisms to survive apparently lethal concentrations of antibiotics when attached to CVCs.[11] For these reasons the use of systemic antibiotics alone cannot be recommended. The use of antibiotic 'locks' – antibiotics left within the lumen of the catheter – to treat suspected CVC-related infection has been mostly investigated in patients with long-term catheters *in situ*. Several workers have reported varying degrees of success using this strategy. This approach assumes that the primary source of infection is from the inner surface of the CVC rather than organisms on the external surface. Despite the appealing simplicity of this approach there is not enough evidence to support its use.

Suspected CVC-related infection

If CVC-related infection is suspected the most practical approaches are guide-wire exchange or removal and *de novo* insertion. Both methods allow culture of the line tip, to establish the diagnosis, but guide-wire exchange reduces mechanical complications. For this reason it is recommended that guide-wire exchange be performed and the line tip cultured (Figure 4.5). If the culture is positive and there are still signs of CVC-related infection, the line should be removed and inserted at a new site. The use of antiseptic-bonded catheters for guide-wire exchanges may reduce the risk of reinfection of the newly inserted CVC.[25]

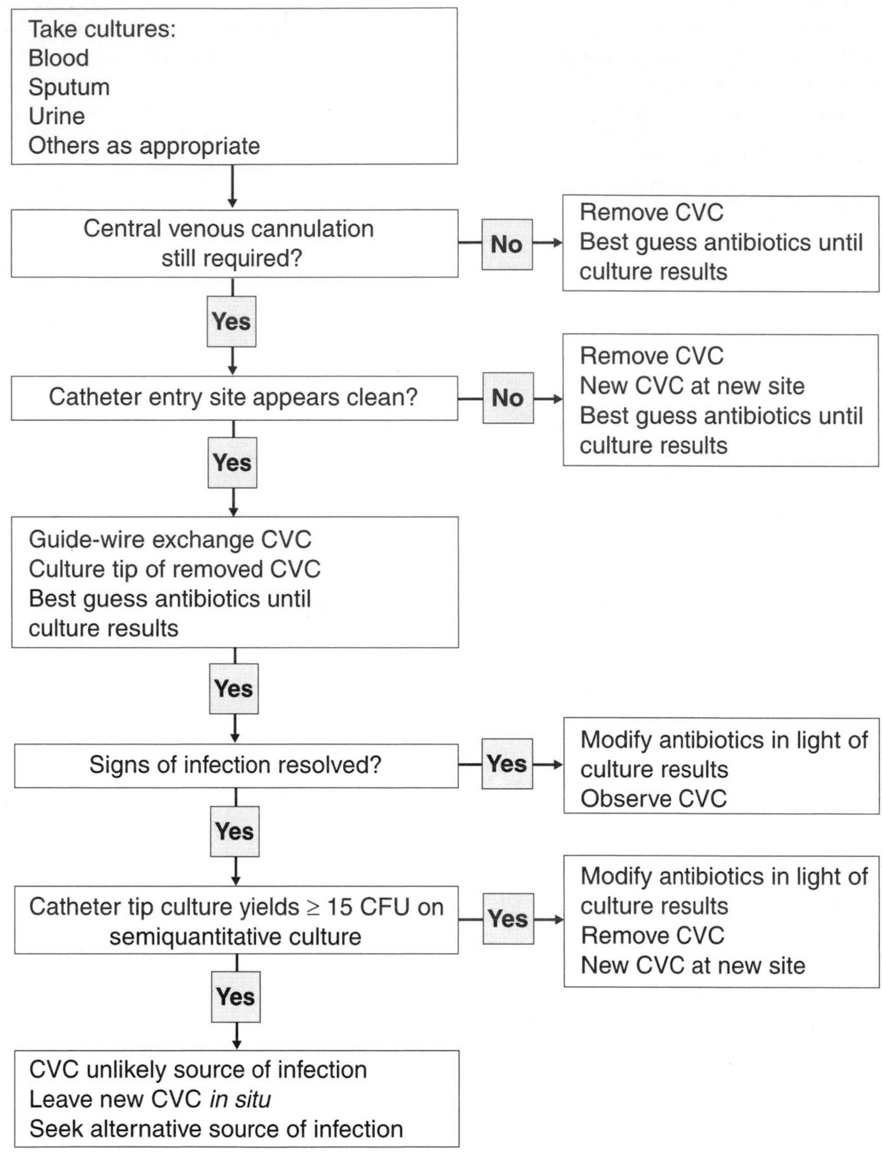

Figure 4.5 Guidelines for the management of suspected CVC-associated infection.

The endoluminal brush, a device that allows sampling of the inner surface of the CVC while *in situ*, has been evaluated as a means of diagnosing CVC-related infection.[51,52] There are only preliminary data concerning this method and so no conclusions can be made as to its value. Some workers have voiced concern that manipulation of the CVC in this manner may lead to bacteraemia and that only the inner surface of the CVC is sampled. Further work is required to evaluate this new method.

KEY POINTS

- There is an unacceptably high rate of nosocomial infections associated with intravascular devices. The skin appears to be the main source of infection and therefore efforts should be made to improve skin disinfection during catheter insertion.
- Scrupulous attention to catheter care needs to become standard practice and clear guidelines for the management of suspected CVC-related infection should be used.
- The advent of novel catheters bonded with antiseptics or antibiotics appears to hold great promise in reducing CVC-related infection but it must be remembered that these are adjunctive methods only.
- Adherence to a strict aseptic technique during insertion and maintenance of catheters remains the most important measure.

References

1. Maki DG. Infections due to infusion therapy. In: Bennett JV, Brachmen PS, eds. Hospital Infections, 3rd edn. Boston: Little, Brown, 1992.
2. Elliott TSJ. Line-associated bacteraemias. Communicable Disease Report 1998; **3**:7.
3. Sznajder JI, Zveibil FR, Bitterman H, Weiner P, Burszteun S. Central vein cannulation. Failure and complication rates by three percutaneous approaches. Archives of Internal Medicine 1986; **146**:259.
4. Bullard KM, Dunn DL. Diagnosis and treatment of bacteraemia and intravascular catheter infections. American Journal of Surgery 1996; **172**:13s.
5. Hampton AA, Sheretz RJ. Vascular access infections in hospitalized patients. Surgical Clinics of North America 1988; **68**:57.
6. Maki DG, Band JD. A comparative study of polyantibiotic and iodophor ointments in the prevention of vascular catheter-related infection. American Journal of Medicine 1981; **70**:739.
7. Reed CR, Sessler CN, Glauser FL *et al.* Central venous catheter infections: concepts and controversies. Intensive Care Medicine 1995; **21**:177.
8. Maki DG, Weise CE, Sarafin HW. A semiquantative culture method for identifying intravenous-catheter-related infection. New England Journal of Medicine 1977; **296**:1305.
9. Cleri DJ, Corrado ML, Seligman SJ. Quantitative culture of intravenous catheters and other intravascular inserts. Journal of Infectious Disease 1980; **141**:781–6.
10. Raad II, Bodey GB. Infectious complications of indwelling vascular catheters. Clinical Infectious Disease 1992; **15**:197.
11. Elliott TSJ. Intravascular device infections. Journal of Medical Microbiology 1988; **27**:161.
12. Tebbs SE, Ghose A, Elliott TSJ. Microbial contamination of intravenous and arterial catheters. Intensive Care Medicine 1996; **22**:272.
13. Elliott TSJ, Moss HA, Tebbs SE *et al.* Novel approach to investigate a source of microbial contamination of central venous catheters. European Journal of Clinical Microbiology and Infectious Diseases 1997; **16**:210.
14. Francois P, Vaudaux P, Nurdin N *et al.* Physical and biological effects of a surface coating procedure on polyurethane catheters. Biomaterials 1996; **17**:667.
15. Tebbs SE, Elliott TSJ. Modification of central venous catheter polymers to prevent in vitro microbial colonisation. European Journal of Clinical Microbiology and Infectious Diseases 1994; **13**:111.
16. Hasaniya NWMA, Angelis M, Brown MR *et al.* Efficacy of subcutaneous silver-impregnated cuffs in preventing central venous catheter infections. Chest 1996; **109**:1030.
17. Flowers RHIII, Schwenzer KJ, Kopel RF *et al.* Efficacy of an attachable subcutaneous cuff for the prevention of intravascular catheter-related infection. Journal of the American Medical Society 1989; **261**:878.
18. Welch GW, McKeel DW, Silverstein P *et al.* The role of catheter composition in the development of thrombophlebitis. Annals of Internal Medicine 1974; **138**:421.
19. Elliott TSJ, Tebbs SE. Intravascular catheters impregnated with benzalkonium chloride. Journal of Antimicrobial Therapeutics 1993; **32**:905.
20. Bach A, Schmidt H, Bottiger B *et al.* Retention of antibacterial activity and bacterial colonisation of antiseptic bonded central venous catheters. Journal of Antimicrobial Therapeutics 1996; **37**:315.
21. Shmitt SK, Knapp C, Hall GS *et al.* Impact of chlorhexidine-silver sulfadiazine-impregnated central venous catheters on in vitro quantitation of catheter-associated bacteria. Journal of Clinical Microbiology 1996; **34**:508.
22. Kamal GD, Pfaller MA, Rempe LE *et al.* Reduced intravascular catheter infection by antibiotic bonding: a prospective, randomised, controlled trial. Journal of the American Medical Association 1991; **265**:2364.
23. Thornton J, Todd NJ, Webster NR. Central venous line sepsis in the intensive care unit – a study comparing antibiotic coated catheters with plain catheters. Anaesthesia 1996; **51**:1018.

24. Raad I, Darouiche R, Dupuis J *et al.* Central venous catheters coated with minocycline and rifampin for the prevention of catheter-related colonisation and bloodstream infections. Annals of Internal Medicine 1997; **127**:267.
25. Maki DG, Stolz SM, Wheeler S *et al.* Prevention of central venous catheter-related bloodstream infection by the use of an antiseptic-impregnated catheter. Annals of Internal Medicine 1997; **127**:257.
26. Bernard RW, Stahl WM, Chase RM. Subclavian vein catheterisations: a prospective study. II. Infectious complications. Annals of Surgery 1971; **173**:191.
27. Farkas JC, Liu N, Bleriot JP *et al.* Single- versus triple-lumen central catheter-related sepsis: a prospective randomised study in a critically ill population. American Journal of Medicine 1992; **93**:277.
28. Snydman DR, Pober BR, Murray SA *et al.* Predictive value of surveillance skin cultures in total parenteral nutrition related infection. Lancet 1982; **ii**:1385.
29. Collingnon P, Soni N, Pearson I *et al.* Sepsis associated with central vein catheters in critically ill patients. Intensive Care Medicine 1988; **14**:227.
30. Pinilla JC, Ross DF, Martin T *et al.* Study of the incidence of intravascular catheter infection and associated septicaemia in critically ill patients. Critical Care Medicine 1983; **11**:21.
31. Maki DG, Ringer M, Alvarado CJ. Prospective randomised trial of povidone-iodine, alcohol, and chlorhexidine for prevention of infection associated with central venous and arterial catheters. Lancet 1991; **338**:339.
32. Ricard P, Martin R, Marcoux JA. Protection of indwelling vascular catheters: incidence of bacterial contamination and catheter related sepsis. Critical Care Medicine 1985; **13**:541.
33. McCredie KB, Lawson M, Marts K *et al.* A comparative evaluation of transparent dressings and gauze dressings for central venous catheters. Journal of Parenteral and Enteral Nutrition 1984; **8**:96.
34. Conly JM, Greives K, Peters B. A prospective, randomised study comparing transparent and dry gauze dressings for central venous catheters. Journal of Infectious Disease 1989; **159**:310.
35. Hoffmann KK, Weber DJ, Samsa GP *et al.* Transparent polyurethane-film as an intravenous catheter dressing: a meta-analysis of the infection rates. Journal of the American Medical Association 1992; **267**:2072.
36. Elliott TSJ. Catheter-associated infections; new developments in prevention. In: Burchardi H, Dobb GJ, Bion J, Dellinger RP (eds) Current Topics in Intensive Care 4. London: WB Saunders 1997; 182.
37. Maki DG, McCormack KN. Defatting catheter insertion sites in total parenteral nutrition is of no value as an infection control measure. American Journal of Medicine 1987; **83**:833.
38. Moyer MA, Edwards LD, Farley L. Comparative culture methods on 100 intravenous catheters: routine, semi-quantative, and blood cultures. Archives of Internal Medicine 1983; **143**:66.
39. Hill RLR, Fisher AP, Ware RJ *et al.* Mupiricon for the reduction of colonisation of internal jugular cannulae – a randomised controlled trial. Journal of Hospital Infection 1990; **15**:311.
40. Zinner SH, Denny-Brown BC, Braun P *et al.* Risk of infection with intravenous indwelling catheters: effect of application of antibiotic ointment. Journal of Infectious Disease 1969; **120**:616.
41. Samsoondar W, Freeman JB. Colonisation of intravascular monitoring devices. Critical Care Medicine 1985; **13**:753.
42. Sitges-Serra A, Linares J, Perez JL *et al.* A randomised trial on the effect of tubing changes on hub contamination and catheter sepsis during parenteral nutrition. Journal of Parenteral and Enteral Nutrition 1985; **9**:322.
43. Snydman DR, Donnely-Reidy M, Perry LK *et al.* Intravenous tubing containing burettes can be safely changed at 72 hour intervals. Infection Control and Hospital Epidemiology 1987; **8**:113.
44. Segura M, Alia C, Valverde J *et al.* Assessment of a new hub design and the semi-quantitative catheter culture method using an in vivo experimental model of catheter sepsis. Journal of Clinical Microbiology 1990; **28**:2551.
45. Falchuk KH, Peterson PK, McNeil BJ. Microparticulate-induced phlebitis: its prevention by in-line filtration. New England Journal of Medicine 1985; **312**:78.
46. Essop AR, Frolich J, Moosa MR *et al.* Risk factors related to bacterial contamination of indwelling vascular catheters in non-infected hosts. Intensive Care Medicine 1984; **10**:193.
47. Cobb DK, High KP, Sawyer RG *et al.* A controlled trial of scheduled replacement of central venous and pulmonary artery catheters. New England Journal of Medicine 1992; **327**:1062.
48. Snyder RH, Archer FJ, Endy T *et al.* Catheter infection: a comparison of two catheter maintenance techniques. Annals of Surgery 1988; **208**:651.
49. Bonawitz SC, Hammel EJ, Kirkpatrick JR. Prevention of central venous catheter sepsis: prospective randomised trial. American Journal of Surgery 1991; **57**:618.
50. Eyer S, Brummitt C, Carossley K *et al.* Catheter-related sepsis: prospective randomised study of three methods of long-term catheter maintenance. Critical Care Medicine 1990; **18**:1073.
51. Markus S, Buday S. Culturing indwelling central venous catheters in situ. Infections in surgery 1989; **5**:157.
52. Tighe MJ, Kite P, Fawley WN *et al.* An endoluminal brush to detect the infected central venous catheter in situ: a pilot study. British Medical Journal 1996; **313**:1528.

5 • The Arm Veins

SHANG NG

Introduction

The most popular technique for inserting central venous catheters has always been through the peripheral arm veins, using a puncture site in the antecubital fossa. The main advantage here is that veins are usually easily seen and palpable, and every clinician has previous experience of venepuncture at this site. Furthermore, because no vital structures lie near these veins, there has been a notable absence of reports of complications arising from the venepuncture.

Nevertheless, the approach through a vein in the antecubital fossa has two main drawbacks. First, studies show that only 65–75% of catheters inserted through these veins reach a suitable central position[1–9] (see Table 5.1). Second, and in contrast to the safety of the initial venepuncture, thrombophlebitis and inflammation at the site ofinsertion quickly develop[10,11] and nearly all patients suffer this complication within 24–48 hours.[8]

In spite of the disadvantages, for short-term use central venous catheterisation through visible palpable peripheral arm veins is safe and remains the method of choice for those with little experience of sophisticated techniques.

Because of the relative ease of cannulation of the antecubital fossa veins, this route has been developed by medical and nursing personnel in particular as a means of gaining central venous access for longer-term (weeks to months) treatments such as chemotherapy. Frequent and sometimes distressing repeated peripheral venous cannulation for treatment courses is reduced. The need for the more invasive Hickman catheters is lessened and patients do not need to attend hospital as much.[12,13]

Commercially produced kits incorporating suitably long (50–60 cm) silicone catheters are available. Although polyurethane catheters are available, the use of silicone material together with other improvements in catheter technology have undoubtedly enhanced the longevity of peripherally inserted central catheters (PICC). The use of peripherally inserted central lines in preference to peripheral cannulae appears to be gaining popularity in a wide variety of clinical settings[14–16]

Some interest has recently centred on the deep brachial veins. When conventional cannulation through visible or palpable antecubital fossa veins is not possible because of obesity or sclerosed veins, deep percutaneous puncture of the venae comitantes of the brachial artery in the antecubital fossa has been used to gain venous access and thereby avoid a venous cut-down.[17] This site of venepuncture has been used for central venous catheterisation, although minor injury to the brachial artery is a risk.[18] Following the description of a cut-down technique on the deep brachial vein at the inner edge of the brachial biceps,[19] a percutaneous method of central venous catheterisation through the deep basilic vein in the groove between the bellies of the biceps and triceps muscles has been successfully tried.[20] These techniques have not yet achieved popular use. They obviously entail more skill than superficial venepuncture and the danger of damage to the brachial artery is ever-present.

In 1967 Spracklen *et al.*[21] described a technique of central venous catheterisation through a percutaneous venepuncture of the proximal basilic or axillary vein. This approach was later described independently by Ayim[22] in 1977. Both papers reported a high success rate with an absence of serious complication.

More recently, a large series involving axillary vein catheterisation in over 300 instances reported favourable results comparable with other techniques.[23] The method was used to insert both central venous lines and pulmonary artery catheters. The authors claim freedom from damage to lung and other structures associated with techniques involving deep veins. The site of insertion was thought to be particularly advantageous in tracheostomised patients as the separation of the catheter from a potentially infected tracheostomy reduced the risk of septicaemia. Another more recent study from the same centre found similar success.[24] These workers recommended the use of a Seldinger guide-wire technique to insert the catheter. However, this approach has not gained popularity, probably because of the high degree of skill required to make the initial venepuncture into a vein that is not readily visible.

The axillary vein can also be reached percutaneously from an infraclavicular approach.[25,26] Based on dissection studies, definitive landmarks have been recommended to trace the course of the axillary vein. Whilst the technique claims to perform venepuncture away from the thoracic inlet, the method does nevertheless involve deep and therefore blind needling of the vein. This technique has not gained popularity but some workers see advantages over other commonly used routes[26] and the axillary approach has been recommended by others as a satisfactory alternative to subclavian and internal jugular catheterisations.[27]

An interesting approach which seeks both to avoid the failings of conventional long arm central venous catheters and the external jugular vein method and at the same time to eliminate the dangers of deep neck vein puncture is the concept of the 'halfway' venous catheter. The rationale and anatomical basis for using this method have been examined in depth.[28,29] In this method the catheter tip is placed within the proximal axillary vein or the distal portion of the subclavian vein. The walls of the proximal axillary vein are held apart by expansions of the coracoclavipectoral fascia so the catheter tip would lie within a large vein which cannot collapse and one that opens into large central veins. The axillosubclavian venous pathway is relatively long so positioning the catheter can be achieved by clinical estimation, making X-ray control unnecessary. The technique has been validated by extensive clinical testing.[30]

Anatomy

The venous blood from the arm drains through two intercommunicating main veins, the basilic and the cephalic. The basilic system runs along the medial side of the arm and the cephalic along the lateral side. There is considerable variation in the anatomy of the arm veins, particularly in the cephalic system. The common arrangement is described below (Figure 5.1).

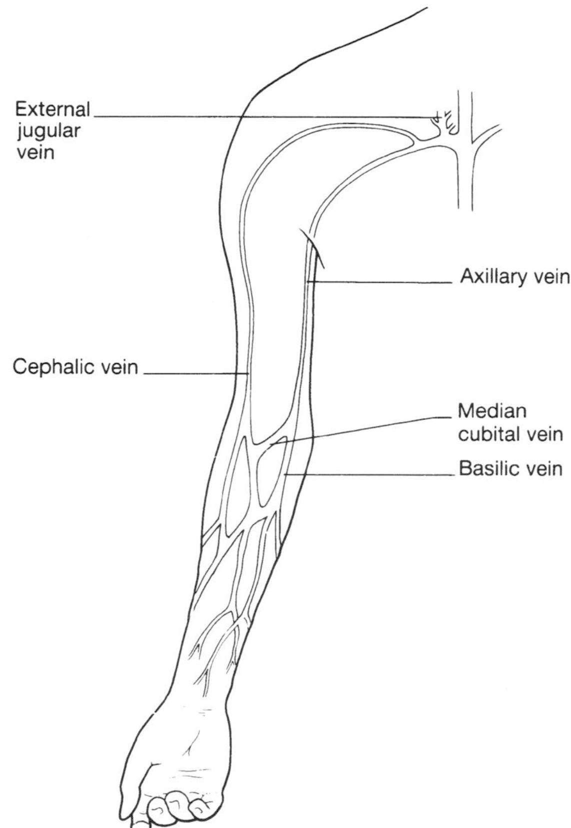

Figure 5.1 Anatomy of the arm veins.

Basilic vein

The basilic vein ascends from the hand along the medial surface of the forearm, often as two channels which unite before they reach the elbow. Near the elbow the vein inclines forwards to run in front of the medial epicondyle, at about which point it is joined by the median cubital vein. It then runs along the medial margin of the biceps to the middle of the upper arm, where it pierces the deep fascia. From here it ascends along the medial side of the brachial artery and becomes the axillary vein on entering the axilla.

Other veins on the posteromedial surface of the forearm ascend to join the basilic vein. Although prominent, they are not firmly supported by the fatty subcutaneous tissue and easily move away from a probing needle point.

Cephalic vein

The cephalic vein ascends on the front of the lateral side of the forearm to the front of the elbow, where it communicates with the basilic vein through the median cubital vein. It then ascends along the lateral surface of the biceps to the lower border of the pectoralis major muscle, where it turns sharply to pierce the clavipectoral fascia and pass beneath the clavicle. It then usually terminates in the axillary vein. The virtual right angle at which the cephalic vein joins the axillary vein is probably one of the main reasons for the obstruction frequently encountered at this point when attempting to pass a catheter through the cephalic vein. Other reasons for obstruction at this site are variations in the anatomy of the termination of the cephalic vein. The vein may join the external jugular vein only or it may bifurcate into two very small veins, one joining the external jugular vein and one the axillary vein. Finally, there are usually valves near its termination.

Axillary vein

The basilic vein continues as the axillary vein on reaching the axilla (Figure 5.2). Anteriorly, the lateral border of the pectoralis major muscle forms the lateral boundary of the axilla. The axillary vein

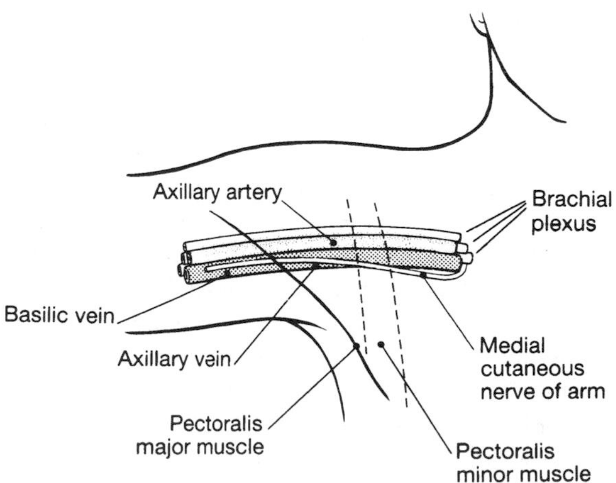

Figure 5.2 Anatomy of the axillary vein.

continues upwards into the apex of the axilla and becomes the subclavian vein on reaching the lower border of the first rib. It usually receives the cephalic vein near its termination.

The axillary vein is divided into three parts by the pectoralis minor muscle, which crosses over the vein to reach its insertion in the coracoid process of the scapula. It is the first (distal) part of the axillary vein which is suitable for venepuncture because it is relatively superficial. This part of the vein is separated from the skin by fascia and fatty tissue; the medial cutaneous nerve of the forearm lies on its surface and separates it from the axillary artery, which lies laterally. Other structures of the brachial plexus are more closely related to the artery than to the vein and are therefore less likely to be damaged during venepuncture.

Median cubital vein

The median cubital vein is a large communicating vein that springs from the cephalic vein just below the bend of the elbow and runs obliquely upwards to join the basilic vein just above the bend of the elbow. It receives veins from the front of the forearm which themselves may be suitable for catheterisation. It is separated from the brachial artery by a thickened portion of the deep fascia (bicipital aponeurosis). Again, variations in this arrangement are commonly seen.

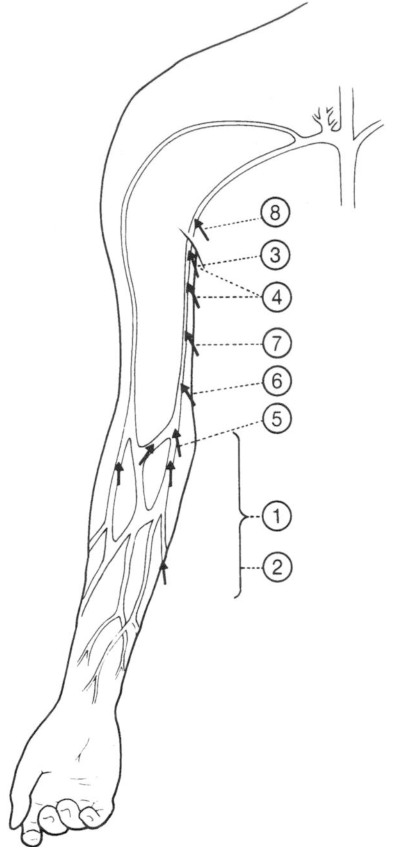

Figure 5.3 Approaches to catheterisation of the arm veins: 1, authors' method; 2, Bridges *et al.* (1979)[38] (basilic vein only); 3, Spracklen *et al.* (1967);[21] 4, Ayim (1977);[22] 5, Linder *et al.* (1985);[30] 6, Saissy *et al.* (1985);[18] 7, Koing-Bo *et al.* (1984);[20] 8, Nickalls (1987).[25] Adults: methods 1, 2, 3 or 4. Infants: methods 1 or 4.

Choice of Technique

A vein in the antecubital fossa is usually the first choice for catheterisation (Figure 5.3). The axillary vein is kept in reserve in case of failure with a more peripheral vein, but may be considered for long-term catheterisation.

Certain recommendations have been made to obtain the best success rate with the peripheral arm vein approach. The advantage of the basilic over the cephalic vein is agreed on by most authors,[1–4,7,31,32] including ourselves, although other studies have revealed no difference in success rate between the two veins.[9,33] With either method the catheter may still not enter the intrathoracic veins. Deitel and McIntyre[3] and Langston[4] suggested turning the head towards the side of venepuncture to reduce the chance of the catheter's entering the ipsilateral internal jugular vein. The value of this manoeuvre was supported by Burgess *et al.*[34] but not by Woods *et al.*,[35] though both of these appear to have been careful studies. When the basilic vein was used, abducting the arm up to 45° from the body improved the success rate.[35]

The value of these various manoeuvres has been assessed while inserting catheters into the basilic vein under fluoroscopic control.[36] The findings and recommendations that follow correspond with our experience of many hundreds of catheters inserted through this route.

(a) Rotation of the head to the side of venepuncture and supraclavicular digital pressure on the same side alter the anatomy of the veins in such a way as to encourage passage of a catheter centrally. Hyperabducting the arm is least helpful.
(b) If resistance is felt after advancing the catheter more than 20 cm then withdrawal of the stylet (if present) 2–3 cm may facilitate the passage of the now more flexible catheter tip.
(c) Withdrawal of the stylet combined with injection of a bolus of saline while advancing the catheter is also worth trying if the catheter appears to be held up.

Kuramoto and Sakabe[37] found that they could more satisfactorily position the catheter tip when the right basilic vein was used, but most authors do not agree with this.[6,9]

Lumley and Russell[9] recommended a neck compression test to detect whether a catheter tip is positioned in the internal jugular vein. Neck compression produces a rise of more than 10 cm H_2O in the venous pressure after inadvertent internal jugular catheterisation, but no such rise occurs when the other side of the neck is compressed. To detect obstruction to the passage of the catheter, Holt[1] measured alterations in the rate of entry of a rapidly running infusion of saline through the catheter. This also indicated whether manoeuvres such as abduction of the arm overcame or reduced the obstruction.

Bridges and his colleagues[38] demonstrated a high success rate when catheterisation was performed with the patient in the sitting position, combined with a special technique for introducing the catheter (described below).

The material or design of the catheter can also influence the success rate. Two groups[6,9] found animproved result with the use of the Drum Cartridge Catheter (Abbott Laboratories), when compared to the I-Catheter (Bardic). That the type of device used appears to be an important factor in determining the success rate of cannulation through arm veins is emphasised by other workers. Wright and Walker[39] obtained a high success rate again using the Drum Cartridge Catheter (Abbott Laboratories). Comparing their results with those obtained with other products, they attributed their 92% success rate to the soft polyurethane catheter stiffened by a flexible wire stylet throughout its length; the stiffening was thought to be significant.

Method preferred by authors

The authors' preferred technique, both for adults and children, is described immediately below. We have found the selection of a medially placed vein (basilic system) to be the most important factor in obtaining successful catheterisation through an arm vein.

The use of a J-tipped guide-wire has been shown to greatly increase the success rate of cannulation through the external jugular vein[40] (see Chapter 8). Similarly, using a J-tipped guide-wire when cannulating the antecubital fossa veins, some workers have achieved 100% successful central venous positioning when using the basilic vein and 78% through the cephalic vein;[41] others are not convinced of the advantage of a J-tipped guide-wire.[42]

The concept of the 'halfway' catheter does not seem to have achieved widespread appeal in spite of its thorough documentation. All the other techniques described involving the axillary vein and the deep brachial veins require a higher degree of skill and in all these methods a vein is punctured in a blind fashion. These techniques have been described in more recent years so it is too early to fully assess their place in this field.

A useful supplementary technique has been suggested to encourage the use of the relatively safe arm veins when these are very small. A guide-wire could be introduced through a small venepuncture needle, followed by a vein dilator and then a sufficiently large introducer for a central catheter.[43]

Whichever technique is used to insert a central venous line through a peripheral arm vein, it should be borne in mind that abduction and adduction of the arm can lead to movement of the catheter tip up to (on average) 2–3 cm. Adduction alone can result in the catheter being drawn into the thorax by as much as 9 cm.[44]

METHODS

ANTECUBITAL FOSSA APPROACH

Authors' method

Patient category

Adults and neonates.

Advantages and disadvantages

Venepuncture is made into a visible and palpable vein, so there is a lower risk of immediate complications compared with puncture of deep veins.

Peripheral veins are unsatisfactory for long-term catheterisation.

Preferred side

Either side may be used. Select the arm with the most favourable vein.

Position of patient

Place the patient in a supine position with the arm to be used held at about 45° from the side of the body. Turn the head towards the side of puncture (Figure 5.4a).

Position of operator

Stand on the same side as the puncture site (Figure 5.4a).

Advice on current equipment

Adults: 14 gauge outside diameter (OD) introducing needle or cannula, length 40 mm (minimum); catheter length 600 mm (minimum).
Neonates: 18 gauge or 20 gauge OD introducing needle or cannula, length 20 mm (minimum); catheter length 200 mm (minimum).

Anatomical landmarks

Apply a tourniquet to the upper arm to distend the veins before selecting a suitable vein (Figure 5.4b). In order of preference, identify:

1. A vein on the medial side of the antecubital fossa – the basilic or median cubital vein. Even when not visible, these veins are often easily palpable when engorged.
2. A vein on the posteromedial aspect of the forearm – a tributary of the basilic vein. An assistant may be needed to rotate the arm externally to display these veins.
3. The cephalic vein if the other arm cannot be used.

Preparation

Perform the puncture under sterile conditions using local anaesthesia if indicated.

Precautions and recommendations

Estimate the length of catheter needed by laying the catheter (in its sterile pack) on the surface of the patient, or by measurement with a tape-measure.

Point of insertion of needle

Close to the chosen vein.

Direction of needle and procedure

After puncturing the vein, advance the catheter a short distance (2–4 cm in adults; 1–2 cm in infants) and release the tourniquet. Keep the arm abducted and the head turned to the side of puncture as the catheter is steadily advanced to the distance estimated beforehand.

If the progress of the catheter is held up, do not use force to advance it and do not attempt to retract it if a catheter-through-needle device is used. If other devices are used, the following 'trial and error' manoeuvres may help to advance the catheter: withdraw the catheter 2–3 cm and attempt reinsertion; rotate the catheter as it is advanced; withdraw the stylet 1 cm and attempt insertion again.

Other useful measures include digital pressure in the supraclavicular fossa on the ipsilateral side and the injection of a bolus of saline while advancing the catheter.

Confirm the position of the catheter tip with a chest X-ray.

Success rate

Success rates were 77.7% (94 catheterisations) using the Drum Cartridge Catheter (Abbott Laboratories) and 52.8% (106 catheterisations) using the I-Catheter (Bardic). No infants were included in this series.

Complications

No complications were associated with the initial venepuncture.

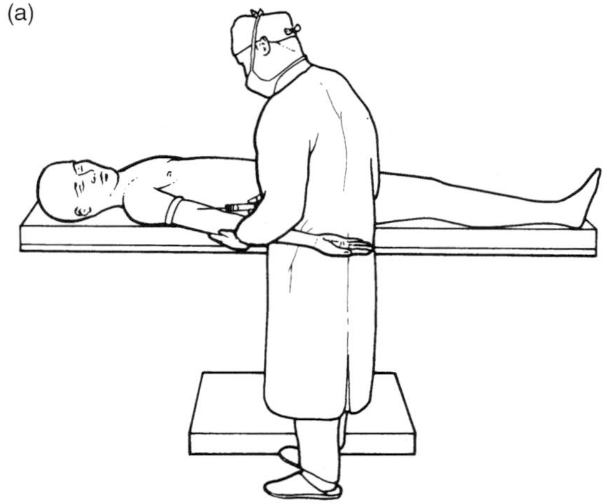

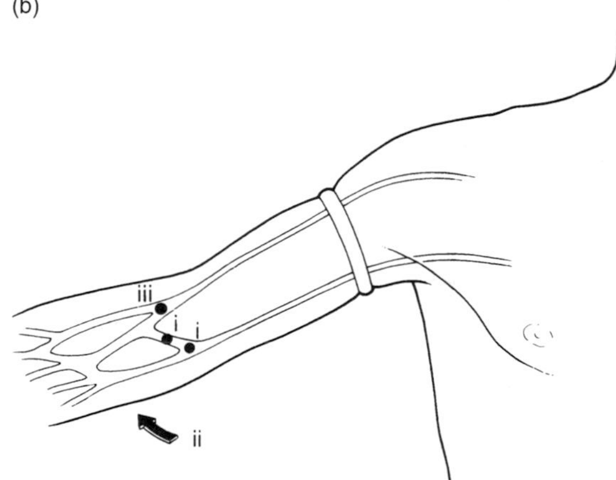

Figure 5.4 Antecubital fossa approach (authors' method).

BRACHIAL VEIN: MIDDLE THIRD OF UPPER ARM

Koing-Bo et al. *(1984)*[20]

Patient category

Adults.

Advantages and disadvantages

Useful when deep neck veins are not suitable. Avoids the need for surgical cut-down. Few complications but the procedure is a blind one so there is a risk of arterial puncture.

Preferred side

Either side.

Position of patient

Place the patient in the supine position. Abduct the arm to be used 45° away from the side with the hand supinated, i.e. palm showing (Figure 5.5).

Position of operator

Stand on the same side as the puncture site.

Equipment used in original description

The guide-wire technique was used, with a 21 gauge introducer needle to locate the vein. A small-diameter guide-wire to pass through this needle (confirmed by pretesting) was introduced into the vein. The vein was then dilated by inserting an 18 gauge cannula over the wire. A stiffer and larger-diameter wire was then introduced, overwhich a large-diameter (13 gauge) cannula was advanced into the dilated vein. The catheter (15 gauge) was finally inserted through this large cannula until a central venous position was reached.

Advice on current equipment

The above technique is recommended.

Anatomical landmarks

Identify the groove between the biceps and triceps muscle in the middle third of the upper arm (Figure 5.5). Palpate the brachial artery. Note from Figure 5.6 the relations of the brachial veins to the brachial artery in this region.

Preparation

Apply a tourniquet high up on the arm. Perform the procedure under aseptic conditions using local anaesthesia if appropriate.

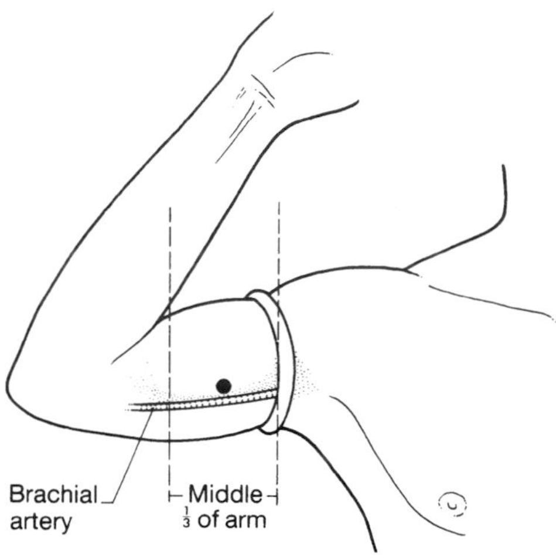

Figure 5.5 Position of the arm for initial venepuncture.

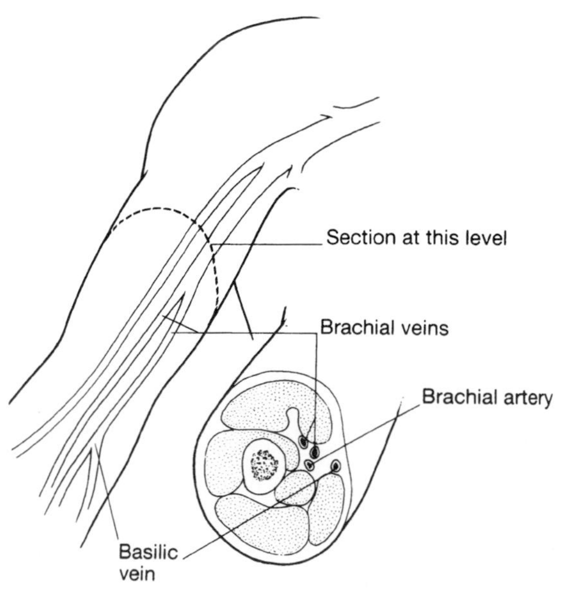

Figure 5.6 Anatomy of veins of the upper arm.

Point of insertion of the needle

The needle is inserted in the groove between the muscle bellies in the middle third of the upper arm. If the brachial artery is palpable the needle is inserted slightly lateral to it (see Figure 5.5).

Procedure

Insert the introducer needle and syringe into the point of insertion and move the syringe about 30–45° away from the skin. Advance while keeping a slight negative pressure in the syringe until a flashback is obtained. Detach the syringe and introduce the small guide-wire into the vein. Release the tourniquet. Proceed as described above. When the catheter appears to be successfully placed, take a chest X-ray for confirmation.

Success rate and complications

Not stated. Apparently successful on a number of occasions with no serious complications.

AXILLARY AND PROXIMAL BASILIC VEIN

Spracklen et al. *(1976)*[21]

Patient category

Adults. The description of the technique by the original authors did not include its application in children, but this does not necessarily exclude its use in this age group.

Advantages and disadvantages

Puncture is made in a 'blind' fashion into the axillary vein or proximal basilic vein, using the axillary artery, identified by palpation, as the landmark. This vein may be patent when more peripheral veins are collapsed, as in circulatory failure. The complications of puncture of deep neck veins are avoided.

Preferred side

Either side may be used.

Position of patient

Place the patient supine with the head in the straight-ahead position and resting on one pillow. The arm to be used is abducted away from the patient's side and the hand placed behind the occiput (Figure 5.7a).

Position of operator

Stand on the same side as the puncture site.

Equipment used in original description

Catheter-through-needle, catheter-through-cannula and guide-wire techniques have been used.

Advice on current equipment

A 14 gauge OD introducing needle or cannula, length 40 mm (minimum); catheter length 600 mm (minimum). Alternatively, a guide-wire technique is recommended.

Anatomical landmarks

Palpate the axillary artery and note its course (Figure 5.7b). Identify the area where the basilic vein continues as the axillary vein.

Preparation

Perform the puncture under sterile conditions using local anaesthesia if indicated.

(a)

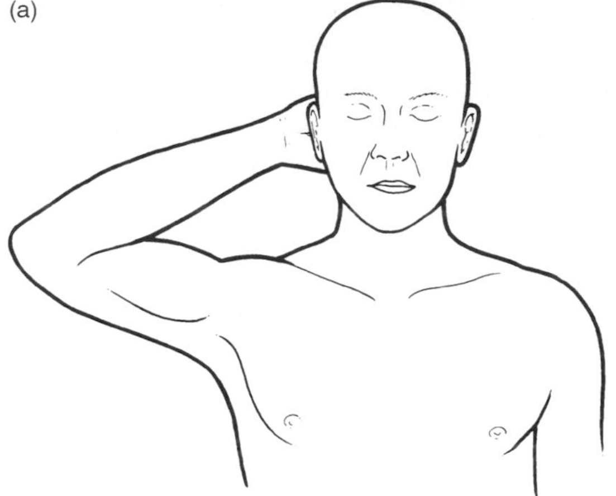

(b)

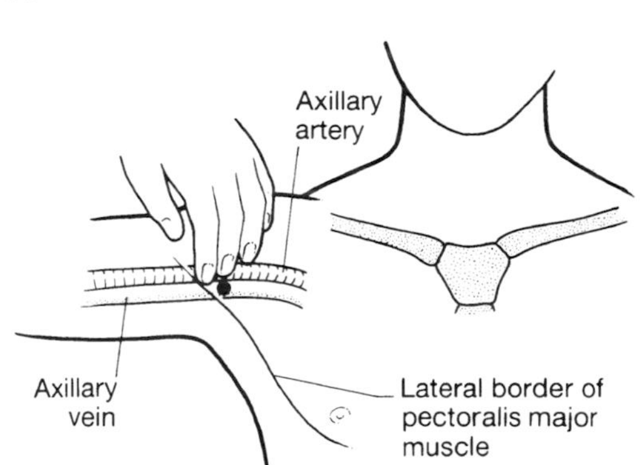

(c)

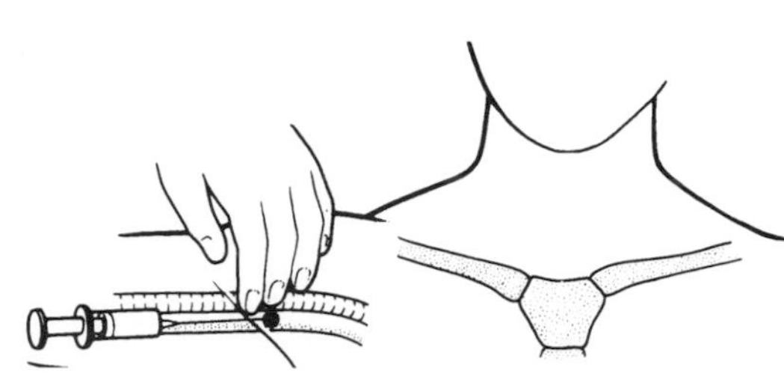

Figure 5.7 Axillary and proximal basilic vein (Spracklen *et al.*, 1976).[21]

Point of insertion of needle

The point of insertion lies 1 cm medial to the artery in the region of the junction of the basilic and axillary veins (Figure 5.7b).

Direction of the needle and procedure

Place the point of the needle on the entry site in the skin and elevate the needle 30° above the skin surface. Direct the needle towards the chest wall keeping the needle parallel to the course of the axillary artery. Keep a finger on the artery during venepuncture to act as a landmark and to protect the artery from inadvertent puncture (Figure 5.9c). An assistant exerting gentle upward pressure in the medial axilla may make venepuncture easier. Maintain a slight negative pressure on the syringe (if used) as the needle is advanced, until the vein is entered. Insert the catheter. Take a chest X-ray to confirm the position of the catheter tip.

Success rate

The success rate was 90% (50 cases). Venepuncture failed at the first attempt in 3 cases but was successful in the opposite arm.

Complications

There were no significant complications. Ten patients (20%) experienced transient local pain or paraesthesiae in the arm. No late neurological injury occurred. Haematomas occasionally formed locally.

AXILLARY AND PROXIMAL BASILIC VEIN

Ayim (1977)[22]

Patient category

Adults and children. No infants younger than 1 year were included in this study.

Advantages and disadvantages

Puncture is made into a visible or easily palpable vein. This technique is claimed to have a lower failure rate than catheterisation through more peripheral veins whilst avoiding the complications of puncture of the deep neck veins. The relative contraindications to the use of this technique include infection at the site of puncture and gross obesity.

Preferred side

Either side may be used.

Position of patient

Place the patient supine with the head in the straight-ahead position. Abduct the arm 45°, or more if possible, away from the patient's side and place the hand under the patient's head (Figure 5.8a).

Position of operator

Stand on the same side as the puncture site.

Equipment used in original description

Adults: catheter-through-cannula and catheter-through-needle (10% of cases).
Infants: 18 gauge OD catheter-over-needle.

Advice on current equipment

Adults: 14 gauge OD introducing needle or cannula, length 40 mm (minimum); catheter length 600 mm (minimum).
Infants: 18 gauge or 20 gauge OD introducing needle or cannula, length 20 mm (minimum); catheter length 200 mm (minimum).

Anatomical landmarks

Identify the lower border of the pectoralis major muscle and the positions of the distal portion of the axillary vein and proximal portion of the basilic vein in the following manner. Palpate the axillary artery; the axillary vein lies medial to the artery (Figure 5.8b). This distal portion of the axillary vein is superficial but becomes inaccessible when it passes deep to a muscle layer in its middle portion. The proximal portion of the basilic vein, which forms the immediate distal continuation of the axillary vein, also lies superficially and has the same relation to its accompanying artery (brachial artery).

Preparation

Perform the puncture under sterile conditions using local anaesthesia if indicated.

Precautions and recommendations

An assistant may be helpful.

Point of insertion of needle

In order to distend the vein, apply a narrow (1–2 cm wide) rubber tourniquet as high up in the axilla as possible and instruct the assistant to pull the tourniquet towards the lateral half of the clavicle (Figure 5.8c). If the armpit is hollow, use a pad of gauze under the tourniquet to help compress the vein. Alternatively, use the thumb or third and fourth fingers of the free hand to compress the vein medial to the pulsation of the axillary artery and as high up in the armpit as possible. Following attempts to distend the vein, enter at the most prominent portion, whether the proximal basilic vein or the axillary vein.

Procedure

Do not proceed with this technique unless one of the veins is visible or easily palpable. Maintain a slight negative pressure in the syringe (if used) as the needle is advanced until the vein is entered. Insert the catheter. Take a chest X-ray to confirm the position of the catheter tip.

Success rate

Axillary vein: 95.9% (73 cases, all adults).
Proximal basilic vein: 93.1% (68 cases, adults and children).

Complications

Haematoma occurred in 3% and probable incipient venous thrombosis in 3.9%. There were no paraesthesiae or evidence of nerve injury. The average duration of catheterisation was, for the axillary vein, 7.8 days (range 1–28 days) and, for the proximal basilic vein, 4.3 days (range 1–14 days).

(a)

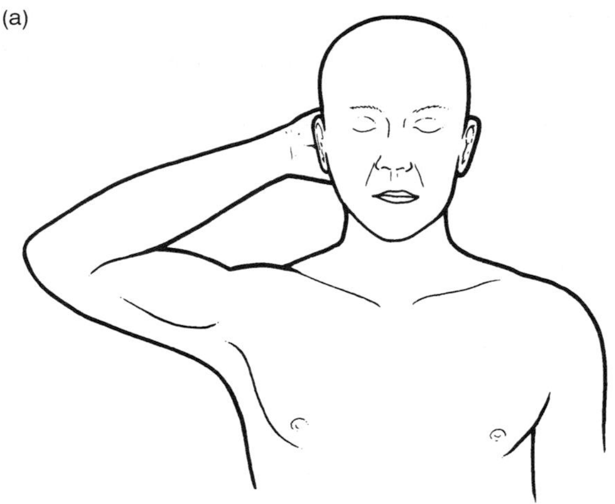

(b)

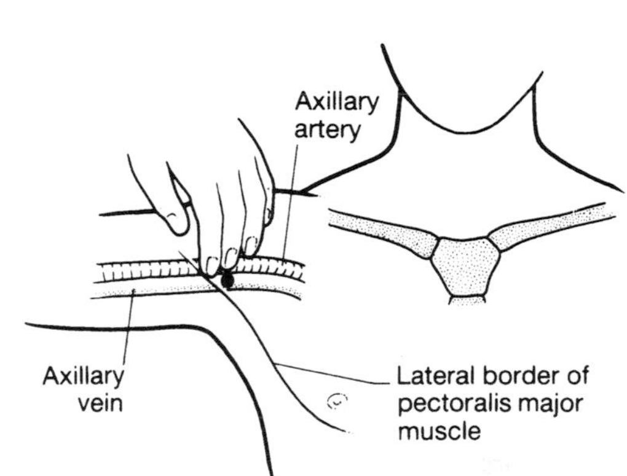

(c)

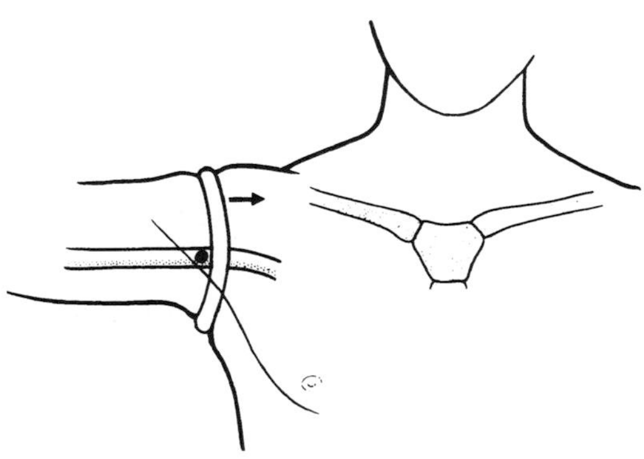

Figure 5.8 Axillary and proximal basilic vein (Ayim, 1977).[22]

AXILLARY VEIN: INFRACLAVICULAR APPROACH

Nickalls (1987),[25] Taylor and Yellowlees (1990)[26]

Patient category

Adults and children.

Advantages and disadvantages

This approach avoids the dangers of trauma to deep structures of the thoracic inlet. There are specific landmarks. Convenience and ease of fixation in the infraclavicular region are further advantages. Since the tip of the needle is always inferior (below) the clavicle, puncture of the pleura is virtually impossible. Furthermore, in the event of inadvertent trauma to a blood vessel, direct pressure is easily applied and surgical exploration is facilitated if this were to become necessary.

Preferred side

No preferred side, but diagrams indicate a right-sided approach.

Position of patient

Place the patient in the supine position and tilt the table 15° head down (Figure 5.9a). Keep the arm straight and move it about 45° away from the patient's side (Figure 5.9b); this manoeuvre straightens out the axillary vein.

Position of operator

Stand on the same side as the puncture site.

Equipment used in original description

Seldinger guide-wire technique (Leader-Cath, Vygon); size 14–16 gauge catheter.

Advice on current equipment

Needle 18 gauge OD, length 60 mm (minimum); guide-wire length 400 mm (minimum); catheter length 200 mm (minimum).

Anatomical landmarks

Mark position A three fingers-breadth (about 5 cm) below the lower border of the coracoid process (Figure 5.9c). In children, the child's own fingers may be used to estimate this landmark.[26] Mark position B where the space between the clavicle and the thorax just becomes palpable: this corresponds to a point immediately below the lower border of the clavicle at the junction of its medial quarter and its lateral three-quarters. Outline the medial border of pectoralis minor by drawing a line starting at the coracoid process and swinging towards the midline, and mark the point at which it crosses the line A–B.

Preparation

Perform the puncture under sterile conditions using local anaesthesia if indicated.

Point of insertion of the needle

The point of insertion is lateral to the medial border of pectoralis minor and on the line A–B (Figure 5.9c).

Initial location of vein with small-gauge needle

Recommended (21 or 22 gauge). If an ordinary needle is too short a similar gauge spinal needle may be used.

Direction of the needle and procedure

Place the point of the needle at the entry site and the syringe on the skin. Elevate the attached syringe about 20° with the needle pointing medially along the line A–B (Figure 5.9c, d). While palpating the axillary artery (ideal, but not always possible) advance the needle slowly, aspirating continuously and aim to enter the vein halfway between the medial border of pectoralis minor and point B. If resistance is met, withdraw the needle and redirect it in an anteroposterior plane parallel to the line A–B. At all times keep the tip of the needle below the lower border of the clavicle to prevent inadvertent puncture of the lung.

After insertion of the catheter a chest X-ray is needed to confirm the position of the catheter tip and to exclude pneumothorax.

Success rate

Nickalls reports a rate of 92% (n = 14);[25] Taylor and Yellowlees 97% (n = 95).[26]

Complications

Nickalls: none in this series but the risk of inadvertent puncture of the axillary artery is noted.[25]
Taylor and Yellowlees: in 92 successful cannulations, the complications were arterial puncture (5 cases) and paraesthesia (2 cases).[26]

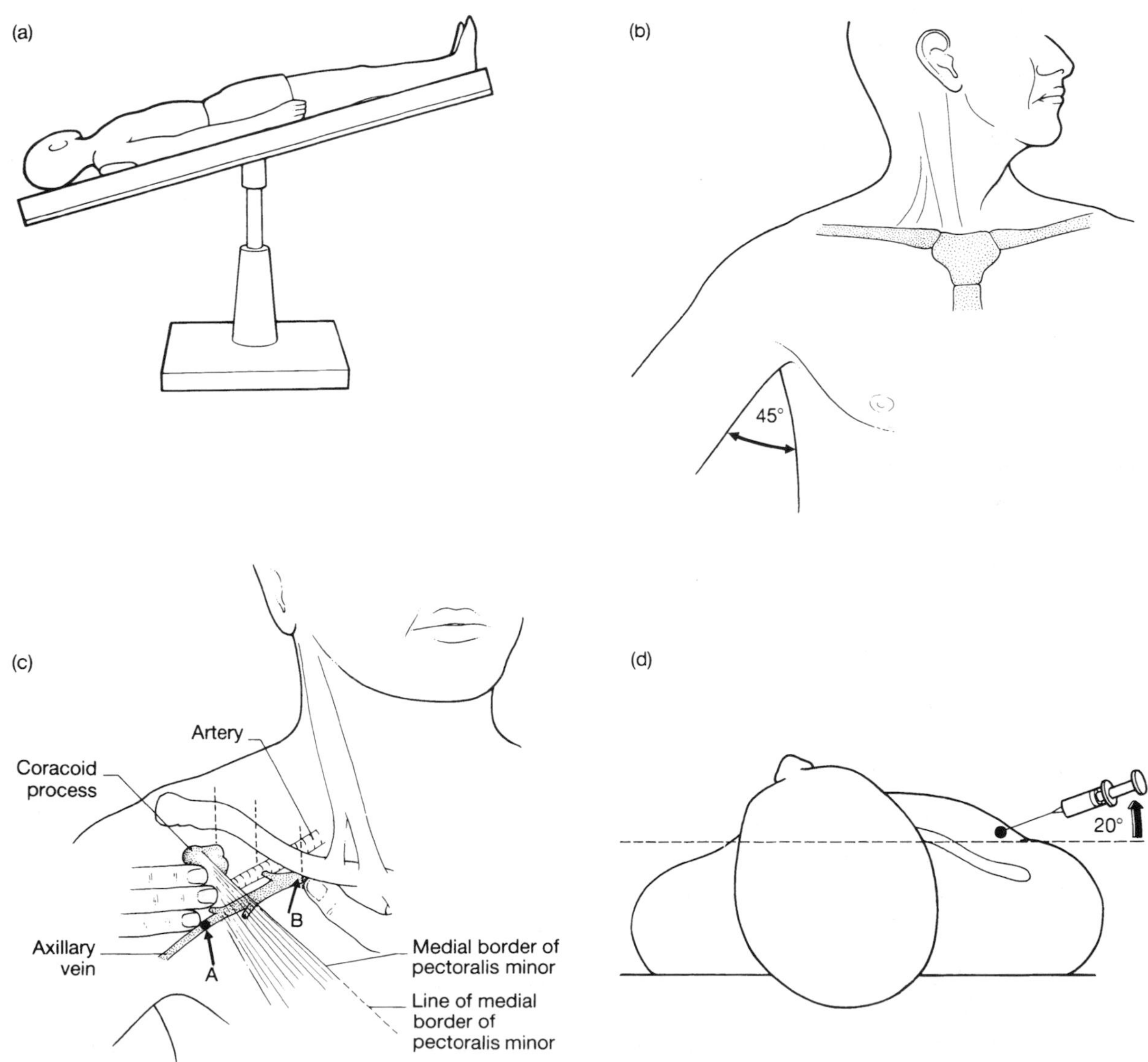

Figure 5.9 Axillary vein: infraclavicular approach (Nickalls, 1987).[25]

ANTECUBITAL FOSSA APPROACH: 'HALFWAY' VENOUS CATHETERS

Linder et al. *(1985)*[30]

Patient category

The original description confines this technique to adults only.

Advantages and disadvantages

Venepuncture into a visible vein is easy and free of the possibility of serious trauma. The dangers of intrathoracic catheters – cardiac arrhythmias and perforation of the vena cava and heart – are avoided. The rate of misplacement of the catheter tip is less than with conventional long catheters although this only applies when insertion is through the basilic vein. Furthermore, radiological confirmation of the catheter tip is usually unnecessary but again, only if the basilic vein has been used.

The main indication for a 'halfway' catheter is for central venous pressure measurement.[45] They are not suitable for long-term parenteral alimentation, central venous blood sampling or for aspiration of air embolus.

Preferred side

Either side may be used.

Position of patient

Establish the patient's height. Place the patient in the supine position with the head in the straight-ahead position. The arm to be used is abducted 90° away from the body and the forearm fully extended (Figure 5.10a).

Position of operator

Stand on the same side as the puncture site.

Equipment used in original description

The Seldinger guide-wire technique was used exclusively to insert soft polyurethane catheters (40 cm long, 1.1 mm inner diameter, 1.7 mm OD).

Advice on current equipment

Introducer cannula 13 gauge or 14 gauge OD, catheter length 600 mm (minimum). Ensure that it is possible to estimate the length of catheter within the vein, e.g. by inspection and measurement of a used or out-of-date catheter of the same type.

Anatomical landmarks

Apply a tourniquet to the upper arm to distend the veins in the antecubital fossa. Identify the basilic

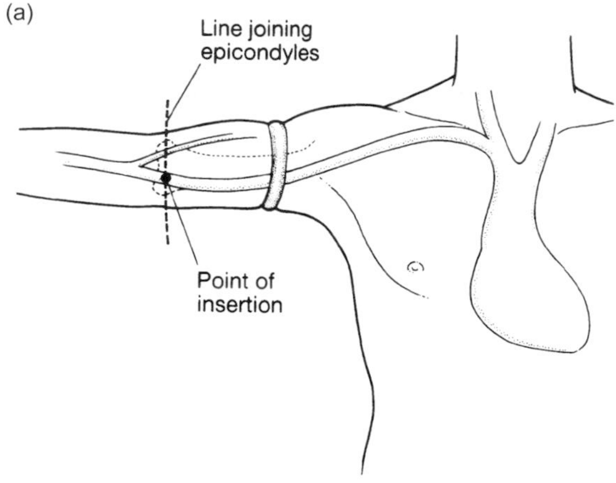

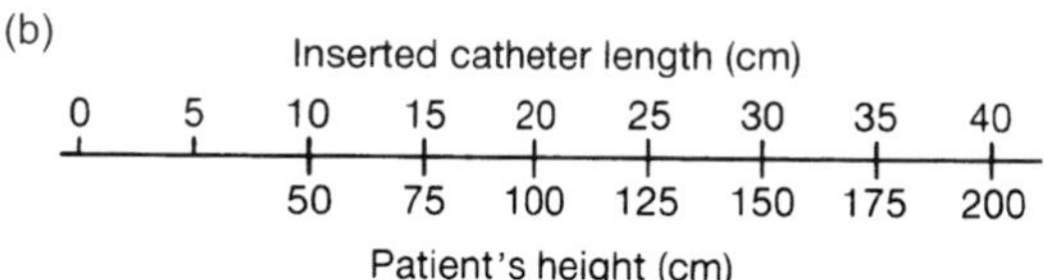

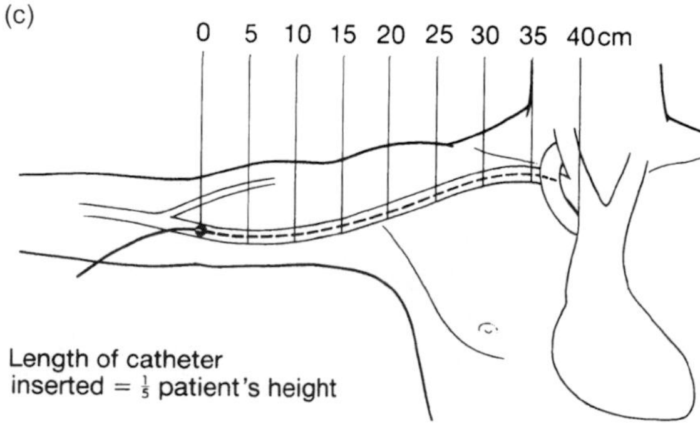

Figure 5.10 Antecubital fossa approach: 'Halfway' venous catheters.[30]

vein (preferable to the cephalic vein). Identify and visualise a line drawn between the epicondyles of the humerus with the arm in the abducted position (Figure 5.10a).

Preparation

Perform the procedure under aseptic conditions using local anaesthesia if indicated.

Precautions and recommendations

Mark off a distance (on the catheter or protective sheath if one is provided) equal to one-fifth of the patient's body height. A useful nomogram is shown in Figure 5.10b.

Point of insertion of the needle

Into the basilic vein where it is crossed by a line joining the two epicondyles.

Procedure

Advance the catheter to the position previously marked on the catheter or sheath (Figure 5.10c). Fix the catheter firmly in this position. If the basilic vein is used, no resistance to advancement is noted and blood can be freely aspirated from the catheter, then no radiological confirmation is necessary. However, if in doubt confirm the position with a chest X-ray.

Success rate

From 113 cases (basilic vein 83, cephalic vein 30) 65% tips were in the proximal axillary vein, 34% in the distal subclavian vein, and 1% in the internal jugular vein on radiological examination.

Complications

Serious: nil. Minor: temporary interruption of intravenous infusion flow with arm movements, 12 cases; partial/total occlusion of flow, 16; leakage of infusate at puncture site, 1; pain along vein during infusion (potassium solution, cytotoxic drug), 2; thrombophlebitis developing in 2–10 days, 5.

ANTECUBITAL FOSSA APPROACH: PATIENT IN THE SITTING POSITION

Bridges et al. *(1979)*[38]

Patient category

Adults. The description of the technique by the original authors did not include its application in children, but this does not necessarily exclude its use in this age group.

Advantages and disadvantages

Because the patient is placed in the sitting position, the catheter is encouraged to bend downwards under the influence of gravity and hence to enter the intrathoracic veins.

Preferred side

Not stated.

Position of patient

Place the patient in the sitting position (45° to 90° above the horizontal). Turn the head towards the side of the puncture. Abduct the arm to be used 30° away from the patient's side (Figure 5.11a).

Position of operator

Stand on the same side as the puncture site (Figure 5.11b).

Equipment used in original description

Catheter through 14 gauge OD needle. Bardic catheters were used after testing a range of catheters for 'softness and tendency to bend'. The catheters were held at an angle of 45° to the horizontal and allowed to bend under their own weight. The angle to which the catheter bent was then taken as a measure of its softness and tendency to bend.

Advice on current equipment

A 14 gauge OD introducing needle or cannula, length 40 mm (minimum); catheter length 600 mm (minimum).

Anatomical landmarks

Apply a tourniquet to the upper arm to distend the veins (Figure 5.11b). Identify a vein on the medial side of the antecubital fossa (basilic or median cubital vein). The vein may be easily palpable even if not visible.

If there is no suitable vein in the antecubital fossa, rotate the arm laterally (an assistant is helpful) and identify a suitable tributary of the basilic vein on the posteromedial surface of the forearm.

Preparation

Perform the procedure under aseptic conditions using local anaesthesia if indicated.

Precautions and recommendations

Estimate the length of catheter needed for its tip to reach:

- the junction of the cephalic and basilic veins
- the junction of the internal jugular and innominate veins
- a satisfactory position in the central veins.

Point of insertion of needle

Insert the needle into the chosen vein (Figure 5.11b).

Procedure

After successful venepuncture, release the tourniquet and insert the catheter until the tip is judged to be in the subclavian vein distal to its junction with the internal jugular vein (indicated by a cross in Figure 5.11c). Withdraw the stylet (if present) 150 mm and advance the catheter slowly 12 mm at a time with intervals of 2 seconds between each 12 mm insertion, until it is judged that the catheter has reached its correct intrathoracic position. Confirm the position of the catheter with a chest X-ray.

Success rate

The success rate was 98% (50 cases).

Complications

Not stated.

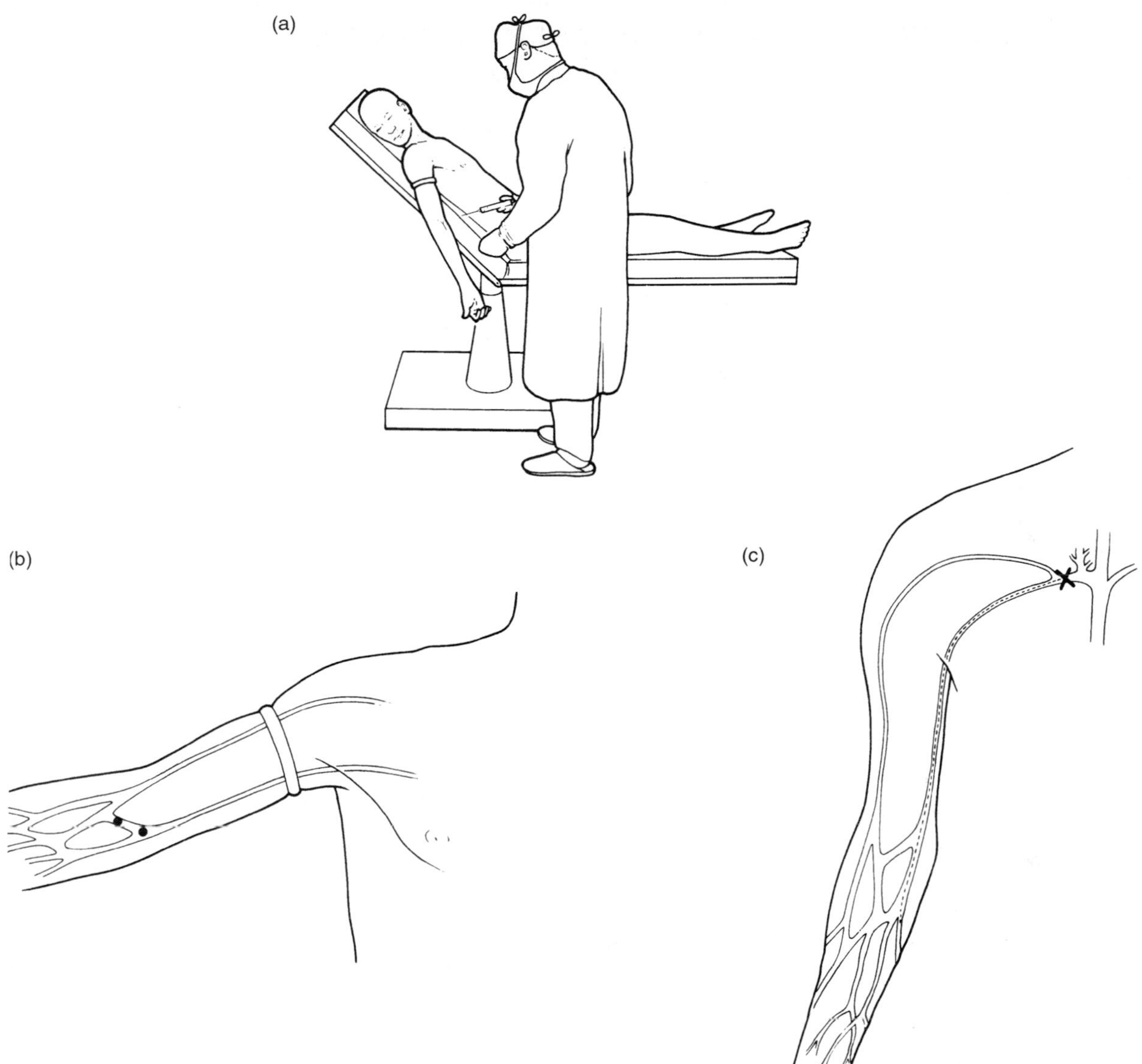

Figure 5.11 Antecubital fossa approach (Bridges *et al*., 1979).[38]

DEEP BRACHIAL VEIN: LOWER THIRD OF UPPER ARM

Saissy et al. *(1985)*[18]

Patient category

The method was described in patients aged 16–70 years.

Advantages and disadvantages

The technique is indicated when superficial veins are unuseable and deep neck venepuncture is dangerous or impossible. Only a moderate success rate together with the risk of injury to the brachial artery are the main disadvantages.

Preferred side

Either side may be used.

Position of patient

Place the patient in the supine position. Turn the head to the same side as the puncture side. Abduct the arm to be used 45° from the trunk and rotate it externally.

Position of operator

Same side as the puncture site.

Equipment used in original description

Introducer needle 15 gauge; 17 gauge polyethylene catheter of 500 mm length.

Advice on current equipment

A Seldinger technique in conjunction with a vein dilator is recommended to minimise potential injury to the artery. Initial needling of vein should be carried out with a small (21–22 gauge) needle.

Anatomical landmarks

Palpate the brachial artery 1 cm above the skin crease in the antecubital fossa. Apply a tourniquet to the upper arm.

Preparation

Perform the procedure under aseptic conditions using local anaesthesia if appropriate.

Point of insertion of the needle

The needle is inserted to the medial side of the palpated brachial artery.

Procedure

Insert the introducer needle to which a 10 ml syringe is attached. Elevate the syringe 45° away from the skin surface. While maintaining a negative pressure on the syringe, advance the needle to the medial side of the brachial artery. A 'flashback' of venous blood confirms successful venepuncture. Remove the syringe and insert the catheter. Take a chest X-ray to confirm the position of the catheter tip.

Success rate

Successful venepuncture 88% (50 attempts); successful catheterisation 72%; successful central venous catheterisation 60%.

Complications

Inadvertent puncture of the brachial artery occurred in 6 cases (12%) with no serious consequence.

Table 5.1 Catheterisation of the arm veins – results and complications.

Author and year	Classification of technique (vein used)	Success rate (%)	No. cases (*n*)	Complications	No. complications (*n* (%))	Personnel	Comments
Holt (1967)[1]	Basilic	71	56	Local	11 (8.2)	Authors	Duration of catheterisation 3 days (mean), 0–9 days (range)
	Cephalic	44	78	Phlebitis, cellulitis of upper arm	2 (1–5)		
Gilday and Downs (1969)[2]	Mainly basic	66·5	200	Not stated			Cephalic vein found to be unsatisfactory
Deitel and McIntyre (1971)[3]	Basilic	75·3	130	Not stated			Duration of catheterisation up to 25 days
	Cephalic	14	7				
Langston (1971)[4]	Basilic (207)	62	300	Not stated		Various residents	
	Cephalic (93)	(75.3 if catheter in right atrium or right ventricle withdrawn)					
Johnston and Clark (1972)[5]	Basilic and cephalic	64	73	Thrombophelbitis at puncture site	2 (2.7)	One operator	Arm abducted 90° Strict aseptic technique
		(77.5 if catheters in right atrium or right ventricle withdrawn)					
Ng and Rosen (1973)[6]	Basilic (I-Catheters and Drum	52.8	106	Not stated		Mainly authors but some	
	Cartridge Catheters)	77.7	94			residents	supervised
Webre and Arens (1973)[7]	Basilic	65	71	Not stated			Most of the unsatisfactory catheters were in the internal jugular vein
Lumely and Russell	Cephalic	45	29				
(1975)[9]	Basilic	75.6	82	Not stated		Various	
Sorensen and	Cephalic	73.9	23				
Sonne-Holm (1975)[8]	Basilic (left)	69	55	None intially			
				Later: swelling of arm	5 (9.1)		
				Inflammation at site of insertion	3 (5.4)		
				Speticaemia	1 (1.8)		
Burgess *et al.* (1977)[34]	Basilic (head in mid position,	58–80	50	Not stated			
	turned towards arm of insertion)		50				

Author and year	Classification of technique (vein used)	Success rate (%)	No. cases (*n*)	Complications	No. complications (n (%))	Personnel	Comments
Bridges *et al.* (1979)[38]	Basilic	72·5	51	Not stated		Authors	
	Cephalic	76	25				
	Basilic vein, sitting position, special technique, 'soft' catheter	98	50				
Smith *et al.* (1984)[41]	Basilic	70					
	Cephalic	30		Unable to cannulate	4 (5)		
	J-tipped guide-wire used	91	77	Unable to advance wire	3 (3.8)		
				Malposition but intrathoracic	3 (3.8)		
				Premature ventricular beat	3 (3.8)		
Spracklen *et al.* (1976)[21]	Proximal basilic or axillary vein	90	50	Transient pain or paraesthesiae during venepuntcture	10 (20)		Duration of catheterisation not stated
				No cases of local infection or thrombophlebitis			
Ayim (1977)[22]	Axillary vein	95.9	73 (4–80 years)	? Venous thrombosis	1 (1.4)		Duration of catheterisation 7·8 days (mean)
	Proximal basilic	93.1	54 (1–75 years)	Venous haematoma	3 (5.5)		Duration of catheterisation 4·3 days (mean)
				?Thrombosis	1 (1.8)		
Gouin *et al.* (1985)[23]	Axillary vein	87	323	Malposition	22 (9)		
Martin *et al.* (1986)[24]	Axillary vein	87.5	63	Arterial puncture (no sequelae)	(11)		
				Thrombosis of axillary and subclavian veins. Used for PA catheters in all patients	1 (1.8)		
Nickalls (1987)[25]	Axillary vein	92	14				
Taylor and Yellowlees (1990)[26]	Axillary vein	97.8	102	Pneumothorax	1 (1.2)	Author only	45 referred by other operators who had failed to cannulate through other routes
				Malposition	1 (1.2)		
				Could not thread catheter	1 (1.2)		
				Overall	0.56%		

KEY POINTS

- Easiest and safest central venous access.
- Antecubital fossa veins are the first choice.
- Other approaches described require more skill and expertise.

References

1. Holt HM. Central venous pressure via peripheral veins. Anesthesiology 1967; **28**:1093.
2. Gilday DL, Downs AR. The value of chest radiography in the localization of central venous pressure catheters. Canadian Medical Association Journal 1969; **101**:363.
3. Deitel M, McIntyre JA. Radiographic confirmation of site of central venous pressure catheters. Canadian Journal of Surgery 1971; **14**:42.
4. Langston CS. The aberrant central venous catheter and its complications. Radiology 1971; **100**:55.
5. Johnston AOB, Clark RG. Malpositioning of central venous catheters. Lancet 1972; **ii**:1395.
6. Ng WS, Rosen M. Positioning central venous catheters through the basilic vein. A comparison of catheters. British Journal of Anaesthesia 1973; **45**:1211.
7. Webre DR, Arens, JF. Use of cephalic and basilic veins for introduction of central venous catheters. Anesthesiology 1973; **38**:389.
8. Sorensen, TIA and Sonne-Holm, S. Central venous catheterization through the basilic vein or by infraclavicular puncture. Acta Chirurgica Scandinavica 1975; **141**:323.
9. Lumley J, Russell, WJ. Insertion of central venous catheters through arm veins. Anaesthesia and Intensive Care 1975; **3**:101.
10. Christensen KH, Nerstrom B, Baden H. Complications of percutaneous catheterization of the subclavian vein in 129 cases. Acta Chirurgica Scandinavica 1967; **133**:615.
11. Colvin MP, Blogg CE, Savege TM, Jarvis JD, Strunin L. A safe long term infusion technique? Lancet 1972; **2**:317.
12. Todd J. Peripherally inserted central catheters. Professional Nurse 1998; **5**:297.
13. Goodwin ML, Carlson I. The peripherally inserted central catheter: a retrospective look at three years of insertions. Journal of Intravenous Nursing 1993; **16**:92–103.
14. Aston V, Maugham T. Techniques in oncology: peripherally inserted central catheters (PICC Lines). CME Oncology 1998; **1**:19.
15. Kearns PJ, Coleman S, Wehner JH. Complications of long arm-catheters: a randomized trial of central vs peripheral tip location. Journal of Parenteral and Enteral Nutrition 1996; **20**:20.
16. Mauro MA, Jaques PF. Radiologic placement of long-term central catheters: a review. Journal of Vascular and Interventional Radiology 1993; **4**:127.
17. Roseman JM. Deep, percutaneous antecubital venipuncture: an alternative to surgical cutdown. American Journal of Surgery 1983; **146**:285.
18. Saissy JM, Driss-Kamili N, Berdouz S, Atmani M, Dimou M. Percutaneous catheterization of the deep brachial vein. Annales Francais d'Anesthesie et de Reanimation 1985; **4**:316.
19. Gilette JF, Susini J. Deep brachial vein catheterization for total parenteral nutrition – an alternate approach: review of 154 cases. Journal of Parenteral and Enteral Nutrition 1984; **8**:49.
20. Koing-Bo K, Gorfine S, Berman M, *et al.* Percutaneous catheterization of the brachial vein for central venous access. Surgery, Gynecology and Obstetrics 1984; **159**:287.
21. Spracklen FHN, Niesche F, Lord PW, Beterman EMM. Percutaneous catheterisation of the axillary vein. Cardiovascular Research 1967; **1**:297.
22. Ayim EN. Percutaneous catheterisation of the axillary vein and proximal basilic vein. Anaesthesia 1977; **32**:753.
23. Gouin F, Martin C, Saux P. Central venous and pulmonary artery catheterizations via the axillary vein. Acta Anaesthesiologica Scandinavica 1985; (suppl.)**81**:27.
24. Martin C, Auffray JP, Albanese J, *et al.* Pulmonary artery catheterization via the axillary vein. Annales Francais d'Anesthesie et de Reanimation 1986; **5**:64.
25. Nickalls, RWD. A new percutaneous infraclavicular approach to the axillary vein. Anaesthesia 1987; **42**:151.
26. Taylor BL, Yellowlees I. Central venous cannulation using the infraclavicular axillary vein. Anesthesiology 1990; **72**:55.
27. Smith MB, Till CWB. The axillary vein as an alternative. Anaesthesia 1994; **49**:741.
28. Gustavsson B, Linder LE, Hultman E, Curelaru I. 'Half-Way' venous catheters. 1. Theoretical premises and aims. Acta Anaesthesiologica Scandinavica 1985; (suppl.)**81**:30.
29. Curelaru I, Gustavsson B, Wojciechowski J, *et al.* 'Half-Way' venous catheters. 2. Anatomoradiological basis. Acta Anaesthesiologica Scandinavica 1985; (suppl.)**81**:32.
30. Linder LE, Wojciechowski J, Zachrisson BF, *et al.* 'Half-Way' venous catheters. 4. Clinical experience and thrombogenicity. Acta Anaesthesiologica Scandinavica 1985; (suppl.)**81**:40.
31. Zohman LR, Williams MH. Percutaneous right heart catheterization using polyethylene tubing. American Journal of Cardiology 1959; **4**:373.
32. Jaikaran SMN, Sagay E. Normal central venous pressure. British Journal of Surgery 1968; **55**:609.
33. Kellner GA, Smart JF. Percutaneous placement of catheters to monitor 'central venous pressure'. Anesthesiology 1972; **36**:515.
34. Burgess GE, Marino RJ, Peuler MJ. Effect of head position in the location of venous catheter inserted via basilic veins. Anesthesiology 1977; **46**:212.
35. Woods DG, Lumley J, Russell WJ, Jacks RD. The position of central venous catheters inserted through arm veins: a preliminary report. Anaesthesia and Intensive Care 1974; **2**:43.
36. Ragasa J, Shah N, Watson R, Bedford MD. Where antecubital CVP catheters go: a study under fluoroscopic control. Anesthesiology 1988; (suppl. 3A),**69**:A231.

37. Kuramoto T, Sakabe T. Comparison of success in jugular versus basilic vein technics for central venous pressure catheter positioning. Anesthesia and Analgesia: Current Researches 1975; **54**:696.
38. Bridges BB, Carden E, Takacs FA. Introduction of central venous pressure catheters through arm veins with a high success rate. Canadian Anaesthetists Society Journal 1979; **26**:128.
39. Wright PJ, Walker DAJ. Central venous cannulation in neurosurgical patients. Intensive Therapy and Clinical Monitoring 1989; **82**:84.
40. Blitt CD, Wright WA, Petty WC, Webster TA. Central venous catheterisation via the external jugular vein. A technique employing the J-wire. Journal of the American Medical Association 1974; **229**:817.
41. Smith SL, Albin MS, Ritter RD, Bunegin L. CVP catheter placement from the antecubital veins using a J-wire catheter guide. Anesthesiology 1984; **60**:238.
42. Colley PS, Artru AA. ECG-guided placement of Sorensen CVP catheters via arm veins. Anesthesia and Analgesia 1984; **63**:953.
43. Editorial. Central venous catheterisation. Lancet 1986; **2**:669.
44. Kalso E, Rosenberg PH, Vuorialho M, Pietila K. How much do arm movements displace cubital venous catheters? Acta Anaesthesiologica Scandinavica 1982; **26**:354.
45. Ricksten SE, Medegard A, Curelaru I, *et al.* Estimation of central venous pressure by measurement of proximal axillary venous pressure using a 'half-way' catheter. Acta Anaesthesiologica Scandinavica 1986; (suppl.)**30**:13.

6 • The Subclavian Vein

SHANG NG

Introduction

Aubaniac first described the technique of infraclavicular subclavian venepuncture in 1952. He pointed out that the vein was large and was prevented from collapsing by the surrounding tissue. Wilson and his colleagues,[2] in 1962, used the infraclavicular route to introduce a catheter into the superior vena cava. Since the catheterisation of the subclavian vein has been widely used for a large range of diagnostic and therapeutic procedures. In addition to its widespread use in central venous pressure monitoring, the technique has been used in cardiac pacing[3,4] and pulmonary artery angiography.[5] Equally the technique has gained a recognised and important place in rapid fluid and blood replacement therapy[2,6] and especially in long-term parenteral nutrition.[7] Potent cardiovascular drugs and agents that are irritant to veins, such as those used in chemotherapy, are now invariably administered through central veins and the subclavian route is often favoured especially when longer-term administration is envisaged.

Yoffa[8] introduced the technique of supraclavicular subclavian venepuncture for central venous catheterisation and parenteral nutrition in 1965. This approach has never attained anything like the popularity of the infraclavicular technique, perhaps it is because it is thought to be more dangerous. When confronted with the need to catheterise in the neck, most operators would perceive the internal jugular vein to be easier and safer. However, the supraclavicular approach should not be overlooked. In one study a high proportion of the successful supraclavicular procedures were performed on patients referred after failure of attempts to catheterise through the infraclavicular subclavian or internal jugular routes.[9]

Subsequently, several modifications to both infraclavicular and supraclavicular techniques as originally described have been put forward to improve the success rate and to reduce the risks. The subclavian vein therefore established itself as a route applicable when peripheral veins are either unavailable or unsuitable. The subclavian route was especially indicated in shock conditions because of the vein's large diameter and because it remained patent even in such poor haemodynamic states. Many occasional users of the subclavian technique have probably been encouraged to use this method because of the relatively low rate of complications reported by authors who have become skilled in the technique. Not surprisingly, when subclavian cannulation is carried out by a wide range of physicians with varied levels of experience a much higher incidence of complications is manifest. Pneumothorax reached an incidence of 12.4% in one such group.[10] The popularity of the subclavian route in adults was maintained for many years in spite of numerous reports of a significant incidence of serious complications and death (see Tables 6.1, 6.2 and 6.3). The same popularity has never been achieved for subclavian vein catheterisation in infants and small children. Although some workers have used the infraclavicular subclavian approach with good success and few complications, it is generally accepted that with infants and small children there is a much greater potential for serious harm, so the newcomer to the technique should carry out the procedure in these patients only under the strictest supervision by an experienced operator.[7,11,12] The subclavian route has been overtaken in popularity by the internal jugular approach because it has been perceived as a safer method and no more technically demanding than subclavian vein catheterisation. Indeed, in the anaesthetic field most other techniques appear to have been abandoned in favour of the internal jugular approach. However, in intensive care and other critical care areas the subclavian vein remains the route for many of the longer-term uses of central lines, notably for prolonged parenteral nutrition.

Anatomy

The subclavian vein lies in the lower part of the supraclavicular triangle (Figure 6.1). This triangle is bounded medially by the posterior border of the sternomastoid muscle, caudally by the middle third of the clavicle, and laterally by the anterior border of the trapezius muscle.

The subclavian vein is the continuation of the axillary vein and begins at the lower border of the first rib. Initially the vein arches upwards across the first rib and then inclines medially, downwards, and slightly forwards across the insertion of the scalenus anterior muscle in the first rib to enter the thorax, where it unites with the internal jugular vein behind the sternoclavicular joint. From here, as the innominate vein, it turns towards the mediastinum and unites with its counterpart from the other side to form the superior vena cava.

Anteriorly, the vein is separated from the skin throughout its entire course by the clavicle. It attains its highest point just medial to the midpoint of the clavicle, where it rises to the upper border of the bone. The lateral portion of the vein lies anterior to and below the subclavian artery as both these structures cross the upper surface of the first rib. Medially the fibres of the scalenus anterior muscle separate the vein in front from the artery behind. Behind the artery is the cervical pleura. The cervical pleura rises above the sternal end of the clavicle. The subclavian vein crosses in front of the phrenic nerve. The thoracic duct arches over the apex of the pleura on the left side to enter the

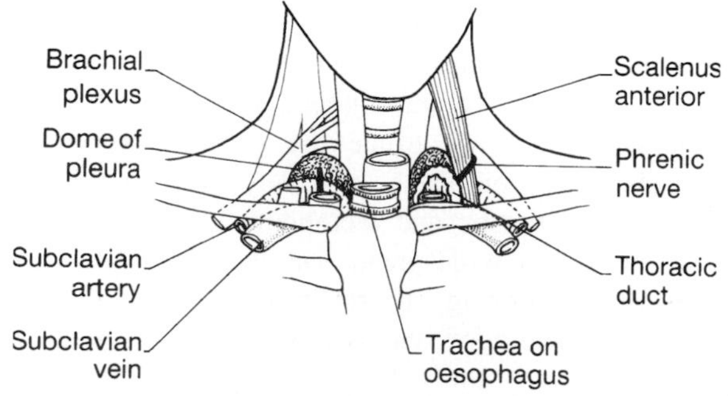

Figure 6.1 Anatomy of the subclavian vein.

angle made by the junction of the internal jugular and subclavian veins.

Choice of Technique

No clear choice between supraclavicular and infraclavicular approaches (Figure 6.2) can be recommended from a comparison of their success and complication rates (Tables 6.1 and 6.2). The few trials that have been undertaken show no difference in success and complication rates.[20] However, several reports suggest that the supraclavicular approach leads to a much higher success rate in satisfactory positioning of the catheter tip.[20,21] This is particularly apparent when central venous catheterisation is being performed during the rather special circumstances of cardiopulmonary resuscitation.[22] Nevertheless, the infraclavicular approach is much more popular judging by the far greater volume of reports in the literature; this may, however, be due to its earlier introduction into medical practice. For central venous catheterisation in infants and small children, only the infraclavicular approach (approach 3 in Figure 6.2) has been used[2,7,11,12,23] and all authors urge great caution on the operator.

Consideration of some practical points will assist in making a choice. With either approach, accurate identification of the landmarks may be difficult in obese patients and the choice may then be influenced by which landmarks can be determined.

The supraclavicular approach offers some practical advantages. The distance from skin to vein is shorter and the needle has only to pierce skin and fascia;[8] the catheter is also more likely to reach a satisfactory central position.[16,22] During operations the supraclavicular area is usually accessible to the anaesthetist at the head of the patient. Many would advocate using the internal jugular vein under these circumstances. Nevertheless, in some cases the subclavian vein may be chosen. Certainly, there is less interruption of cardiopulmonary resuscitation manoeuvres when the supraclavicular approach to cannulating the subclavian vein is chosen, because the operator stands at the head of the patient away from those carrying out airway management and chest compression.[22] However, because of the hollow contour of the supraclavicular

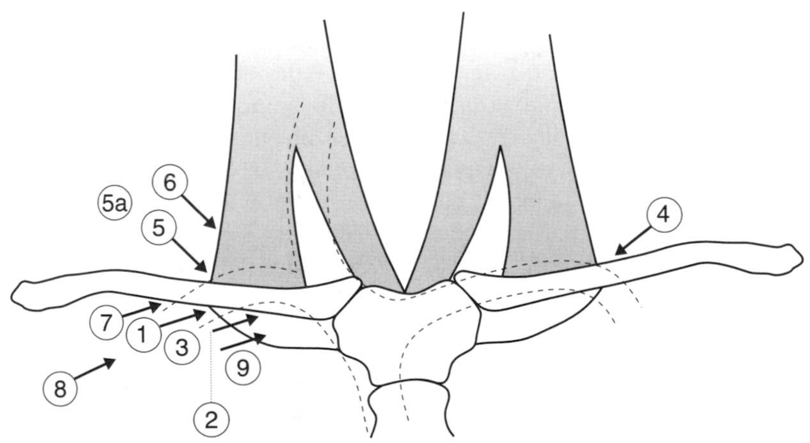

Figure 6.2 Approach to the catheterisation of the subclavian vein: 1, Aubaniac (1952);[1] Wilson *et al.* (1962);[2] 2, Mogil et al. (1967);[13] 3, Morgan and Harkins (1972);[11] 4, Yoffa (1965);[8] 5, James and Myers (1973);[14] 5A, Brahos (1977);[15] 6, Haapaniemi and Slatis (1962);[16] 7, Tofield (1969);[17] 8, Untracht (1988);[18] 9, Tripathi and Tripathi (1996);[19] Adults: methods 1–9. Infants: method 3. Methods preferred by authors: Aubaniac (1952);[1] Wilson ***et al***. (1962);[2] for adults. Although the only approach described by the authors as performed on children that of Morgan and Harkins (1972);[11] this does not necessarily imply that the others are unsuitable

fossa, securely fixing the catheter and surgical dressing may be difficult. Furthermore, it is not easy to keep the site dry and free from infection, since perspiration tends to collect in the hollow.

With the infraclavicular approach, a longer needle may be necessary since it has to pass through a muscle layer as well as skin and fascia before reaching the vein. However, the method is preferable for long-term catheterisation because the catheter and surgical dressing can be more easily and securely fixed. There is also less chance of infection.

There are differences in technique with both approaches. Accounts of the supraclavicular route usually describe the same point for insertion of the needle, but the landmarks used to guide the direction of the needle differ. Haapaniemi and Slatis[16] advocate a point of insertion somewhat higher up in the neck so that the venepuncture is made into the junction of the internal jugular and subclavian veins. They claim that the catheter passes more easily, but their results are no different from those of other techniques (see Table 6.2).

Six techniques have been described for the infraclavicular approach. They differ on the point of insertion of the needle in relation to the midpoint of the clavicle. Most authors use the midpoint or a position slightly lateral to this. A much more lateral point of insertion was advocated by Tofield[17] to reduce the risk of producing a pneumothorax, but no results were given. A modification to the infraclavicular route[18] recommends a point of insertion more laterally and using the palpable axillary artery as a definite and reliable landmark. The method appears to warrant more study. Other authors[23–25] claim that a more medial point (at the junction of the medial and middle thirds of the clavicle) is safer in avoiding trauma to the subclavian artery, brachial plexus and pleura. The results again do not appear to be markedly different (see Table 6.1). There are many anatomical differences between left- and right-sided approaches to the central veins through the subclavian vein but the choice of which side to use remains uncertain since success rates and complication rates are not related to the side of puncture in most reported series. Most authors recommend the right side whether through a supraclavicular or infraclavicular approach as this gives a more direct route to the superior vena cava, avoids trauma to the thoracic duct and facilitates the procedure for a right-handed operator.

Some authors have found no difference in failure and complication rates when left- and right-sided infraclavicular catheterisations were compared[26] but others[27–29] have shown a significantly higher rate of misplacement of the catheter tip in right-sided catheterisations – 15% compared with 2% in one report.[30] Catheter tips which were considered unsatisfactory lay in the ipsilateral internal jugular vein and the innominate vein (right-sided) or contralateral subclavian vein. Much the same findings were reported in a study of over 13 000 cannulations, of which 98% were through the infraclavicular route.[31]

Retracting the shoulders and turning the head away from the side of puncture are often recommended to improve the rates of successful cannulation but such manoeuvres are probably inconsequential.[29] Indeed, distortion of the anatomy may lead to more difficult catheterisation.[26]

Method preferred by authors

We favour the infraclavicular approach to the subclavian vein as described by Aubaniac[1] and Wilson *et al.*[2] (see below). The technique for infants, described later by Morgan and Harkins,[11] is essentially the same. The infraclavicular technique employs more definite landmarks and has been safer in our hands. Subclavian vein catheters are popular for long-term use and catheters inserted into the infraclavicular site are more readily kept free from infection than those inserted into the supraclavicular fossa.

Locating the Vein with an Ultrasound Blood Flow Detector

The position of the subclavian vein as it passes below the clavicle can be detected with an ultrasound flow probe such as the Sonicaid (Sonicaid Ltd, Bognor Regis, UK).[32] A characteristic venous hum is heard, which is accentuated when the arm on the same side is firmly squeezed. The venous hum ceases abruptly when a sudden Valsalva effect is produced (a cooperative patient is instructed to breathe out sharply against a closed glottis; in a patient connected to a breathing circuit the inspiratory phase is briefly held). The position of the subclavian artery is given by detecting its pulsatile flow sounds.

An ultrasound probe is easy to use and can be recommended as a preliminary step when cannulating the subclavian vein by any approach, especially in obese and heavily built patients. Its use does not guarantee success or eliminate complications, although it is likely to increase the former and diminish the latter.

Modern, sophisticated real-time ultrasound technology can make all forms of deep vein catheterisation more successful and safer. High-resolution imaging enables accurate delineation of all the anatomical structures together with visualisation of the needle and catheter. The technique is not appropriate to all clinical situations but is particularly suited for training the inexperienced and in catheterisation where the anatomy is abnormal or distorted.[33–35]

METHODS

INFRACLAVICULAR APPROACH

Aubaniac (1952)[1], *Wilson* et al. *(1962)*[2]

Patient category

Adults and children.

Preferred side

Not stated. Most other authors using this technique prefer the right side.

Position of patient

Place the table in a 25° head-down position. Place the patient in the supine position with both arms at the side. Turn the head away from the side of the puncture. Position a pillow under the chest to thrust up the clavicular area above the shoulders (Figure 6.3a).

Position of operator

Stand on the same side as the puncture site (Figure 6.3b).

Equipment used in original description

Adults: 14 gauge outside diameter (OD) introducing needle; catheter-through-needle.
Infants: 17 gauge OD introducing needle; catheter-through-needle; catheter length 200 mm.

Advice on current equipment

Adults: guide-wire technique strongly recommended using an 18 gauge or 16 gauge introducer needle. Catheter-through-cannula, 14 gauge or 16 gauge OD needle or introducer, length 60 mm (minimum). Catheter length 200 mm (minimum). Long cannula on long needle, length 130 mm (minimum).
Neonates: 20 gauge OD needle or introducer, length 30 mm (minimum). Catheter length 80 mm (minimum). Long cannula on long needle, length 40 mm (minimum).

Anatomical landmarks

Anatomical landmarks are the midclavicular point; the lower border of the clavicle; and the triangle formed by the sternal and clavicular heads of the sternomastoid muscle with the upper border of the clavicle (Figure 6.3c).

Preparation

Perform the puncture under sterile conditions using local anaesthesia if indicated.

Precautions and recommendations

Ensure that the syringe can be removed easily from the needle.

Point of insertion of needle

The point of insertion lies 1 cm below the midpoint of the lower border of the clavicle in adults, and immediately below the midpoint of the lower border of the clavicle in neonates (Figure 6.3c).

Direction of the needle and procedure

Place the point of the needle at the entry site on the skin and point the needle and syringe towards the head (A in Figure 6.3d). Then swing the syringe laterally so that the needle points medially towards the small triangle formed by the sternal and clavicular attachments of the sternomastoid muscle and the upper border of the clavicle (A to B). If this landmark is not clearly defined, point the needle towards the suprasternal notch, keeping a fingertip in the notch to act as a target. Advance the needle posterior to the clavicle keeping close to its posterior aspect, maintaining the needle and syringe parallel to the coronal plane (Figure 6.3e). Maintain a slight negative pressure in the syringe as the needle is advanced until the vein is entered. Introduce the catheter.

Take a chest X-ray to confirm the position of the catheter tip and to exclude pneumothorax.

Success rate

Rate not stated in a total of 250 catheterisations.

Complications

The authors stated that there were no complications in the 250 cases, but that a 'number of pneumothoraces' occurred in subsequent cases performed by residents.

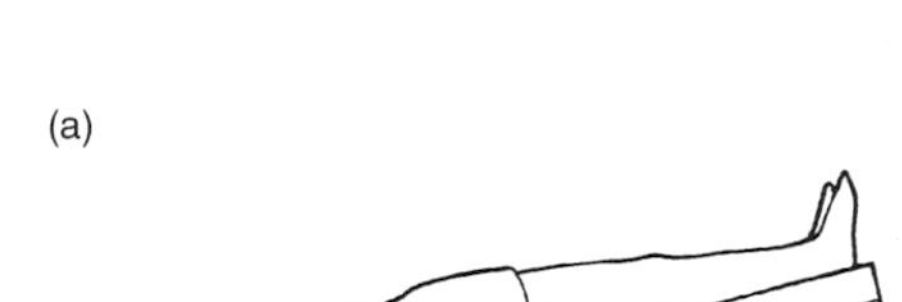

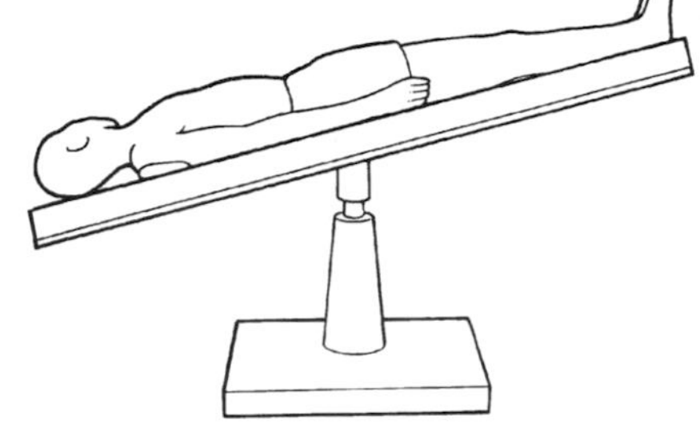

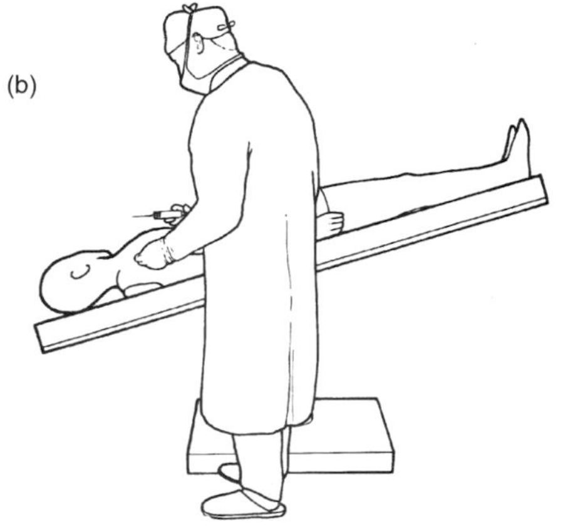

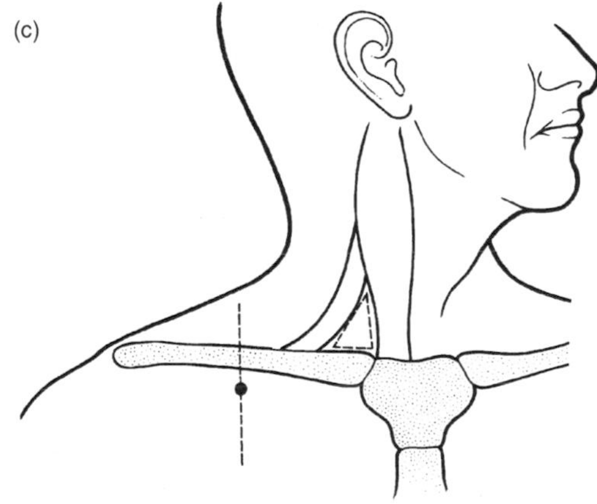

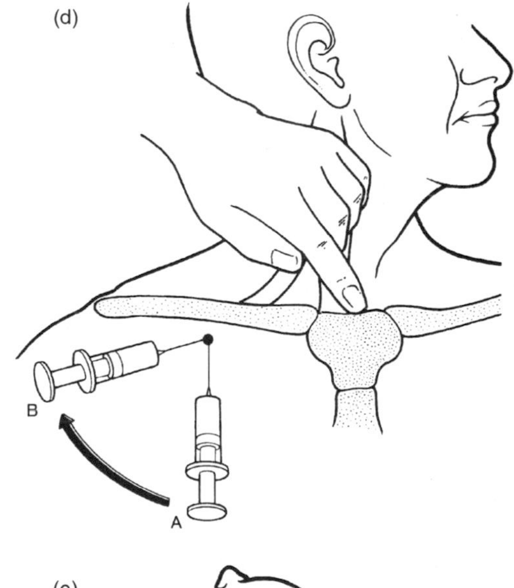

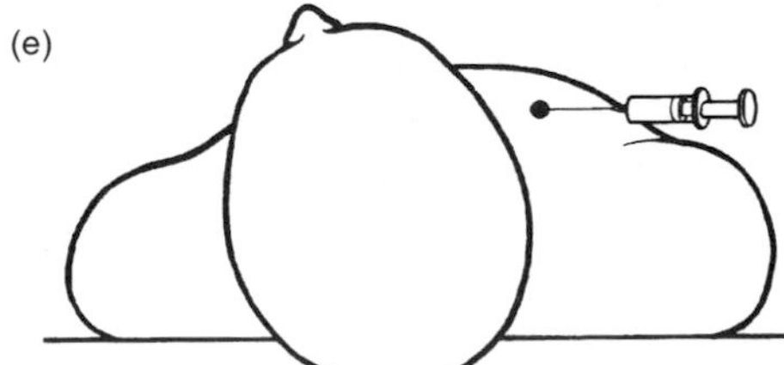

Figure 6.3 Infraclavicular approach: Aubaniac (1952),[1] Wilson *et al.* (1962).[2]

INFRACLAVICULAR APPROACH

Morgan and Harkins (1972)[11]

Patient category

Adults and neonates. This series included neonates.

Preferred side

The left side is preferred. The right side may, nevertheless, be used.

Position of patient

Place the table in a 25° head-down position. Place the patient supine with arms at the sides. Turn the head away from the side of puncture. A rolled towel placed beneath the vertebral column thrusts the clavicular area upwards and opens up the small space between the clavicle and first rib (Figure 6.4a).

Position of operator

Stand on the side of the puncture site (Figure 6.4b).

Equipment used in original description

Neonates: Catheter through 17 gauge OD needle.
Older infants: catheter through 14 gauge OD needle.

Advice on current equipment

Neonates: 20 gauge OD needle or introducer, length 30 mm (minimum); catheter length 80 mm (minimum). Guide-wire technique strongly recommended.
Older infants: larger size equipment may be appropriate.

Anatomical landmarks

Landmarks are the midpoint of inferior border of clavicle and the suprasternal notch – alternatively the small triangle formed by the sternal and clavicular heads of the sternomastoid muscle (Figure 6.4c).

Preparation

Perform the puncture under sterile conditions using local anaesthesia if indicated.

Precautions and recommendations

An operator unfamiliar with this technique and proposing to use it in infants should be strictly supervised by an experienced clinician. The technique should be performed in an operating room environment. Immobilise infants and take measures to prevent excessive heat loss (for instance, use an overhead radiant heater).

Point of insertion of needle

The needle is inserted just below the midpoint of the clavicle (Figure 6.4c).

Direction of the needle and procedure

Place the point of the needle at the entry site on the skin and point the needle cephalad (A in Figure 6.4d). Then swing the needle and syringe laterally so that the needle points towards the tip of a finger of the free hand pressed firmly into the suprasternal notch (A to B).

Advance the syringe behind the clavicle keeping the syringe and needle parallel to the coronal plane (Figure 6.4e). Maintain a slight negative pressure in the syringe while advancing the needle.

If no 'flashback' is obtained, withdraw the needle slowly to the subcutaneous tissue before attempting venepuncture using a slightly different direction. As the syringe is withdrawn maintain the negative pressure, since the needle tip may enter the lumen of the vein during withdrawal. After inserting the catheter take a chest X-ray to confirm its position and to exclude a pneumothorax.

Success rate

'Almost invariably successful' in over 400 infants and older children. Operators were experienced or closely supervised.

Complications

One hundred consecutive catheterisations were analysed: 74 were performed in patients less than

12 months of age. Of these, 37% were performed in infants less than 6 weeks old, including 15 premature babies weighing less than 1.5 kg. No complications occurred in the younger infants. In the older infants there were two instances of arterial puncture with local bleeding and one case each of the catheter entering the pericardial cavity and the pleural cavity. Both the latter cases were detected radiologically before the infusion was started and in both the catheter was withdrawn immediately and produced no clinical problem.

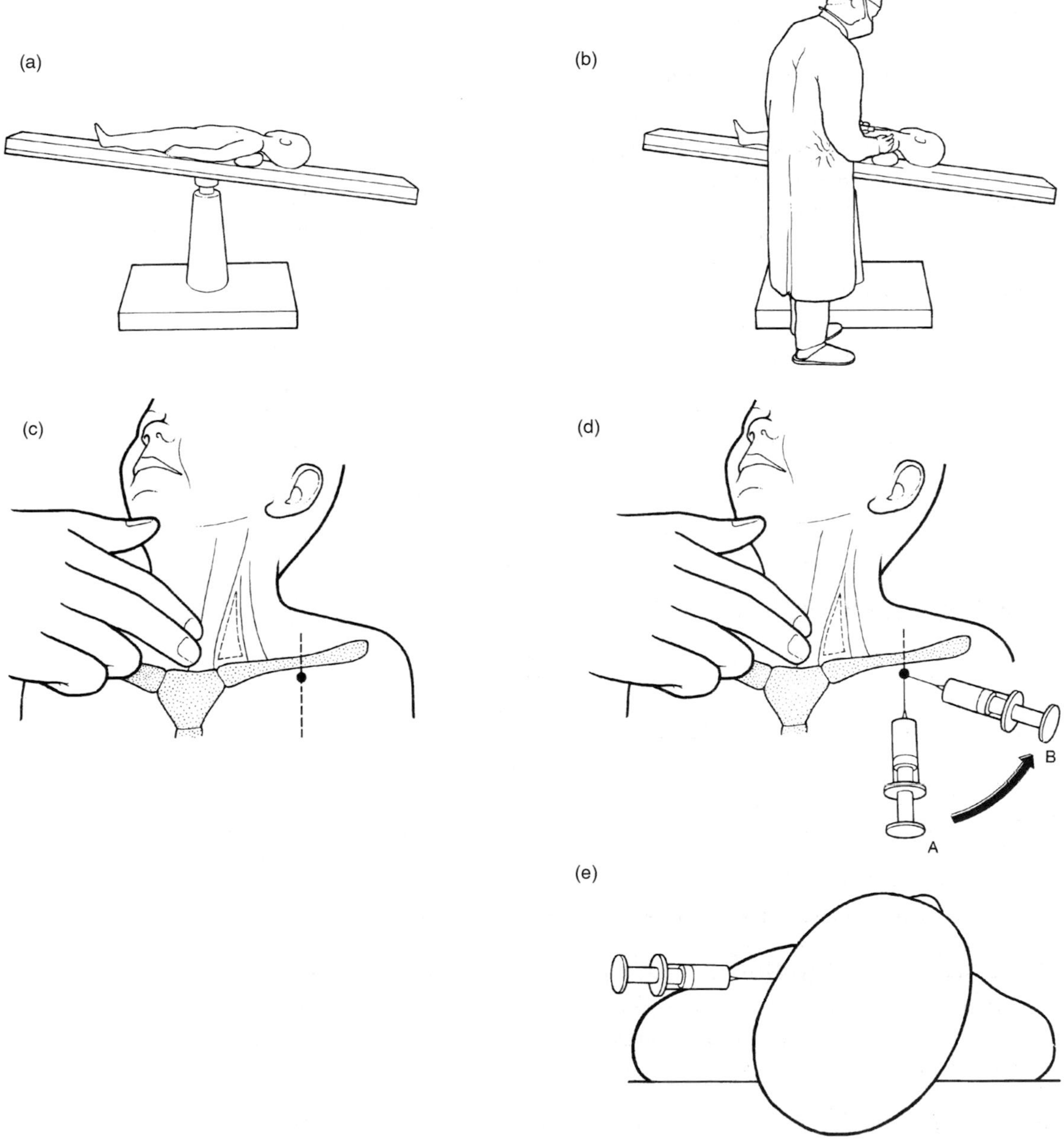

Figure 6.4 Infraclavicular approach: Morgan and Harkins (1972).[11]

INFRACLAVICULAR APPROACH

Mogil et al. *(1967)*[13]

Patient category

Adults. The description of the technique by the original authors did not include its application in children, but this does not necessarily exclude its use in this age group.

Advantages and disadvantages

The original authors claimed that this technique is safer than techniques using a more lateral approach, where the subclavian artery, brachial plexus, and pleura are in danger from the needle.

Preferred side

The right side, in order to avoid injury to the thoracic duct: it is also technically easier for a right-handed operator.

Position of patient

Place the table in a 25° head-down position. Place the patient in the supine position with both arms by the sides (Figure 6.5a). Do not place a pillow under the head, but a pillow under the back may be used to let the shoulders fall back so that the head of the humerus is not in the way.

Position of operator

Stand on the same side as the puncture site (Figure 6.5b).

Equipment used in original description

Adults: 14 gauge or 16 gauge OD introducing needle; 200 mm or 300 mm catheter-through-needle.

Advice on current equipment

Adults: guide-wire technique strongly recommended using an 18 gauge or 16 gauge introducer needle. Catheter-through-cannula, 14 gauge OD introducing needle or cannula, length 60 mm (minimum). Catheter length 200 mm (minimum). Long cannula on long needle, 130 mm length (minimum).

Anatomical landmarks

Junction of the medial and middle thirds of the lower border of the clavicle; small triangle formed by the two heads of the sternomastoid muscle and the clavicle (Figure 6.5c).

Preparation

Perform the puncture under sterile conditions using local anaesthesia if needed.

Precautions and recommendations

If a syringe is used, ensure that it can easily be detached from the needle.

Point of insertion of needle

Insert the needle just below the lower border of the clavicle at the junction of the medial and middle thirds of the clavicle (Figure 6.5c).

Direction of the needle and procedure

Place the point of the needle at the entry site on the skin and point the needle cephalad (A in Figure 6.5d). Then swing the needle and syringe laterally so that the needle points towards the small triangle formed by the two heads of the sternomastoid muscle and the upper border of the clavicle (A to B).

Advance the syringe behind the clavicle, keeping the syringe parallel to the coronal plane (Figure 6.5e). Maintain a slight negative pressure in the syringe while advancing the needle, until the vein is entered. A finger placed in the sternal notch is a useful guide to the landmarks, especially in obese patients. Do not alter the direction of the needle without first withdrawing its tip to the subcutaneous tissue. Having inserted the catheter take a chest X-ray to confirm the position of the catheter tip and to exclude a pneumothorax.

Success rate

There was a success rate of 95.9% in 219 attempts at catheterisation made by the authors.

Complications

There were 6 complications (an incidence of 2.7%): pneumothorax (1); haematoma (3); bleeding at puncture site (2).

(a)

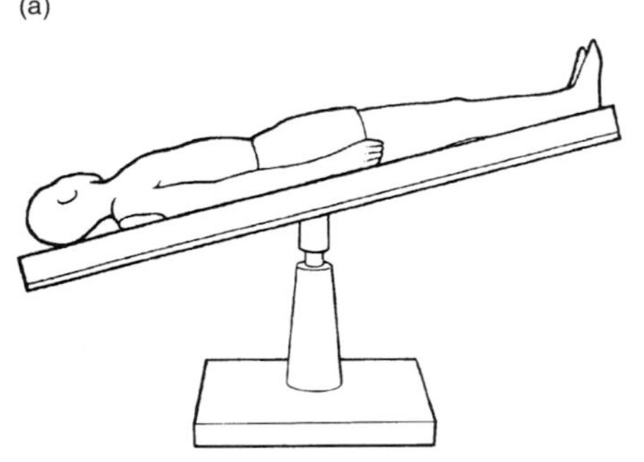

(b)

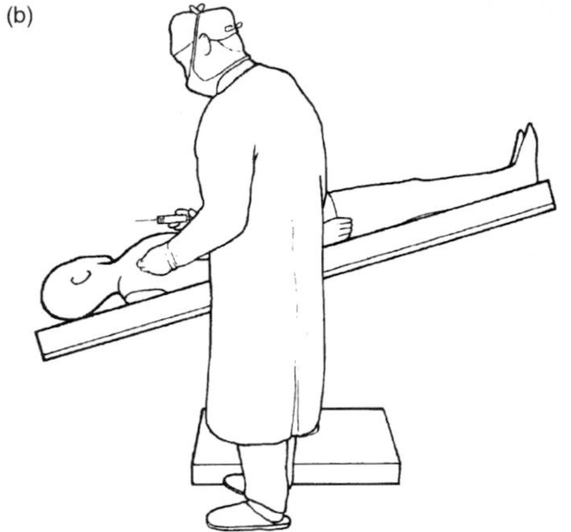

(c)

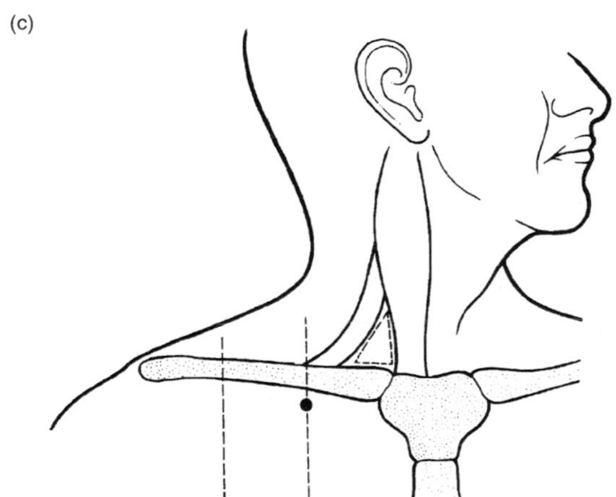

(d)

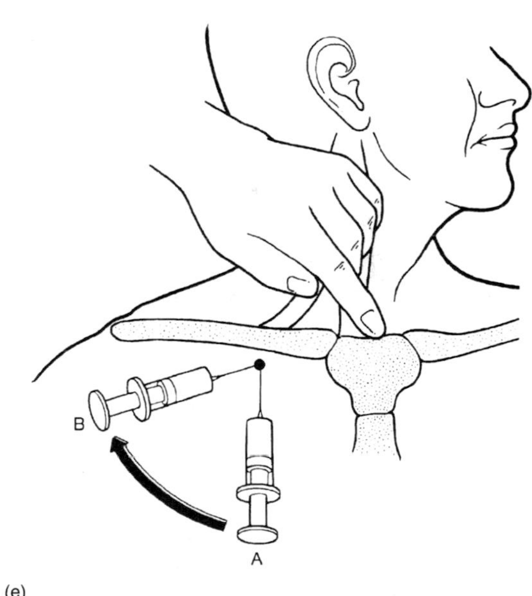

(e)

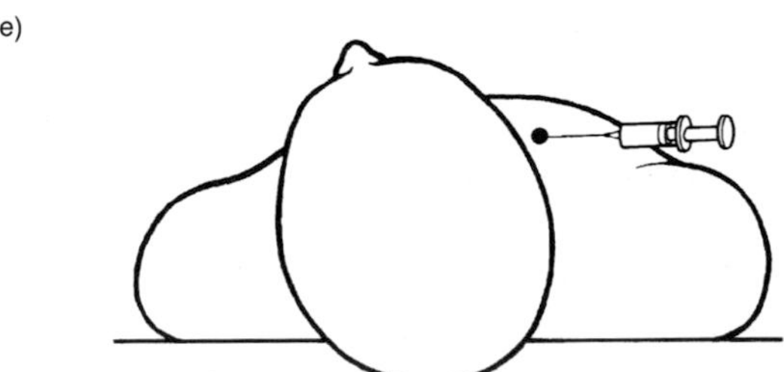

Figure 6.5 Infraclavicular approach: Mogil *et al.* (1967).[13]

INFRACLAVICULAR APPROACH

Tofield (1969)[17]

Patient category

Adults. The description of the technique by the original authors did not include its application in children, but this does not necessarily exclude its use in this age group.

Advantages and disadvantages

The more lateral and oblique approach is claimed to reduce the risk of pneumothorax and puncture of the subclavian artery.

Preferred side

Not stated.

Position of patient

Place the table in a 25° head-down position. Place the patient in the supine position with both arms by the sides. Turn the head away from the side of the puncture (Figure 6.6a).

Position of operator

Stand on the same side as the puncture site (Figure 6.6b).

Equipment used in original description

Catheter-through-needle. Size not stated.

Advice on current equipment

Adults: guide-wire technique strongly recommended using an 18 gauge or 16 gauge introducer needle. Catheter-through-cannula, 14 gauge or 16 gauge OD needle or introducer, length 70 mm (minimum). Catheter length 200 mm (minimum). Long cannula on long needle, length 130 mm (minimum).

Anatomical landmarks

Anatomical landmarks are the midclavicular point, the lower border of the clavicle and the suprasternal notch (Figure 6.6c).

Preparation

Perform the puncture under sterile conditions using local anaesthesia if indicated.

Precautions and recommendations

Ensure that the syringe can be removed easily from the needle.

Point of insertion of needle

Needle insertion is lateral (precise distance not stated) to the midclavicular point, 1 cm below the lower border of the clavicle (Figure 6.6c).

Direction of the needle and procedure

Place the point of the needle at the entry site on the skin and point the needle and syringe towards the head (A in Figure 6.6d). Then swing the needle and syringe laterally so that the needle points medially towards the tip of the index finger of the free hand, firmly pressed into the suprasternal notch (Figure 6.6e). Advance the needle posterior to the clavicle, keeping close to its posterior aspect and aiming all the time for the tip of the index finger in the suprasternal notch. Maintain a slight negative pressure in the syringe as the needle is advanced until the vein is entered. Insert the catheter.

Take a chest X-ray to confirm the position of the catheter tip and to exclude a pneumothorax.

Success rate

Not stated.

Complications

Not stated.

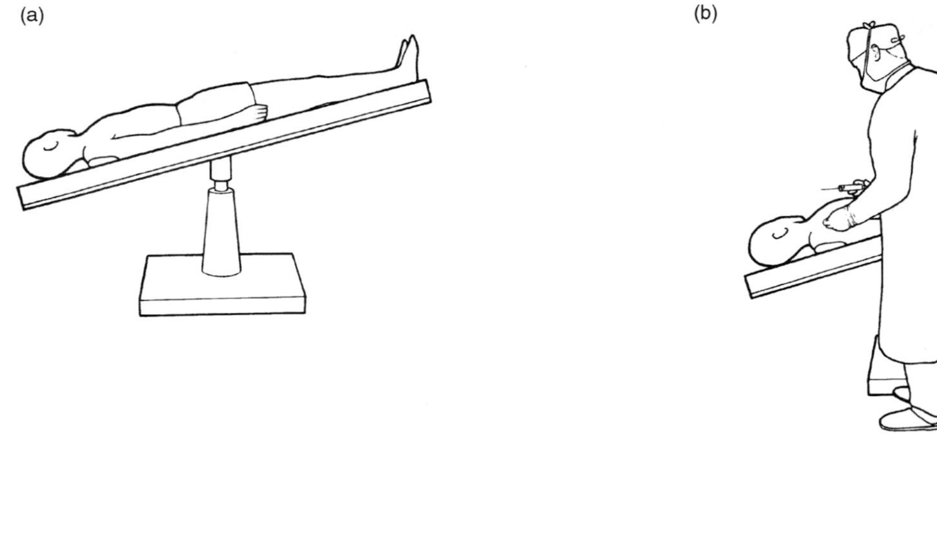

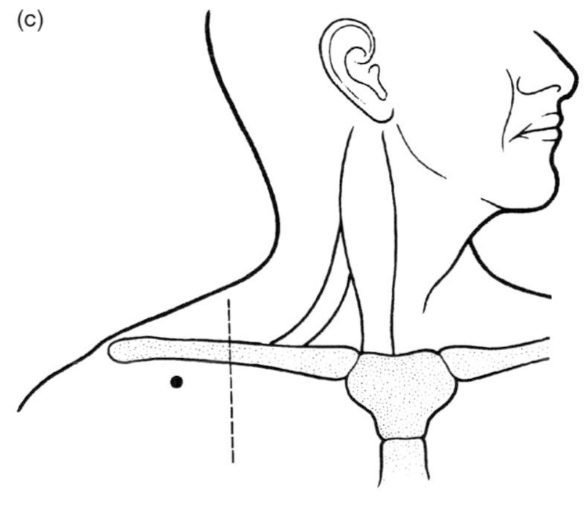

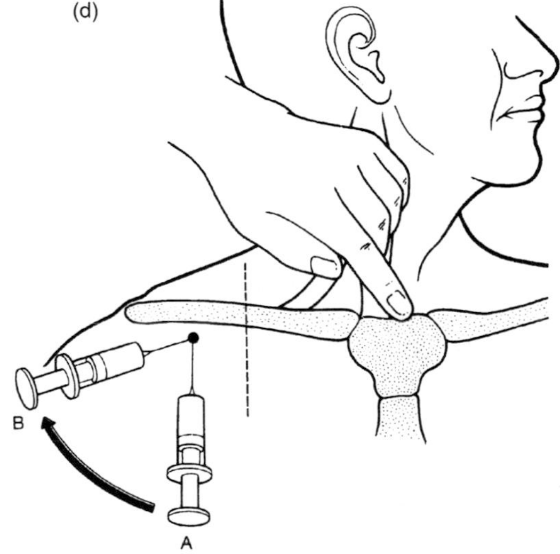

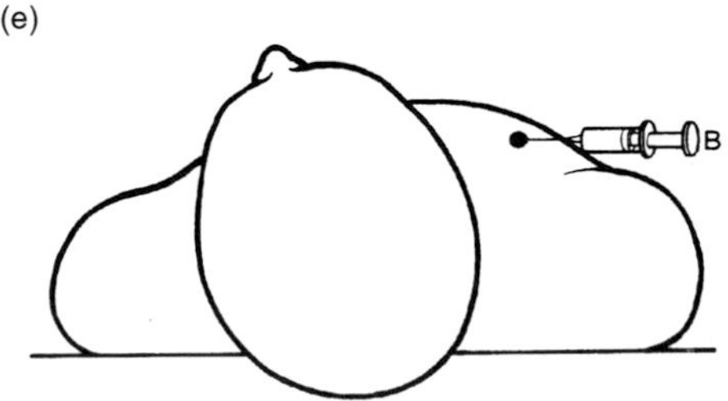

Figure 6.6 Infraclavicular approach: Tofield (1969).[17]

INFRACLAVICULAR APPROACH: THE AXILLARY ARTERY AS A LANDMARK

Untracht (1988)[18]

Patient category

Adults.

Advantages and disadvantages

In most other infraclavicular methods there are no clear landmarks; also, because the needle must be inserted almost directly backwards towards the spine in order to initially pierce the tissues immediately below the clavicle, the pleura is at risk. The axillary artery is a more constant relative landmark and the path of the needle is more parallel to the pleura so reducing the risk of pneumothorax. An added advantage is that after successful catheterisation, a long skin tunnel confers extra security.

Preferred side

Not stated, but a left-sided approach is described.

Position of patient

Place the patient in the 25° head-down position with arms by the side. Place a rolled towel under the spine at the thoracic level so that the shoulders fall away towards the table. Turn the head away from the side of venepuncture (Figure 6.7a).

Position of operator

Stand on the same side as the venepuncture (Figure 6.7b).

Equipment used in the original description

Not stated.

Advice on current equipment

Adults: guide-wire technique highly recommended. Small-diameter (18 gauge or 16 gauge) needle, length 70 mm minimum, to introduce wire. Catheter length 200 mm minimum. Long catheter on long needle 130 mm (minimum).

Anatomical landmarks

Landmarks (Figure 6.7c) are the suprasternal notch, lower border of the clavicle and the midclavicular line. Palpate the axillary artery lateral to the midclavicular line.

Preparation

Perform the procedure under sterile conditions using local anaesthesia if indicated.

Point of insertion of needle

The point of insertion lies approximately 2.5 cm below the axillary pulse and lateral to the midclavicular line (A in Figure 6.7c).

Direction of the needle and procedure

If local anaesthetic solution is used, it is infiltrated along a line between the skin puncture site and suprasternal notch (line a–b in Figure 6.7c, d) up to and including the periosteum of the clavicle. The introducer needle is advanced along the same track as described below.

With the needle at the entry point, aim the needle and syringe towards the head. Then swing the needle laterally so that the needle points medially towards the suprasternal notch, keeping a finger in the notch to act as a target. Advance the needle parallel to the coronal plane (Figure 6.7e) which keeps the needle parallel to the pleura as it passes under the lower border of the clavicle usually, but not always, between the middle and medial thirds. Maintain a slight negative pressure in the syringe to identify entry into the vein, which occurs as the needle point passes under the clavicle. Proceed with the catheterisation. Take a chest X-ray to confirm position of the catheter tip and to exclude a pneumothorax.

Success rate

There were 80 successful cannulations, usually at the first or second pass. No failure rate was stated.

Complications

No pneumothorax; one case of axillary artery puncture.

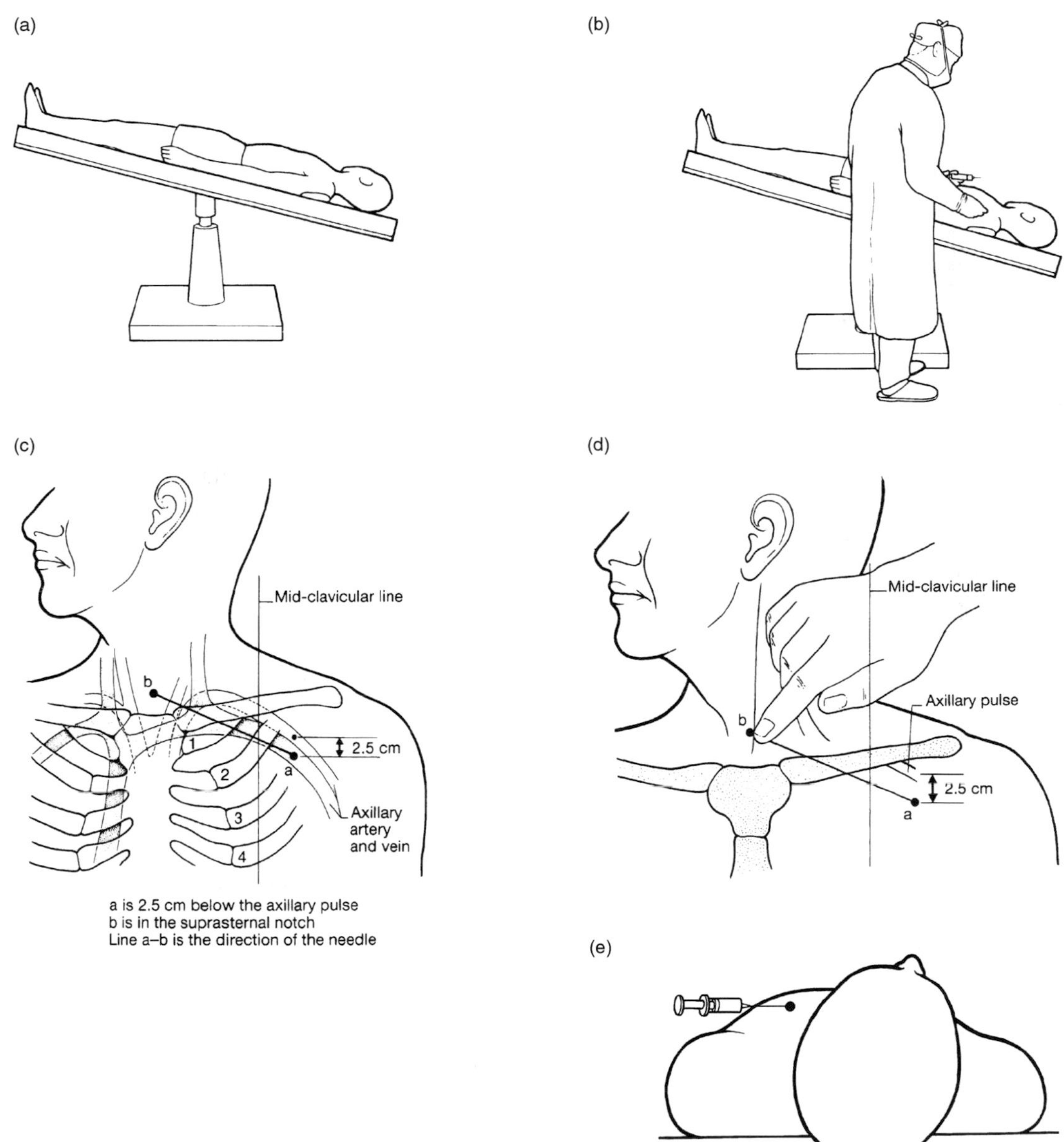

Figure 6.7 Infraclavicular approach: Untracht (1988).[18]

INFRACLAVICULAR APPROACH: USING DEFINITE LANDMARKS

Tripathi and Tripathi (1996)[19]

This approach claims to use more definite landmarks and guides to needle direction. It is based on the observation that the coracoclavicular line (from the lower border of the coracoid process to the upper border of the medial head of the clavicle) lies parallel to the radiologically observed indwelling subclavian catheter.

Preferred side

The right side.

Position of patient

With the table in a 15° head-down position, place the patient with arms by the sides and the left side of the body raised by 10–15° (by tilting the table or inserting a wedge under the left shoulder). The head is turned to the left.

Position of operator

Stand on the same side as the venepuncture.

Equipment used in original description

A 23 gauge 'finder' (seeker) needle; guide-wire technique or catheter-over-needle device.

Advice on current equipment

The guide-wire technique is recommended by the authors.

Anatomical landmarks

Mark the lower border of the clavicle. Mark the lower border of the coracoid process (C in Figure 6.8a). Mark the upper end of the medial head of the clavicle (M). Draw a line joining these points.

Preparation

Perform the procedure under sterile conditions using local anaesthesia if indicated.

Point of insertion of the needle

On the line CM (Figure 6.8a), insert the needle 1.5 cm below the point at which the two lines cross (P).

Direction of the needle and procedure

Locate the vein with a small-gauge needle. Advance the needle below the clavicle along the direction of the line CM (Figure 6.8b, c). Keep the needle in the horizontal plane until flashback occurs. Venous puncture is usually about 2.5 cm and 4 cm. If flashback is not obtained, the needle is withdrawn to the skin and reinserted after elevat-ing the syringe a few degrees above the horizontal.

Success rate

The overall success rate in a group of 205 patients was 100%, with 95.6% of catheterisations successful at the first attempt.

Complications

Arterial puncture by the seeker needle in 4 patients (1.9%); no other complications occurred.

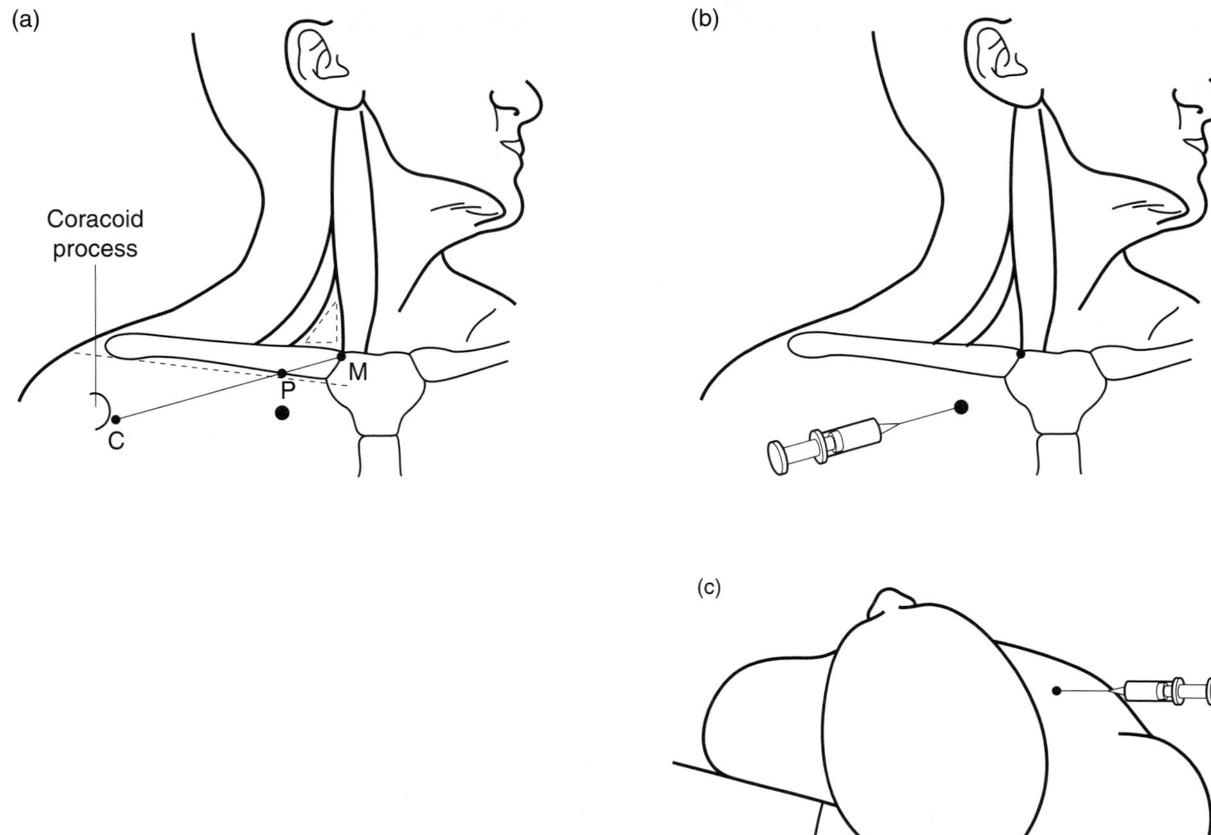

Figure 6.8 Infraclavicular approach: Tripathi and Tripathi (1996).[19]

SUPRACLAVICULAR APPROACH

Yoffa (1965)[8]

Patient category

Adults. The description of the technique by the original authors did not include its application in children, but this does not necessarily exclude its use in this age group.

Advantage and disadvantages

Several advantages over the infraclavicular approach are claimed. There is a reduced risk of pneumothorax because the needle points away from the pleura. There is a definite skin landmark. The distance from skin to vein is shorter (0.5–4.0 cm). Only fascial tissue has to be pierced.

Preferred side

The left side for the right-handed operator.

Position of patient

Place the table in a 25° head-down position (Figure 6.9a). Place the patient in the supine position with no pillow and with both arms by the sides. Turn the head slightly away from the side of the puncture.

Position of operator

Stand at the head of patient on the side of the puncture site (Figure 6.9b).

Equipment used in original description

Catheter through 14 gauge OD introducing needle.

Choice of current equipment

Adults: guide-wire technique strongly recommended, using an 18 gauge or 16 gauge introducer needle. Catheter-through-cannula, 14 gauge or 16 gauge OD needle or introducer; length 60 mm (minimum). Catheter length 200 mm (minimum). Long cannula on long needle, length 130 mm (minimum).

Anatomical landmarks

Lateral border of the clavicular head of the sternomastoid muscle just above the clavicle (Figure 6.9b). A patient who is conscious can be asked to raise his or her head against the resistance of a hand placed on the forehead to make the muscle stand out.

Preparation

Perform the puncture under sterile conditions using local anaesthesia.

Precautions and recommendations

Ensure that the syringe, if used, can be easily disengaged from the needle.

Point of insertion of needle

Insert the needle precisely into the angle between the clavicular head of sternomastoid and the upper border of the clavicle (Figure 6.9b).

Direction of the needle and procedure

Place the point of the needle at the entry site on the skin and point the needle and syringe caudally (A in Figure 6.9c). Then swing the needle and syringe 45° laterally (A to B). Depress the needle and syringe 15° below the coronal plane (B to C in Figure 6.9d, e). Maintain a negative pressure in the syringe as the needle is advanced. The vein is entered usually 1.0–1.5 cm from the skin (perhaps as little as 0.5 cm). If the catheter does not pass freely, its passage may be assisted by rotating the needle or introducer slightly while advancing the catheter. Take a chest X-ray to confirm the position of the catheter tip and to exclude a pneumothorax.

Success rate

The success rate was 97% (130 cases).

Complications

None, although there was one pneumothorax in a later series.

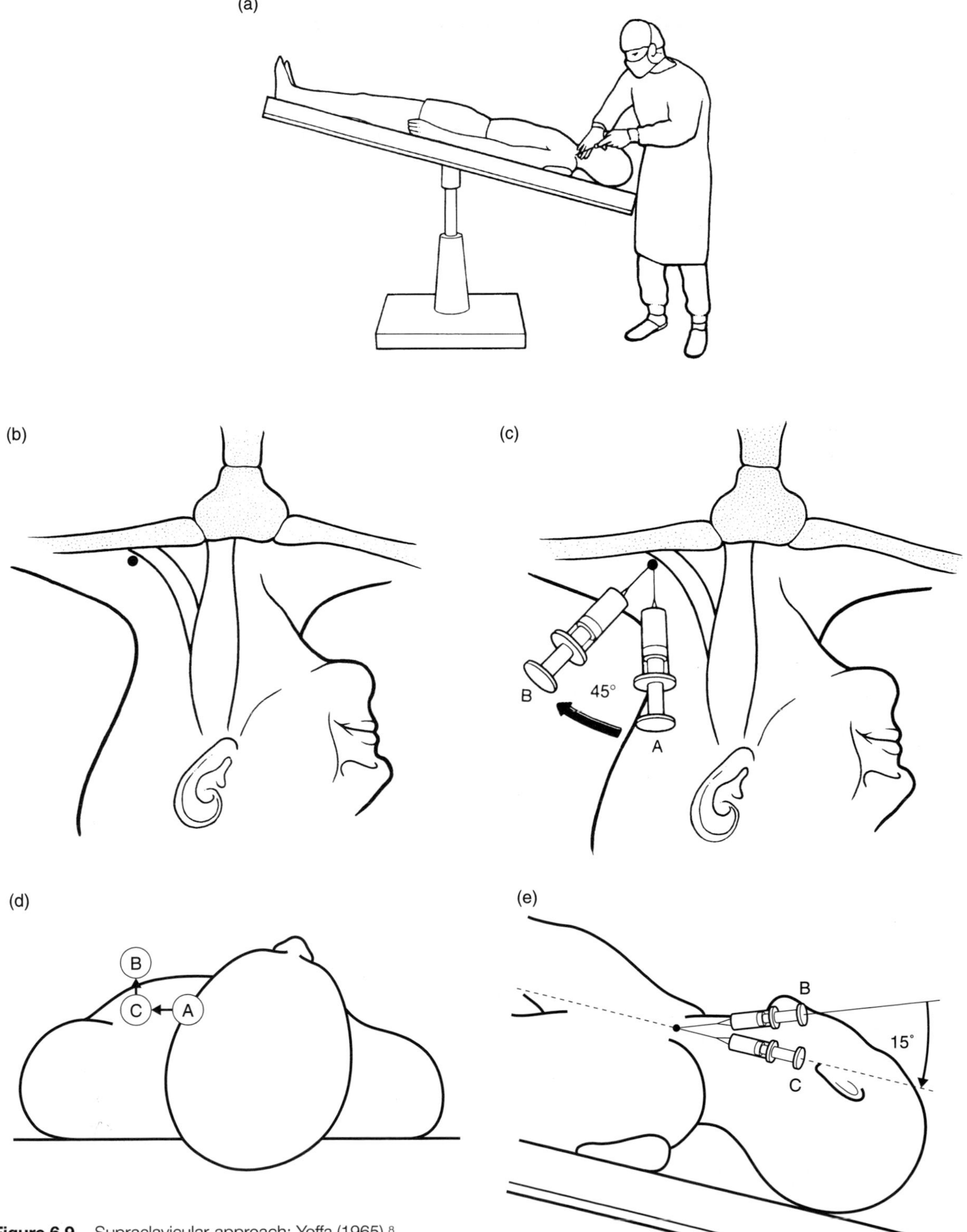

Figure 6.9 Supraclavicular approach: Yoffa (1965).[8]

SUPRACLAVICULAR APPROACH

James and Myers (1973)[14]

Patient category

Adults. The description of the technique by the original authors did not include its application in children, but this does not necessarily exclude its use in this age group.

Preferred side

Not stated.

Position of patient

Place the patient in the supine position with no pillow and with arms by the sides. Tilt the table 25° head-down. Turn the head away from the side of the puncture (Figure 6.10a).

Position of operator

Stand at the head of the patient (Figure 6.10a).

Equipment used in original description

Introducing needle 14 gauge OD; catheter-through-needle.

Choice of current equipment

Adults: guide-wire technique strongly recommended, using an 18 gauge or 16 gauge introducer needle. Catheter-through-cannula, 14 gauge OD needle or introducing cannula, length 60 mm (minimum). Catheter length 200 mm (minimum). Long cannula with long needle, length 130 mm (minimum).

Anatomical landmarks

Landmarks are the posterior border of the sternomastoid muscle and the superior border of the clavicle (Figure 6.10b).

Preparation

Perform the puncture under sterile conditions using local anaesthesia if indicated.

Precautions and recommendations

The borders of the sternomastoid can be made more prominent by asking the patient, if conscious, to tense the muscle by raising his or her head against resistance. Fill the syringe with saline to eject small plugs of fat and tissue to keep the needle patent. Ensure that the syringe can be easily detached.

Point of insertion of the needle

Insert the needle into the angle made by the posterior border of the clavicular head of the sternomastoid muscle and the clavicle (Figure 6.10b).

Direction of needle and procedure

Place the point of the needle at the entry site on the skin and point the needle caudally (A in Figure 6.10c). Then swing the needle and syringe laterally so that the needle lies along the line bisecting the angle between the clavicle and the clavicular head of the sternomastoid muscle (A to B). Depress the needle and syringe 10° below the coronal plane (B to C in Figure 6.10d, e). Advance the needle – its direction will be towards the retromanubrial area at the level of the sternal angle – until the vein is entered. Keep the needle clear by injecting a small volume of saline; otherwise maintain a slight negative pressure in the syringe as the needle is advanced. Insert the catheter if venepuncture is successful. If venepuncture and catheterisation are unsuccessful, delay any attempt on the other side if possible.

A chest X-ray should be performed to exclude a pneumothorax in all cases.

Success rate

A 95% success rate was achieved in 3000 attempted catheterisations. The operators were experienced or closely supervised.

Complications

In the 3000 cases the overall complication rate was 11.2%: 1.2% major and 10% minor. The major complications included pneumothorax (0.4%), hydrothorax (0.09%), subclavian thrombophlebitis (0.06%), haemorrhage (0.06%), air embolus (0.03%), and arteriovenous fistula (0.03%).

Minor complications included failure to puncture the vein or to thread the catheter.

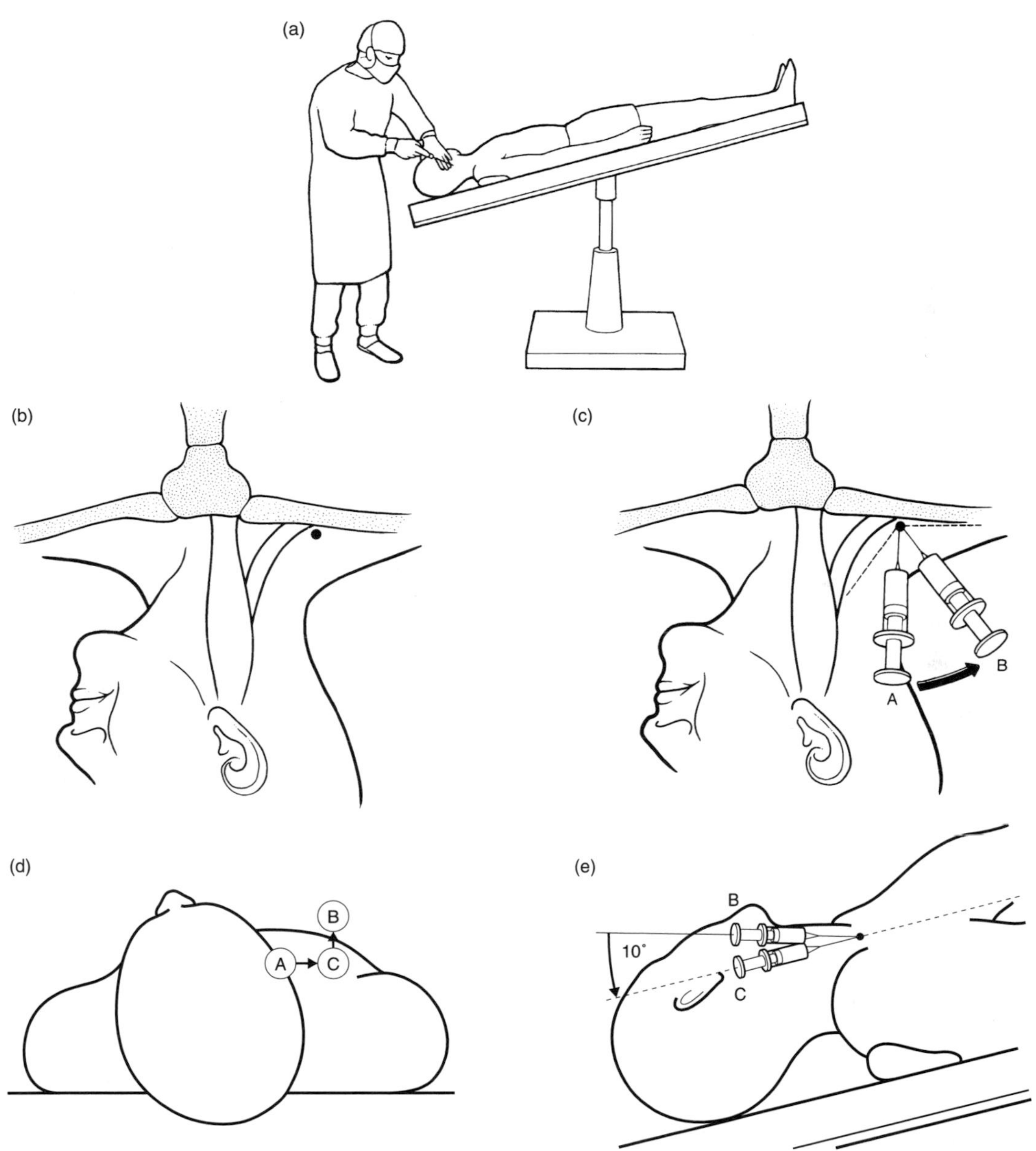

Figure 6.10 Supraclavicular approach: James and Myers (1973).[14]

SUPRACLAVICULAR APPROACH

Brahos (1977)[15]

The approach is similar to that of James and Myers (see previous page) but there are small differences.

Patient category

Adults and children aged 8 years and over.

Preferred side

Either side may be attempted but the right side is preferable because the vein is usually larger and has a more direct route to the superior vena cava. Avoids the thoracic duct.

Position of patient

Tilt the patient to the 20–25° head-down position. Turn the patient's head to the opposite side (Figure 6.11a).

Position of operator

Stand at the head of the patient (Figure 6.11a).

Equipment used in original description

Introducer needle 14 gauge, length 2 inches (5 cm); catheter 16 gauge, length 8–9 in (20–22 cm) for the right side, 10 in (25 cm) for the longer path of the left side.

Advice on current equipment

The use of a guide-wire technique is strongly recommended. Long cannula on long needle, length 130 mm minimum.

Anatomical landmarks

Identify the angle between the clavicle and the lateral border of the sternomastoid muscle – usually just medial to the external jugular vein (Figure 6.11b). In a conscious patient the landmarks are more easily seen in the obese if the patient actively lifts his or her head.

Preparation

Perform the procedure under sterile conditions using local anaesthesia if indicated.

Point of insertion of needle

Insert the needle in the angle between the lateral border of the sternomastoid muscle and the upper border of the clavicle (Figure 6.11b).

Direction of the needle and procedure

Place the needle point at the entry site and point the needle and syringe towards the feet. Then swing the needle and syringe laterally so that it lies along a line which bisects the clavisternomastoid angle (Figure 6.11c). The line points just caudad to the opposite nipple. Depress the needle about 10° below the horizontal plane and advance along the line described, just beneath the sternomastoid muscle. If no flashback occurs when about 5 cm of needle has been inserted, withdraw and and depress the needle a little more and repeat the insertion. Increase the angle step by step to a maximum of 25° below the coronal plane. Flashback usually occurs when the needle is about 15–20° below the coronal plane with about 3–4 cm of the needle inserted. Proceed with the rest of the catheterisation. Take a chest X-ray to confirm that the catheter tip is correctly placed and to exclude pneumothorax.

Success rate

All procedures were carried out by residents supervised by the author. No more than two attempts in any case were allowed. Success rates were: right-sided attempts 100% (68 cases); left-sided attempts 100% (32 cases).

Complications

Inability to thread catheter or unsatisfactory placement 5%; arterial puncture 1%; pneumothorax 1%.

(a)

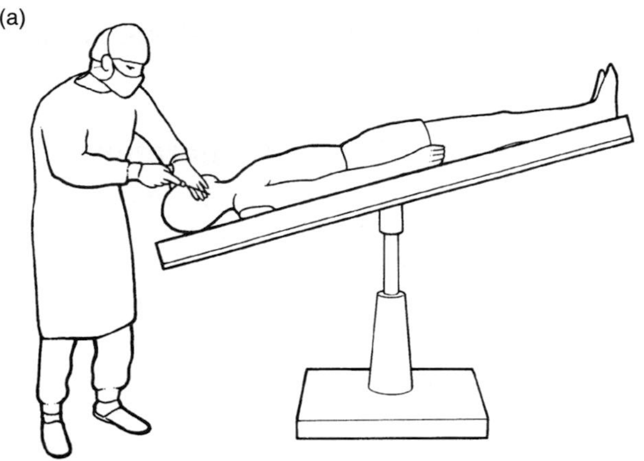

(b)

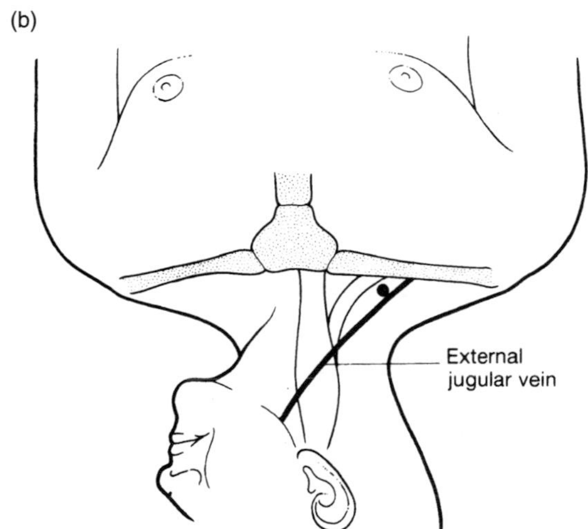

(c)

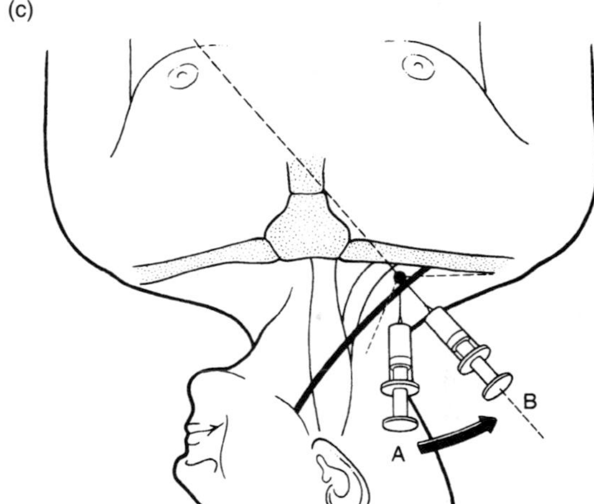

(d)

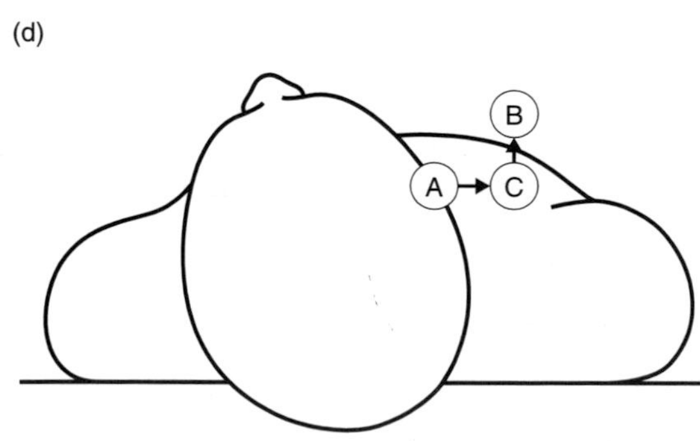

(e)

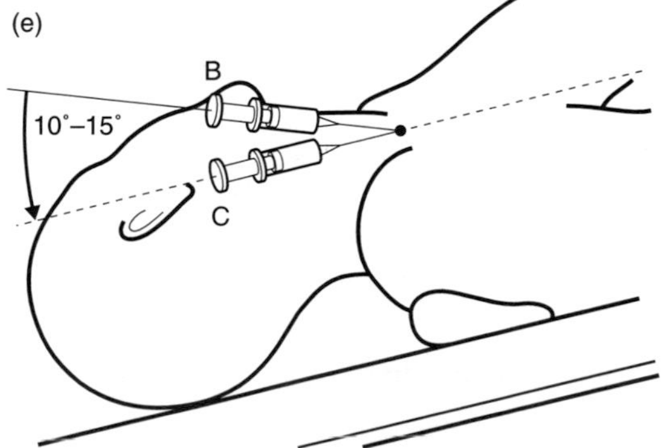

Figure 6.11 Supraclavicular approach: Brahos (1977).[15]

SUPRACLAVICULAR APPROACH

Haapaniemi and Slatis (1974)[16]

Patient category

Adults. The description of the technique by the original authors did not include its application in children, but this does not necessarily exclude its use in this age group.

Advantages and disadvantages

The authors claim that advancing the catheter is easier because there is a less obtuse angle between the needle and the vessel wall than in other supraclavicular and infraclavicular techniques. Furthermore, they claim that there is less risk of introducing the catheter into neck veins compared with the infraclavicular route.

Preferred side

The right side. The left side may be used, however.

Position of patient

Place the table in a 10° head-down position. Place the patient supine with arms by the sides and with shoulders depressed. Turn the head slightly away from the side of the puncture (Figure 6.12a).

Position of operator

Stand at the head of the patient or on the opposite side to the puncture site (Figure 6.12a).

Equipment used in original description

Polypropylene catheter through 14 gauge OD needle.

Advice on current equipment

Adults: guide-wire technique strongly recommended using an 18 gauge or 16 gauge introducer needle; 14 gauge or 16 gauge OD needle or introducer; length 60 mm (minimum). Catheter length 200 mm (minimum). Long cannula with long needle, length 130 mm (minimum).

Anatomical landmarks

The posterior border of the sternomastoid muscle (Figure 6.12b).

Preparation

Perform puncture under sterile conditions using local anaesthesia if indicated.

Precautions and recommendations

Maintain positive intrathoracic pressure during venous cannulation to distend the vein.

Point of insertion of needle

Insert the needle, 2–3 cm above the clavicle close to the posterior border of the sternomastoid muscle.

Initial location of vein with small-gauge needle

Locate the vein with a fine needle (21 or 22 gauge) using the directions given below. Then remove the fine needle and insert the large needle attached to a saline-filled syringe along the same path.

Direction of the needle and procedure

Place the point of the needle at the entry site on the skin and point the needle caudally (A in Figure 6.12c, d). Then swing the needle and syringe laterally 35° (A to B). Depress the syringe slightly below the coronal plane (B to C in Figure 6.12e). Maintain a slight negative pressure in the syringe as the needle is advanced. The vein is entered 2–3 cm (occasionally up to 5 cm) from the puncture site. The needle enters the vein behind the medial portion of the clavicle 1–2 cm lateral to the sternoclavicular joint. The point of entry into the vein corresponds to the junction of the subclavian and internal jugular veins. Advance the needle 3–4 mm into the vein and then introduce the catheter. Take a chest X-ray to confirm the position of the catheter and to exclude a pneumothorax.

Success rate

Catheterisations were reported to be 85.4% successful in the first 171 cases; 97% successful in the subsequent 429 cases.

Complications

The overall complication rate was 5%. There was a 0.6–1.0% incidence each of arterial puncture, haematoma, local infection, and puncture of the thoracic duct. The incidence of pneumothorax, air embolus, sepsis and thrombophlebitis was 0.1–0.5% each.

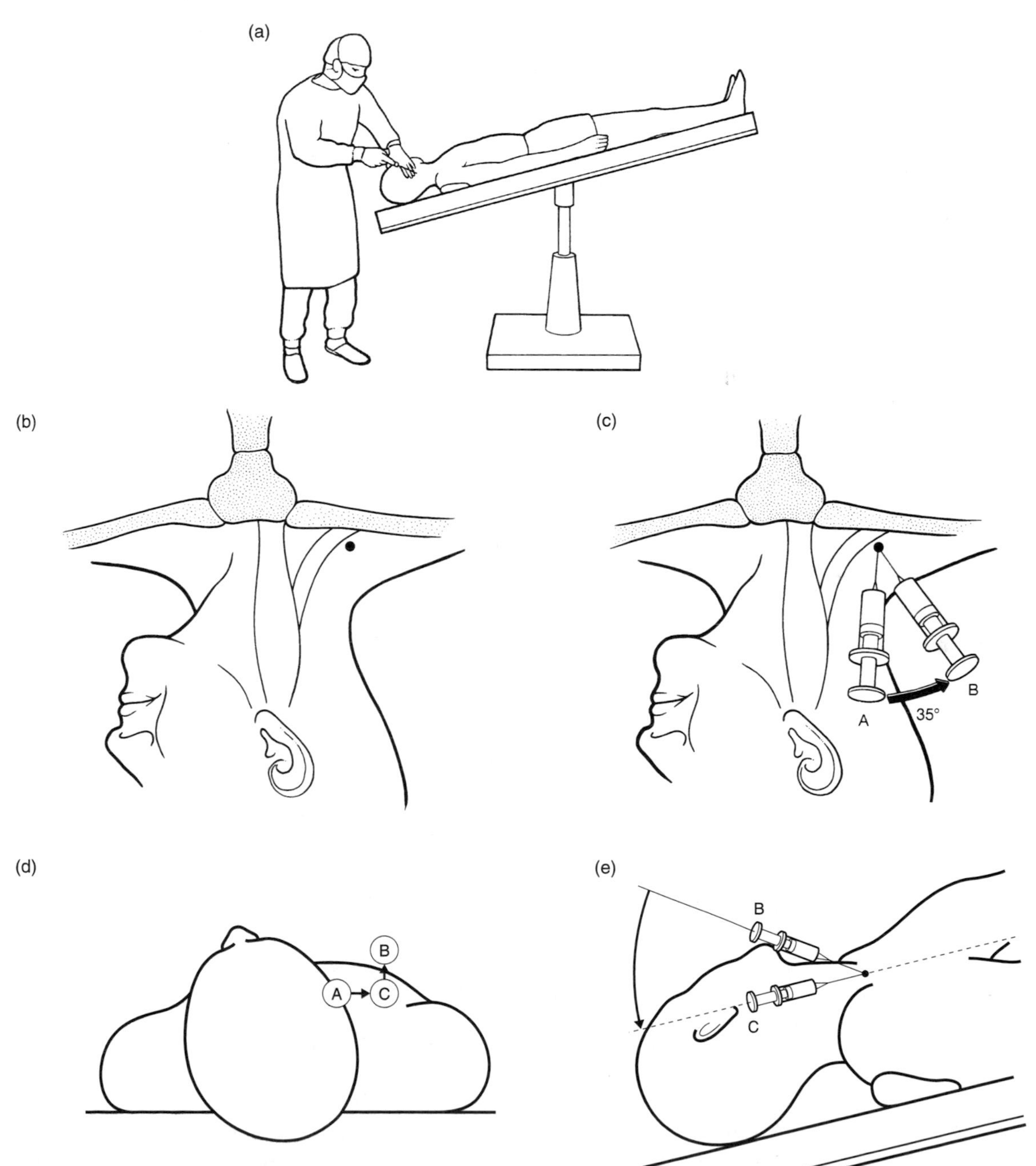

Figure 6.12 Supraclavicular approach: Haapaniemi and Slatis (1974).[16]

Case Reports of Complications Related to the Subclavian Vein Route

The commonly occurring hazards of central venous catheterisation through the subclavian vein are now well known (Table 6.3). The case reports set out below illustrate some unusual presentations of common complications as well as descriptions of some rare problems. Some cases include instructive as well as salutary lessons in diagnosis and management.

Pleural space and lung

The hazard of pneumothorax complicating subclavian venepuncture is the most well-known and obvious risk and is well documented in numerous series (see Table 6.1). The incidence ranges from 0% to 4.7% and up to 12.4% in certain physician groups.[10] Several case reports have warned of the apparent onset of a pneumothorax after some delay, sometimes days later. The chest X-ray taken immediately after the venepuncture has been clear.

Other types of respiratory tract complications appear to be rare.

Delayed pneumothorax[36,37]

The significance of 'difficult' subclavian catheterisation is illustrated in three cases where pneumothorax from a slow pleural air leak only became manifest later.[36] A repeat chest X-ray is worth considering in such cases. The diagnosis may be anticipated if air was aspirated at the time of venepuncture or if subcutaneous emphysema develops. Pleuritic or any persistent chest pain should alert to the possibility. Chest X-ray in such patients about to undergo surgery is advised.

In another study,[37] subclavian catheterisation was attempted properatively in three patients about to undergo major abdominal surgery in which intermittent positive pressure ventilation was used. One case ended in failure to cannulate, and in another case multiple attempts were made. In one case 2 days elapsed between cannulation and operation. In all cases the chest X-ray taken immediately after catheterisation was normal. In all three cases hypotension had developed during surgery, and in all cases subsequent X-rays revealed an obvious pneumothorax.

It is probable that the small laceration of the visceral pleura accidentally made at the time of attempted venepuncture is insufficient to produce immediately detectable air embolus but with the passage of time and especially in the presence of positive pressure ventilation the problem becomes manifest.

Late appearance of pneumothorax[38]

An immediate chest X-ray taken after a difficult catheterisation showed a correctly placed tip and no pneumothorax. Five days later, because of persistent shoulder tip pain and proposed surgery requiring positive pressure ventilation, a repeat X-ray revealed a pneumothorax. The value of a preoperative film in such patients is obvious.

Pneumothorax[39]

Three cases of pneumothorax following attempted subclavian puncture illustrate two points. Firstly, additional safety results from adequate monitoring and having an awake patient. In one case, during awake insertion of a subclavian line, the patient complained of sudden pleuritic pain and cough; oxygen saturation fell. Chest X-ray showed 25% apical pneumothorax. Secondly, two cases manifested pneumothorax only after surgery. Late presentation of pneumothorax has been well described by Williamson *et al.*[40] and see above.

Other cases were reported by Spiliotis *et al.*[41]

Bilateral pneumothorax[42]

A common pleural space was produced by inadvertent entry of both pleural cavities at median sternotomy. Subsequently pneumothorax complicated a subclavian venepuncture. The air leak was able to spread bilaterally with life-threatening effect.

Hydrothorax[43]

Perforation of the central vein wall occurred after apparently successful subclavian catheterisation in two patients (children). In both patients the line was used to administer fluid therapy which was followed by deterioration of the patients' general condition instead of the expected improvement. Progressive respiratory distress accompanied by dullness to percussion and diminished breath sounds led to the diagnosis, which was confirmed radiologically. Pleurocentesis produced clear (i.e. the infused) fluid.

Perforation of the central vein is more likely to be related to the catheter material and the design of its tip and its position in the central veins rather than to the route of insertion.

Bilateral hydrothorax and hydromediastinum[44]

A patient developed bilateral hydrothorax. However, injection of radio-opaque medium through the catheter demonstrated only a leak into the mediastinum. It was thought that the hydrothorax resulted from a shift of fluid from the mediastinum due to pressure differences in the two compartments.

Contralateral haemothorax[45]

The case demonstrates the difficulty in diagnosis when late and especially contralateral manifestations follow central venous catheterisation. In this case two subclavian catheters had been inserted, the right-sided one several days later than the left catheter. Haemorrhage into the right chest was interpreted as a complication of the right-sided catheterisation. However, chyle-like fluid continued to flow from the right chest drain, and anaesthetic drugs (methohexitone and suxamethonium) injected through the left catheter failed to be effective. Eventually, contrast studies established that perforation of the left-sided catheter into the right pleural cavity had occurred. The erosion of the superior vena caval wall was attributed to the stiff material of the catheter and the use of a left-sided approach. Cannulation from the left side allows the catheter to take an approximately horizontal course, its tip coming to abut at about 90° to the wall of the superior vena cava.

Late development of hydrothorax[46]

A left-sided subclavian line was inserted for long-term parenteral nutrition. Dyspnoea developed 47 days after insertion. The cause was a life-threatening hydrothorax. The catheter tip had inadvertently turned upwards and was in constant contact with the wall of the superior vena cava and eventually perforated the vessel. Dye studies confirmed this.

Massive haemothorax[47]

Massive haemorrhage due to laceration of the vein wall is the usual cause. Conservative measures are not likely to be effective. In this case, thoracotomy and complex surgical procedures were needed to resolve the problem.

Contralateral effusions[48]

Two cases are presented. Radiological studies were performed to elucidate the mechanisms.

Contralateral hydrothorax following guide-wire catheter replacement[49]

Fatal contralateral hydrothorax followed replacement of a central venous catheter using the guide-wire technique.

Venopulmonary fistula[50]

Two weeks after insertion of a silicone parenteral nutrition catheter into a 13-year-old child through the subclavian vein, pneumonitis and life-threatening respiratory failure developed. Removal of the catheter was followed by complete resolution.

Puncture of the trachea[51]

Puncture of the trachea occurred during infraclavicular subclavian catheterisation using a 14 gauge diameter needle of 7 cm length. The injury was revealed by leakage of inflated gases from around the tracheostomy tube through which the patient was receiving positive pressure ventilation. Changing the tube solved the problem; the original tube had a puncture of 1 mm diameter. The trachea lies in close relation to subclavian venepuncture, but in this case the puncture was made more likely by the tracheal wall reaching much more laterally. This resulted from dilatation of the trachea after prolonged tracheal intubation.

Acute airway obstruction[52]

During an emergency resuscitation of a shocked patient in pulmonary oedema, attempts were made at infraclavicular venepuncture with a large-bore 14 gauge needle. At the fourth attempt arterial blood was aspirated. Twenty minutes later a swelling appeared in the suprasternal notch and the neck also became swollen. Intense cyanosis appeared and total airway obstruction supervened only relieved by tracheal intubation. This proved extremely difficult because of the stiffness of the tissues which were distended with blood together with obstruction to passage of the tube. Radiological studies performed later showed a marked widening of the retropharyngeal space (by haematoma) and tracheal deviation. The subclavian artery was almost certainly lacerated because of its proximity to the venepuncture site.

Once again the danger inherent in needling of deep veins with a large-bore device is illustrated.

Vascular System

Punct ure of the ascending aorta[53]

In this case of attempted left infraclavicular subclavian venepuncture, an 80 mm needle was of sufficient length and size (12 gauge) to puncture the ascending aorta within 2 cm of the aortic root causing a fatal haemopericardium. It was thought that gross abdominal distension together with the head-down tilt position adopted during cannulation resulted in the mediastinum being distorted upwards. This was supported at post-mortem examination. A Seldinger guide-wire technique using a small, short introducer needle is advised in cases of marked abdominal distension.

Pulmonary artery puncture[54]

Infraclavicular subclavian venepuncture was performed with a long cannula-over-needle (140 mm) and illustrates the danger of this type of device. Although the vein can be reached by a needle of 60–70 mm length, the extra length of the long cannula-over-needle device means that it can reach and injure mediastinal structures if it is inserted too deeply. In this patient, at emergency sternotomy, the apex of the pulmonary artery was found to be punctured together with holes in the anterior pericardium and a large haemopericardium. The author stressed the need to consider cardiac tamponade in a patient presenting with cardiovascular collapse after central venous catheterisation.

Intercostal artery laceration[55]

Severe pneumothorax followed subclavian venepuncture with injury to the first intercostal artery. Emergency thoracotomy and intensive care saved the patient.

Subclavian arteriovenous fistula[56]

Inadvertent puncture of the subclavian artery was noted when infraclavicular venepuncture was carried out using a 14 gauge needle. Ten days after discharge the patient became aware of a loud murmur over the subclavian area. At operation a fistula was found encased in a 3 cm fibrous mass; a vein graft was used to bypass the fistula. The danger of using wide-bore venepuncture needles is commented upon.

Vertebral artery pseudoaneurysm[57]

Stridor and dysphagia followed 5 days after a difficult attempt at subclavian catheterisation. A computed tomographic scan showed a superior mediastinal, contrast-enhancing mass in the region of the right subclavian artery with the 'bull's-eye' sign suggestive of a pseudoaneurysm. Arteriography proved the aneurysm to originate from the vertebral artery which had presumably been lacerated at the time of venepuncture. The aneurysm was successfully ligated.

Benign intracranial hypertension[58]

This resulted from an arteriovenous fistula complicating subclavian catheterisation.

Spurious central venous pressure[59]

During an operation in a very ill patient, two markedly different central venous pressure measurements were obtained from two different sites of cannulation. A falsely elevated pressure (30 cmH_2O versus only 15 cmH_2O in the other catheter) recorded from one catheter inserted through the subclavian vein was related to the increased blood flow and pressure in a patent arteriovenous shunt which had been previously inserted for haemodialysis. There could have been errors in fluid management if the higher figure had been accepted. In addition the high and fluctuating pressure in the catheter which was in communication with the arteriovenous fistula produced dangerous fluctuations in vasoactive drugs being administered through the same line.

Arteriovenous fistula of the internal mammary artery and innominate vein[60]

Some days following a difficult subclavian vein catheterisation a machinery-like murmur was heard over the right clavicle. Further studies demonstrated an arteriovenous fistula. To avoid surgical exploration in an ill patient, transcatheter intravascular coil occlusion was successfully attempted. The steel coil prevents arterial blood from entering the arterial to venous fistula.

Pacemaker malfunction due to subcutaneous emphysema[61]

A pacemaker-dependent patient presented with pacemaker malfunction 2 days after its insertion. Subcutaneous emphysema developed at subclavian venepuncture and accumulation of air within the generator pocket of the pacemaker resulted in insulation of the unipolar anodal plate and consequent dysfunction of the device.

Malposition of catheter in a left anomalous pulmonary vein[62]

An anteroposterior radiograph taken immediately after catheterisation showed the catheter to have apparently entered the lung but aspiration of blood confirmed that the catheter was not extravascular.

Subclavian aneurysm and brachial plexus injury[63]

Complications only became apparent 8 hours after removal of a left subclavian catheter which had been *in situ* for 6 days for intermittent plasma exchange. The patient complained of left shoulder pain. Examination revealed a swelling in the left suprascapular region extending into the left side of the neck. Within 2 hours the patient had lost power and tendon reflexes in the left arm. Magnetic resonance scan showed a mass in the region of the left subclavian artery which was compressing the brachial plexus. Angiography confirmed the mass to be a false aneurysm arising from the subclavian artery. After surgical repair the patient was left with residual weakness of the arm. It was likely that the damage to the subclavian artery had occurred at insertion of the catheter but had been masked by the 'tamponading' effect of the catheter on the damaged artery. When the catheter was removed, the problem was revealed. Close scrutiny of the patient after removal of central venous devices is recommended by the author.

Perforation of a major vessel during placement of a central line[64]

A review of central cannulation over a 7-year period revealed a 1% incidence (10 cases) of perforation of a great vessel. These cases were mainly associated with right-sided subclavian venepuncture, which is the route most commonly chosen. Nearly half the patients died immediately or of subsequent complications. The study implicated guide-wire kinking during advancement of a vessel dilator as the main cause, linked to lack of adequate training in some operators.

Fatal subclavian artery haemorrhage[65]

Post-mortem examination revealed a 3 mm laceration of the first part of the right subclavian artery which had led to fatal haemorrhage after attempted subclavian vein catheterisation. The result in this case was surprising because the operator was experienced and had used a relatively small-gauge needle (19 gauge, 0.8–1.1 mm) to perform the venepuncture. Nevertheless, subclavian artery puncture was noted and cannulation performed on the other side without incident. Signs of severe blood loss were delayed until the next day; the bleeding appeared to be into the soft tissues of the chest wall. No haemothorax was discovered at post-mortem.

If the subclavian artery is known to have been punctured, then vigilance should be exercised, watching for signs such as enlarging haematoma, bruit, distal pulse quality, brachial plexus signs or hoarseness as well as for signs of haemothorax and hypovolaemia.

Innominate vein stenosis[66]

The patient presented with left upper arm swelling which was related to acute exercise. The patient had undergone repeated and prolonged central venous catheterisation 10 months previously. Phlebography revealed left innominate vein stenosis. There was no subclavian vein thrombosis.

Heart and mediastinum

Cardiac tamponade[67]

A case reported in 1975 is a classic example of the ease with which the correct diagnosis of perforation of a central venous catheter into the mediastinum is overlooked. The patient was recovering from cardiac surgery and although the clinical features were rightly interpreted as those of cardiac tamponade this was never attributed to inadvertent pericardial infusion through a central venous line that had perforated into the mediastinum. This was only too apparent at emergency thoracotomy. Interestingly, the anaesthetist noted that drugs injected through the line had no effect. The authors pointed out that if perforation had been considered, injection of radio-opaque dye would have easily confirmed the diagnosis and the patient would have been spared exploratory thoracotomy.

Other cases are reported by Adar and Mozes[68] and Defalque.[69]

Radiological demonstration of cardiac tamponade[70]

Radiological demonstration of a central venous catheter which had perforated into the pericardial sac explained why a patient developed a shocked state some hours after commencement of intravenous alimentation administered through the same line. A post-insertion chest X-ray had not permitted a clear view of the terminal portion of the catheter which was 'lost' amongst the equally radio-opaque mediastinal structures. The true position of the tip only became apparent after the injection of radio-opaque dye. When the correct diagnosis is made, the authors recommend aspiration of tamponade fluid through the line before its withdrawal.

Perforation of heart by a guide-wire[71]

A straight soft-tipped guide-wire used to insert a subclavian dialysis catheter perforated the heart. The use of a J-tipped wire is advised to avoid this life-threatening complication.

Massive mediastinal haematoma caused by a double-lumen catheter[72]

A special subclavian double-lumen catheter inserted to gain temporary access for extracorporeal circulation had worked perfectly well on the first occasion. At the start of the second treatment, the patient experienced excruciating pain and was found to have developed a massive mediastinal haematoma. While the proximal orifice remained inside the vein so that blood could still move freelyinto the circuit, blood was forcibly pumped through the distal orifice of the catheter tip, which had perforated the vein wall, into the mediastinum.

Cardiac tamponade with a multilumen catheter[73]

In two cases the possibility of perforation of the central vein by the catheter and subsequent infusion through the line causing a pericardial collection was not considered as the cause of acute hypotension and cardiac arrest. However, at emergency thoracotomy the catheter tip was found to have penetrated the posterior aspect of the heart and was lying in a fluid-filled pericardium. The position of the catheter tip is all-important and in these cases the catheters were inserted well beyond the 20 cm mark recommended by the manufacturers. The check X-ray should confirm that the catheter tip is lying no further than 2 cm below a line joining the inferior borders of the clavicles. The temptation to insert excess catheter to be sure that the most proximal orifice of the multilumen catheter is within the central vein should be guarded against.

'Ring around the artery' sign in pneumomediastinum[74]

Following subclavian catheterisation, a small pneumomediastinum resulted in the collection of a thin layer of gas around the right pulmonary artery, which on lateral chest X-ray produced a distinctive oval shadow at the right hilum.

Hydromediastinum from perforation of the innominate vein[68,69,75]

Reports of fatal hydromediastinum following subclavian catheterisation warned of the delay in onset of symptoms and signs for over 24 hours. The possibility of the catheters advancing spontaneously was suggested, emphasising the need for secure fixing of the catheters at the time of insertion. Any sudden unexpected deterioration in a patient's condition should throw suspicion on the central venous catheter. Radiographic and ECG changes may be absent. Timely aspiration of the mediastinum or pericardium can be life-saving.

Lymphatic system

Laceration of the thoracic duct[4]

Trauma to the thoracic duct occurred at an attempt to insert a pacing electrode through the track previously occupied by an electrode wire (which had failed and been removed) into the left subclavian vein. Lymph drainage stopped spontaneously after 4 days.

Lymphatic fistula[76]

The thoracic duct or one of its branches must have been inadvertently punctured at left subclavian venepuncture. Chylous fluid (confirmed by its high fat content and lymphocyte content) was leaking from the skin entry site one week later. The fistula healed spontaneously in 36 hours. The authors correctly point out that injury to the thoracic duct cannot occur with right subclavian puncture, but this does not eliminate the danger of damage to the lymphatic system as shown in the next report.

Lymph leakage after right-sided catheterisation[77]

Two days after easy right-sided infraclavicular subclavian venepuncture to insert a pacing electrode in a 6-year-old child, milky fluid (confirmed to be lymph) leaked out from around the catheter. No chylothorax developed and after 4 days the leak stopped spontaneously. Right-sided subclavian venepuncture is often recommended in order to avoid thoracic duct injury. However, the right lymphatic duct enters the superior margin of the subclavian vein near its junction with the internal jugular vein so the lymphatic system is still vulnerable although to a far lesser degree.

Neurological complications

Neurological sequelae of subclavian cannulation are uncommon. Unless the possibility of the clinical features being related to injury from venepuncture is borne in mind, the correct diagnosis must be difficult to arrive at.

Phrenic nerve paralysis due to local anaesthesia[78]

Left-sided infraclavicular puncture preceded by 5 ml 2% lignocaine infiltration was performed with a guide-wire technique. Respiratory distress and cyanosis developed immediately. Radiological studies revealed elevation of the left hemidiaphragm, deviation of the trachea to the right and paradoxical movement of the left hemidiaphragm. The paralysis lasted for 3 hours and was attributed to block of the phrenic nerve by the local anaesthetic agent. The authors comment that such cases appear to be rare although the phrenic nerve lies so closely related, behind the subclavian vein, to the site of venepuncture.

Permanent phrenic nerve palsy[79]

The very rare complication of phrenic nerve palsy followed successful and uneventful cannulation of the left subclavian vein for insertion of a pacemaker. The needle and sheath used in this procedure were large (12 F sheath). Dyspnoea and shoulder pain were complained of about 2 weeks later. Radiological studies revealed paralysis of the left hemidiaphragm. Follow-up confirmed its permanent nature. The conclusion was that the phrenic nerve was directly traumatised at venepuncture and had become scarred so explaining the dyspnoea and referred shoulder pain from the C3–C5 dermatome.

Diaphragmatic paralysis[80]

Two cases of hemidiaphragmatic paralysis following right-sided supraclavicular subclavian puncture are described after apparently easy catheterisations. In both cases there were no symptoms and diaphragmatic paralysis was only seen on routine chest X-rays some days later. Extensive investigations were performed to determine the cause of this finding but were negative. The abnormal hemidiaphragm remained in both cases up to 3 years later. It was concluded that the phrenic nerve which lies in close proximity at subclavian venepuncture had been damaged at the time of catheterisation.

Recurrent laryngeal nerve paralysis[81]

Recurrent laryngeal nerve paralysis followed pacemaker insertion through the subclavian vein.

Brown-Séquard's syndrome[82]

This syndrome followed spinal cord infarction following subclavian vein catheterisation. Pain in the left arm and leg was experienced immediately at the time of attempted infraclavicular venepuncture. No flashback of blood was obtained. Left hemiplegia was severe and accompanied by Horner's syndrome partially affecting the left side. There was diminished sensation on the right side corresponding to a lesion between C8 and T4 spinal segments. These signs persisted over 3 months.

It was thought that needling at the time of attempted subclavian venepuncture induced severe spasm of one of the arteries of the costocervical plexus and consequent ischaemia to the left anterior part of the lower spinal cord leading to infarction of the cervicothoracic spinal cord. Apparently spasm of arteries in this area due to the mechanical irritation of needling is sometimes seen during angiographic studies.

Transient paralysis of the upper arm[83]

In two elderly patients transient motor and sensory paralysis of the upper limb was attributed to excessive amounts of lignocaine infiltrated too deeply and too laterally. The amounts of lignocaine 2% used were 16 ml and 25 ml respectively and had produced a brachial plexus block.

Injury to the lower cord of the brachial plexus[84]

Clinical evidence supported by electrophysiological tests confirmed injury to the brachial plexus after cannulation through the infraclavicular route. The rarity of brachial plexus injuries with infraclavicular catheterisation can be attributed to the anatomical distance between the plexus and the point of insertion of the catheter. However, minor neurological deficits may easily escape detection.

Brachial plexus neuropathy was reported by Trentman *et al.*[85]

Unsuspected cerebral perfusion[86]

During an emergency, drugs were infused into a line the position of which had not been confirmed radiologically. The tip, in fact, lay deep in the internal jugular vein so that the drugs administered produced cerebral effects by retrograde perfusion of the intracranial venous sinuses. Adrenaline produced severe headache; lignocaine led to an increased clouding of consciousness. Yet there was virtually no therapeutic effect on the heart from either of these drugs.

Cortical blindness[87]

After subclavian venepuncture, the patient became acutely confused and developed a transient left hemiplegia. Loss of vision followed. Pupillary reflexes and examination of the optic fundi were normal so the disorder was attributed to an acute cortical lesion produced by an air embolus.

Air embolism

Air embolism: a lethal but preventable complication[88]

Fourteen cases of air embolism related to subclavian vein catheterisation are reported. In 13 of these, a sudden catastrophe was associated with inadvertent disconnection of the catheter. Four patients died; nine had profound neurological impairment, of whom five recovered. Five patients had severe cardiorespiratory complications. Lack of integrity of catheter connections was the overwhelming cause of this serious but preventable hazard and the authors stress the need to ensure secure connection between the catheter and intravenous tubing.

Air embolism in the sitting position[89]

With the patient in the sitting position during neurosurgery, downward traction of the cannula enlarged the opening around the puncture site of the subclavian catheter, so allowing air to enter. Air embolism was diagnosed by the appearance of typical precordial Doppler sounds, fall of end-tidal $P\text{CO}_2$ and acute hypotension. Packing and pressure over the puncture site effected a temporary cure. A through-needle catheter had been used which means that the puncture would have been larger than the catheter. A guide-wire technique would have been safer, because the puncture would have been smaller than the catheter.

Air embolism causing acute pulmonary oedema[90]

Immediately after the removal of a triple-lumen subclavian catheter, while in the sitting position, the patient suddenly developed a sense of retrosternal oppression and became acutely dyspnoeic. Consciousness was lost for 5 minutes. An hour later symptoms and signs developed and chest X-ray confirmed the clinical diagnosis of bilateral pulmonary oedema. All these features were attributed to venous air embolism which must have entered along the large (2.3 mm diameter) catheter track aided by the patient being in the sitting position.

Other cases were reported by Flanagan *et al.*,[91] Aulenbacher,[92] Johnson *et al.*[93] and Levinsky.[94]

Non-cardiogenic pulmonary oedema[95]

A patient suffering from irregular palpitations was treated by medication and pacing. The pacing wires were inserted through a Swan–Ganz catheter placed in the right subclavian vein. A post-insertion chest X-ray was normal. Six days after insertion, the patient developed clinical and radiological signs of pulmonary oedema which deteriorated although no myocardial dysfunction could be demonstrated. However, on transthoracic echocardiography frequent streams of air bubbles could be seen which confirmed the diagnosis of central venous air embolism. Inspection of the insertion site of the subclavian line showed cyclical ballooning of the occlusive plastic dressing and incomplete apposition of the skin and subcutaneous tissue to the introducer. Air was being aspirated into the subclavian vein during respiration. The dressing formed a tent with the side arm of the introducer and seemed to be acting as a one-way valve. Immediate removal of the introducer and application of an occlusive dressing resulted in rapid improvement of the patient's condition and resolution over the following 2 days.

Acute pulmonary oedema occurring secondary to venous air embolism has rarely been reported. Its development seems to depend on a steady stream of bubbles entering the pulmonary circulation which produces an acute inflammatory response in the pulmonary vasculature, manifesting itself as pulmonary oedema.

This case demonstrates the value of echocardiographic detection of air embolus. Ultrasonography is also an effective means of detecting haemodynamically silent air embolus. Lessons from this case include the need for care and vigilance both during and after the insertion and dressing of central venous catheters.

Infection

Catheter-related infections and septicaemia are common and important sequelae to central venous catheterisation especially in relation to long-term use. These problems have received extensive attention. However, some rare and unusual infective conditions have also been reported.

Osteomyelitis of the first rib[96]

A patient presented with a cold chest-wall mass 9 months after subclavian catheterisation for insertion of temporary pacing wires. Investigation revealed a staphylococcal osteomyelitis of the first rib.

Breast 'abscess'[97]

Eight days after successful insertion of an infraclavicular subclavian catheter, the patient developed severe pleuritic pain in the right chest. Injection of drugs into the catheter induced severe right-sided chest pain. Simultaneously a fluctuant right 'breast abscess' was drained. Fluid emerged from the drain in this lesion at the same rate as infusion into the venous line. Contrast studies showed inadvertent catheterisation of the right internal mammary vein from which a track had formed leaking into the right breast tissues.

Clavicular periostitis[98]

Three children developed this benign condition following percutaneous subclavian catheterisation.

Osteomyelitis of both clavicles[99]

Osteomyelitis of both clavicles occurred with no systemic signs of infection, but simply local pain and tenderness over the affected area.

Sternoclavicular septic arthritis[100]

Four weeks after subclavian catheterisation, the patient slowly developed a painful shoulder, chest discomfort and painful swelling over the sternoclavicular joint accompanied by low-grade pyrexia. Diagnosis was confirmed by blood cultures and an abnormal bone scan. Antibiotic therapy cured the condition. The authors estimate the incidence of this complication to be as common as 1 in 500.

Acute pharyngitis[101]

Seven days after subclavian vein catheterisation to facilitate intravenous hyperalimentation, a 60-year-old patient developed a sore throat, neck pain and fever. Examination showed a marked swelling in the right posterior wall of the oropharynx and hypopharynx. Radiography of the neck revealed that the tip of the catheter was in the internal jugular vein, so in effect the patient was suffering from acute phlebitis of the internal jugular vein and not pharyngitis. Resolution occurred within 2 days of removing the catheter.

Miscellaneous complications

Intravascular knot formation[102]

Suspicion was aroused when after several attempts, resistance to withdrawal was noted and the catheter appeared kinked. If knotting is suspected further pulling should be avoided as this may tighten the knot and make attempts to remove the catheter by unravelling the knot with a pigtail catheter impossible, in which case surgical exploration is necessary.

Extravascular knotting of a guide-wire[103,104]

Although the Seldinger technique is usually recommended for catheterisation of deep veins, the technique itself can lead to problems. Wang and Einarsson reported that although the wire was advanced with ease, the catheter could not be.[103] Attempts to withdraw the wire were unsuccessful. Surgical exploration revealed that the wire had perforated the posterior wall of the subclavian vein and knotted itself outside the vein. Undoubtedly, the vein was abnormal from many previous catheterisations for chemotherapy. Although no resistance was encountered when the wire was introduced in this case, when resistance is felt, it should always be a signal to withdraw or to proceed with extreme caution. This especially applies when there is a history of previous central venous catheterisations. Almost certainly, a J-tipped wire should be used in these cases.

A similar case was reported by Nicholas *et al.*[104]

Catheter embolism[105,106]

Intravascular foreign body[107]

Infraclavicular subclavian catheterisation was being attempted by an experienced operator using a Seldinger technique when difficulty was encountered in advancing the straight guide-wire. When the wire was retracted it broke. Immediate chest X-ray showed the wire. At exploration under local anaesthesia the tip of the fractured wire was found under the clavicle where it had become caught in the clavicular periosteum. Perhaps use of a J-tipped guide-wire would have avoided this problem.

Misplacement of guide-wire and loop formation[108]

During attempted insertion of a catheter using the guide-wire technique, resistance was felt in trying to advance the wire. Catheterisation was impossible, but attempts to remove the wire failed. Chest X-ray demonstrated loop and knot formation. At surgical exploration, the wire was seen to have perforated the wall of an almost occluded subclavian vein and buried itself in the scalenus anterior muscle. In this case the patient had received numerous previous catheterisations for chemotherapy which no doubt had led to a partially thrombosed and softened vein wall.

Contact dermatitis[109]

In this case contact dermatitis arose from a subclavian catheter.

Extravasation from a multilumen catheter[110]

In this case a five-lumen central venous catheter was inserted 18 cm through the right subclavian vein. Correct positioning was confirmed by equal aspiration of blood through all ports and by chest X-ray. In this catheter the most external lumen is 8.75 cm from the tip. Extravasation became manifest by increasing swelling of the neck. Blood could not be aspirated, and chest X-ray showed no migration of the catheter; nevertheless, dye studies confirmed extravasation.

Preventive measures include aspirating the proximal lumen at intervals and possibly using this channel for isotonic crystalloids only. The outermost port (nearest the skin) of multilumen catheters may be some distance from the catheter tip. Care is needed to ensure that sufficient length of catheter is inside the lumen of the vein to avoid extravasation from this port.

Fracture of catheter[111]

This report describes the compression of a subclavian catheter between the clavicle and first rib.

KEY POINTS

- The subclavian vein is an effective approach to gaining access to central veins.
- This vein is still the preferred route for very long-term venous access.
- The potential exists for serious complication at time of cannulation.
- Gaining expertise must be conducted under supervision.
- Ultrasound guidance is useful in training and in difficult cases.
- Serious complications are often associated with a history of difficulty in atheterisation.
- Pneumothorax may not be evident on early chest X-ray.

Table 6.1 Subclavian vein catheterisation by the infraclavicular approach – results and complications.

Author and year	Classification of technique (point of insertion)	Success rate (%)	No. of cases	Complication: Type	Complication: No. (%)	Personnel	Comments
Wilson *et al.* (1962)[2]	Midclavicular point	Not stated	250	None (pneumothorax in some later cases performed by residents)	0	Authors	Series included infants
Davidson *et al.* (1963)[23]	Junction of middle and medial thirds of clavicle	94	100	Pneumothorax	1 (1)	Adults and children; youngest patient 3 1/2 years	
				Haematoma	3 (3)		
Smith *et al.* (1965)[112]	Midclavicular point	Not stated	200	Lacerated subclavian vein communicating with pleura (both patients died)	2 (1)		
				Severe subcutaneous emphysema – tracheostomy needed	2 (1)		
				Brachial plexus palsy	1 (0.5)		
				Haemothorax	1 (0.5)		
				Septicaemia	1 (0.5)		
Mogil *et al.* (1967)[13]	Just lateral to the junction of middle and medial thirds of clavicle	95.9	219	Overall	6 (2.7)	Main author only	
				Pneumothorax	1 (0.4)		
				Haematoma	3 (1.3)		
				Bleeding at puncture site	2 (0.9)		
Christensen *et al.* (1967)[24]	Medial to midclavicular point	80	90	Tension pneumothorax	1 (1.1)		
Defalque (1968)[113]	Slightly medial to mid-clavicular point	98.8	1000	Arterial puncture	1 (0.1)		Some catheterisations performed by supraclavicular approach
				Pneumothorax	3 (0.3)		
Morgan and Harkins (1972)[11]	Midclavicular point	Not stated	100	*Infants* (< 12 m):		Probably closely supervised personnel	74 catheterisations in children aged < 12 m; 37% of these were < 6 wk old
				None	0		
				Older children:			
				Arterial puncture with local bleeding	2 (2)		
				Catheter in pericardium	1 (1)		
				Catheter in pleural cavity	1 (1)		
James and Myers (1973)[14]	Midclavicular point	94	511	Overall	85 (16.6)		
				Major	38 (7.44)		
				Pneumothorax	15 (2.93)		
				Hydrothorax	6 (1.17)		
				Sepsis	8 (1.56)		
Ryan *et al.* (1974)[114]	Not stated	Not stated	355	Pneumothorax	6 (1.7)		Some catheters not inserted by the subclavian route
				Brachial plexus injury	2 (0.6)		
				Pleural effusion	1 (0.3)		
				Carotid artery laceration	1 (0.3)		
				Mediastinal haemorrhage from innominate vein laceration	1 (0.3)		
				Death (catheter sepsis)	1 (0.3)		

Groff and Ahmed (1974)[12]	Midclavicular point		< 1 yr, 67 < 2 yr, 36	Hydrothorax Haemothorax Pneumothorax Catheter sepsis Death (haemorrhage)	2 (1.9) 1 (0.9) 1 (0.9) 1 (0.9) 1 (0.9)	Experienced	
Blackett *et al.* (1978)[115]	Midclavicular point	84.3	211	Overall Subclavian artery puncture Bilateral pneumothorax	5 (2.3) 3 (1.4) 1 (0.4)		All patients catheterised for intravenous feeding
Craig *et al.* (1969)[116]	Not stated	Not stated	453	Pneumothorax Subcutaneous haematoma Subcutaneous infiltration with fluids	3 (0.6) 14 (3) 6 (1.3)		
Dudrick *et al.* (1969)[7]	Midclavicular point	Not stated	400	None (pneumothorax in later cases performed by residents)	0	Author	Series included infants
Feiler and de Alva (1969)[117]	Not stated	Not stated	704	Pneumothorax Subclavian vein thrombosis	2 (0.3) 1 (0.1)		This series covered 41/2 years. Complications) occurred in the first 11/2 years only
Tofield (1969)[17]	Lateral to midclavicular point	Not stated	Not stated	Not stated			More lateral approach said to avoid the risk of pneumothorax
Borja and Hinshaw (1970)[25]	Junction of medial and middle thirds of clavicle	Not stated	Not stated	Not stated			More medial approach said to be safer than lateral approach to avoid subclavian artery, brachial plexus, and pleural damage
Williams and McDonald (1971)[118]		93.3	75	Haematoma Pneumothorax Septicaemia	2 (2.6) 1 (1.3) 6 (8)	Included medical students and residents	Average age 64 yr (range 20–87 yr)
Matthews and Worthley (1982)[30]		88	R 126	Malposition Pneumothorax Subclavicular artery puncture	16 (12.6) 5 (3.9) 3 (2.3)	Experienced	Choice of side left to operator Malposition greater on right side
		88	L 111	Malposition Pneumothorax Artery puncture Haemothorax (died)	3 (2.3) 4 (3.1) 2 (1.5) 1 (0.8)		
Eerola *et al.* (1985)[31]		88	13 857 (98% infraclavicular; 76% right-sided; 24% left-sided)	Malposition into internal jugular vein Other malposition Pneumothorax	(10) (0.5) (0.1)	Mainly experienced physicians	

Table 6.1 *Continued*

Author and year	Classification of technique (point of insertion)	Success rate (%)	No. of cases	Complication		Personnel	Comments
				Type	No. (%)		
Untracht (1988)[18]		100	80	Axillary artery puncture	1 (1.2)		
Mansfield *et al.* (1994)[119]	Ultrasound identification of vein before puncture but not at puncture		411	Overall (not failed)	(9.7)		
				Failed attempts	(12.4)		
	Normal anatomical identification of vein		410	Overall	(9.8)		
		87	All Cases	Failed	(12)		
				Overall	(9.7)		
				Misplacement	49 (6)		
				Arterial puncture	30 (3.7)		
				Pnemothorax	12 (1.5)		
				Mediastinal haematoma	5 (0.6)		
				Patrents with >1 complication	1.9		
				Failure to pass catheter	28 (28)		
Gualtieri (1995)[120]	Anatomical landmark	44	12	Overall	11 (4)	Previously inexperienced with <30 successful attempts	
				All minor – arterial puncture, haematoma, malposition			
				Arterial puncture			
				Arterial puncture			
	Ultrasound	92	23	with seeker needle	1 (4)		
Tripathi (1996)[19]	Insertion point on coracoclavicular line	100	205		4 (1.9)	Authors only (experienced)	

Table 6.2 Subclavian vein catheterisation by the infraclavicular approach – results and complications.

Author and year	Success rate (%)	No. of cases	Complications: Type	Complications: No. (%)	Personnel	Comments
Yoffa (1965)[8]	97.6	130	None		Author only	Successful venepuncture at first attempt in 80% of cases
Christensen *et al.* (1967)[24]	38	21	Subclavian artery puncture	1 (4.7)	Experienced surgeons	Supraclavicular route attempted only after failure by infraclavicular route
			Pneumothorax	1 (4.7)		
			Subcutaneous emphysema	1 (4.7)		
Freeman (1968)[121]	99	300	Arterial puncture	2 (0.6)		
			Pneumothorax	3 (1.0)		
Defalque and Nord (1970)[122]	98.9	1500	Pneumothorax	4 (0.26)		
			Haematoma	1 (0.06)		
James and Myers (1973)[14]	95	3000	Overall	337 (11.2)		Experienced or supervised
			Major complication	36 (1.2)		
			Subclavian thrombophlebitis	2 (0.06)		
			Haemorrhage	2 (0.06)		
			Air embolus	1 (0.03)		
			Pneumothorax	12 (0.4)		
			Hydrothorax	3 (0.09)		
			Arteriovenous fistula	1 (0.03)		
Brahos (1977)[15]	95	R 68	Unable to thread catheter	4 (4)		Residents supervised by author
		L 32	Malposition of catheter	1 (1)		
			Arterial puncture	1 (1)		
			Pneumothorax	1 (1)		
Haapaniemi and Slatis (1974)[16]	85.4	First 171	Overall	30 (5)		
	97	Later 429	Malposition	10 (1.7)		
			Arterial puncture	4 (0.6)		
			Pneumothorax	2 (0.3)		
			Haematoma	4 (0.6)		
			Local infection	6 (0.9)		
			Sepsis	3 (0.5)		
			Thrombophlebitis	3 (0.5)		
			Puncture of thoracic duct	6 (0.9)		
			Air embolism	1 (0.2)		
Nevarre and Domingo (1997)[9]	97.8	178	Pneuomothorax	1	Author only	45 referred by other operators who had failed to cannulate through other routes
			Malposition	1		
			Could not thread catheter	1		
			Overall	0.56%		

L, R, left, right, side.

Table 6.3 Complications of subclavian venous catheterisation: case reports.

Pleural space and lung	
	Delayed pneumothorax
	Bilateral pneumothorax
	Hydrothorax
	Bilateral hydrothorax
	Contralateral haemothorax
	Contralateral effusion, venopulmonary fistula
	Puncture of trachea
	Airway obstruction
Vascular	
	Puncture of aorta
	Puncture of pulmonary artery
	Puncture of intercostal artery
	Arteriovenous fistula
	Benign intracranial hypertension
	Spurious central venous pressure measurement
Heart and mediastinum	
	Cardiac tamponade
	Perforation of heart by guide-wire
	Pneumomediastinum
	Arrhythmia
Lymphatic system	
	Laceration of thoracic duct
	Lymphatic fistula
	Lymph leak after venepuncture on right
Neurological	
	Phrenic nerve paralysis
	Diaphragmatic paralysis
	Recurrent laryngeal nerve paralysis
	Brown-Sequard syndrome
	Brachial plexus injury
	Unsuspected cerebral perfusion
	Blindness
Air embolus	
Infection	Osteomyelitis of ribs
	Osteomyelitis of clavicle
	Breast 'abscess'
Miscellaneous	
	Intravascular foreign body
	Intravascular knot formation
	Catheter embolus
	Contact dermatitis

References

1. Aubaniac R. L'injection intraveineuse sousclaviculaire; advantages et technique. Presse Médicale 1952; **60**:1456.
2. Wilson JN, Grow JB, Demong CV, Prevedel AE, Owens JC. Central venous pressure in optimal blood volume maintenance. Archives of Surgery 1962; **85**:563.
3. Mobin-Uddin K, Smith PE, Lombardo C, Jude J. Percutaneous intracardiac pacing through the subclavian vein. Journal of Thoracic and Cardiovascular Surgery 1967; **54**:545.
4. Vellani CW, Tildesley G, Davies LG. Endocardial pacing: a percutaneous method using the subclavian vein. British Heart Journal 1969; **31**:106.
5. Lemole GM, Soulen RL, Swartz BE. Technique of rapid pulmonary angiography by percutaneous subclavian vein catheterization. Radiology 1971; **100**:179.
6. Defalque RJ. The subclavian route. A critical review of the literature up to 1970. Anaesthesist 1972; **21**:325.
7. Dudrick SJD, Wilmore DW, Vars HM, Rhoads JE. Can intravenous feeding as the sole means of nutrition support growth in the child and restore weight loss in an adult. Annals of Surgery 1969; **169**:974.
8. Yoffa D. Supraclavicular subclavian venepuncture and catheterisation. Lancet 1965; **2**:614.
9. Nevarre DR, Domingo OH. Supraclavicular approach to subclavian catheterization: review of the literature and results of 178 attempts by the same operator. Journal of Trauma 1997; **42**:305.
10. Lockwood AH. Percutaneous subclavian vein catheterisation: too much of a good thing? Archives of Internal Medicine 1984; **144**:1407.
11. Morgan WW, Harkins GA. Percutaneous introduction of long-term indwelling venous catheters in infants. Journal of Pediatric Surgery 1972; **7**:538.
12. Groff DB, Ahmed N. Subclavian vein catheterization in the infant. Journal of Pediatric Surgery 1974; **9**:171.
13. Mogil RA, Delaurentis DA, Rosemond GP. The infraclavicular venepuncture. Archives of Surgery 1967; **95**:320.
14. James PM, Myers RT. Central venous pressure monitoring: complications and a new technic. American Surgeon 1973; **39**:75.
15. Brahos GJ. Central venous catheterization via the supraclavicular approach. Journal of Trauma 1977; **17**:872.
16. Haapaniemi L, Slatis P. Supraclavicular catheterisation of the superior vena cava. Acta Anaesthesiologica Scandinavica 1974; **18**:12.
17. Tofield JJ. A safer technique of percutaneous catheterisation of the subclavian vein. Surgery, Gynecology and Obstetrics 1969; **128**:1069.
18. Untracht SH. Axillary artery as a landmark in cannulating the subclavian vein. Surgery, Gynecology and Obstetrics 1988; **166**:565.
19. Tripathi M, Tripathi M. Subclavian vein cannulation: an approach with definite landmarks. Annals of Thoracic Surgery 1996; **61**:238.
20. Sterner S, Plummer DW, Clinton J, Ruiz E. A comparison of the supraclavicular approach and the infraclavicular approach for subclavian vein catheterization. Annals of Emergency Medicine 1986; **15**:421.
21. Malatinsky J, Faybik M, Griffith M, Majek M, Samel M. Venepuncture, catheterization and failure to position correctly during central venous cannulation. Resuscitation 1983; **10**:259.
22. Dronen S, Thompson B, Nowak R, Tomlanovich M. Subclavian vein catheterization during cardiopulmonary resuscitation. Journal of the American Medical Association 1982; **247**:3227.
23. Davidson JT, Ben-Hur N, Nathen H. Subclavian venepuncture. Lancet 1963; **2**:1139.
24. Christensen KH, Nerstrom B, Baden H. Complications of percutaneous catheterisation of the subclavian vein in 129 cases. Acta Chirurgica Scandinavica 1967; **133**:615.
25. Borja AR, Hinshaw JR. A safe way to perform infraclavicular subclavian vein catheterisation. Surgery, Gynecology and Obstetrics 1970; **130**:673.
26. Jesseph JM, Conces DJ, Augustyn GT. Patient positioning for subclavian vein catheterization. Archives of Surgery 1987; **122**:1207.
27. Malatinsky J, Kadlic T, Majek M, Samel M. Misplacement and loop formation of central venous catheters. Acta Anaesthesiologica Scandinavica 1976; **20**:237.
28. Padberg FT, Ruggiero J, Blackburn GL, Bistrian BR. Central venous catheterization for parenteral nutrition. Annals of Surgery 1981; **193**:264.
29. Sanchez R, Halck S, Walther-Larsen S, Heslet L. Misplacement of subclavian venous catheters: importance of head position and choice of puncture site. British Journal of Anaesthesia 1990; **64**:632.
30. Matthews NT, Worthley LIG. Immediate problems associated with infraclavicular subclavian catheterisation; a comparison between left and right sides. Anaesthesia and Intensive Care 1982; **10**:113.
31. Eerola R, Kaukinen L, Kaukinen S. Analysis of 13 800 subclavian vein catheterizations. Acta Anaesthesiologica Scandinavica 1985; **29**:193.
32. Peters JL, Kenning BR, Garrett CPO, Kurzer M. Percutaneous central venous cannulation. British Medical Journal 1980; **281**:618.
33. Machi J, Takeda J, Kakegawa T. Safe jugular and subclavian venipuncture under ultrasonographic guidance. American Journal of Surgery 1987; **153**:321.
34. Kawamura R, Okabe M, Namikawa K. Subclavian vein puncture under ultrasonic guidance. Journal of Parenteral and Enteral Nutrition 1987; **11**:505.
35. Nolse C, Nielsen L, Karstrup S, Lauritsen K. Ultrasonically guided subclavian vein catheterization. Acta Radiologica 1989; **30**:108.

36. Slezak FA, Williams GB. Delayed pneumothorax: a complication of subclavian vein catheterization. Journal of Parenteral and Enteral Nutrition 1984; **10**:542.
37. Cronen MC, Cronen PW, Arino P, Ellis K. Delayed pneumothorax after subclavian vein catheterization and positive pressure ventilation. British Journal of Anaesthesia 1991; **67**:480.
38. Mitchell A, Steer H. Late appearance of pneumothorax after subclavian vein catheterisation: an anaesthetic hazard. British Medical Journal 1980; **281**:1339.
39. Singleton RJ, Webb RK, Ludbrook GL, Fox MA. Problems associated with vascular access; an analysis of 2000 incident reports. Anaesthesia and Intensive Care 1993; **21**:664.
40. Williamson JA, Webb RK, Van der Walt JH. Pneumothorax: an analysis of 2000 incident reports. Anaesthesia and Intensive Care 1993; **21**:642.
41. Spiliotis J, Kordossis T, Kalfarentzos F. The incidence of delayed pneumothorax as a complication of subclavian vein catheterization. British Journal of Clinical Practice 1992; **46**:171.
42. Schorlemmer GR, Khouri RK, Murray GF, Johnson G. Bilateral pneumothoraces secondary to iatrogenic buffalo chest. An unusual complication of median sternotomy and subclavian vein catheterization. Annals of Surgery 1984; **199**:372.
43. Rudge CJ, Bewick M, McColl I. Hydrothorax after central venous catheterization. British Medical Journal 1973; **3**:23.
44. Naguib M, Farag N, Joshi RN. Bilateral hydrothorax and hydromediastinum after a subclavian line insertion. Canadian Anaesthetists Society Journal 1985; **32**:412.
45. Bardosi L, Mostafa SM, Wilkes RG, Wenstone R. Contralateral haemothorax: a late complication of subclavian vein cannulation. British Journal of Anaesthesia 1988; **60**:463.
46. Tayama K, Inoue T, Yokoyama H, Yano T, Ichinose Y. Late development of hydrothorax induced by a central venous catheter: report of a case. Surgery Today 1996; **26**:837.
47. Harrer J, Brtko M, Zacek P, Knap J. Hemothorax – a complication of subclavian vein cannulation. Acta Medica (Hradec Kralove) 1997; **40**:21.
48. Ciment LM, Rotbart A, Galbut RN. Contralateral effusions secondary to subclavian venous catheters. Report of two cases. Chest 1988; **93**:926.
49. Armstrong CW, Mayhall CG. Contralateral hydrothorax following subclavian catheter replacement using a guidewire. Chest 1988; **94**:231.
50. Demey HE, Colemont LJ, Hartoko TJ, *et al.* Venopulmonary fistula: a rare complication of central venous catheterization. Journal of Parenteral and Enteral Nutrition 1982; **11**:580.
51. Breen MT, Kageler WV. Puncture of the trachea during catheterization of the subclavian vein. New England Journal of Medicine 1989; **320**:1148.
52. O'Leary AM. Acute airway obstruction due to arterial puncture during percutaneous central venous cannulation of the subclavian vein. Anesthesiology 1990; **75**:780.
53. Childs D, Wilkes RG. Puncture of the ascending aorta – a complication of subclavian venous cannulation. Anaesthesia 1986; **41**:331.
54. Hirsch NP, Robinson PN. Pulmonary artery puncture following subclavian venous cannulation. Anaesthesia 1984; **39**:727.
55. Bergmann J, Gok Y, Smague E. Haemothorax caused by an injury of the first intercostal artery after the trial of a vena subclavian aspiration. Der Anaesthetist 1984; **33**:592.
56. Hagley SR. Subclavian arteriovenous fistula from central venous catheterisation. Anaesthesia and Intensive Care 1985; **13**:103.
57. Amaral JF, Grigoriev VE, Dorfman GS, Carney WI. Vertebral artery pseudoaneurysm. Archives of Surgery 1990; **125**:546.
58. Rotellar C. Benign intracranial hypertension: a complication of subclavian vein catheterization and arteriovenous fistula. American Journal of Kidney Disease 1987; **9**:242.
59. Barrowcliffe MP. Spurious central venous pressure. Anaesthesia 1987; **42**:293.
60. Nakamura T, Nakashima Y, Yu K, *et al.* Iatrogenic arteriovenous fistula of the internal mammary artery. Transcatheter intravascular coil occlusion. Archives of Internal Medicine 1985; **145**:140.
61. Giroud D, Goy JJ. Pacemaker malfunction due to subcutaneous emphysema. International Journal of Cardiology 1990; **26**:234.
62. Hoka S, Murakami M, Nagata T, *et al.* Unusual placement of a central venous catheter. Journal of Anesthesia 1995; **9**:115.
63. Walden FM. Subclavian aneurysm causing brachial plexus injury after removal of a subclavian catheter. British Journal of Anaesthesia 1997; **79**:807.
64. Robinson JF, Robinson WA, Cohn A, Garg K, Armstrong JD. Perforation of the great vessels during central venous line placement. Archives of Internal Medicine 1995; **155**:1225.
65. Mercer-Jones MA, Wenstone R, Hershman MJ. Fatal subclavian artery haemorrhage. A complication of subclavian vein catheterisation. Anaesthesia 1995; **50**:640.
66. Fourestie V, Godeau D, Lejonc JL, Schaeffer A. Left innominate stenosis as a late complication of central venous catheterization. Chest 1985; **88**:636.
67. Dosios TJ, Magovern GJ, Gay TC, Joyner CR. Cardiac tamponade complicating percutaneous catheterization of subclavian vein. Surgery 1975; **78**:261.
68. Adar R, Mozes M. Fatal complications of central venous catheter. British Medical Journal 1971; **3**:746.
69. Defalque RJ. Fatal complication of subclavian catheter. Canadian Anaesthetists Society Journal 1971; **18**:681.
70. James OF, Tredrea CR. Cardiac tamponade caused by caval catheter – a radiological demonstration of an unusual complication. Anaesthesia and Intensive Care 1979; **7**:174.
71. Blake PG, Uldall R. Cardiac perforation by a guide wire during subclavian catheter insertion. International Journal of Artificial Organs 1989; **12**:111.

72. Vaziri ND, Maksy M, Lewis M, Martin D, Edwards K. Massive mediastinal hematoma caused by a double lumen subclavian catheter. Artificial Organs 1984; **8**:223.
73. Maschke SP, Rogove HJ. Cardiac tamponade associated with a multilumen central venous catheter. Critical Care Medicine 1984; **12**:611.
74. Hammond DI. The 'ring around the artery' sign in pneumomediastinum. Journal of the Canadian Association of Radiologists 1984; **35**:88.
75. Adar R, Mozes M. Hydromediastinum. Journal of the American Medical Association 1970; **214**:372.
76. Ng YC, Walls J. Lymphatic fistula after subclavian vein cannulation. British Medical Journal 1983; **287**:1264.
77. Ryan DW. Lymph leakage following catheterization of the right subclavian vein. Anesthesia and Analgesia 1978; **57**:123.
78. Obel IWP. Transient phrenic-nerve paralysis following subclavian venipuncture. Anesthesiology 1970; **33**:369.
79. Lip GYH, Jane-Hogg K. Permanent phrenic nerve palsy: a rare complication of pacemaker insertion. British Journal of Cardiology, 1994; **1**:275.
80. Epstein EJ, Quereshi MSA, Wright JS. Diaphragmatic paralysis after supraclavicular puncture of subclavian vein. British Medical Journal 1976; **1**:693.
81. Copperman YJ, Daiser M, Samuel Y, *et al.* Recurrent laryngeal nerve paralysis following pacemaker introduction. Pacing and Clinical Electrophysiology 1982; **5**:505.
82. Koehler PJ, Wijngaard PRA. Brown-Sequard syndrome due to spinal cord infarction after subclavian vein catheterisation. Lancet 1986; **2**:914.
83. Bastani B, Bolton WK, Westervelt FB. Transient paralysis of upper extremity after percutaneous cannulation of the subclavian vein for hemodialysis. American Journal of Kidney Disease 1987; **10**:376.
84. Joyce DA, Stewart Wynne EG. Brachial plexopathy complicating central venous catheter insertion. Medical Journal of Australia 1983; **1**:82.
85. Trentman TL, Rome JD, Messick JM. Brachial plexus neuropathy following attempt at subclavian vein catheterization. Case report. Regional Anesthesia 1996; **21**:163.
86. Klein OH, Segni ED, Kaplinsky E. Unsuspected cerebral perfusion. Chest 1978; **74**:109.
87. Acalovschi I, Corbaciu D, Paraianu I. Cortical blindness after subclavian catheterization. Journal of Parenteral and Enteral Nutrition 1988; **12**:526.
88. Coppa GF, Gouge TH, Hoffstatter SR. Air embolism: a lethal but preventable complication of subclavian vein catheterization. Journal of Parenteral and Enteral Nutrition 1981; **5**:166.
89. Kloosterboer TB, Springman SR, Coursin DB. Subclavian vein catheter as a source of air emboli in the sitting position. Anesthesiology 1986; **64**:411.
90. Kuhn M, Fitting JW, Levenberger P. Acute pulmonary edema caused by venous air embolism after removal of a subclavian catheter. Chest 1987; **92**:364.
91. Flanagan JP, Gradisar JA, Gross RJ, Kelly TR. Air embolus. A lethal complication of subclavian venipuncture. New England Journal of Medicine 1969; **281**:488.
92. Aulenbacher CE. Hydrothorax from subclavian vein catheterization. Journal of the American Medical Association 1970; **214**:372.
93. Johnson CL, Lazarchick J, Lynn HB. Subclavian venipuncture: preventable complications. Report of two cases. Mayo Clinic Proceedings 1970; **45**:712.
94. Levinsky WJ. Fatal air embolism during insertion of CVP monitoring apparatus. Journal of the American Medical Association 1969; **209**:1721.
95. Fitchet A, Fitzpatrick AP. Central venous air embolism causing pulmonary oedema mimicking left ventricular failure. British Medical Journal 1998; **316**:604.
96. Rosenfeld LE. Osteomyelitis of the first rib presenting as a cold abscess nine months after subclavian venous catheterization. Pacing and Clinical Electrophysiology 1985; **8**:897.
97. Rowley S, Downing R. Breast 'abscess': an unusual complication of catheterisation of the subclavian vein. British Journal of Radiology 1987; **60**:773.
98. Friedman AP, Velcek FT, Haller JO, Nagar H. Clavicular periostitis: an unusual complication of percutaneous subclavian venous catheterization. Radiology 1983; **148**:692.
99. Klein B, Mittelman M, Katz R, Djaldetti M. Osteomyelitis of both clavicles as a complication of subclavian venipuncture. Chest 1988; **86**:140.
100. Aglas F, Gretler J, Rainer P, Krejs GJ. Sternoclavicular septic arthritis: a rare but serious complication of subclavian venous catheterization. Clinical Rheumatology 1994; **13**:507.
101. Sakaguchi M, Taguchi K, Ishiyama T. Acute pharyngitis, an unusual complication of intravenous hyperalimentation. Journal of Laryngology and Otology 1994; **108**:159.
102. Handsworth JL. An uncommon complication of central venous catheterization. Anaesthesia and Intensive Care 1981; **9**:67.
103. Wang LP, Einarsson E. A complication of subclavian vein catheterisation. Extravascular knotting of a guidewire. Acta Anaesthesiologica Scandinavica 1987; **31**:187.
104. Nicholas F, Fenig J, Richter RM. Knotting of subclavian central venous catheter. Journal of the American Medical Association 1970; **214**:373.
105. Longerbeam JK, Vannix R, Wagner W, Joergenson E. Central venous pressure monitoring. A useful guide to fluid therapy during shock and other forms of cardiovascular stress. American Journal of Surgery 1965; **110**:220.
106. Massumi RA, Ross AM. A traumatic non-surgical technic for removal of broken catheters from cardiac cavities. New England Journal of Medicine 1967; **277**:195.

107. Johansen JR, Jakobsen H. Intravascular foreign body in subclavian vein catheterization by the Seldinger technique. Acta Chirugica Scandinavica 1982; **148**:297.
108. Kjeldsen L. Transvenous misplacement and loop formation of spring guide wire. Anaesthesia 1987; **42**:216.
109. Guin JD, Hutchins L, Johnson JL. Contact dermatitis from a subclavian catheter. International Journal of Dermatology 1990; **29**:58.
110. Walker C, Jackson D, Dolan S. The potential for extravasation using a new five lumen catheter [letter]. Anaesthesia 1997; **52**:716.
111. Ramsden WH, Cohen AT, Blanshard KS. Case report: central venous catheter fracture due to compression between the clavicle and first rib. Clinical Radiology 1995; **50**:59.
112. Smith BE, Modell JH, Gaub ML, and Moya F. Complications of subclavian vein catheterisation. Archives of Surgery 1965; **90**:228.
113. Defalque RJ. Subclavian venipuncture – a review. Anesthesia and Analgesia: Current Researches 1968; **47**:677.
114. Ryan JA, Abel RM, Abbott WM, *et al.* Catheter complications in total parenteral nutrition. New England Journal of Medicine 1974; **290**:757.
115. Blackett RJ, Bakran A, Bradley JA, Halsall A, Hill GL, McMahon MJ. A prospective study of subclavian vein catheters used exclusively for the purpose of intravenous feeding. British Journal of Surgery 1978; **65**:393.
116. Craig RG, Jones RA, Sproul GJ, Kinyot GE. Alternate methods of central venous system catheterisation. American Surgeon 1968; **34**:131.
117. Feiler EM, de Alva WE. Infraclavicular percutaneous subclavian vein puncture: a safe technic. American Journal of Surgery 1969; **118**:906.
118. Williams RW, McDonald JC. A prospective study of the dangers of central venous pressure monitoring. American Surgeon 1971; **37**:719.
119. Mansfield PF, Hohn DC, Fornage BD, *et al.* Complications and failures of subclavian-vein catheterization. New England Journal of Medicine 1994; **331**:1735.
120. Gualtieri E, Deppe SA, Sipperly ME, Thompson DR. Subclavian venous catheterization: greater success rate for less experienced operators using ultrasound guidance. Critical Care Medicine 1995; **23**:692.
121. Freeman J. Subclavian vein catheterisation. Medical Journal of Australia 1968; **2**:979.
122. Defalque RJ, Nord HJ. Supraclavicular Technik der V. subclavia Punktion fur den Anaesthesisten. Anaesthesist 1970; **19**:197.

7 • The Internal Jugular Vein

PETER LATTO

Introduction

The internal jugular vein is a large vessel which may be used (a) to introduce central venous catheters, (b) to obtain blood samples from infants and young children, or (c) to administer intravenous infusions through short cannulae.

Benotti *et al.*[1] advocated internal jugular vein cannulation for parenteral nutrition and used a subcutaneous tunnel so that the catheter's skin exit site was below the clavicle. Civetta and Gabel[2] introduced Swan–Ganz catheters via the internal jugular vein, using a spinal needle (22 gauge) to locate the vein. Hess and Tarnow[3] described a method for inserting both a central venous and a Swan–Ganz catheter into one internal jugular vein. In the UK, English and his colleagues[4] popularised the use of the internal jugular vein for central venous cannulation. Numerous alternative techniques have been described, sometimes with added refinements. Internal jugular vein cannulation has become more popular recently following reports of serious complications associated with subclavian vein cannulation.

The techniques can be classified as high or low. A high approach has the advantage of minimising the risks of pneumothorax and damage to other structures at the root of the neck.

We have arbitrarily defined the high approach as being at or above a line drawn level with the cricoid cartilage. The head is turned to the side when the line is drawn. This point is close to the apex of the triangle formed by the two heads of the sternomastoid muscle (Figure 7.1). The apex of the triangle formed by the two heads of the muscle is, however, frequently not visible (Figure 7.2). The cricoid cartilage is therefore a much easier landmark to identify in many patients.

A low approach is below the apex of the triangle. The cricoid cartilage is approximately level with the apex of the triangle. Techniques can also be classified as medial, lateral or central, depending upon their relation to the sternomastoid muscle.

Anatomy

The sigmoid sinus passes through the mastoid portion of the temporal bone, emerging from the jugular foramen at the base of the skull as the internal jugular vein. Behind the sternal end of the clavicle it joins the subclavian vein to become the innominate vein. The internal jugular vein dilates at a valve 1 cm above the clavicle.

The internal jugular vein, the carotid artery and the vagus nerve are contained together in the carotid sheath. The internal jugular vein at first lies posterior to the internal carotid artery, before becoming lateral and then anterolateral to the artery. The vein is thus capable of expanding mainly on its lateral aspect to accommodate an increase in blood flow. The lower part of the vein lies behind the junction of the sternal and clavicular insertions of the sternomastoid muscle, loosely attached to the posterior surface of the muscle with fascia. Behind the vein are the prevertebral fascia, the prevertebral muscles, and the cervical transverse processes, and posteriorly, at the root of the neck, are the subclavian artery and its branches, the phrenic and vagus nerves, and the cupola of the pleura. On the left the thoracic duct and on the right the lymphatic duct drain into the junction of the internal jugular and subclavian veins.

The larger right jugular vein is believed to drain most of the blood from the cerebral hemispheres. Blood from the posterior fossa contents drains into the vein on the left.[5]

A number of authors have shown that there is a wide variation in internal jugular vein anatomy in life.[6–8] In one study in 200 patients it was shown that the anatomy was sufficiently aberrant in 8.5% of cases to complicate access when using a blinded method.[6] The vein was not in its predicted position in 5.5% of patients and in another 3% the vein was very small. In another study the vein was shown to lie over the carotid artery in 54% of patients.[8] This information would appear to support the use of a technique that minimises the chance of transfixing the vein. This wide variation in anatomy does not, however, appear to prevent the achievement in experienced hands of high success rates for venous cannulation without the advantage of using ultrasound equipment. The choice of an appropriate technique, appropriate apparatus and a sensible fall-back plan if the first attempt is unsuccessful are all of paramount importance.

Using computed tomography and magnetic resonance techniques it was also demonstrated that the internal jugular vein is located 1.5 cm lateral to the sternal end of the clavicle;[9] it lies parallel to the skin surface of the neck. The mean distance from the skin surface to the axis of the vein at this point is 22.4 mm (in 36 patients). There is a valve in the vein 0.5–2.0 cm above the junction of the subclavian and internal jugular veins.[10] The competence of the valve is important because it prevents retrograde flow of blood to the brain. The valve becomes incompetent if a hole is made in it with a needle. Insertion of a needle near the clavicle could damage the valve. This would be less likely to occur if the needle insertion point is above the cricoid cartilage.

The Site-Rite ultrasound machine (Jade Medical, Reading, UK) has been used to determine vascular anatomy prior to cannulation.[11] It was not used during the actual cannulation as it needs a sterile cover to avoid problems with sepsis. The patients were anaesthetised and placed in a 10° head-down position. There was a wide variation in vein diameter ranging from 5 mm to greater than 20 mm. In 92% of cases the vein was anterolateral to the carotid artery and 1–1.5 cm deep to the skin. In 3% the vein was small and fixed in size; in 1% it was more lateral; in 2% more medial; and in 2% of cases (who had had previous internal jugular vein cannulation) it was absent.

In another study using the Site-Rite an inverse correlation between the diameters of the internal and external jugular veins was demonstrated.[12] Patients were placed in a 10° head-down position and were anaesthetised. It was shown that if the external jugular vein diameter was 7 mm or greater then the internal jugular vein diameter was less than 15 mm. If the external jugular vein diameter was less than 7 mm then the internal jugular vein diameter was greater than 20 mm. It was postulated that because the internal and external veins may communicate, the blood normally passing through one system may be diverted to the other causing an inverse relationship in the size of the two vessels.

In another study the diameter and area of the vein were shown to be influenced by posture in volunteers.[13] The mean anteroposterior diameters of the vein were 6.5 mm and 10.3 mm with the subjects in the flat and 20° head-down positions respectively. Values for the mean area of the veins were 32.8 mm^2 and 70.4 mm^2 in the flat and 20° head-down positions respectively. Intermediate values were found with the subjects in a 10° head-down position. The value of posture in facilitating venepuncture is clearly indicated and this effect should be used whenever there is difficulty in venous cannulation.

There is a wide variation in surface neck anatomy in different patients. The distance between the sternal notch and the cricoid cartilage varies widely. In patients with short, 'bull' necks the distance is much less than in patients with long, 'swan-like' necks. There is more potential for causing trauma to the structures at the root of the neck in patients with short necks.

History

English noted that major advances in cardiac surgery were being made from about 1955 onwards.[14] He believed, however, that it took several years for those involved in these developments to recognise the value and importance of central venous pressure monitoring. At that time pressure transducers were unavailable and the water manometers that were in use had slow response times. Blood replacement was often made on the basis of complicated weighing of swabs rather than on the response to changes in central venous pressure.

There were drawbacks to the use of the arm, subclavian, femoral and external jugular routes. English and his colleagues first elected to use the internal jugular vein in a cardiac patient in whom the vein was observed to be very prominent.[14] The technique developed by this team was published in 1969[4] and has remained in use in their unit with minor modifications. The elective method described by English involved palpating the carotid artery as an aid to venous placement, and variations on this method have stood the test of time. Since 1969 a bewildering number of alternative methods of internal jugular vein cannulation have been described. In this chapter we have attempted to provide guidance on the selection of an internal jugular technique that is firstly as safe as possible, secondly has a high success rate and thirdly is easy both to teach and to learn.

The arm veins continued to be used almost exclusively by the majority of anaesthetists in the UK for a number of years after the internal jugular technique was described by English in 1969. It was normal practice to insert two Drum Cartridges (Venisystems, Sligo, Ireland) into arm veins for management of cardiac anaesthesia. Most anaesthetists in the UK were unable to use any other technique. Cut-downs were required when it proved impossible to cannulate the arm veins and radiographs were taken routinely to establish the position of the tip of the catheters. One of the two catheters frequently failed to function during the cardiac surgical procedures.

The use of the jugular route was slow to catch on and it was rarely used in the UK when the first edition of this book was published in 1981. The introduction of short double- and triple-lumen catheters was a major influence in persuading clinicians to use the internal jugular vein. In our hospital, however, attempts were made to prevent anaesthetists using triple-lumen catheters when these first became available. The rationale for this decision was cost curtailment. Fortunately, common sense eventually prevailed. The same restraints were in operation in other centres in 1990 and the use of three separate long catheter-over-needle devices in one vein resulted in life-threaten-

(a)

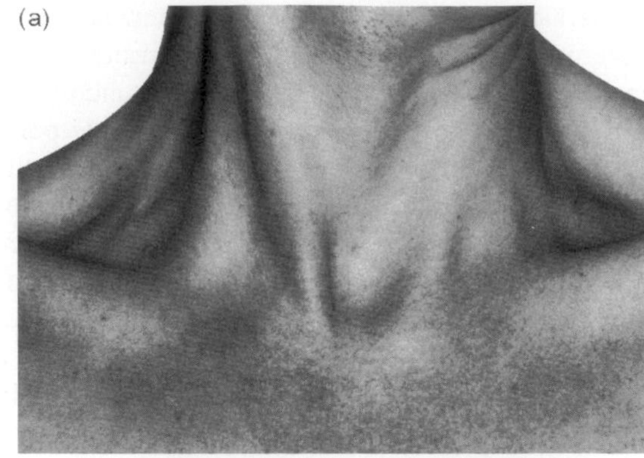

(b)

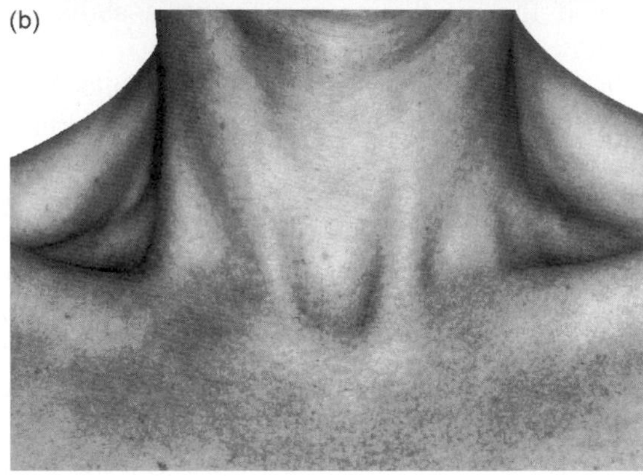

Figure 7.1 Anatomical landmarks – the sternal and clavicular heads of the sternomastoid muscle: (a) with the head turned to the left; (b) from the front.

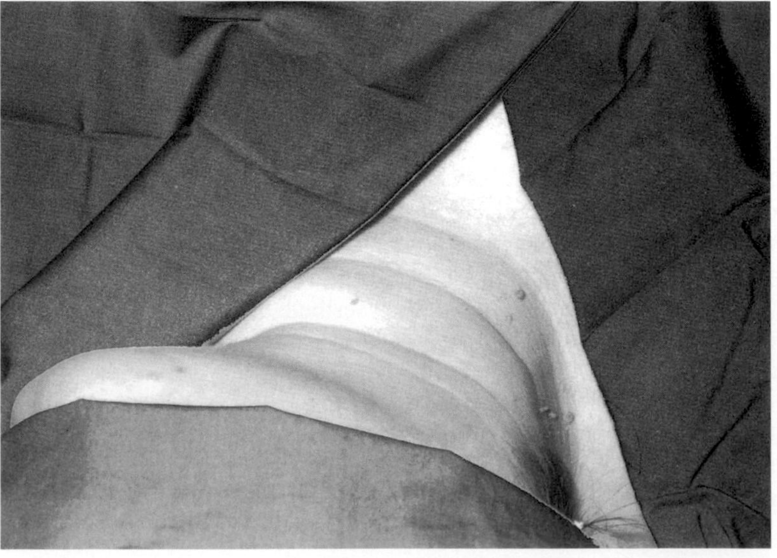

Figure 7.2 In the obese patient, or one with a short 'bull' neck, the sternomastoid muscle may not be readily visible.

ing arterial haemorrhage in a cardiac surgery patient.[15] It was estimated that the additional cost per case at that time of using a triple-lumen catheter was £7; the extra costs incurred in the treatment of complications in the above case exceeded £5000. It was implied that the complication would have been avoided if a Seldinger wire technique had been used.

The internal jugular route is firmly established and is used by most anaesthetists in the majority of patients presenting for major surgical procedures. Indeed, the arm veins are now used only in the most unusual circumstances in cardiac surgery patients.

Technical Considerations

Teaching internal jugular vein cannulation: confirmation that the needle is in the vein

Both Jobes[16,17] and Hayashi *et al.*[18] concluded that it was possible to teach central venous cannulation without influencing the success or complication rate of the technique. Jobes concluded that only a little practice is required to achieve proficiency in needle manipulation. If carefully supervised the trainee should quickly acquire the knowledge of the supervisor. It is certainly important to teach an inherently safe technique and to avoid teaching techniques that are likely to be dangerous. Jobes also concluded that more knowledge is required rather than continued practice to avoid carotid artery puncture. The use of ultrasound allows both the highest success and the lowest complication rates (see below).

It is usually easy for an experienced clinician to recognise that a needle is in the internal jugular vein both by observation of the colour of the blood aspirated into the syringe and by observation of the way the blood comes out of the end of the needle when the syringe is removed. If there is any doubt, and particularly if it is decided that a large introducer is to be placed in the vein, then the pressure in the vein should be measured with a pressure transducer. If no transducer is available then the Finucaine technique can be used.[19] A 60 cm length of sterile tubing is connected to the needle in the vein. The end of the tube is lowered allowing blood to flow into the tubing. The following observations confirm venous placement:

(a) Non-pulsatile filling of the tube.
(b) Venous blood is dark in colour and darker than an arterial sample (particularly if the patient is given additional oxygen).
(c) The tube will not fill if held vertically.
(d) Blood leaves the tubing when the tubing is held vertically.
(e) There is variation in the height of the column of blood with respiration or when a Valsalva manoeuvre is performed.

Most clinicians do not routinely measure the pressure in the vessel before inserting the central venous catheter. They are confident (occasionally mistakenly) that the needle is in a vein and not an artery. Pressure measurements should be made if there is doubt about the situation of the needle. This is of the utmost importance if the clinician intends to insert a sheath or large cannula into the vessel.

Time required

A number of authors have examined the time needed to cannulate the vein. One study compared a catheter-over-needle method with a technique using a seeker needle followed by a Seldinger method.[20] In anaesthetised patients the mean times to cannulate the vein were 28.2 seconds and 141.6 seconds respectively. These differences are of no particular clinical significance (speed is only essential during resuscitation of patients who have suffered cardiac arrest). Cannulating the right or left vein made no difference to the time of insertion. In another study 82% of cannulations were performed in less than 60 seconds; only 18% took from 60 seconds to several minutes.[21]

A different study investigated the time required to perform cut-downs under local anaesthesia on the internal jugular and subclavian veins.[22] The mean time to insert internal jugular catheters was 28.7 minutes compared with 48.5 minutes for the subclavian catheters. The internal jugular catheters were not only quicker and easier to insert but also resulted in smaller and less conspicuous scars.

In an emergency in the absence of suitable apparatus a short catheter (5 cm) can be used to catheterise the internal jugular vein. This is adequate for infusions of drugs and will provide accurate measurements of central venous pressure.[23] Such catheters should not be left *in situ* for longer than necessary because of the risk of air embolus.

Our experience is that internal jugular catheterisation is usually a quick and easy procedure. Nevertheless, insertion can be unpredictably difficult in some patients and in some patients cannulation may not be possible at all.

Number of stabs to cannulate the vein

It is widely recognised that it is sensible to limit the number of stabs required to cannulate the vein. The upper limit is arbitrary and will depend on the size of the needle used, the urgency of the procedure, the availability of alternative veins and the equipment available. Many clinicians allow up to five attempts with a seeker needle but only three with the much larger introducer needle.

It is perhaps surprising that even after successful venepuncture with the seeker needle there may still be problems in locating the vein with the introducer needle[24] (see page 159). Some authors believe that hitting the vein with a seeker needle may induce venospasm.

Other authors have suggested that abandoning venepuncture after only three failed attempts is premature if the carotid artery has not been inadvertently punctured. In a study of patients with coagulopathies, three or more attempts were made in over 40% of 1000 cannulations without apparent serious consequences.[25] In another series one or two punctures were required in 82% of cases and in the others it was stated that more than five attempts at cannulation were rarely required.[21]

Use of ultrasound

Ultrasound has been used to facilitate internal jugular vein cannulation[26–32] and to study different techniques of cannulation.[33]

Use of Doppler ultrasonography facilitates cannulation and results in fewer passes per cannulation, a shorter time to cannulation and a lower incidence of carotid artery puncture.[28,32] Early use of ultrasound enabled localisation of the internal jugular vein; cannulation was subsequently performed blindly.[26–29] It is now possible to use a real-time technique to view the needle as it advances through the neck tissues and then through the vein wall.[31] The method would seem to be useful in facilitating venous cannulation if the anatomy is grossly abnormal.

Some points of practical value have emerged from the use of ultrasound.[27,33] The right internal jugular vein is usually bigger than that on the left. Palpation of the carotid artery and extreme head rotation can decrease vein diameter. The vein is wider below the cricoid cartilage than above it. Head-down tilt increases vein diameter. The mean skin-to-vein distance travelled by the needle was only 2.59 cm in a study comparing 15 different techniques.[33] The findings appear to recommend that palpation of the carotid artery should be performed routinely prior to cannulation and the arterial pulse used as a guide.

In clinical practice venous cannulation is usually a simple procedure and ancillary complex equipment is superfluous. Most clinicians on encountering difficulty with internal jugular vein cannulation would use an alternative vein. Ultrasound would seem to be helpful in cases of special difficulty and in training procedures.

Scott, in a recent editorial, has predicted that ultrasound guidance will soon be a prerequisite both before and during central venous cannulation.[169] In another study ultrasound was used in patients whom there had been previous difficult or failed attempts. Other inclusion criteria included obesity, limited availability of access sites, uncorrected coagulopathy and inability to tolerate the supine position. Successful central venous cannulation was achieved in all 33 patients studied.[170]

Improve your technique: avoid venous transfixion

Mangar *et al.*[34] demonstrated when using a thin-walled Seldinger needle (Arrow International Inc., Reading, Pa, USA) that the vein was transfixed in 50% of cases. The depth of the vein had in all cases been initially determined with a seeker needle.

Thus no blood was demonstrable on advancing the needle in 50% of cases; blood was demonstrable only when withdrawing the needle. Rapid removal of the needle can cause the needle point to pass in error through the posterior wall of the vein, the lumen and the anterior wall. To avoid this problem it was recommended that the needle should be withdrawn slowly while negative pressure is maintained on the syringe. It was stressed that this is a particularly important lesson for trainees to learn.

Ultrasound observations demonstrated that slow needle withdrawal allows the vein to re-expand with the needle tip remaining in the lumen.[35] Ultrasound examination should also demonstrate if the carotid artery is lying behind the internal jugular vein and will thus allow a different angle of approach to be taken in order to minimise the risk of arterial puncture.[36] In another study on 12 volunteers it was recommended that the neck should be kept in as neutral a position as possible (less than 40° rotation) during cannulation in order to decrease the degree of overlap of the vein over the artery.[37]

Later work has shown that the vein is only transfixed in 5% of cases with the main needle (even when the patient is in a horizontal position). A seeker needle was used in all cases and this never transfixed the vein. It was stressed that both the the seeker needle and the main needles should be advanced very slowly.[38] The depth of the vein from the skin surface is indicated by the length of the seeker needle that is visible after venous cannulation. This information should help to prevent the main needle being advanced too far into the tissues and minimise the risk both of pneumothorax and damage to the structures in the root of the neck.

It is imperative to avoid inserting a long needle to its full length if the vein is not entered as the needle is advanced. This approach is a recipe for disaster. The use of a seeker needle should help to prevent this happening and minimise trauma to the structures at the root of the neck. In order to enter the vein it should never be necessary to advance the main needle further than 40 mm from the skin surface (the length of a green seeker needle). Ideally all needles longer than this should be avoided; the use of long catheter-over-needle devices is an invitation to disaster.

Use of multilumen catheters

Some clinicians routinely use two or even three catheters in a single internal jugular vein.[39] This practice is likely to become less common with the introduction of double- and triple-lumen catheters. The disadvantage associated with the use of some multilumen catheters is that the introducer needle may be of large diameter. When using more than one catheter in a vein there is a possibility that the first catheter can be damaged by the second needle.

How to avoid arterial puncture and its sequelae

Choice of equipment

Ryan *et al.* reported a number of fatalities following central venous catheterisation using catheter-over-needle systems.[40] It was recommended that the Seldinger technique should be used in preference to catheter-over-needle devices. A number of authors have described techniques of multiple entry into a single vein.[39,41] There is an increased risk of complications with multiple entry into a single vein.[42] Such techniques were described when multilumen catheters were not always widely available; these catheters are now easily obtainable and should be used in preference to multiple-puncture techniques, which should now be used only when multilumen catheters are unavailable – this is likely to be unusual in the UK. A short, fine needle, narrow wire and a vein dilator should ideally be used for the Seldinger techniques.[43] It was noted that some ‘Seldinger’ kits provided a large needle, a large guide-wire and a large-bore catheter, which clearly removes the advantage of an ideal Seldinger technique. A long needle can cause trauma even when a Seldinger technique is used.[44]

Oshima *et al.* described a technique using a curved needle which prevented transfixion of the vein and penetration of the posterior vein wall.[9] The vein was first located using a seeker needle. The skin insertion point was 0.5 cm cephalad to the notch on the superior surface of the clavicle[45] and the needle was inserted perpendicular to the skin surface. This needle acted as a guide and the curved needle was then introduced at right angles to the neck, parallel to the sagittal plane and advanced until the vein was entered (see Figure 7.10). As soon as the vein was entered the needle was tilted posteriorly. The catheter was inserted using a Seldinger technique. The vein was hit at the first attempt with the seeker needle in 129 of 130 attempts. The vein was entered in 112 patients at the first attempt and at the second attempt in 16 patients. There were no cases of arterial puncture or pneumothorax and it was claimed that the shape of the curved needle means that it penetrates only the anterior wall of the vein.

Choice of technique

In a study on 40 patients it was shown that the vein was entered on advancing a thin-walled needle in half the patients and on withdrawing the needle in the other half.[34] It was recommended that the needle should be withdrawn very slowly so that if the needle has transfixed the vein the tip will enter the lumen as it is retracted. It is clearly better not to penetrate the posterior wall of the vein and cause two punctures of the vessel – particularly because the artery may be lying behind the vein. Similar results have been reported by other authors.[46]

Later work has shown that the vein lumen is entered without transfixion in 95% of cases if the vein is first located with a seeker needle and the main needle is then advanced slowly to the depth of the seeker needle.[38] Transfixion of the vein is more likely to occur when a large needle is used because the tissues will be pushed backwards more easily. The vein was not transfixed with the seeker needle in any patient in the above study.

It is important to use a seeker needle and to have an alternative plan if the vessel is not entered with the first pass of the seeker needle. Any technique in which the needle is pointed in a medial direction is inherently dangerous. Once the vein is entered with the seeker needle, information is available regarding the depth and location of the vein. This information should minimise the risk of arterial puncture with the larger needle. If the vein is not entered with the first pass of the seeker needle important information is also provided indicating where the vein is not located.

Any technique in which the needle is inserted low in the neck runs the risk of causing a pneumothorax or subclavian artery damage; this is particularly likely if a long catheter-over-needle device is used. Techniques where the needle insertion point is high in the neck are preferable. External pressure can be maintained on a puncture site that is higher in the neck but this will not be possible if arterial damage occurs behind the clavicle when a low technique is used. There has been no instance of a fatality following puncture of the carotid artery with a seeker needle;[47] however, fatalities have been reported following the use of large-diameter needles or sheaths.[48,49] It is therefore of vital importance that correct venous placement is accurately confirmed before placing a large-diameter dilator in the vessel.

In one study there was shown to be an increased risk of the jugular vein overlapping the carotid artery when the head was rotated laterally.[37] It was recommended that in order to decrease the risk of arterial puncture the head should be kept in as neutral a position as possible (certainly less than 40° rotation) during cannulation. This advice becomes less relevant if the technique adopted minimises the risk of transfixion of the vein. A technique using lateral head rotation is probably adopted by the majority of anaesthetists. It is sensible to choose routes of venous access which are safe, although the ease of venous access and the incidence of central placement must also be considered. The external jugular vein was advocated as a route that should be used in used in preference to the internal jugular when possible in order to avoid arterial puncture and other serious sequelae.[50]

Occasionally it may not be possible to obtain peripheral venous access for the purpose of fluid replacement, and under these circumstances a large catheter may be placed in the internal jugular or subclavian vein. This should only be done if peripheral venous access is unobtainable because of the obvious potential risks.

Ultrasound-aided cannulation

It is clear that ultrasound (if available) is an important aid to increasing the success of internal jugular puncture and to decreasing the incidence of arterial puncture (see below). In one study the carotid artery was shown to lie completely behind the internal jugular vein in one patient.[51] The skin insertion point of the needle was at the apex of the triangle formed by the sternomastoid muscle. The needle accidentally transfixed the vein and then entered the carotid artery. The needle was withdrawn while aspirating blood into a syringe. Initially bright red arterial blood and then darker venous blood was obtained as the lumen of the vein was entered. The catheter was then successfully advanced into the vein. In a further two patients the artery was shown to be behind the vein at the apex of the sternomastoid triangle: in these patients a needle insertion point was chosen which was caudad to the apex of the triangle. At this point the vein was shown to be lateral rather than in front of the artery. Arterial puncture was avoided in both these patients. Others have recommended that ultrasound should be used routinely.[8] If the vein lies in front of the artery then ultrasound can be used to demonstrate a more favourable skin entry site. A laterally directed needle and avoiding digital compression of the vein (after initial localisation of the artery) should help to avoid arterial puncture in such cases. Attempts should also be made to increase the diameter of the vein to minimise the chance of transfixion. Such manoeuvres are particularly important because it has been shown that the vein lies in front of the artery in 54% of patients.[8] The authors of this study showed that it was not possible to predict on the basis of clinical examination the patients in whom the vein is lateral to the artery (safe) and the patients in whom the vein is in front of the artery (potentially dangerous). In the latter group it is particularly important to avoid transfixing the vein.

The patient

Research into the risks of internal jugular vein catheterisation in patients on heparin is confusing.[52] Peterson found, however, that there was no increased risk of haematoma formation in his hospital when the catheterisation was undertaken by anaesthetists who routinely performed cardiac anaesthesia.[52] It is becoming increasingly common for patients with unstable angina to present for surgery with long-term infusions *in situ* of both heparin and isosorbide dinitrate. Jugular lines are regularly inserted into such patients without problems.

Choice of Technique

It is generally accepted that the incidence and severity of complications associated with cannulation of the internal jugular vein are lower than those for the subclavian vein. Consequently, internal jugular vein cannulation is now being employed with increasing frequency. If cannulation fails on one side, many clinicians then try the vein on the opposite site. This is an advantage not shared by the subclavian approach, where it is generally recommended that attempts should be restricted to one side to avoid the risk of bilateral pneumothorax.

The technique chosen is usually the one with which the operator is most familiar. However, it is not always possible or desirable to employ this approach. Most techniques rely on identifying the sternomastoid muscle and its sternal and clavicular insertions (see Figure 7.1), but this muscle may not be readily visible in obese patients or in patients with short, 'bull' necks (Figure 7.2). In these circumstances a technique may be required which relies on palpation of an additional structure such as the thyroid cartilage,[53] the carotid artery,[54] the internal jugular vein and the carotid artery,[4] or the notch on the superior surface of the medial end of the clavicle.[45]

Techniques in which the needle is inserted well above the clavicle – a high approach – are less likely to cause major complications and are therefore preferable. Nevertheless, a pneumothorax can result from a high approach if a long needle is inserted at a shallow angle to the skin; the use of a short needle makes venous cannulation easier and decreases the frequency of carotid artery puncture.[55] With a low approach it is important to avoid hyperventilation during the cannulation so as to decrease the risk of a pneumothorax. Venous cannulation may be facilitated in the high approach by keeping the lung inflated for a short period or asking the patient to perform a Valsalva manoeuvre, thus distending the vein with minimal risk of pneumothorax.

This chapter sets out a representative selection of previously described techniques for internal jugular vein cannulation. Some of these were originally described only for use in adults, although this does not necessarily preclude their use in children.

Method preferred by authors

In our preferred technique the carotid artery is palpated to facilitate location of the internal jugular vein.[54,63] Despite the original authors' recommendation to use the left side,[54] we find it much easier for a right-handed operator to cannulate the internal jugular vein on the patient's right side.

Method for describing the direction of the needle after positioning the patient for venepuncture

The approximate direction and points of insertion of the needle for some of the techniques that have been described are shown in Figure 7.3. For each technique, the directions have five steps (see Figure 7.4):

1. Identify the point of insertion of the needle on the skin.
2. Place the needle tip on the skin at that point and direct the needle caudally (position A).
3. Swing the needle and syringe laterally or medially as instructed (A to B).
4. Elevate or depress the syringe to an appropriate degree above the coronal plane (the same plane as the surface of the operating table) or the skin (B to C).
5. Penetrate the skin with the needle and advance the needle into the vein. Then remove the syringe and thread the catheter centrally.

Points of management common to all techniques

To avoid unnecessary trauma, the vein can first belocated with a fine needle using the chosen technique. The fine needle is then removed and the larger needle introduced. Alternatively, the fine needle can be left in the vein and the larger needle introduced alongside, using the fine needle as a guide. Saline should be injected through the larger needle after puncturing the skin to clear the needle of any tissue. The catheter is fixed securely to the skin with a stitch to prevent movement. Alternatively, the catheter with its connection is looped down and fixed to the chest to allow free neck movement. A chest X-ray enables the position of the catheter to be determined.

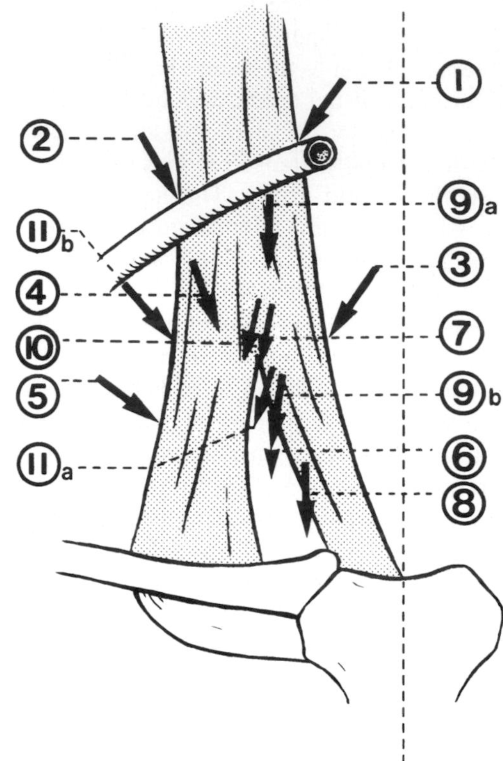

Figure 7.3 A selection of approaches to the catheterisation of the internal jugular vein. 1, Boulanger *et al*. (1976);[53] 2, Brinkman and Costley (1973);[56] 3, Mostert *et al*. (1970);[54] 4, Civetta and Gabel (1972);[2] 5, Jernigan *et al*. (1970);[57] 6, Daily *et al*. (1970);[58] 7, Vaughan and Weygandt (1973);[59] 8, Rao *et al*. (1977);[45] 9a, English *et al*. (1969),[4] elective method; 9b, English *et al*. (1969),[4] alternative method; 10, Prince *et al*. (1976);[60] 11a, Hall and Geefhuysen (1977),[61] elective method; 11b, Hall and Geefhuysen (1977),[61] lternative method. Routes 1, 2, 3, 4 and 5 were originally described for adults; routes 6, 7, 8 and 9 for adults and children; and routes 10 and 11 for children.

How to Maximise the Chances of Success and Minimise the Incidence of Complications

Examine and position the patient before scrubbing up

1. Place patient in a head-down position.
2. Slight extension of the head of the table head may be helpful if the patient has a short or 'bull' neck. Remove the pillow from behind the head. In children place a pillow or bolster behind the shoulders.
3. Mark the position of the cricoid and thyroid cartilages with a marker pen. Draw a line across the neck at the level of proposed catheterisation.
4. Examine the carotid artery to assess ease of palpation (if this is used as part of technique).
5. See if the external jugular vein on same side will be suitable if failure occurs with internal jugular catheterisation.

Equipment

1. Use a seeker needle to locate the vein.[171]
2. Use a short, fine needle and a Seldinger technique.
3. Avoid long catheter-over-needle devices.
4. Avoid using large-diameter needles to puncture the vein initially.
5. Avoid rigid catheters, particularly on the left side.
6. Use ultrasound when possible.

Operator and technique

1. For the Seldinger technique the clinician should use gown and gloves and full aseptic technique. Inexperienced clinicians should initially be carefully supervised.
2. Use a high approach in the neck to minimise risk of damage to the pleura.
3. Stay in the 'safe area' (see Oda's technique). Avoid going too far medially (damage to artery, trachea or oesophagus). Avoid going too far posteriorly (damage to vertebral vessels and nerves).
4. If the patient is conscious perform catheterisation while a Valsalva manoeuvre is performed. If the patient is anaesthetised and ventilated perform venepuncture during inspiration.
5. Limit the number of stabs with both the seeker needle (maximum five) and the definitive needle (maximum three).
6. Have a plan for failure, i.e. try:
   external jugular vein same side
   internal jugular vein other side
   external jugular vein other side.

How to Minimise the Chances of Success and Maximise the Incidence of Complications

Failure to examine and to position the patient before scrubbing up

This makes catheterisation more difficult and may prolong what could in any case be a difficult procedure.

Equipment

1. Failure to use a seeker needle.
2. Use of long catheter over long needle devices.
3. Use of rigid catheters, particularly on the left side.
4. Failure to use ultrasound when available.

Operator and technique

1. Careless scrubbing up and lack of sterile precautions.
2. Failure to use a seeker needle.
3. Use of low approaches in the neck and straying outside the 'safe area', i.e. posteriorly and medially.
4. Unsupervised inexperienced clinicians who persevere beyond the permitted number of attempts.
5. Experienced clinicians who persevere beyond the permitted number of attempts.
6. Not having a plan for failure if the initial attempt fails.

METHODS

A number of methods advocated by various authors are described in the following pages. It is certainly not necessary for the reader to study all these in detail. It is appropriate for an experienced clinician to have expertise in more than one method. The inexperienced clinician should first gain experience and confidence with a single suitable method. We recommend that a method in which the *carotid artery* is used as a primary landmark should be used initially, such as the techniques of Mostert *et al.*[54], Oda *et al.*[21] and Latto *et al.*[63]

Detailed descriptions of four methods that were included in the second edition of this book have been omitted: those of Civetta *et al.*[62], Jernigan *et al.*,[57] Hall and Geefhuysen[61] and Daily *et al.*[58] Four new techniques have been included: those of Latto *et al.*,[63] Messahel and Al-Mazroa,[64] Oshima *et al.*[65] and Willeford and Reitan.[66] These new techniques have one feature in common which commends them: they all use palpation of the carotid artery *plus* utilisation of bony landmarks.

Readers unfamiliar with any technique for internal jugular vein cannulation will need to make a rational choice as to which method to learn first. Others wishing to change and improve their technique or learn a new technique will similarly need to make a rational decision as to which alternative methods to choose. We have not been impressed with techniques that employ palpation or observation of the internal jugular vein as a primary feature.[24] These methods may work well in expert hands but they do not appear to be easy to teach or to learn.

The choice of technique that is learned to start with (preferably a carotid artery plus bony landmark method) should be determined by its ease of use in the average patient and the inherent simplicity of the technique. Most clinicians do not accept techniques that are needlessly complex – they can never remember them.

In Cardiff we have found that the technique in which both the larynx and the carotid artery are palpated has been both easy to teach and free of serious complications. Use of a seeker needle is an important safety feature irrespective of the method that is finally chosen.

HIGH TECHNIQUE: MEDIAL APPROACH

Mostert et al. *(1970)*[54]

Patient category

Adults. The description of the technique by the original authors did not include its application in children, but this does not necessarily exclude its use in this age group.

Advantages and disadvantages

This method relies on palpating the carotid artery, thus eliminating the need to identify the two heads of insertion of the sternomastoid muscle. The method was used successfully under local anaesthesia in conscious, critically ill patients. It was found to be acceptable to patients, who did not find it unduly painful. The stiff catheter was easily threaded beyond the bevel of the needle because the shaft of the needle was pointed in the same axis as the vein. This is the only approach which indicates preference for the vein on the left side, and in which the patient remains horizontal. We have found this method successful in adults under general anaesthesia and in children.

Preferred side

The left side. We find it easier for a right-handed operator to use the vein on the right side.

Position of patient

Place the table in a 25° head-down position. Extend the patient's neck by placing a small towel under the shoulders and turn the head away from the side of the puncture. Place the arms by the sides (Figure 7.4a).

Position of operator

Stand at the head of the patient or on the opposite side to the puncture site (Figure 7.4a).

Equipment used in original description

A 14 gauge outside diameter (OD) needle with a 15 gauge OD 525 mm radio-opaque catheter (catheter-through-needle).

Advice on current equipment

A guide-wire technique is strongly recommended. Long, rigid catheter-over-needle devices should be avoided, especially on the left side.

Anatomical landmarks

The carotid artery and the midpoint of the sternomastoid muscle.

Preparation

Perform the puncture under sterile conditions using local anaesthesia if indicated.

Precautions and recommendations

It is technically easier for a right-handed operator to cannulate the patient's right internal jugular vein.

Point of insertion of needle

The insertion point lies along the medial border of the sternomastoid muscle at its midpoint just lateral to the carotid artery (Figure 7.4b). This is above the level of the cricoid cartilage. In an adult this point should be at least 5 cm above the clavicle.

Initial location of vein with a small needle

Locate the vein with a fine (21 gauge) needle using the following directions. Then using the fine needle as a guide, puncture the skin with the larger needle attached to a saline-filled syringe.

Direction of needle and procedure

Separate the sternomastoid muscle and the common carotid artery with the index and middle fingers of the left hand. The arterial pulsations should be felt by the tips of these fingers. Place the point of the needle at the entry site on the skin and point

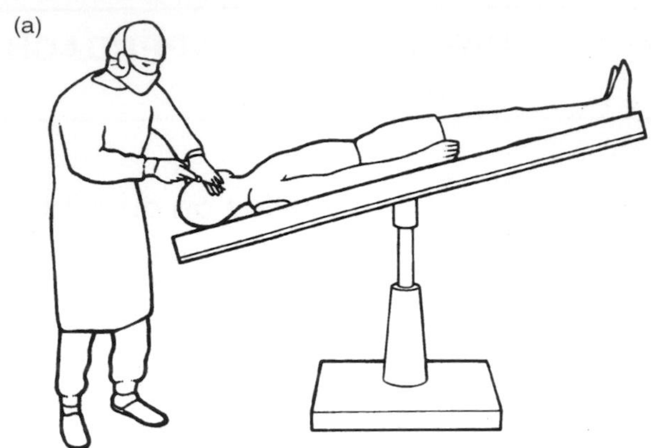

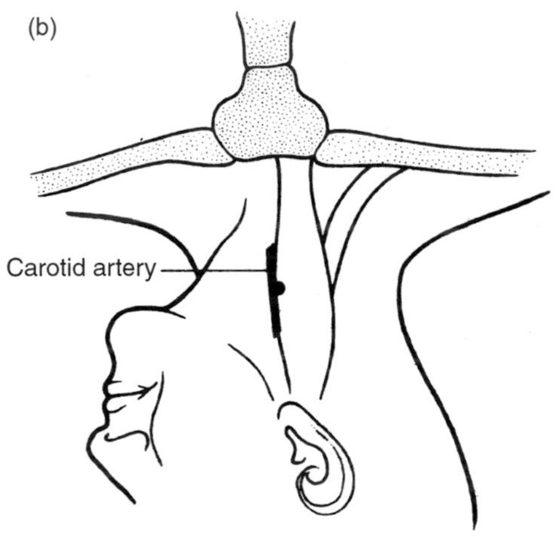

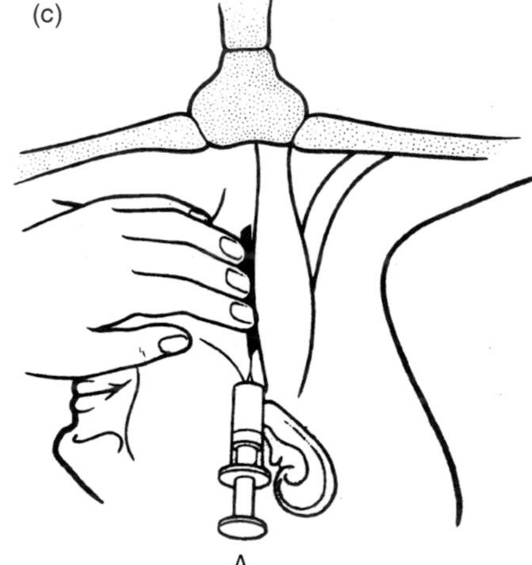

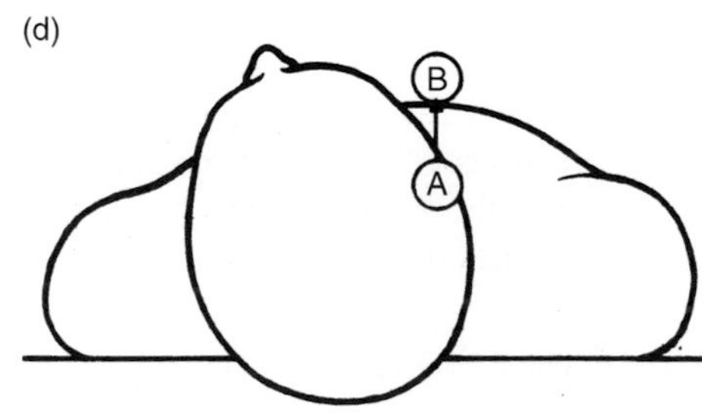

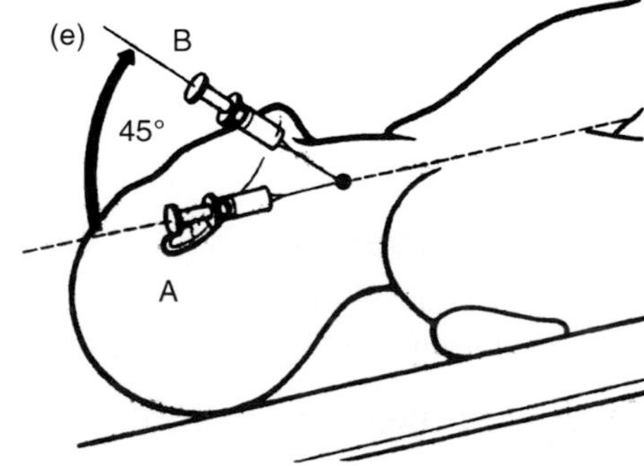

Figure 7.4 High technique, medial approach: Mostert *et al*. (1970).[54]

the needle and syringe caudally (A in Figure 7.4c). Elevate the syringe 45° above the coronal plane (A to B, Figure 7.4d, e). Swing the needle and syringe to point the needle towards the junction of the medial and middle thirds of the ipsilateral clavicle. Advance the needle, maintaining a slight negative pressure in the syringe until the vein is entered. *We prefer to keep the needle in the midline or pointing only slightly laterally as recommended by Hermosura and his colleagues.*[67] On some occasions the vein may be transfixed and the lumen is entered only when the needle is slowly withdrawn. Once the lumen is entered remove the syringe and thread the wire centrally. Then remove the needle from the vein and thread the catheter centrally.

Success rate

A success rate of 97.7% was reported in 133 patients aged 15–81 years (130 out of 133). On three occasions the catheter could not be advanced beyond the hub of the needle and the subclavian vein was used instead.

Complications

The carotid artery was punctured twice (1.5%). There was a 34.5% incidence of tenderness at the catheter site when this was examined 24 hours after removal of the catheter. The incidence of tenderness was greater in patients in whom the catheter had been left *in situ* for at least 36 hours.

HIGH TECHNIQUE: MEDIAL APPROACH

Latto et al. *(1992)*[63]

Patient category

Adults. The description of the technique by the original authors did not include its application in children. The authors have, however, used the method successfully on children since publication of the original paper.

Advantages and disadvantages

Many techniques advocate palpation of the carotid artery. The artery is, however, not always easy to feel and indeed may be impalpable. This technique combines palpation of the artery (when possible) with palpation of the lateral border of the larynx (easy to feel, and a constant landmark). The technique can be used both when it is not possible to turn the head to the side and with the patient in a horizontal position. The technique can also be used successfully when the artery is impossible or difficult to feel. Before starting it is important to draw a cross on the skin; this indicates the insertion point of the needle.

Preferred side

The right side.

Position of patient

Place the table in a 15° head-down position. Remove the pillow and extend the patient's neck approximately 10° by adjusting the end of the table. Turn the head of the patient to the left. Both arms are placed by the sides.

Position of operator

Stand at the head of the patient.

Equipment used in the original description

Lignocaine was injected subcutaneously. A 21 gauge seeker needle was used to locate the vein. The catheter was then inserted into the vein using an 18 gauge needle and a Seldinger technique. All the patients were awake during the procedure.

Advice on current equipment

A seeker needle should be used to locate the vein; then a guide-wire technique is strongly recommended. A suitable 12 cm triple-lumen catheter should be used if indicated. Long, rigid catheter-over-needle devices should be avoided, especially on the left side.

Anatomical landmarks and skin markings

The patient should be carefully examined *before* starting the procedure. The positions of the suprasternal notch, the cricoid cartilage and the top of the thyroid cartilages are marked on the skin (Figure 7.5a). A transverse line is then drawn across the neck between the cricoid and the top of the thyroid cartilages. This transverse line is drawn parallel to the end of the table (D in Figure 7.5a).

The position of the carotid artery is then determined. The pads of the fingers of the left hand are placed on the lateral surface of the larynx with the tips of the fingers pointing vertically backwards. If the carotid artery is felt under the finger-tips (which happens in most cases) then a vertical line is drawn just lateral to the artery at right angles to the transverse line (E in Figure 7.5b). If the artery is not palpable then the finger-tips are moved further laterally in an attempt to palpate the artery and a vertical line is drawn lateral to the artery. If the artery cannot be palpated the vertical line is drawn one finger's-breadth lateral to the larynx. The use of a vertical line has been shown to be a valuable addition to the original technique. The needle is inserted at the point of intersection of the two lines (Figure 7.5c).

Preparation

Perform the puncture under sterile conditions using local anaesthesia if indicated.

Precautions and recommendations

It is technically easier for a right-handed operator to cannulate the internal jugular vein on the right side.

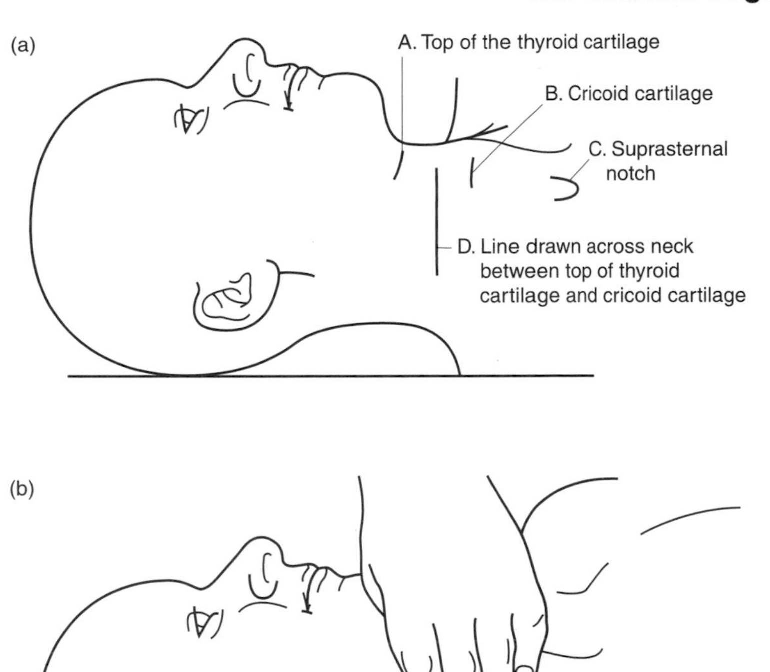

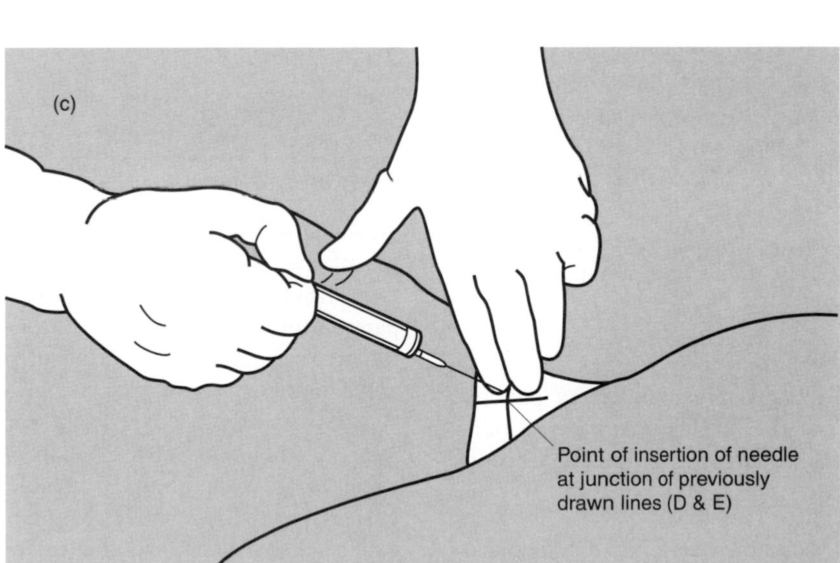

Figure 7.5 High technique, medial approach: Latto *et al.* (1992).[63]

Point of insertion of needle

The point lies at the intersection of the vertical and horizontal lines drawn on the neck (Figure 7.5c).

Initial location of vein with a small needle

Locate the vein with a fine (21 gauge) needle using the following directions. Then using the fine needle as a guide, puncture the skin with the larger needle attached to a saline-filled syringe.

Direction of needle and procedure

Place the fingers of the left hand over the carotid artery. Place the point of the needle at the entry site on the skin and point the syringe and needle caudally. The needle is in the sagittal plane and at 30–40° to the coronal plane. Advance the needle *slowly* maintaining a slight subatmospheric pressure in the syringe until the vein is entered. If the vein is not entered with the first pass of the needle, pull the needle back and readvance it in a more lateral direction (15°, 30°, 45°, 60° or 75° if required). The seeker needle is left in the vein and acts as a guide for the Seldinger needle. The Seldinger needle is then advanced slowly to the same depth and in the same direction as the seeker needle.

Success rate

The results given in Tables 7.1 to 7.3 were obtained when inexperienced registrars used the technique often for the first time. The outcome is likely to be much better in the hands of more experienced doctors. The technique was used successfully in 5 patients in whom the carotid artery was impalpable. The value of identifying and marking reference points *before* draping the patients was commented on by 40% of the operators. It was claimed that this was a safe technique which was easy to learn.

Complications

There were 2 instances of carotid artery puncture using the seeker needle. No case of arterial puncture occurred with the 18 gauge introducing needle.

Comment

This technique is particularly useful if palpation of the carotid artery is used as a method for locating the vein and the artery is either impalpable or difficult to feel. The technique has been used both in infants and in adults who are unable to turn their heads to the side; it has also been used in patients in whom the neck was not extended. The method can therefore be used in patients with cervical injuries.

There is a wide variation in neck anatomy. This method is appropriate for patients with short necks (it gives a high point of needle insertion). For patients with long necks the line across the neck can be drawn level with the cricoid cartilage. This variation works well and makes the technique easier to remember.

Table 7.1 Ease of palpation of the carotid artery with the head facing 45° to the left.

Ease of palpation	Number	%
Impalpable	5	10
Just palpable	24	48
Easily palpable	18	36
Bounding	3	6
Total	50	100

Table 7.2 Location of carotid artery in relation to the larynx.

Carotid artery position	Number	%
Directly below fingers with pads of fingers resting on side of larynx	29	58
One finger's breadth lateral to the above position	15	30
More than one finger's breadth lateral	1	2
Impalpable artery	5	10
Total	50	100

Table 7.3 Number of attempts required to locate the internal jugular vein with the seeker needle and the introducing needle.

Number of attempts	Seeker needle (no.)	Seeker needle (%)	Introducing needle* (no.)	Introducing needle* (%)
1	31	62	41	82
2	14	28	6	12
3	3	6	2	4
4	0		—	
5	2	4	—	
Failure	0	0	1	2
Total	50	100	50	100

* Only three tries allowed.

HIGH TECHNIQUE: MEDIAL APPROACH

Boulanger et al. *(1976)*[53]

Patient category

Adults. The description of the technique by the original authors did not include its application in children, but this does not necessarily exclude its use in this age group.

Advantages and disadvantages

The high approach eliminates the risk of pneumothorax. The needle is pointed laterally, thus greatly decreasing the risk of puncturing the carotid artery. The vein is not transfixed with this method, which is claimed to be easy to teach and to learn. The internal jugular vein is at its widest (13–15 mm diameter) at this point. The method was also used to insert Swan–Ganz catheters.

Preferred side

The right side.

Position of patient

Place the table in a 25° head-down position. Extend the patient's neck by placing a small towel under the shoulder and turn the head away from the side of the puncture. Place the patient's arms by the sides (Figure 7.6a).

Position of operator

Stand at the head of the patient or on the opposite side to the puncture site (Figure 7.6a).

Equipment used in original description

Catheter-through-needle.

Advice on current equipment

A guide-wire technique is strongly recommended. Long, rigid catheter-over-needle devices should be avoided, especially on the left side.

Anatomical landmarks

The sternomastoid muscle, the thyroid cartilage and the external jugular vein.

Preparation

Perform the puncture under sterile conditions using local anaesthesia if indicated.

Precautions and recommendations

If possible, maintain positive intrathoracic pressure during venous cannulation to distend the vein.

Point of insertion of needle

The needle is inserted at the superior border of the thyroid cartilage (level with the fourth cervical vertebra) on the medial border of the sternomastoid muscle (Figure 7.6b).

Initial location of vein with a small needle

Locate the vein with a fine (21 gauge) needle using the following directions. Then using the fine needle as a guide puncture the skin with the larger needle attached to a saline-filled syringe.

Direction of needle and procedure

Pinch the sternomastoid muscle to determine its thickness. Place the point of the needle at the entry site on the skin and point the needle and syringe caudally (A in Figure 7.6c). Then swing the needle and syringe and point the needle laterally to make an angle of approximately 45° with the medial border of the sternomastoid (A to B). Elevate the syringe 10° above the skin (B to C, Figure 7.6d, e). Direct the needle just underneath the sternomastoid, keeping close to its posterior aspect. The needle is directed superficially as if to come out 2 cm beyond the lateral border of the muscle. Maintain a slight negative pressure in the syringe as the needle is advanced. The vein is entered 2–4 cm from the puncture site. On entering the vein, direct the syringe and needle in the axis of the vein (that is, towards the midline) and advance the needle 1–2 cm into the vein. Introduce the wire centrally and remove the needle. Then thread the catheter centrally.

Success rate

A 94% success rate was achieved by nine supervised residents with their first 100 attempted cannulations.

Complications

There was a 2% incidence of puncture of the carotid artery.

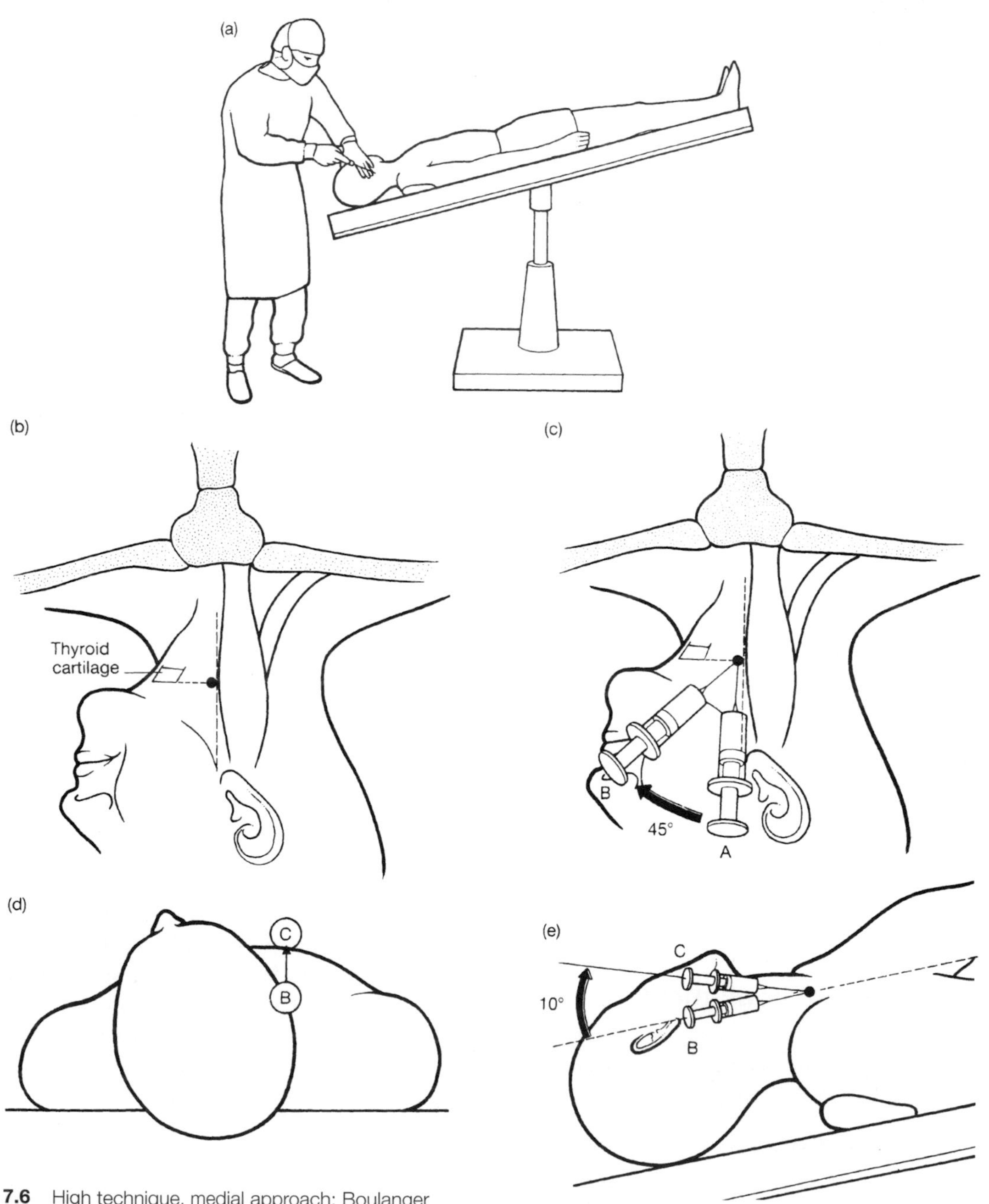

Figure 7.6 High technique, medial approach: Boulanger *et al*. (1976).[53]

HIGH TECHNIQUE: LATERAL APPROACH

Brinkman and Costley (1973)[56]

Patient category

Adults. The description of the technique by the original authors did not include its application in children, but this does not necessarily exclude its use in this age group.

Advantages and disadvantages

The high approach eliminates the risk of a pneumothorax. This technique cannot be used if the external jugular vein is not visible. If the approach via the internal jugular vein fails, the external jugular vein can be cannulated through the same skin puncture. The puncture in the vein wall is completely filled by a catheter outside a needle. This method was developed in response to failures with the method described by Jernigan and his colleagues.[57]

Preferred side

The right side.

Position of patient

Place the table in a 25° head-down position. Extend the patient's neck by placing a small towel under the shoulders and turn the head away from the side of the puncture. Place the patient's arms by the sides (Figure 7.7a).

Position of operator

Stand at the head of the patient (Figure 7.7a).

Equipment used in original description

A 14 gauge 150 mm catheter over long needle.

Advice on current equipment

A guide-wire technique is strongly recommended. Long, rigid catheter-over-needle devices should be avoided, especially on the left side.

Anatomical landmarks

The lateral border of the sternomastoid muscle, the external jugular vein and the sternal notch.

Preparation

Perform the procedure under sterile conditions using local anaesthesia if indicated.

Precautions and recommendations

If possible, maintain positive intrathoracic pressure during venous cannulation to distend the vein.

Point of insertion of needle

Insert the needle at a point along the lateral border of the sternomastoid muscle cephalad to the junction of the external jugular vein and the muscle (Figure 7.7b).

Initial location of vein with a small needle

Locate the vein with a fine (21 gauge) needle using the following directions. Then using the fine needle as a guide, puncture the skin with the larger needle attached to a saline-filled syringe.

Direction of needle and procedure

Place the point of the needle at the entry site on the skin and point the needle and syringe caudally (A in Figure 7.7c). Then swing the needle and syringe and point the needle towards the sternal notch (A to B). Elevate the syringe 10° above the coronal plane (B to C, Figure 7.7d, e). Advance the needle, maintaining a slight negative pressure in the syringe, just beneath the belly of the sternomastoid muscle, aiming towards the sternal notch. The internal jugular vein is usually entered within 5–7 cm. Introduce the wire centrally and remove the needle. Then thread the catheter centrally.

Success rate

The technique was used in 180 punctures. The success rate was not specifically reported.

Complications

The carotid artery was punctured on 4 occasions (2.2%).

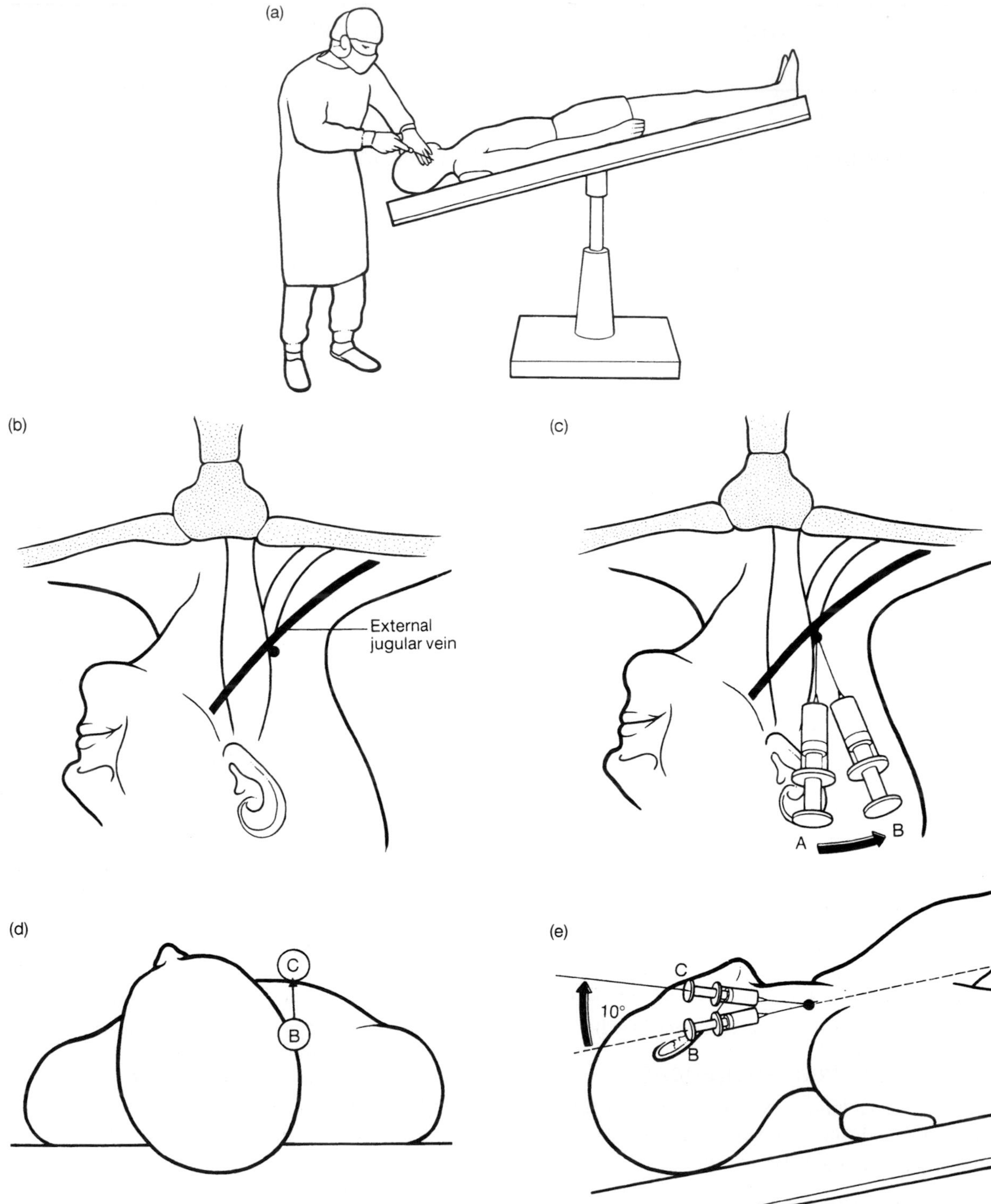

Figure 7.7 High technique, lateral approach: Brinkman and Costley (1973).[56]

HIGH TECHNIQUE: MEDIAL APPROACH

Oda et al. *(1981)*[21]

Patient category

The subjects were 456 consecutive patients aged from less than 6 months to adults.

Advantages and disadvantages

The technique was used successfully in neonates, children and adults. It was used by junior trainees as well as senior anaesthetists. The carotid artery is palpated with the bare hand before skin preparation is undertaken to identify the course and depth of the artery and its lateral wall. Palpation is applied by the finger-tips perpendicular to the carotid artery. The method was used successfully in patients who were in the lateral position.

Preferred side

The right side.

Position of patient

Place the patient in a slightly head-down position. The head is either not rotated or only slightly rotated to the contralateral side. Small children need hyperextension of the neck and a small pillow or towel is placed under the shoulders.

Position of operator

Stand at the head of the table.

Equipment used in original description

Hakko over-the-needle catheters – 18 gauge, 130 mm catheters for adults; 21 gauge, 60 mm or 19 gauge, 50 mm catheters for small children. A 12 or 14 gauge, 80 mm catheter introducer was used for passing cardiac pacemakers or pulmonary artery catheters in adults. A flexible Teflon catheter guide was inserted into the 12, 14 and 18 gauge catheters after removal of the needle to facilitate catheter advancement.

Advice on current equipment

A guide-wire technique is strongly recommended. Long, rigid catheter-over-needle devices should be avoided, especially on the left side.

Anatomical landmarks

The carotid artery and the laryngeal prominence of the thyroid cartilage (the cephalad portion).

Preparation

Perform the puncture under sterile conditions using local anaesthesia if indicated.

Precautions and recommendations

It is technically easier for a right-handed operator to cannulate the patient's right internal jugular vein. Avoid inserting the needle more deeply than the transverse processes of the cervical vertebrae to avoid damage to vertebral vessels and the cervical nerve plexus. Keep the needle in the safe puncture area (Figure 7.8a). Do not make more than five attempts at cannulation to minimise complications.

Point of insertion of needle

The point of insertion lies just lateral to the carotid artery and level with the laryngeal prominence of the thyroid cartilage.

Initial location of vein with a small needle

A fine (21 gauge) needle can be used to locate the vein using the following directions. The fine needle is then removed and the skin punctured with the large needle attached to a saline-filled syringe.

Direction of needle and procedure

Make a small incision in the skin at the needle insertion point. Palpate the right carotid artery with the tips of the fingers of the left hand pointing perpendicularly to the coronal plane (Figure 7.8b). Place the tip of the needle on the skin entry site and point the needle caudally. Then elevate the needle 30–45° to the skin. Advance the needle into the vein. If the initial puncture fails, withdraw the needle and direct subsequent attempts gradually more laterally. Clicks may be noted on penetrating the cervical fascia, carotid sheath and the vein wall.

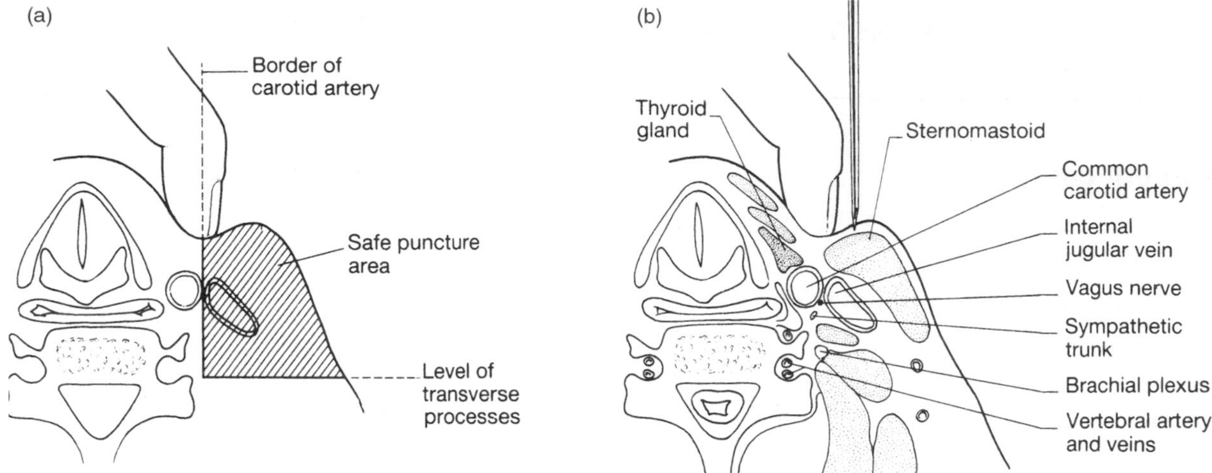

Figure 7.8 Cross-section of the neck. The direction of the fingers during palpation is perpendicular to the coronal plane. The direction of the catheter is parallel with the patient's sagittal plane. The catheter should not be directed medially and should not be advanced deeper than the transverse process of the cervical vertebra. The safe puncture area is also indicated schematically by hatching. Reproduced with kind permission of Oda *et al.* (1981).[21]

Table 7.4 Success rates for Oda's method in favourable clinical circumstances.

Age distribution	Number of cases	Success	Success rate (%)
15 yr–adult	408	396	97.1
5–15 yr	20	18	90.0
1–5 yr	14	13	92.9
6 mo–1 yr	7	6	85.7
Less than 6 mo	7	4	57.1
Total	456	437	95.8

Table 7.5 Success rates for Oda's method in unfavourable clinical circumstances.

	Number of cases	Success	Success rate (%)
Neuroanaesthesia patients (in horizontal position)	46	41	89.1
Patients in preshock state	15	14	93.3
Patients with extreme dehydration	12	11	91.6
Patients in lateral or kidney position	8	8	100
Cannulation with a 14 or 12 gauge catheter	13	11	84.6

Success rate

Success rates in favourable clinical circumstances are shown in Table 7.4; the rates in unfavourable clinical circumstances are shown in Table 7.5.

Complications

There were 5 (1.1%) carotid artery punctures. Haematomas occurred in 2 of these after prolonged cardiopulmonary bypass.

HIGH TECHNIQUE: CENTRAL APPROACH

Sharrock and Fierro (1983)[24]

Patient category

Adults aged 22–95 years. Most were elderly and had either cardiac or respiratory problems.

Advantages and disadvantages

The authors claimed a low incidence of complications and a high success rate. They used a 'no touch' technique which is helpful for asepsis and avoids palpation of the carotid artery with its attendant complications.

Preferred side

The right side.

Position of patient

Place the table in a slightly head-down position. If the vein is seen to collapse on expiration apply more head-down tilt. Turn the patient's head approximately 30° to the left. Examine the neck for venous pulsations. These are usually visible in the middle of the neck beneath the sternomastoid. The vein was located by inspection only.

Position of operator

Stand at the head of the table.

Equipment used in original description

A 22 gauge or 23 gauge seeker needle; a 14F or 8F catheter.

Advice on current equipment

Suitable Seldinger wire equipment.

Anatomical landmarks

The pulsating internal jugular vein.

Preparation

Perform the punctures under sterile conditions using local anaesthesia if indicated. All patients in this series were anaesthetised and ventilated.

Precautions and recommendations

Always use a seeker needle. The fingers of the left hand are placed beneath the body of the mandible to retract the skin and stabilise the neck. Needle insertion should take place during the inspiratory phase of artificial ventilation when the vein is distended. This method should only be used if the vein is visible; if it is not visible use an alternative technique. Macdonald noted that compression and release of the neck with three fingers in the anticipated line of the vein often demonstrated the vein as it refilled.[68] (See also English *et al.*[4]: elective method, page 170.)

Point of insertion of needle

Insert the needle directly over the venous pulsation (in the middle of the neck under the sternomastoid).

Direction of needle and procedure

Place the point of the 23 gauge or 22 gauge seeker needle on the skin entry and point the needle

Table 7.6 Number of needle insertions before successful internal jugular venous entry (a) or cannulation (b).

	No. of patients	%
a) 'Seeker' 22 or 23 gauge needle		
First attempt	186	87.7
Second attempt	14	6.6
Third attempt	4	1.9
> 3 attempts	7	3.3
Failures	1	0.5
Total	212	
(b) 14 F or 8 F catheters		
First attempt	175	82.5
Second attempt	13	6.1
Third attempt	13	6.1
> 3 attempts	7	3.3
Failures	1	0.5
Carotid punctures	3	1.4
Total	212	

caudally. Elevate the syringe to an angle of 45° to the neck. Advance the needle maintaining a slightnegative pressure in the syringe until the vein isentered. Then repeat this procedure using the definitive needle, and thread the catheter centrally.

Success rate

Successful venous cannulation was performed in 210 out of 212 patients (Table 7.6).

Complications

Cartoid artery puncture occurred in 3 patients.

VERY HIGH TECHNIQUE: MEDIAL APPROACH

Messahel and Al-Mazroa (1992)[64]

Patient category

Adults. The description of the technique by the original authors did not include its application in young children, but this does not necessarily exclude its use in this age group.

Advantages and disadvantages

A combination of palpation of the angle of the mandible and palpation of the carotid artery is used. It was claimed that the use of the high technique would avoid major complications. The technique can be used once surgery has started. Conscious patients were easily able to move their necks with the catheter *in situ*.

Preferred side

The right side.

Position of patient

Place the table in a 20° head-down position. Extend the patient's neck by placing a small towel under the shoulders and turn the head to the left. Place both arms by the sides.

Position of operator

Stand at the head of the patient.

Equipment used in the original description

Lignocaine was injected subcutaneously and a 2 mm incision was made in the skin using a pointed scalpel. A seeker needle was used to locate the vein and then the catheter was inserted into the vein using a Seldinger technique.

Advice on current equipment

A guide-wire technique is strongly recommended. A suitable 12 cm triple-lumen catheter should be used if indicated. Long, rigid catheter-over-needle devices should be avoided, especially on the left side.

Anatomical landmarks

The carotid triangle is limited posteriorly by the sternomastoid muscle, superiorly lie the stylohyoid and the posterior belly of the digastric muscle, and anteriorly and inferiorly lies the omohyoid muscle (Figure 7.9a). It was claimed that the triangle was an obvious feature in the non-obese patient and was visible as a small, triangular depression which was most evident when the head was rotated to the other side. The triangle contains the common carotid artery as it bifurcates into its internal and external branches; the internal jugular vein lies lateral to the artery.

Preparation

Perform the puncture under sterile conditions using local anaesthesia if indicated.

Precautions and recommendations

If possible maintain positive intrathoracic pressure during venous cannulation to distend the vein.

Point of insertion of needle

The needle is inserted lateral to the carotid artery and as high as possible and below the angle of the mandible. The point of insertion is 1–1.5 cm from the angle of the mandible.

Initial location of vein with a small

needle

Locate the vein with a fine (21 gauge) needle using the following directions. Then using the fine needle as a guide, puncture the skin with the larger needle attached to a saline-filled syringe.

Direction of needle and procedure

The larger needle is advanced through the 2 mm skin incision. The needle is passed in a caudad direction in the sagittal plane and advanced at 75–85° to the coronal plane (Figure 7.9c). Advance the needle maintaining a slight negative pressure in the syringe. Once the needle enters the vein, remove the syringe and thread the wire centrally. If there is difficulty in threading the wire centrally reduce the angle of the needle to the skin until there is easy passage of the wire. The catheter is attached to an extension tube that is looped round the pinna of the ear. The reported distance between the skin and the vein was 0.5–1 cm.

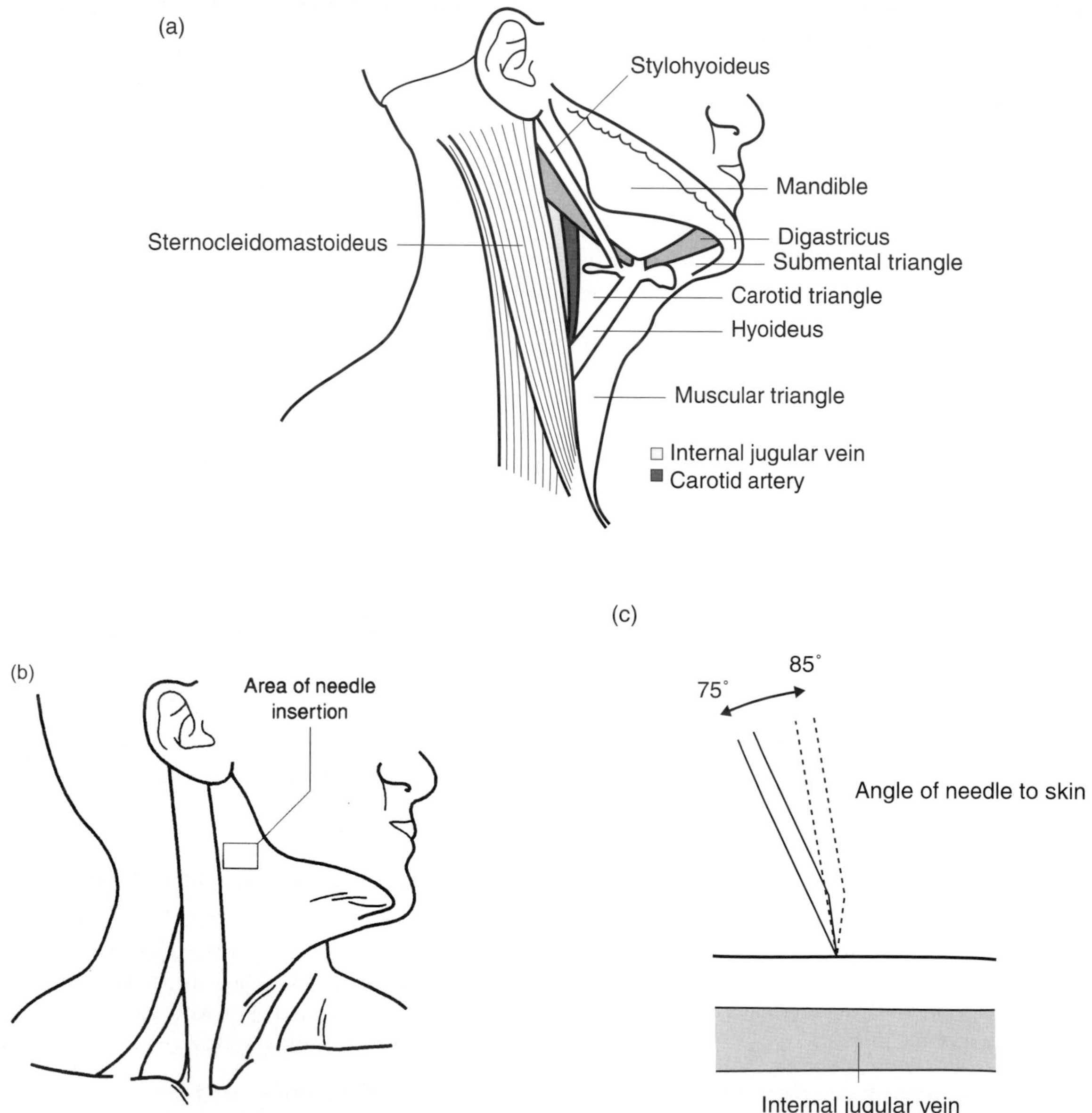

Figure 7.9 (a) Anatomy of the carotid triangle; (b) site of needle insertion; (c) angle of needle during insertion. Reproduced with kind permission of Messahel and Al-Mazroa (1992).[64]

Success rate

First attempt at cannulation was successful in 286 (85.4%) of 335 patients (aged 12–91 years). The remainder of patients were successfully cannulated after a second attempt.

Complications

Catheters were left *in situ* for 1–11 days (average 3.8 days) and there were no complications.

Comment

The authors claimed that the ease of use and lack of complications for this very high approach rendered many other methods obsolete. These authors did not describe the change in their technique when the first pass of the needle was unsuccessful. A high approach is preferable to a low approach. We believe that other techniques where the skin entry point is level with or above the cricoid cartilage are also safe.

HIGH TECHNIQUE: MEDIAL APPROACH

Oshima et al. *(1991)*[65]

Patient category

Adults. The description of the technique by the original authors did not include its application in children, but this does not necessarily exclude its use in this age group.

Advantages and disadvantages

It was noted that the sternomastoid muscle, the carotid artery and the internal jugular vein can all be used as part of techniques to cannulate the internal jugular vein. However, these anatomical structures may be unrecognisable. A technique using bony landmarks was therefore developed. This technique used both palpation of the carotid artery and four bony landmarks. Although three attempts were permitted on each side with the seeker needle no comment was made aboutchange in direction of the needle if the vein was not entered at the first pass. There was no change in the skin entry position if the first attempt failed.

Preferred side

The right side.

Position of patient

Place the table in a 20° head-down position. Extend the patient's neck (if required) by placing a small towel under the shoulders and turn the head to the left. Place the arms by the sides.

Position of operator

The operator stands at the patient's head.

Equipment used in the original description

A 23 gauge (32 mm long) seeker needle was used to locate the vein. The vein was then cannulated with a 16 gauge, 57 mm cannula.

Advice on current equipment

Always use a seeker needle. Then a guide-wire technique is strongly recommended. A suitable 12 cm triple-lumen catheter should be used if indicated. Long, rigid catheter-over-needle devices should be avoided, especially on the left side.

Anatomical landmarks

An axial line level with the cricoid cartilage is drawn across the neck (Figure 7.10). A second line is then drawn from the mastoid process to the medial end of the clavicle, crossing the first line. The notch described by Rao *et al.*[45] on the superior surface of the clavicle (0.25–1 cm from the medial end of the clavicle) is also identified.

Preparation

Perform the puncture under sterile conditions using local anaesthesia if indicated. All punctures in the original description were performed under general anaesthesia.

Precautions and recommendations

If possible maintain positive intrathoracic pressure during venous cannulation to distend the vein. A positive end-expiratory pressure of 2–5 cmH_2O was used by the authors.

Point of insertion of needle

The point of insertion lies at the intersection of the two lines shown in Figure 7.10. The carotid artery was noted to be 1–1.5 cm medial to the insertion point in all patients and was usually beneath the medial border of the sternomastoid muscle. The point of insertion varied but was always between the apex of the triangle formed by the two heads of the sternomastoid and the clavicle.

Initial location of vein with a small needle

Locate the vein with a fine (21 gauge) needle using the following directions. Then using the fine needle as a guide (leave the seeker needle in the vein), puncture the skin with the larger needle attached to a saline-filled syringe. The vein was entered within 3 cm of the skin surface and was usually 1.5–2 cm from the surface.

Direction of needle and procedure

Although the lines and the notch on the superior surface of the clavicle (Figure 7.10) were not marked on the skin in the original description we believe that it would be helpful to do so. The needle is advanced towards the notch on the superior surface of the clavicle at an angle of 30–45° to the coronal plane. Advance the needle maintaining a slight negative pressure in the syringe. Once the needle enters the vein, remove the syringe and thread the wire centrally.

Success rate

A total of 134 patients were prospectively evaluated. The vein on the right side was entered with the seeker needle at the first attempt in 120 patients (89.6%). It was entered at the second attempt in 10 patients. In 4 patients it was not possible to enter the vein at the third attempt. The vein on the left was entered at the first attempt in 3 of these patients but could not be entered after three tries in the fourth patient. In the 133 patients in whom the vein was located with the seeker needle cannulation with the 16 gauge cannula was accomplished within three attempts (range not given). The overall success rate was 99.3%.

Complications

Arterial puncture occurred in 2 patients (it was not clear whether this was with the seeker needle or the main needle).

Comment

This technique has the advantage of relying on bony landmarks. It was noted that the carotid artery was medial to the puncture site in all patients. The technique was used in anaesthetised paralysed patients and it was suggested that the technique might be useful in cardiac arrest patients. These authors did not describe the change in their technique when the first pass of the needle was unsuccessful. We believe that it is essential to have a sensible plan if the first pass with any needle fails to locate the vein. They suggested that the four failures on the right side might be due to variation in the anatomical relationship between the carotid artery and the internal jugular vein.

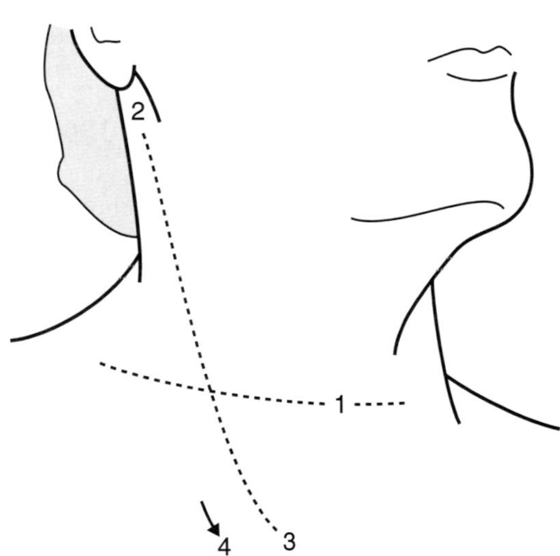

Figure 7.10 High technique, medial approach: Oshima *et al.* (1991).[65] 1, Line drawn across neck level with cricoid cartilage; 2, mastoid process; 3, medial end of clavicle; 4, notch on surface of clavicle.

HIGH TECHNIQUE: LATERAL APPROACH

Willeford and Reitan (1994)[66]

Patient category

Adults. The description of the technique by the original authors did not include its application in children, but this does not necessarily exclude its use in this age group.

Advantages and disadvantages

The head is kept in the neutral position and the technique is particularly indicated in patients with suspected cervical spine injuries: turning the head as is usual for internal jugular cannulation would pose unacceptable additional risks to these patients. In addition to palpation of the carotid artery the technique uses simple bony and cartilaginous landmarks.

Preferred side

The right side.

Position of patient

The head was placed in the neutral position in the first group of 55 patients. In the second group of 20 patients suspected of sustaining cervical trauma a two-piece (anterior and posterior) immobilising hard cervical collar was in place. The anterior portion of the collar could be removed by releasing Velcro straps which fastened it to the posterior portion. The posterior portion of the collar extended under the shoulders and cradled the occiput to keep the head in the neutral position. Sandbags were placed on either side of the head to immobilise the neck during catheter placement. The patients were placed in a 10° head-down position.

Position of operator

Stand at the head of the patient.

Equipment used in the original description

A 22 gauge 'finder' needle and then a Seldinger technique with a thin-walled 18 gauge needle, wire and 6 inch (15 cm) catheter.

Advice on current equipment

A guide-wire technique is strongly recommended. A suitable 12 cm triple-lumen catheter should be used. Long, rigid catheter-over-needle devices should be avoided, especially on the left side.

Anatomical landmarks

There is a bony indentation at the point of insertion of the clavicular head of the sternomastoid muscle (Figure 7.11). Run a finger along the superior border of the clavicle to find the indentation. Also identify the cricoid cartilage. The carotid artery is palpated to ensure it is not directly under the insertion point. The artery is not palpated during the procedure.

Preparation

Perform the puncture under sterile conditions using local anaesthesia if indicated.

Precautions and recommendations

If possible maintain positive intrathoracic pressure during venous cannulation to distend the vein.

Point of insertion of needle

Insert the needle at the level of the cricoid cartilage vertically above the lateral border of the bony depression caused by the clavicular insertion of the sternomastoid muscle (Figure 7.11).

Initial location of vein with a small needle

Locate the vein with a fine (21 gauge) needle using the following directions. Then using the fine needle as a guide, puncture the skin with the larger needle attached to a saline-filled syringe.

Direction of needle and procedure

Palpate the carotid artery prior to insertion of the 'finder' needle to ensure that the artery is not directly under the insertion point; the artery is *not* palpated during the procedure. Locate the bony clavicular depression with the thumb of the non-

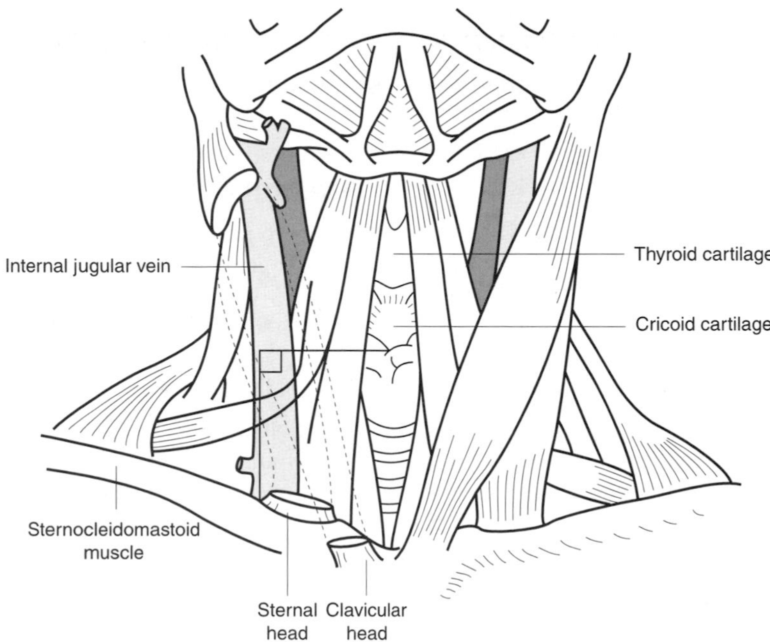

Figure 7.11 High technique, lateral approach. With kind permission of Willeford and Reitan (1994).[66]

Table 7.7 Success rates for location of the internal jugular vein using the high lateral approach of Willeford and Reitan.[66]

	Operators	Success rate
Initial study		
General patients (55)	5 residents	24 (1st or 2nd attempt) (more than 2 attempts)
	1 senior anaethetist	26/29 (1st attempt)
Depth of insertion to locate vein	2.5–3.7cm (mean 2.9 cm)	
Second study		
Trauma patients (20)	residents and 1 senior anaesthetist	17/18 (1st attempt) for senior average for all 1.2 (range 1–3)

dominant hand. The finder needle is kept in the sagittal plane and advances at 60–90° to the frontal plane. Maintain a slight negative pressure in the syringe as the needle is advanced. The vein is located with the finder needle. Jugular cannulation is then performed with the Seldinger equipment. If the first attempt with the finder needle is unsuccessful, reinsert the needle at a point 2 mm lateral to the original entry site (an alternative not described by the authors would be to keep the same skin insertion point but to direct the needle more laterally).

Results are presented in Table 7.7 *for the seeker needle* using the right internal jugular vein when possible and the left only when the right side is not appropriate.

Complications

In the initial study the carotid artery was hit with the finder needle in 1 patient. A haematoma developed in 1 patient in whom it was not possible to pass the Seldinger wire after entry into the vein with the 18 gauge needle. There were no complications in the trauma patients.

HIGH TECHNIQUE: CENTRAL APPROACH

Vaughan and Weygandt (1973)[59]

Patient category

Adults and children.

Advantages and disadvantages

A very high failure rate (86.5%) with this technique in children under age 2 years led the authors to use a cut-down and abandon this percutaneous technique. It is recommended that the electrocardiograph be monitored during cannulation to detect dysrhythmias caused by the catheter tip. In some patients an intravascular ECG was used to check the position of the catheter tip.

Preferred side

The right side.

Position of patient

Place the table in a 15–20° head-down position. Extend the patient's neck by placing a small towel under the shoulders. These authors position the head in the *midline*, with the patient's arms by the sides (Figure 7.12a).

Position of operator

Stand at the head of the patient or on the opposite side to the puncture site (Figure 7.12a).

Equipment used in original description

Catheter-through-needle.

Advice on current equipment

A guide-wire technique is strongly recommended. Long, rigid catheter-over-needle devices should be avoided, especially on the left side.

Anatomical landmarks

The sternal and clavicular heads of the sternomastoid muscle and the clavicle.

Preparation

Perform the puncture under sterile conditions using local anaesthesia if indicated.

Precautions and recommendations

Avoid hyperinflation of the lung to minimise the risk of pneumothorax.

Point of insertion of needle

The needle is inserted at the apex of the triangle bounded below by the inner edge of the sternal insertion and the outer edge of the clavicular insertion and above by the junction of the two heads of the sternomastoid muscle (Figure 7.12b).

Initial location of vein with a small needle

A fine (21 gauge) needle can be used to locate the vein using the following directions. Then, using thefine needle as a guide, puncture the skin with the larger needle attached to a saline-filled syringe.

Direction of needle and procedure

Place the point of the needle at the entry site on the skin and point the needle caudally (Figure 7.12c). Elevate the syringe about 30° above the skin (A to B, Figure 7.12d, e). Inject 0.5 ml of saline after the needle has punctured the skin. Advance the needle maintaining a slight negative pressure in the syringe. A click is noted both when the cervical fascia and when the vein wall are punctured. When the vein is entered, remove the syringe and thread the wire centrally. Then remove the needle and thread the catheter centrally. If the first attempt fails, redirect the needle more laterally.

Success rate

The technique was used by junior and senior anaesthetists on 242 cardiac patients aged 0–65 years with an overall success rate of 93.8% (15 failures). Thirteen failures occurred in 15 attempts (86.5% failure rate) in children aged 1–2 years, and the authors now avoid percutaneous cannulation in this age group. In 14 adults, right-sided cannulation was unsuccessful but an attempt on the left side succeeded.

Complications

There were 4 (1.6%) major complications, 3 of which required surgical correction. In 2 adults there was persistent bleeding from the left internal jugular vein requiring exploration postoperatively. A 13-month-old child bled from the right pleura as a result of a pulmonary puncture. In a 4-year-old child with a ventricular septal defect the catheter tip precipitated a supraventricular tachycardia. In 26 patients (11%) the carotid artery was punctured.

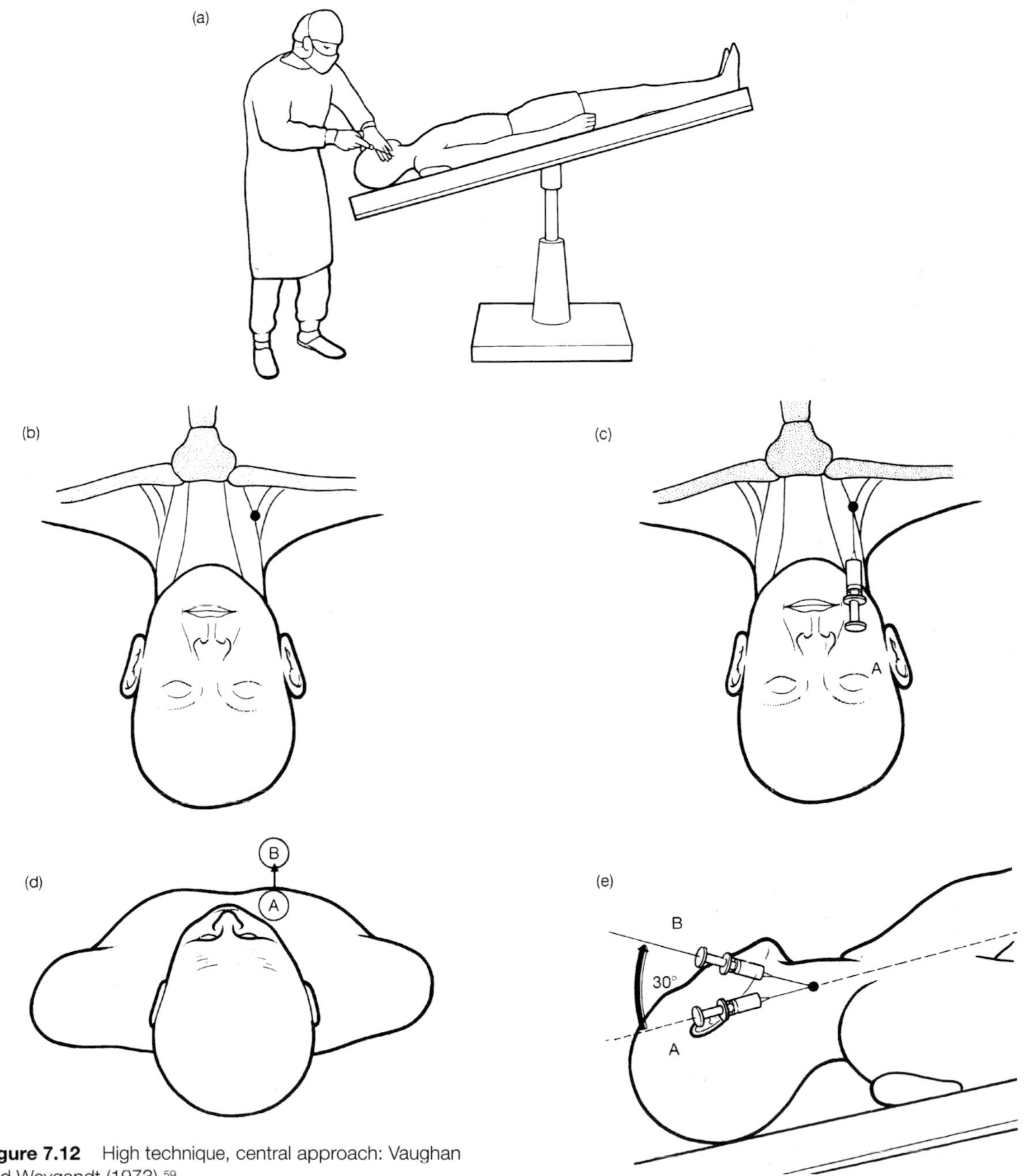

Figure 7.12 High technique, central approach: Vaughan and Weygandt (1973).[59]

HIGH TECHNIQUE: CENTRAL APPROACH

English et al. *(1969)*[4]*: elective method*

Patient category

Adults. This technique is not often used in infants as it is difficult to feel the vein.

Advantages and disadvantages

The elective technique requires muscle relaxation and is the preferred method with general anaesthesia. Both the carotid artery and the internal jugular vein should be palpated. If the vein was not palpable the authors used the alternative technique (see below). In some patients two catheters were inserted into the vein, one by the elective technique and one by the alternative technique.

Preferred side

The right side.

Position of patient

Place the table in a 25° head-down position. The neck is extended by placing a small towel under theshoulders and the head is turned away from the side of the puncture. Both arms are placed by thesides (Figure 7.13a).

Position of operator

Stand at the head of the patient (Figure 7.13a).

Equipment used in original description

A 200 mm catheter through 14 gauge needle. Catheters without stylets are recommended for observing the immediate reflux of blood into the catheter.

Advice on current equipment

A guide-wire technique is strongly recommended. Long, rigid catheter-over-needle devices should be avoided, especially on the left side.

Anatomical landmarks

The internal jugular vein, the carotid artery and the sternomastoid muscle.

Preparation

Perform the puncture under sterile conditions using local anaesthesia if indicated.

Precautions and recommendations

Make sure there is full muscle relaxation. Maintain positive intrathoracic pressure during venous cannulation to distend the vein.

Point of insertion of needle

The needle is inserted cephalad and medial to where the vein is most clearly felt (Figure 7.13b).

Initial location of vein with a small needle

Locate the vein with a fine (21 gauge) needle using the following directions. Then, using the fine needle as a guide, puncture the skin with the larger needle attached to a saline-filled syringe.

Direction of needle and procedure

First palpate the carotid artery and the internal jugular vein with the fingers of the left hand. Place the point of the needle at the entry site on the skin and point the needle caudally (A in Figure 7.13c). Swing the syringe and point the needle slightly laterally (A to B). Elevate the syringe 30–40° above the skin surface (B to C, Figure 7.13d, e). The needle may pierce the sternomastoid muscle if the internal jugular vein is palpated lateral to its medial edge. Advance the needle, maintaining a slight negative pressure in the syringe. A sensation of 'give' is usually noted both as the deep cervical fascia is pierced and as the vein is entered. Once the needle enters the vein, remove the syringe and thread the wire centrally. Then remove the needle and thread the catheter centrally.

Success rate

The results of the elective and alternative techniques are presented together. The techniques were used for 500 cannulations of the internal jugular vein in unselected cases of all ages by all members of the anaesthetic department. There were 26 failures (5.2%): 8 (9.4%) failures in 85 patients aged 0–15 years and 18 (4.3%) failures in 415 patients over 15 years. The failure rate was reduced with increasing experience. In 12 cases the vein was entered but the catheter could not be threaded down it.

Complications

Three arterial punctures occurred (0.6%). There was one pneumothorax (0.2%). Internal jugular vein thrombosis did not occur. In one patient the vein was cannulated on four occasions and appeared undamaged by the procedure. The average duration of venous cannulation was 48 hours.

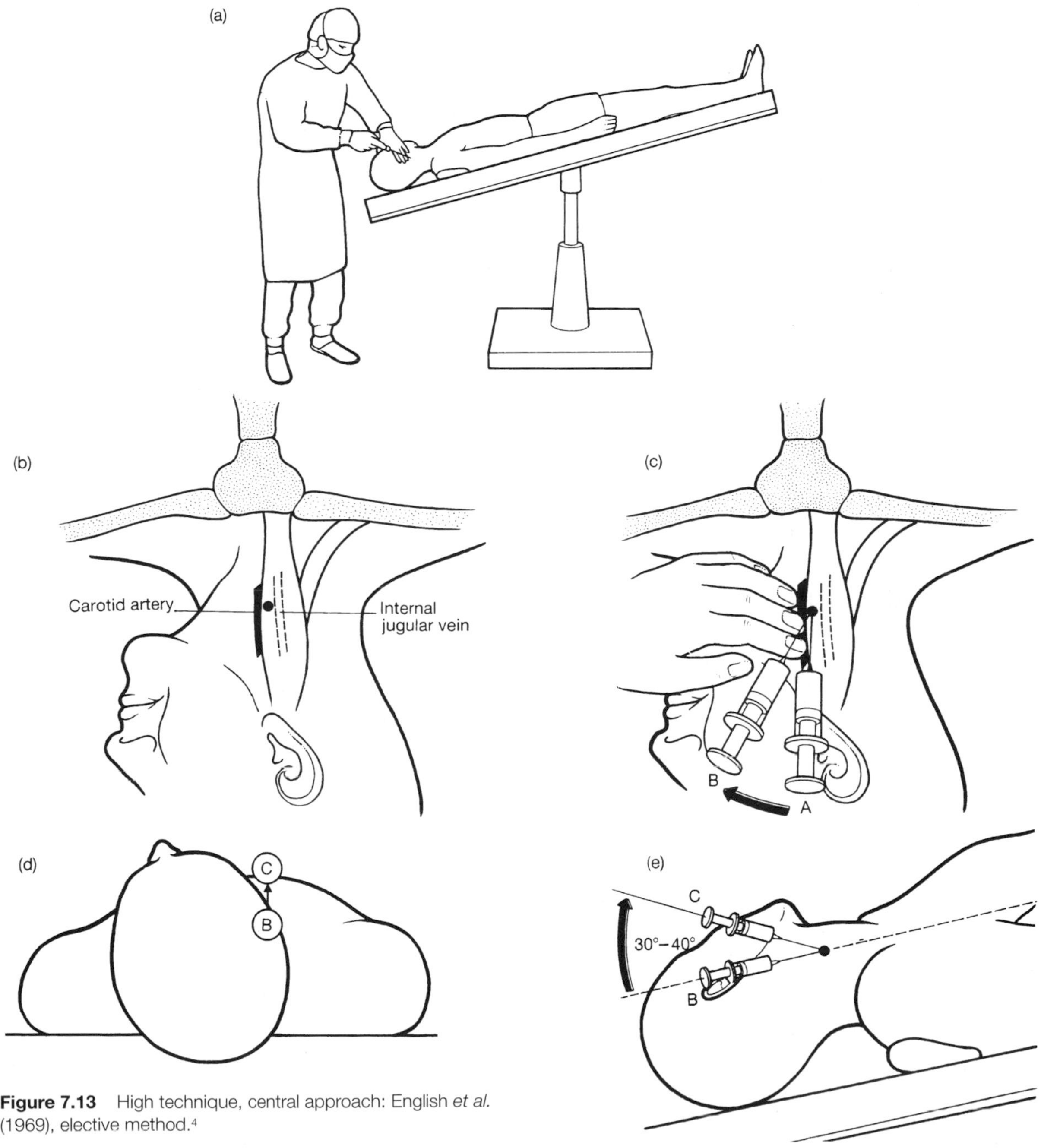

Figure 7.13 High technique, central approach: English *et al.* (1969), elective method.[4]

LOW TECHNIQUE: CENTRAL APPROACH

English et al. *(1969)*[4]*: alternative method*

Patient category

Adults and children.

Advantages and disadvantages

This method does not require muscular relaxants or palpation of the vein and is used under local anaesthesia in awake patients and in emergencies such as cardiac arrest. It is used when the elective technique has failed or the internal jugular vein is not palpable. It is normally used in children as the vein is difficult to palpate.

Preferred side

The right side.

Position of patient

Place the table in a 25° head-down position. The neck is extended by placing a small towel under theshoulders and the head is turned away from the side of the puncture. Both arms are placed by thesides.

Position of operator

Stand at the head of the patient (Figure 7.14a).

Equipment used in original description

A 20 mm catheter (without stylet) through needle; 14 gauge needle for adults and most children; 17 gauge needle for small children, infants and neonates.

Advice on current equipment

A guide-wire technique is strongly recommended. Long, rigid catheter-over-needle devices should be avoided, especially on the left side.

Anatomical landmarks

The clavicle and the sternal and clavicular heads of insertion of the sternomastoid muscle.

Preparation

Perform the puncture under sterile conditions using local anaesthesia if indicated.

Precautions and recommendations

Avoid hyperventilation of the lung to decrease the risk of pneumothorax.

Point of insertion of needle

The point of insertion lies near the apex of the triangle formed by the sternal and clavicular heads of the sternomastoid muscle and the clavicle (Figure 7.14b).

Initial location of vein with a small needle

Locate the vein with a fine (21 gauge) needle using the following directions. Then using the fine needle as a guide, puncture the skin with the larger needle attached to a saline-filled syringe.

Direction of needle and procedure

Place the point of the needle at the entry site on the skin and point the needle caudally (A in Figure 7.14c). Swing the syringe and point the needle laterally (A to B). Elevate the syringe 30–40° above the skin surface (B to C, Figure 7.14d, e). Advance the needle towards the inner border of the anterior end of the first rib behind the clavicle. Once the vein is entered, introduce the wire. Then remove the needle and thread the catheter centrally.

Success rate

See under elective method.

Complications

See under elective method.

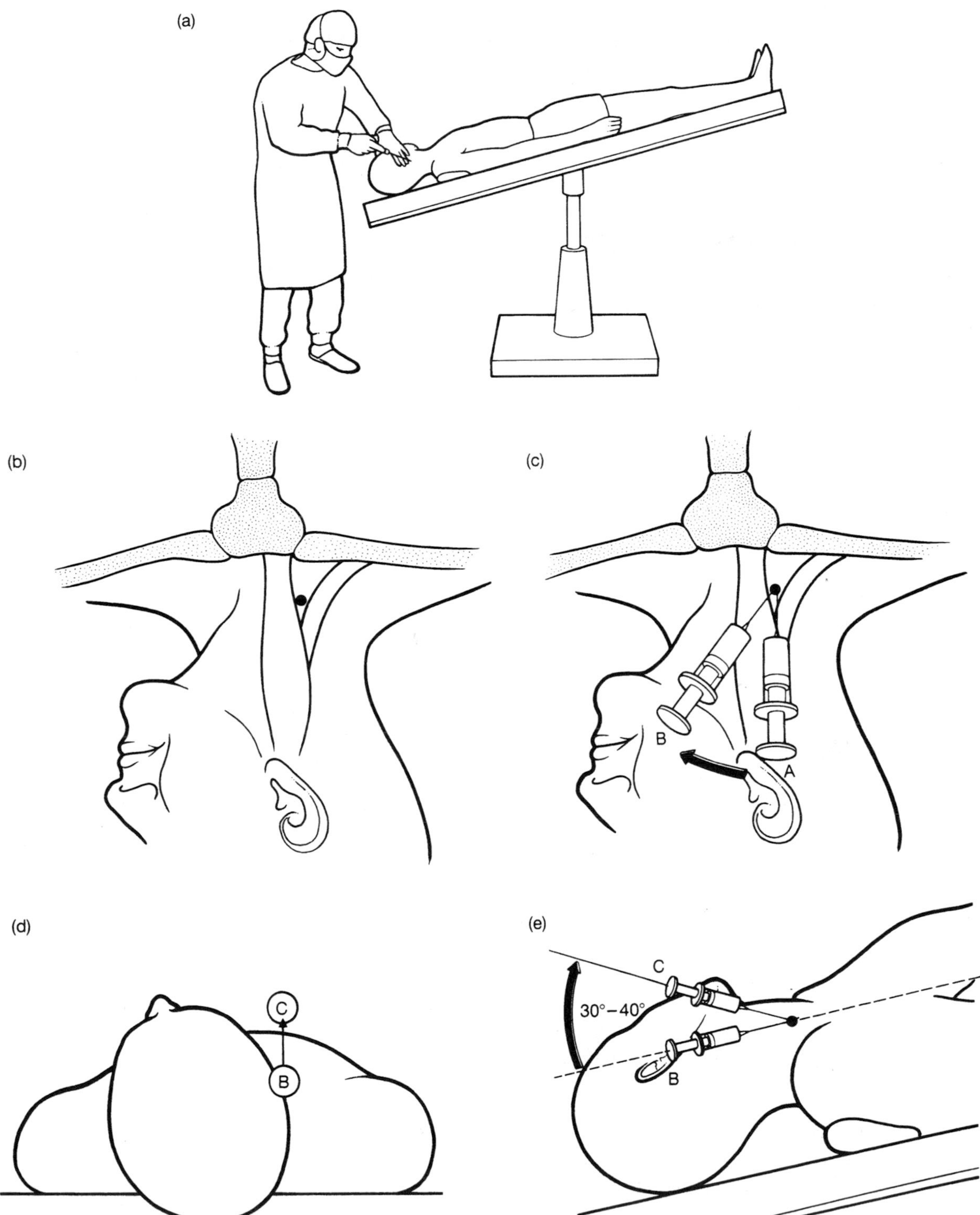

Figure 7.14 Low technique, central approach: English *et al*. (1969), alternative method.[4]

HIGH TECHNIQUE: CENTRAL APPROACH

Prince et al. *(1976)*[60]

Patient category

Infants and children.

Advantages and disadvantages

This technique was performed under general anaesthesia. Puncture of the internal jugular vein is more difficult in infants than in older children as the landmarks are less apparent and there is often difficulty in threading the catheter into the vein. Internal jugular vein cannulation is considered to be preferable to subclavian vein cannulation in infants. The technique is similar to that used by Daily and his colleagues,[58] who strongly recommended using a fine needle to locate the vein.

Preferred side

The right side.

Position of patient

Place the table in a 15° or 20° head-down position. Extend the patient's neck by placing a small towel under the shoulders and turn the head away from the side of the puncture. Place both arms by the sides (Figure 7.15a).

Position of operator

Stand at the head of the patient or on the opposite side to the puncture site (Figure 7.15a).

Equipment used in original description

Catheter-through-needle.

Advice on current equipment

A guide-wire is strongly recommended. Long, rigid catheter-over-needle devices should be avoided, especially on the left side.

Anatomical landmarzks

The sternal and clavicular heads of insertion of the sternomastoid muscle, and the clavicle.

Preparation

Perform the puncture under sterile conditions.

Precautions and recommendations

Avoid hyperinflation of the lung to minimise the risk of pneumothorax. Care should be taken to avoid the prevertebral area as trauma here can cause Horner's syndrome.

Point of insertion of needle

The point of insertion lies at the apex of the triangle formed by the two heads of the sternomastoid muscle and the clavicle (Figure 7.15b).

Initial location of vein with a small needle

Locate the vein with a fine (21 gauge) needle using the following directions. Then, using the fine needle as a guide, puncture the skin with the larger needle attached to a saline-filled syringe.

Direction of needle and procedure

Place the point of the needle at the entry site on the skin and point the needle caudally (A in Figure 7.15c). Swing the syringe and needle and point the needle laterally towards the ipsilateral nipple (A to B). Elevate the syringe 45° above the skin surface (B to C, Figure 7.15d, e). Then advance the needle, maintaining a slight negative pressure in the syringe. A loss of resistance is frequently noted on entering the vein, usually within 1–2 cm of the skin surface. Remove the syringe and thread the wire centrally. Then remove the needle and thread the catheter centrally.

Take a chest X-ray to check the position of the catheter tip.

Success rate

The technique was performed by supervised residents familiar with the technique of internal jugular vein cannulation in adults. If cannulation of the right internal jugular vein failed, an attempt was made on the left side. If this failed, an attempt was made to cannulate the external jugular vein. This technique was used on 52 patients aged from 6 weeks to 14 years. Cannulation of right or left vein was successful in 40 patients (77%); 31 on the right and 9 on the left. The success rate in 19 infants aged 6 weeks to 2 years was 68% and in 33 patients aged 2–14 years was 82%.

A higher but statistically insignificant success rate was achieved in infants weighing over 10 kg and in patients with a central venous pressure higher than 10 cm H_2O.

In 9 of the 12 failures the external jugular vein was then cannulated. One of the left internal jugular vein catheters passed down the left subclavian vein. All the others passed to the superior vena cava or right atrium.

Complications

The carotid artery was punctured in 12 patients (23%) and resulted in a cervical haematoma in 3 instances (5.7%). Horner's syndrome developed in 2 patients (4%) but both recovered completely.

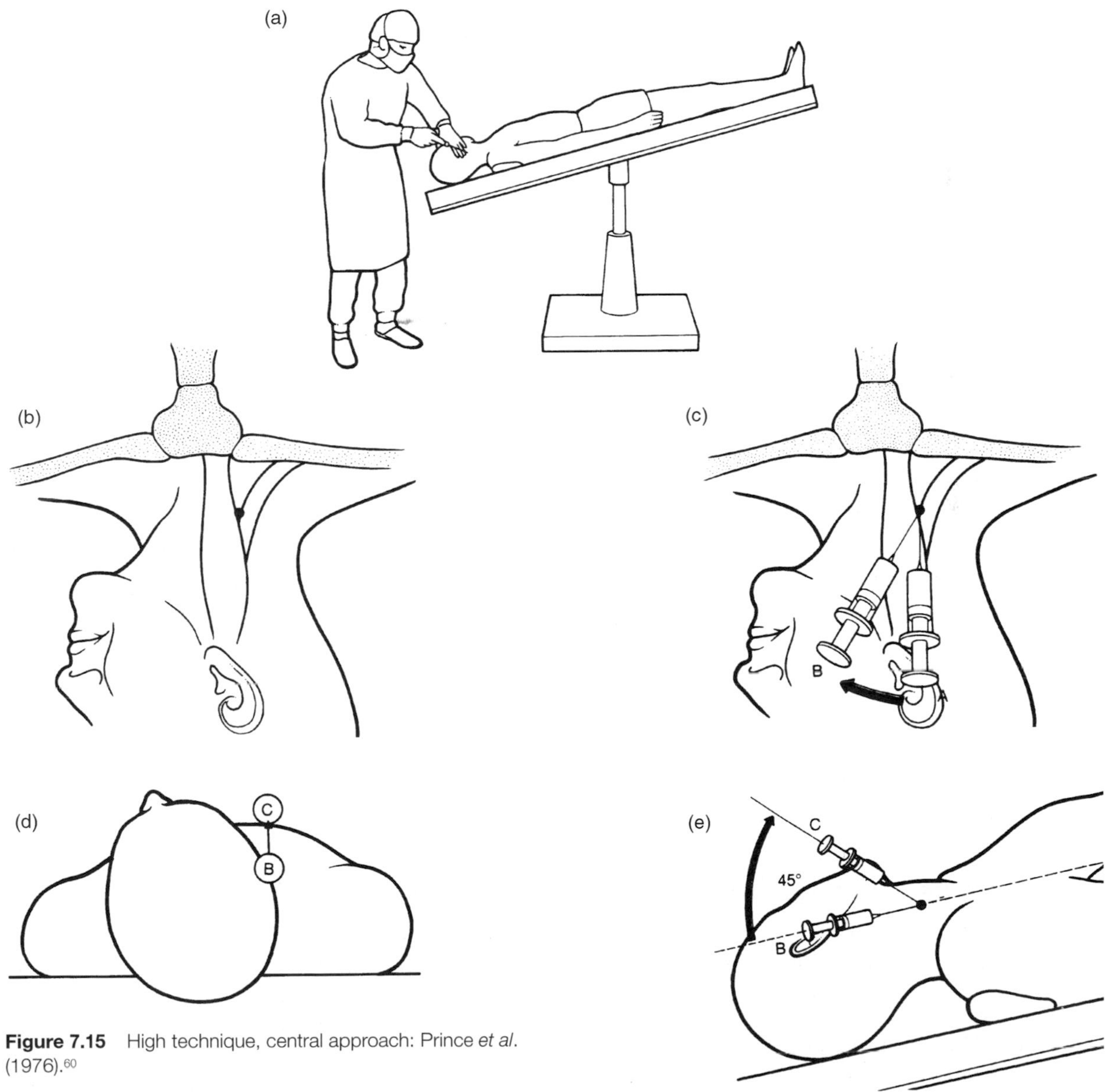

Figure 7.15 High technique, central approach: Prince *et al.* (1976).[60]

LOW TECHNIQUE: CENTRAL APPROACH

Rao et al. *(1977)*[45]

Patient category

Adults and children.

Advantages and disadvantages

This technique avoids the need to identify the sternomastoid muscle, which may be difficult to see or to palpate in obese patients and children. An easily palpable notch on the superior surface of the medial end of the clavicle must be identified. This method gives the highest success rate of all published methods but the low approach introduces a risk of pneumothorax and trauma. In a comparative trial of this low technique with two high techniques in children,[4,60] the authors recommended using a high approach as it was associated with a lower incidence of significant clinical morbidity.[69] Coté and his colleagues,[69] using this low technique, reported a lower success rate and a higher incidence of major complications than were found by Rao and his colleagues.[45] One death in a child was reported with the use of the low approach.

Preferred side

The right side.

Position of patient

Place the table in a 25° head-down position. Extend the patient's neck by placing a small towel under the shoulders and turn the head away from the side of the puncture. Place both arms by the sides (Figure 7.16a).

Position of operator

Stand at the head of the patient or on the opposite side to the puncture site (Figure 7.16a).

Equipment used in original description

A 19 gauge OD needle and 22 gauge OD catheter for infants younger than 3 months; 17 gauge OD needle and 19 gauge OD catheter in children between 4 months and 6 years old; 14 gauge OD needle and 17 gauge OD catheter for patients older than 6 years.

Advice on current equipment

A guide-wire technique is strongly recommended. Long, rigid catheter-over-needle devices should be avoided, especially on the left side.

Anatomical landmarks

A notch, 0.25–1 cm from the medial end of the clavicle, is bounded medially by the upward curve of the clavicle and below by its superior surface (Figure 7.16f).

Preparation

Perform the puncture under sterile conditions using local anaesthesia if indicated. All catheterisations in this series were performed under anaesthesia.

Precautions and recommendations

Ventilate the lungs manually and avoid hyperinflation to minimise the risk of pneumothorax.

Point of insertion of needle

The point is just above the notch on the upper surface of the clavicle (Figure 7.16b).

Initial location of vein with a small needle

A fine needle can be used to locate the vein using the following directions. Then, using the fine needle as a guide, puncture the skin with the larger needle attached to a saline-filled syringe.

Direction of needle and procedure

Identify the notch on the clavicle with the left thumb. Place the point of the needle at the entry site on the skin and point the needle caudally (A) with the needle bevel facing medially (Figure 7.16c). Elevate the syringe 30–40° above the coronal plane (A to B, Figure 7.16d, e). Then advance the needle caudally and posteriorly. A clicking sensation may be noted as the needle penetrates the cervical fascia and also as it penetrates the vein at a depth of 2–4 cm. Remove the syringe and thread the wire centrally. Then remove the needle and thread the catheter centrally.

If the vein is not located, redirect the needle in a slightly lateral direction to the sagittal plane. Take a chest X-ray after insertion to exclude a pneumothorax.

Success rate

The procedures were performed both by anaesthesia trainees and by consultants. There was a 93% success rate on the first attempt in 192 children (ages 21 days to 12 years), and a 97% success rate on the second attempt. A 94% success rate was achieved on the first attempt in 124 adults, and a 99% success rate on the second attempt.

Complications

The overall complication rate was 2% (6 out of 315). One patient (0.3%) developed a pneumothorax. In 2 patients (0.6%) the thoracic duct was punctured. In 3 patients (1%) the carotid artery was punctured.

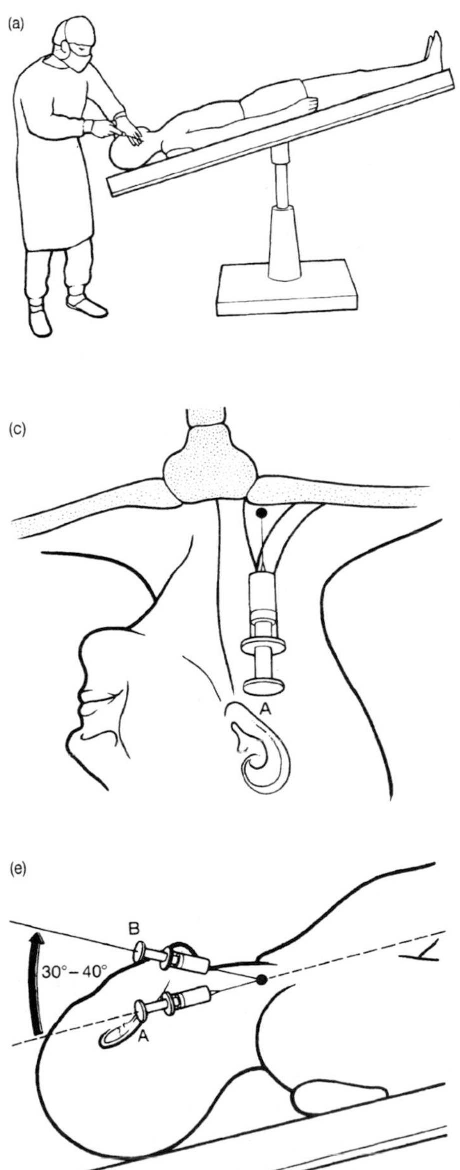

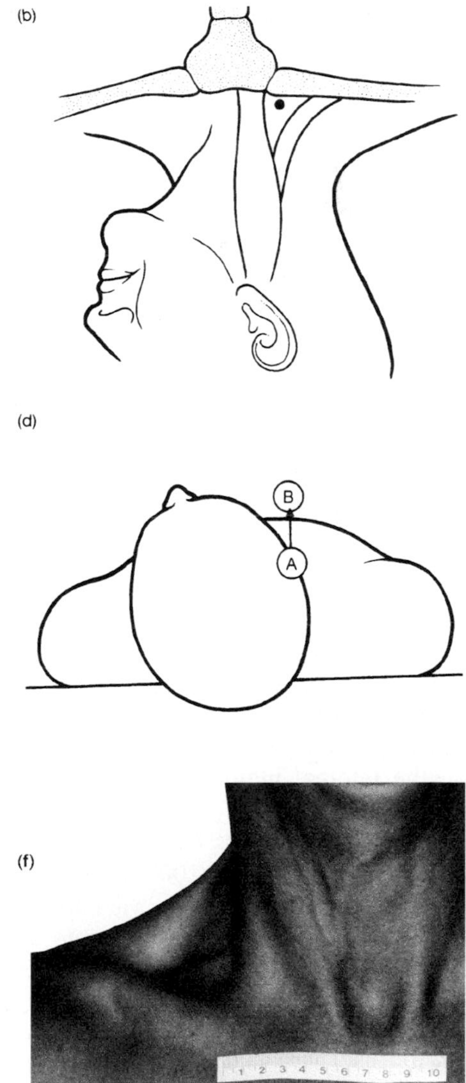

Figure 7.16 Low technique, central approach: Rao *et al.* (1977).[45]

Summary of Techniques

The techniques are summarised for comparison in Tables 7.8, 7.9 and 7.10. Although some techniques are described for use in the anaesthetised patient, there is no obvious reason why they cannot be used in conscious patients under local anaesthesia. Other techniques have been described for cannulation of the internal jugular vein.[29,67,69–77]

Factors influencing the incidence of successful cannulation

A number of factors have been described as increasing the chance of successful venous cannulation and catheter replacement. These include the increasing experience of the operator,[4] cannulation in adults as compared with children,[4,59,70] particularly in children more than 2 years old,[59] and in patients over 10 kg,[60] if the central venous pressure is greater than 10 cm H_2O,[60] using a short 4 cm 18 gauge needle and the Seldinger wire technique,[55] in anaesthetised patients,[71] using the right side,[55,60,70] and using an ultrasound Doppler blood flow detector.[29]

Some factors have been reported to make venous cannulation and central catheter placement less easy. These include severe obesity,[72,73] a short thick neck,[73,74] the presence of a tracheostomy,[72] cannulation of the left side,[55,60,70,75] hypovolaemia[75] and lack of clinical experience. The route has, however, been successfully used in severe hypovolaemia.[76]

Central placement of the catheter tip

Many techniques have been described for cannulating the internal jugular vein. In only a few of these has the position of the catheter tip been fully documented (Table 7.11). The success rate for central placement varies from 100% to 66%. For right-sided cannulation, success rates vary from 100% to 94.3%. The right internal jugular route appears to give the highest incidence of central placement of all routes.

Function of central catheters

It is not uncommon with arm vein catheters inserted centrally to find that either blood cannot be aspirated or the catheters stop giving accurate measurements of the central venous pressure. These catheters have a single distal orifice and in such cases it is probable that this is occluded by the vessel wall. Once the position of the catheter has been adjusted, blood can often be aspirated. In one report 10% of external jugular vein catheters inserted centrally did not give satisfactory pressure readings until the position was adjusted.[78] We have not found this to be a problem with catheters introduced through the right internal jugular vein, possibly because the catheter comes straight down into the superior vena cava and the distal end does not press against the vein wall. The problem is less likely to occur with catheters possessing side holes as well as a distal orifice.[79]

Complications

The complications and their incidences in some of the techniques described are shown in Tables 7.8–7.10 and 7.12. The most common complication is puncture of the carotid artery; this has an average incidence of approximately 2% but ranges with different techniques from 0–30% of catheters inserted. Pneumothorax occurred with only two of the techniques and in both of these the site of insertion of the needle was low. The incidence of pneumothorax with the two techniques was 0.2%[4] and 0.3%[45] respectively. Other complications reported with these techniques included malposition of the catheter, air embolus, catheter-related infection, thrombophlebitis of the internal jugular vein, infusion of fluid into the mediastinum or pleural cavity, trauma to the lung, supraventricular tachycardia, puncture of the thoracic duct, Horner's syndrome and postoperative venous bleeding.

There have been other case reports of complications associated with internal jugular cannulation.[80–104] Since the second edition of this book appeared in 1992 numerous additional case reports of complications have been published. It is not appropriate or possible to include all these reports of complications, but a few extra pertinent cases are described. A brief description of the selected complications is given in Table 7.12. The reports are described in five different sections: arterial, venous, pleural, neurological and miscellaneous. It is clearly important to classify the various case reports in a logical manner. It is important to be aware that these complications can occur, to be able to recognise them, and to be able to institute prompt and effective treatment if required. Some can be avoided by a knowledge and understanding of their aetiology and by using a technique in which the needle has a high point of insertion. As with any technique of central venous cannulation, the distal end of the catheter should not be more than 2 cm below a line joining the lower end of the clavicles, to avoid the possibility of cardiac tamponade.

The list of complications described is formidable. It is noteworthy, however, that we very rarely see major or significant complications in our clinical practice. We believe that this is because guide-wire techniques are now widely used and attention is paid to the recommendations in Table 7.12.

Conclusion

The internal jugular vein can be successfully cannulated both as an elective procedure and in emergency circumstances. Catheters can be left *in situ* either for the short term or for the long term. The incidence of central placement of the catheter is greater when the vein on the right, rather than the left, is used.

The overall complication rate for internal jugular vein techniques is much lower than with the subclavian route and the incidence of major complications is very low. Nearly all major complications can be avoided by using a technique in which the needle is inserted high above the clavicle. Proficiency in the selected technique is easily acquired. The internal jugular vein is now used confidently, routinely and safely by anaesthetists all over the world.

KEY POINTS

- In the UK the internal jugular vein is now probably the most commonly selected vein for insertion of central venous catheters during anaesthesia.
- The anaesthetist is presented with a bewildering number of choices of technique.
- An ideal technique would be inherently safe, have a high incidence of success and have a low incidence of complications. It should be easy to teach and perform.
- The technique selected should be intrinsically simple and be easy to remember.
- Soft tissue landmarks may be variable. The two heads of sternomastoid may not be visible; the carotid artery may be difficult or impossible to feel. The vein itself is not always visible after digital compression and spontaneous re-expansion.
- It is sensible to use a technique that uses both the carotid artery and either a bony or a cartilaginous landmark.
- Careful examination and optimal positioning of the patient before starting the technique are important.
- The use of a seeker needle is strongly advised. No one is able to hit the vein first time on every patient. Multiple attempts at locating the vein with a large needle are a certain cause of largely avoidable morbidity and mortality. Legal proceedings are likely to result from such behaviour.
- A fine, short Seldinger needle should be used. The use of long catheter-over-needle devices is intrinsically dangerous and should be avoided at all times.
- Both the seeker needle and the main needle should be advanced slowly. A sensible alternative plan should be adopted if the seeker needle fails to enter the vein at the first attempt.
- If there is undue difficulty in locating the vein an alternative technique should be used.
- Ultrasound technology should be used if available.
- The incidence of morbidity and mortality can be minimised by adopting sensible procedures and avoiding obvious dangers.
- The work surface that has been used for venepuncture and radial artery lines should not be used for Seldinger wire techniques: it is no longer sterile. Seldinger techniques should always be performed under sterile conditions.

Table 7.8 Internal jugular vein cannulation – results and complications of techniques used in adults.

Author and year	Point of insertion of needle		Distance between skin and vein (cm)	No. of patients or cannulation attempts	Successes No. (%)	Complication		Personnel	Comments	State of consciousness
	Height	Position				Type	No. (%)*			
Boulanger *et al.* (1976)[53]	High	Medial	2–4	100 cannulation attempts	94 (94)	Carotid artery puncture	2 (2.1)	Supervised inexperienced residents	Method claimed easy to learn	Not stated. Probably both awake or under anaesthesia
Brinkman and Costley (1973)[56]	High	Lateral	5–7	180 cannulation attempts	Not given	Carotid artery puncture	4 (2.2)	Authors	Technique can be used when access to arm and subclavian veins is limited	Awake or under anaesthesia
Mostert *et al.* (1970)[54]	High	Medial	NS	133 patients	130 (97.7)	Carotid artery puncture Local tenderness following puncture	2 (1.5) 45 (35.4)	Authors	Technique relies on palpation of carotid artery.	Awake; we have frequently used this technique under anaesthesia
Civetta *et al.* (1972)[62]	High	Central	NS	NS	NS	NS		Authors and residents	Spinal needle used as alternative to using needle to locate the vein Technique has also been used for introducing Swan–Ganz catheters	Awake
Jernigan *et al.* (1970)[57]	Low	Lateral	NS	1000 patients	NS	3 non-fatal major complications in 3 yr: Air embolus Thrombophlebitis of the IJV with septicaemia Mediastinal widening and fluid in left pleural space	3 (0.3) 1 (0.1) 1 (0.1) 1 (0.1)	Authors	These authors consider the IJV the first choice for central cannulation	Probably awake
Sharrock and Fierro (1983)[24]	High	Central	NS	212 patients	210 (99)	3 carotid artery punctures	3 (1.4)	Authors	Used a technique in which the vein was located by inspection only	Under anaesthesia

* Percentage of catheters inserted.
IJV, internal jugular vein; NS, not stated.

Table 7.9 Internal jugular vein cannulation – results and complications of techniques used in adults and children.

Author and year	Point of insertion of needle		Distance between skin and vein (cm)	No. of patients or cannulation attempts	Successes No. (%)	Complications		Personnel	Comments	State of consciousness
	Height	Position				Type	No. (%)*			
Daily *et al.* (1970)[58]	Low	Central	NS	100 patients, ages not given	91 (91) after 1st attempt 99 (99) after 2nd attempt	Carotid artery puncture Mediastinal fluid Infusion due to use of short catheter	NS 1 (1)	Authors	Recommended that use of short catheters be avoided	Awake or under anaesthesia
Vaughan and Weygandt (1973)[59]	High	Central	NS	242 patients, ages 0–65+ yr	227 (93.8)	Carotid artery puncture	26 (11)	Authors	Head positioned in midline	Awake or under anaesthesia
				15 patients, ages 1–2 yr	2 (13.3)	Bleeding from IJV postoperatively (adult) Supraventricular tachycardia (child) Trauma to right lung (child)	2 (0.9) 1 (0.45) 1 (0.45)		These authors had high failure rate in children under 2 yr old and subsequently introduced catheters using surgical cut-down	
Rao *et al.* (1977)[45]	Very Low	Central	2–4	316 patients: 124 adults 192 children (0–11 yr)	311 (98) 123 (99) 188 (97) same after 2nd attempt	Arterial puncture Pneumothorax Thoracic duct puncture	3 (1.0) 1 (0.3) 2 (0.6)	Authors and residents	Bony landmark used. This technique has highest success rate of all methods reviewed Avoid hyperventilation during insertion	Under anaesthesia
English et al. (1969)[4]										
Elective technique	High	Central	NS	500 patients:	474 (94.8)	Arterial puncture with haematoma	3 (0.6)	All members of anaesthetic department	Elective technique requires profound muscle relaxation for palpation of vein. Artery should also be palpated. Alternative technique recommended in small children	Under anaesthesia for elective technique. Awake or under anaesthesia for alternative technique
Alternative technique	Low	Central	NS	415 adults 85 children	397 (95.6) 77 (90.6)	Pneumothorax	1 (0.2)			
Oda *et al.* (1981)[21]	High	Medial	NS	408 (15 y–adults) 20 (5–15 yr) 14 (1–5 yr) 7 (6 mo–1 yr) 7 (0–6 mo) 456 Total	396 (97) 18 (90) 13 (92.9) 6 (85.7) 4 (57.1) 437 (95.8)	Carotid artery puncture	5 (1.1)	Authors	A safe puncture area was described lateral to the carotid artery	NS

*Percentage of catheters inserted; NS, not stated.

Table 7.10 Internal jugular vein cannulation – results and complications of techniques used in children.

Author and year	Point of insertion of needle		Distance between skin and vein (cm)	No. of patients or cannulation attempts	Successes	Complication				
	Height	**Position**			**No. (%)**	**Type**	**No. (%)***	**Personnel**	**Comments**	**State of consciousness**
Prince *et al.* (1976)[60]	High	Central	1–2	52 patients:	40 (77)	Carotid artery puncture	12 (30)	Residents supervised by anaesthesiologist	These authors argued strongly against the use of subclavian catheterisation in children	Under anaesthesia
				19 aged 6 wks–2 yr	13 (68)	Haematoma	3 (7.5)			
				33 aged 2–14 yr	27 (82)	Horner's syndrome	2 (5)			
Hall and Geefhuysen (1977)[61]										
Elective technique	Low	Central	NS	100 patients ages 2 wk–9 yr	90 (90)	Carotid artery puncture	3 (3.3)	Authors	Positive bacterial culture in more than 10% of catheter tips removed. These authors avoid the use of rigid cannulae. No serious complications occurred in this series	Awake
Alternative technique	High	Lateral								

*Percentage of catheters inserted.
NS, not stated.

Table 7.11 Success rate for central placement of the catheter tip.

Author and year	Attempted cannulations No.	Successful cannulations No. (%)	Right (R) or left (L)	Central placements* No. (%)	Non-centrally placed catheters Position	No.
English *et al*. (1969)[4]	500	474 (94.8)	NS	472 (99.6)	Subclavian vein	2
Belani *et al*. (1980)[55]	125	114 (91.2)	111 R 3L	111 (100) 2 (66)	Left superior intercostal vein	1
Prince *et al*. (1976)[60]	52	40 (76.9)	31 R 9 L	31 (100) 8 (88.9)	Subclavian vein	1
McConnell and Fox (1972)[72]	NS	70 (–)	NS	70 (100)		
Baker and Wallace (1976)[73]	100	88 (88)	88 R	83 (94.3)	NS	5
Korshin *et al*. (1978)[70]	168	156 (92.9)	145 R 11 L	141 (97.2) 9 (81.8)	Subclavian vein Loop in innominate vein Subclavian vein Internal thoracic vein	2 2 1 1
Coté *et al*. (1979)[69]	122	97 (79.5)	NS	97 (100)	None	0
Malatinsky *et al*. (1976)[105]	NS	87 (–)	NS	82 (94.3)	Loop formation left right	 3 2
Kuramoto and Sakabe (1975)[106]	NS	50 (–)	25 R 25 L	24 (96) 20 (80)†	Axillary vein Catheter coiled	1 5
Fischer *et al*. (1977)[107]	NS	262 (–)	247 R 15L	231 (93.5) 9 (60)	Subclavian vein Internal jugular vein Subclavian vein Internal jugular vein	6 10 4 2

*Central position defined as right atrium, superior vena cava, innominate vein. Values in parentheses are percentage of successful venous cannulations.

† Central position definition includes right atrium, superior vena cava, inferior vena cava, innominate vein, subclavian vein.

Table 7.12 Complications following internal jugular vein cannulation.

Complication	Comments
ARTERIAL COMPLICATIONS	
Carotid artery puncture	Carotid artery puncture is the most common complication associated with internal jugular cannulation and occurs in 0.6%[4] to 30%[60] of catheters inserted. In most series the incidence varies between 1% and 5%. The severity of ensuing complications is related to the size of the needle entering the artery. If a small-gauge seeker needle is used initially the chances of sequelae are minimised. With larger needles severe damage may result. Use if possible a short, fine needle and a Seldinger wire technique. If the pleura is also damaged there is the possibility of massive haemorrhage and the formation of a haemothorax. If the pleura is not damaged the blood loss will be less and restricted to the tissues in the neck. There also exists the hazard of unappreciated arterial cannulation which occurred in approximately 0.5% of cases in two reported series[108,109]
Carotid artery laceration[48]	The carotid artery was entered in two patients with a 16 gauge cannula. In one patient direct repair of the laceration was required. In the other the large haematoma slowly reabsorbed spontaneously. It was recommended that if the artery is damaged with a large needle the patient should not be heparinised and any cardiopulmonary bypass procedure be postponed for a few days. The needle should be left *in situ*, the area explored and the defect repaired before the definitive surgical procedure is commenced
Subclavian artery laceration[15]	Three long catheter over long needle devices were inserted into the right internal jugular vein. Massive haemorrhage ensued and the patient's life was saved only because cardiac bypass was used for a coronary vein graft. The right subclavian artery was lacerated. The traumatic lesion was successfully repaired and the patient recovered
Carotid artery cannulation with 8 F catheter sheath[108]	Out of 1021 attempted internal jugular cannulations there were 43 (4.2%) arterial punctures. In 5 patients this was unrecognised and an 8 F catheter sheath was threaded into the carotid artery. Three patients underwent the proposed surgery after respective delays of 2 h, 5 days and 13 days. One died 48 ;h later of his ischaemic heart disease (perhaps owing to the delay), and the other died of haemorrhage (a haemothorax) 12 h later. It was recommended that a pressure wave form should initially be obtained before passing the sheath. If an 8 F sheath is accidentally placed in the carotid artery the neck should be explored and any arterial damage repaired. However, in three other patients accidental carotid artery puncture with a 7.5F introducer sheath was treated by 5 min compression over the artery after immediate removal of the sheath. The patients were heparinised within 2 h and no adverse sequelae were observed[110]
Avoidance of carotid artery puncture sequelae[109]	Following the above study the authors used the external jugular vein as the first choice route and the internal jugular vein as the second choice. In addition when using the internal jugular vein the intravascular wave form was monitored from the 20 gauge catheter before inserting the 8 F introducer sheath. The incidence of carotid artery puncture was 4.5%. There were 4/710 clinically inapparent carotid artery punctures in which carotid artery damage with the 8 F introducer was avoided by detection of arterial placement of the 20 gauge catheter by waveform monitoring
Carotid artery aneurysm[111]	Cannulation of the right internal jugular vein of a patient with an abdominal aortic aneurysm was performed during resuscitation. The cannulation was apparently uneventful but the patient developed a dissecting aneurysm of the common carotid artery. This was thought to have been due to the catheterisation procedure
Vertebral artery pseudoaneurysm[112]	Vertebral artery pseudoaneurysm followed arterial puncture with a 22 gauge needle. The vascular lesion was later repaired but the patient died of pulmonary insufficiency on the eleventh postoperative day
Transverse cervical artery pseudoaneurysm[113]	Transverse cervical artery pseudoaneurysm followed an initially unrecognised placement of a 7 F triple-lumen catheter into the carotid artery prior to cardiac surgery. The catheter was removed and a pseudoaneurysm (diagnosed by digital subtraction angiography) developed postoperatively which resolved spontaneously. It was noted that the use of a Raulerson syringe may reduce the recognition of arterial puncture

Fistula between the common carotid artery and the internal jugular vein[114]	The fistula was treated surgically and there were no further complications
Cervical arteriovenous fistulae following internal jugular vein catheterisation[115]	Five cases were treated by percutaneous transarterial occlusion with a detachable balloon. Such fistulae are most common between the vertebral artery and vein but may also form between the inferior thyroid artery and internal jugular vein. Such fistulae can also be closed by surgical ligation
Fistula between right vertebral artery and vertebral venous plexus[116]	Produced by unsuccessfully attempting to thread 14 gauge needle over a spinal needle as described by Civetta *et al.*[62] The patient complained of tinnitus postoperatively and a continuous to-and-fro murmur was audible in the neck. A surgical repair was required
Severed thyrocervical artery[117]	Carotid artery puncture occurred at attempted internal jugular catheterisation and resulted in haematoma formation. After open heart surgery anticoagulants were given and the haematoma increased in size and became tense. At surgical exploration the thyrocervical artery was found to be severed
Laceration of vertebral artery near its origin with the subclavian artery[49]	An unsuccessful attempt was made to cannulate the right internal jugular vein with a 14 gauge introducer needle. At the end of the operation there was cervical bruising and a large haematoma was drained. Two hours later the patient collapsed and internal cardiac massage was performed. The patient also required large-volume infusions of blood, colloid and crystalloid. Exploration of the neck revealed the lacerated vertebral artery, which was tied off. The patient recovered
Disconnected right subclavian artery[118]	Three Wallace cannulae inserted into one internal jugular vein caused a large right-sided haemothorax. The patient required large quantities of blood, FFP and platelets. Surgical exploration revealed that the subclavian artery was disconnected at its junction with the common carotid. This was repaired and the patient spent 8 days on intensive care. The use of Seldinger techniques was advocated
Damage to ascending cervical artery[90]	The ascending cervical artery was damaged prior to cardiac surgery when an unsuccessful attempt was made to cannulate the right internal jugular vein. Fatal postoperative haemorrhage occurred. Early surgical exploration is mandatory if this complication is suspected
Aortic catheterisation[99]	Aortic catheterisation occurred in child with transposition of great arteries through the use of a low approach to the vein on the right side
Aortic dissection[100]	Aortic dissection followed a number of attempts at venous catheterisation when using a 7 cm needle and catheter
Pseudoaneurysm of the brachiocephalic arteries[80]	Three cases of cervical arterial pseudoaneurysms occurred due to arterial laceration following the low lateral approach for cannulation of vein. Pseudoaneurysms were treated surgically. It appears that this approach should be avoided
Cardiac arrest[101]	Compression of carotid artery following accidental arterial puncture resulted in cardiac arrest; ECG monitoring is recommended during cannulation for early diagnosis
Ventricular fibrillation[102]	Ventricular fibrillation occurred during carotid artery palpation prior to internal jugular vein cannulation. Care during arterial palpation was advocated
VENOUS COMPLICATIONS	
Valve injury[10]	There is a valve located 0.5–2 cm above the junction of the internal jugular and subclavian veins. The valves are important in preventing retrograde blood flow to the brain. If punctured with a needle the valve becomes imcompetent. This is an indication to avoid low techniques with a long needle when damage to the valve could occur
Avulsion of the right facial vein[119]	This occurred during double cannulation of the jugular vein
Postoperative cervical haematoma requiring surgical evacuation[95]	The haematoma occurred after an unsuccessful attempt at internal jugular vein cannulation in a patient who underwent coronary artery surgery. The haematoma was removed 6 weeks postoperatively
Respiratory obstruction due to cervical haematoma[96]	A large cervical haematoma followed venous cannulation in a patient with coagulation defects. It was recommended that arm veins should be used in such patients for central venous cannulation

Table 7.12 Continued

Complication	Comments
Cervical haematoma[120]	Cervical haematoma occurred in 10 out of 1000 patients with coagulopathies after internal jugular vein cannulation. It was not stated if the carotid artery had been punctured in any of these 10 patients. In one patient the haematoma compressed the airway and required surgical drainage. The carotid artery had not been punctured in this patient
Superior vena cava thrombosis[97]	This complication developed 5 days after venous cannulation in a 72-year-old woman. Thrombectomy was undertaken using cardiopulmonary bypass
Superior vena cava syndrome[98]	The catheter passed through a narrowed segment of the superior vena cava and symptoms of obstruction developed. These resolved on removal of the catheter
Cardiac tamponade[103]	Cardiac tamponade can be caused by central venous catheters, introduced by any route, if the catheter tip lies below the line of pericardial reflection and perforates the vascular wall. However, this is least likely to arise with the right internal jugular vein route, probably because the catheter tip lies clear of vessel wall
Fatal tamponade after left internal jugular catheter[121]	Five days after a left-sided internal jugular vein catheter was inserted a 74-year-old woman developed a cardiac tamponade and died. A tract was demonstrated linking the superior vena cava with the pericardial cavity which contained 450 ml of blood. *Avoid rigid catheters, particularly on the left side, and keep the tip of the catheter above the line of the pericardial reflection*
Septic internal jugular vein thrombosis[122]	Jugular cannulation is one of the causes of this rare condition. Expert investigation is required to make the diagnosis. The treatment may include surgery plus the use of antibiotics and anticoagulants
Axillary vein thrombosis[123]	Axillary vein thrombosis occurred in 2 of 63 patients with long-term (mean 93 days) Hickman catheters
Internal jugular vein thrombosis following insertion of PA catheters[124]	Chastre *et al.* found a 66% incidence of internal jugular vein thrombosis demonstrated either by venography or at autopsy
Failure to demonstrate internal jugular vein thrombosis following insertion of PA catheters[125–127]	Late studies failed to demonstrate evidence of venous thrombosis using ultrasound or venography after short-term (1–3 days) catheterisation
Venous thrombosis with Silastic haemodialysis catheters[128]	Jugular thrombosis is lower in percutaneous insertions (2/101 cases) than in surgical insertions (5/15 cases). The internal jugular vein should be used preferentially for venous access in these cases. Percutaneous techniques are preferable to surgical techniques
Bilateral thrombosis of internal jugular veins[129]	This complication is very rare and occurred in a 75-year-old man who had both veins catheterised twice in a 14 day period. The patient developed a hemiparesis and died. At autopsy both veins were occluded by thrombosis but there was no obvious cerebral pathology
Atrial thrombus[130,131]	A prospective study of post-mortem findings in patients with a central venous catheter showed a 5% incidence of right atrial thrombus.[130] Diagnosis in vivo is by echocardiography and treatment is by anticoagulation, thrombolysis or surgery.[131] There was a 29% mortality in patients with atrial thrombus diagnosed in vivo
Septic atrial thrombus[132]	This thrombus developed postoperatively in a 77-year-old man and was demonstrated by echocardiography. A PA catheter was inserted postoperatively to facilitate haemodynamic management. Treatment with heparin and antibiotics was successful
Jugular vein thrombosis and hydrocephalus	See Neurological complications

PLEURAL COMPLICATIONS

One of the factors that encouraged the move from subclavian to internal jugular vein catheterisation was the latter's apparent freedom from pleural complications especially pneumothorax. These complications are rare and nearly always avoidable with internal jugular cannulation. A short needle and a high approach in the neck should be used. They are, however, relatively frequent and unavoidable when the subclavian vein is cannulated

Complication	Description
Tension pneumothorax[86]	After preoperative insertion of a cannula into the right internal jugular vein a tension pneumothorax was diagnosed during operation. Nitrous oxide administration should be discontinued if this occurs and the pneumothorax should be released
Bilateral hydrothorax[87]	The internal jugular vein catheter slipped out of the vein and intravenous fluid accumulated in the pleural spaces
Bilateral hydrothorax[88]	It is sometimes possible for fluid under pressure in one pleural cavity to flow into the opposite pleural cavity
Mediastinal fluid extravasation in infants following the use of the infusion pump[89]	Extravasation of fluid into the mediastinum associated with the use of an infusion pump was reported in 2 infants, with 1 fatality. *Only gravity-fed devices for delivering fluid should be used in infants and neonates*
Fatal haemothorax following damage to the ascending cervical artery[90]	The ascending cervical artery was damaged prior to cardiac surgery when an unsuccessful attempt was made to cannulate the right internal jugular vein. Fatal postoperative haemorrhage occurred. Early surgical exploration is mandatory if this complication is suspected
Contralateral effusion of Intralipid[133]	Late perforation of the innominate vein probably occurred following the use of a rigid 5 in (12.5 cm) catheter in the right internal jugular vein
Contralateral hydrothorax[134]	Six cases of delayed right-sided hydrothorax after *left* jugular cannulation were described. All patients recovered uneventfully after removal of the catheters and placement of chest drains. A stiff catheter can produce gradual vein wall erosion and perforation. *Avoid rigid polyethylene or Teflon catheters and use soft polyurethane catheters and Seldinger techniques*. If the perforation occurs below the line of the pericardial reflection tamponade can result. This complication is unlikely to occur with right internal jugular catheter as the catheter goes straight down the lumen of the vein and the tip does not abut against the vein wall
Catheter tip not recognised as being in pleural cavity[135]	The catheter entered the pleural cavity in a patient with a traumatic haemopneumothorax. Blood could be aspirated from the cavity. *Check rate of drainage from the chest against the rate of infusion of fluid via the catheter*
Contralateral hydrothorax[136]	Five out of 8 patients who had a left-sided Teflon (Wallace Flexihub) internal jugular vein catheter inserted showed evidence of venous wall perforation 2 days after insertion of the catheter. None of 9 patients with right-sided catheters showed evidence of perforation. Four of 5 patients who developed confirmed perforations had either no symptoms or mild shoulder tip pain. *Avoid using rigid Teflon catheters on the left side*

NEUROLOGICAL COMPLICATIONS

Complication	Description
Bilateral vocal cord paralysis[91]	This complication occurred after bilateral attempts at internal jugular vein cannulation. Cervical haematomas caused temporary dysfunction of the recurrent laryngeal nerves and a tracheostomy was required
Extensive neurological damage[92]	Lesions of the left cranial nerves IX–XII, anterior primary rami of the left 2–4 cervical nerves and a left Horner's syndrome occurred after jugular cannulation. These were caused by pressure from haematoma or by chemical damage from extravasated fluid and the drugs it contained. These lesions resulted in chronic pulmonary aspiration and contributed to the patient's death
Horner's syndrome[93]	Horner's syndrome was caused by damage to the cervical sympathetic trunk either by needle or from a haematoma. The sympathetic trunk lies behind the carotid artery but outside the carotid sheath
Ipsilateral mydriasis following accidental carotid artery puncture[137]	A dilated pupil unreactive to light was noted 1 h after accidental carotid artery puncture. Pupil size spontaneously returned to normal over the next 10 days. Transient irritation of the sympathetic trunk occurred secondary to needle trauma or haematoma. Such mydriasis could proceed to a typical Horner's syndrome
Permanent right phrenic nerve injury[138]	This nerve injury occurred following repeated unsuccessful attempts to insert a temporary transvenous pacemaker into the right internal jugular vein. The patient developed rapid-onset shortness of breath and hypoxaemia. The symptoms rapidly improved but the paralysis of the right hemidiaphragm persisted

Table 7.12 Continued

Complication	Comments
Transient phrenic nerve paralysis[139]	Right shoulder tip pain was experienced during insertion of a seeker needle. Two ml of 1% lignocaine were injected as the needle was removed. The catheter entered the vein but could not be advanced into the vein. Shortness of breath was noticed 15 min after the lignocaine injection. An X-ray showed an elevated right hemidiaphragm. This had returned to normal 10 h later
Intermittent hiccups for 8 days[55]	Following accidental carotid artery puncture a right paratracheal haematoma developed which caused phrenic nerve irritation. The hiccups ceased when the haematoma resolved
Transient brachial plexus lesions[140]	Paraesthesia or muscle weakness occurs after cardiac surgery in 5–13% of cases. This may be due to sternal retraction, fractured ribs, or to trauma to the phrenic nerve during internal jugular vein cannulation
Paralysis of C5[141]	A flaccid paralysis of the arm developed 24 h after uneventful left-sided internal jugular cannulation; 20 days later EMG analysis showed complete denervation of C5. The possible causes of nerve damage are: needle trauma diffusion of local anaesthetic solution haematoma compressing a nerve action of drugs or fluids escaping from the vein
Isolated hypoglossal nerve palsy[142]	A right hypoglossal nerve palsy was noted after right internal jugular vein cannulation. This resolved spontaneously over 8 weeks. The patient noted difficulties in moving his tongue and in mastication. A high medial approach was used and the cause of the palsy was thought to be direct trauma or haematoma around an aberrant hypoglossal nerve
Internal jugular vein aneurysm and vagal palsy[143]	A traumatic venous aneurysm compressed the vagus nerve and resulted in a vagal palsy
Lesion of vagus nerve[144]	Vagus nerve lesions occurred in 5 patients after internal jugular vein cannulation. The main symptoms were hoarseness, problems with deglutition and aspiration into the respiratory tract
Accessory nerve injury[145]	Accessory nerve injury followed internal jugular vein cannulation
Cerebral infarct following central venous cannulation[146]	The carotid artery, which contained a small calcified plaque, was accidentally punctured with a 21 gauge seeker needle. The patient developed left-sided mortor weakness. A CT scan revealed a cerebral infarct involving the right frontal lobe. There was no residual weakness 3 months after the operation. This is the only known case of a neurological complication purporting to come from arterial puncture with a 21 gauge seeker needle.
Cerebrovascular accident during jugular vein cannulation[147]	Six cases were reviewed where carotid artery puncture occurred followed by manual compression of the puncture site. Contralateral hemiparesis ensued. The cause was thought to have been dissection of the intima of the carotid artery, dislodgment of atheromatous plaques or manual pressure Haematoma compressing the carotid artery was not thought to be a common contributing cause of the problem. One patient developed the hemiparesis immediately and died 8 h later. The mean age of the patients involved was 68 y Stroke has also been reported as a complication of carotid sinus massage and it was recommended that such massage should be avoided in elderly patients[148]
Cerebral embolus resulting in hemiparesis[149]	The right carotid artery was accidentally cannulated with a large French Cordis introducer. Removal was delayed for 96 h and a left hemiparesis developed 18 h after surgery for removal. The authors stressed the need for recognition of arterial puncture and immediate removal of cannulae inadvertently placed in the carotid artery
Fatal brainstem stroke[150]	The patient suffered an accidental injury to the vertebal artery during attempted internal jugular catheterisation. An embolus caused occlusion of the distal basilar and posterior cerebral arteries and resulted in extensive pontine and cerebellar infarction. The patient was declared brain-dead soon after the completion of surgery. The vertebral artery arises from the subclavian artery and lies behind the internal jugular vein in its lower portion.

Superior sagittal sinus thrombosis[151]	Two rigid 125 mm catheters were inserted into the patient's left internal jugular vein. Total parenteral nutrition was administered via a catheter for 5 days postoperatively. Jugular and cerebral sinus thrombosis ensued. The incidence of thrombosis is influenced by the position of the catheter tip, the properties of the catheter and the nature of the infused fluid. Use of rigid catheters, particularly in the left internal jugular vein, should be avoided. Central placement of the catheter tips should help to prevent this complication. The patient was treated with anticoagulants and antibiotics. Fatal superior sagittal sinus thrombosis was reported to follow internal jugular vein catheterisation.[152]
Bilateral thrombosis of internal jugular veins[129]	Bilateral thrombosis is very rare and occurred in a 75-year-old man who had both veins catheterised twice in a 14 day period. The patient developed a hemiparesis and died. At autopsy both veins were occluded by thrombosis but there was no obvious cerebral pathology
Cerebral infarction and death[153]	A retropharyngeal haematoma followed an unsuccessful attempt at venous cannulation. The haematoma compressed an already narrowed carotid artery and resulted in impaired cerebral blood supply. Caution was urged in cases of bleeding diatheses and stenotic carotid artery disease
Air embolus after accidental removal of catheter with cannula left in vein[94]	Cardiac arrest occurred secondary to air embolus. The patient suffered cerebral damage and failed to regain consciousness. Introducing cannulae should be removed from the vein after the catheter has been inserted and the catheter should be securely stitched in place
Emboli into the distal basilar artery resulted in massive brainstem stroke and death[150]	Inadvertent vertebral artery injury followed jugular cannulation. At autopsy thrombosis of the vertebral artery was demonstrated with emboli in the basilar artery
Earache following internal jugular vein cannulation[154] (auricular branch of X, tymphanic branch of IX)	The adventitial sheath of the vein is supplied by unmyelinated nerve fibres that are stimulated if the vein is distended. The proximal jugular vein is supplied by the vagus and the distal part of the vein is supplied by the glossopharyngeal nerve. Venous distension and stimulation of the auricular branch of the vagus and/or the tympanic branch of the glossopharyngeal nerve resulted in referred pain in the ear. The arm vein catheter had gone up into the internal jugular vein and its tip lay level with the mastoid. Pain relief was obtained by withdrawing the catheter a few cm
The 'ear-gurgling' sign[155]	In 5 cases catheters inserted into the infraclavicular subclavian vein went up the internal jugular vein. On administration of fluid an unpleasant gurgling or swishing sound was heard by the patient. The sound was magnified by increasing fluid flow and stopped when the infusion was clamped. A buzzing sensation in the ear on the rapid insertion of 10 ml of saline into such a catheter has been described.[156] This was thought to have been due to turbulence in the internal jugular vein being transmitted to the auditory ossicles. If the neck is compressed when an arm vein catheter goes into the internal jugular vein then there is a rise of central venous pressure of approximately 10 cmH_2O
Unsuspected cerebral perfusion of noradrenaline and lignocaine[157]	This complication occurred following insertion of a subclavian catheter to help in the resuscitation of a 48 year-old woman. The catheter went up into the internal jugular vein. The patient complained of headache prior to a systemic pressor effect with the noradrenaline and later became stuporous following infusion of lignocaine
Unsuspected cerebral perfusion of hyperosmolar alimentation fluid[158]	A subclavian feeding catheter went up into the jugular vein. Six days after starting the infusion the patient developed pain in the ear and neck. Five days later she developed an upper motor neurone lesion of cranial nerves V and VII, and a right parietal infarct was demonstrated associated with a cortical venous thrombosis. It was recommended that the catheter tip should be demonstrated to be in the superior vena cava before infusion of hyperosmolar fluid is started
Pseudotumour cerebri[159]	A left subclavian catheter used for feeding accidentally went into the left internal jugular vein. The patient developed headache, diplopia, bilateral papilloedema and a partial right VI nerve paresis. A thrombosis of the internal jugular vein and the transverse sinus was demonstrated. The patient recovered after treatment with steroids and anticoagulants

Table 7.12 Continued

Complication	Comments
Communicating hydrocephalus related to prolonged TPN and jugular vein thrombosis[160]	Four cases were described of communicating hydrocephalus in very young children. It was believed that this occurred after both internal jugular veins had been used for TPN and the veins had subsequently thrombosed
Accidental insertion of a Swan–Ganz catheter into the intrathecal space[161]	A guide-wire was threaded centrally after an attempt to locate the internal jugular vein. The Swan–Ganz catheter was advanced 20 cm centrally. When the balloon was inflated it was noticed that the patient's right leg twitched. An X-ray showed that the catheter was in the spinal canal and it was immediately removed. No permanent neurological sequelae were noted. Guide-wires should never be advanced unless there is free flow of blood
MISCELLANEOUS	
Infection[61,123,162,163]	The incidence of positive tip culture has been reported as 5.6%[162], 6%[163] and greater than 10%[61] in catheters removed from children. This incidence did not imply catheter-related septicaemia or endocarditis. In a series of long-term catheters (mean 98 days) in adults, 5 out of 71 catheters had to be removed as a result of sepsis[123]
Puncture of cuff of tracheal tube[81]	Puncture of the cuff of the tracheal tube occurred as a result of the needle being directed too far medially. No other complication resulted from puncture of the trachea in this patient
Tracheal perforation and puncture of cuff of tracheal tube[164]	This complication occurred in 2 patients when a posterior approach was used to catheterise the jugular vein. It was recommended that the posterior route should be avoided if possible. Both patients recovered uneventfully. Subcutaneous emphysema, pneumomediastinum or air trapping between the pleura and the chest wall can follow this complication
Oesophageal perforation[165]	A 17-year-old girl had an oesophageal stricture and a prestenotic dilatation. The dilated oesophagus was perforated three times during attempted right-sided venous cannulation. A large amount of thick, clear fluid was aspirated. Eight hours later she developed chest pain, and an elevated temperature. She was treated with antibiotics and recovered
Perforation of introducer with triple-lumen catheter[166,167]	The triple-lumen catheter was inserted 1 cm caudad to the sheath.[166] The complication was only recognised when it proved difficult to remove the introducer. The triple-lumen catheter must be removed prior to removal of the sheath. It was recommended that simultaneous placement of guide-wires should be followed by dilation of both catheter tracks and subsequent catheter insertion. The patient came to no harm as a result of this complication. The same recommendations were made by others following a similar problem[167]
Laryngeal oedema and airway obstruction[168]	Laryngeal oedema occurred after development of a haematoma following attempted jugular cannulation in a pregnant woman. The carotid artery was punctured. It was assumed that blood tracked out of the carotid sheath and into the paratracheal tissues causing venous obstruction and laryngeal oedema. Respiratory obstruction developed without preceding stridor and the patient lost consciousness. It was initially impossible to intubate or ventilate using a face mask so transtracheal ventilation was required. It then proved possible to intubate the patient using a bougie

ECG, electrocardiograph; EMG, electromyograph; FFP, fresh frozen plasma; PA, pulmonary artery; TPN, total parenteral nutrition.

References

1. Benotti PN, Bothe A, Miller JDB, Blackburn GL. Safe cannulation of the internal jugular vein for long term hyperalimentation. Surgery, Gynecology and Obstetrics 1977; **144**:574.
2. Civetta JM, Gabel JC. Flow directed pulmonary artery catheterization in surgical patients: indications and modifications of technic. Annals of Surgery 1972; **176**:753.
3. Hess W, Tarnow J. Ein Verfahren zur gleichzeiter Pazierung von zwei zentralen Katheteren über ein V. Jugularis interna. Anaesthesist 1978; **27**:579.
4. English ICW, Frew RM, Pigott JF, Zaki M. Percutaneous catheterization of the internal jugular vein. Anaesthesia 1969; **24**:521.
5. Andrews PJD, Dearden NM, Miller JD. Jugular bulb cannulation: description of a cannulation technique and validation of a new continuous monitor. British Journal of Anaesthesia 1991; **67**:55.
6. Denys BG, Uretsky BF. Anatomical variations of internal jugular vein location: impact on central venous access. Critical Care Medicine 1991; **19**:1516.
7. Armstrong PJ, Sutherland R, Scott DHT. The effect of position and different manoeuvres on internal jugular vein diameter size. Acta Anaesthesiologica Scandinavica 1994; **38**:229.
8. Troianos CA, Kuwick RJ, Pasqual JR, Lim AJ, Odasso DP. Internal jugular vein and carotid artery anatomic relation as determined by ultrasonography. Anesthesiology 1996; **85**:43.
9. Oshima E, Ishizu K, Urabe N. A newly designed curved needle for percutaneous cannulation of the internal jugular vein. Anesthesiology 1993; **78**:792.
10. Imai M, Hanaoka Y, Kemmotsu O. Valve injury: a new complication of internal jugular vein cannulation. Anesthesia and Analgesia 1994; **78**:1041.
11. Armstrong PJ, Cullen M, Scott DHT. The 'Site Rite' ultrasound machine – an aid to internal jugular vein cannulation. Anaesthesia 1993; **48**:319.
12. Stickle BR, McFarlane H. Prediction of a small internal jugular vein by external jugular vein diameter. Anaesthesia 1997; **52**:220.
13. Davidson A, Blumgart C, Paes ML, Enever G. Posture and internal jugular vein size studied with the 'SiteRite' ultrasound device. British Journal of Anaesthesia 1993; **71**:771P.
14. English ICW. Percutaneous catheterisation of the internal jugular vein. Anaesthesia 1995; **50**:1070.
15. Powell H, and Beechey APG. Internal jugular catheterisation. Case report of a potentially fatal hazard. Anaesthesia 1990; **45**:458.
16. Jobes DR. The element of experience in internal jugular vein cannulation. Anesthesia and Analgesia 1992; **75**:643.
17. Jobes DR, Schwartz AJ, Ellison N. Teaching central venous cannulation of pediatric patients [abstract]. Anesthesiology 1979; **51**:S346.
18. Hayashi Y, Uchida O, Takaki D, *et al*. Internal jugular vein catheterization in infants undergoing cardiovascular surgery: an analysis of the factors influencing successful catheterization. Anesthesia and Analgesia 1991; **74**:688.
19. Arndt GA, Felton F, Finucaine B, Santora A. Confirmation of internal jugular vein cannulation: the Finucaine technique. Canadian Anaesthetists Society Journal 1993; **40**:1220.
20. Escarpa A, Gomez-Arnau J. Internal jugular vein catheterization: time required with several techniques under different clinical situations. Anesthesia and Analgesia 1983; **62**:97.
21. Oda M, Fukushima Y, Hirota T, Tanaka A, Aono M, Sato T. The para-carotid approach for internal jugular catheterization. Anaesthesia 1981; **36**:896.
22. Stotter AT, Sim AJW, Dudley HAF. The insertion of intravenous feeding catheters: comparing internal jugular and subclavian approaches. British Journal of Parenteral Therapy 1994; **4**:193.
23. Reynolds AD, Cross R, Latto IP. Comparison of internal jugular and central venous pressure measurements. British Journal of Anaesthesia 1984; **56**:267.
24. Sharrock NE, Fierro LE. Jugular venous pulsations as the sole landmark for percutaneous internal jugular cannulation. British Journal of Anaesthesia 1983; **55**:1213.
25. Goldfarb G, Lebrec D. Percutaneous cannulation of the internal jugular vein in patients with coagulopathies: an experience based on 1000 attempts. Anesthesiology 1982; **56**:321.
26. Bazaral M, Harlan S. Ultrasonographic anatomy of the internal jugular vein relevant to percutaneous cannulation. Critical Care Medicine 1981; **9**:307.
27. Tryba M, Kleine P, Zenz M. Sonographic studies for optimizing the cannulation of the internal jugular vein. Anaesthetist 1982; **31**:626.
28. Legler D, Nugent M. Doppler localization of the internal jugular vein facilitates central venous cannulation. Anesthesiology 1984; **60**:481.
29. Ullman JI, Stoelting RK. Internal jugular vein location with the ultra-sound Doppler blood flow detector. Anesthesia and Analgesia 1978; **57**:118.
30. Lee KC, Chinyanga M. Use of a modified doppler flow detector for percutaneous cannulation of the internal jugular vein. Canadian Anaesthetists Society Journal 1985; **32**:548.
31. Bond DM, Champion LK, Nolan R. Real time ultrasound imaging aids jugular venipuncture. Anesthesia and Analgesia 1989; **68**:698.
32. Troianos CA, Jobes DR, Ellison N. Ultrasound guided cannulation of the internal jugular vein. Anesthesiology 1990; **72**:A450.
33. Metz S, Horrow JC, Balcar I. A controlled comparison of techniques for locating the internal jugular vein using ultrasonography. Anesthesia and Analgesia 1984; **63**:673.
34. Mangar D, Turnage WS, Mohamed SA. Is the internal jugular vein cannulated during insertion or withdrawal of

the needle during central venous cannulation? Anesthesia and Analgesia 1993; **76**:1375.
35. Ellison N, Jobes DR. Internal jugular vein cannulation. Anesthesia and Analgesia 1994; **78**:190.
36. Denys BG, Uretsky BF, Reddy PS. Ultrasound-assisted cannulation of the internal jugular vein. Circulation 1993; **87**:1557.
37. Sulek CA, Gravenstein N, Blackshear RH, Weiss L. Head rotation during internal jugular vein cannulation and the risk of carotid artery puncture. Anesthesia and Analgesia 1996; **82**:125.
38. Latto IP. Internal jugular vein cannulation. Avoid venous transfixion. Anaesthesia 1999; **54**:400.
39. Latto IP, Hilton PJ. Multiple cannulation of a single vein. Anaesthesia 1986; **41**:559.
40. Ryan DW, Guy AJ, Weldon OGW, Wai PTJ. Route for major vein cannulation. Anaesthesia 1991; **45**:1086.
41. Skowronski GA, Pearson IY. A technique for insertion of two intravascular catheters via a single vein puncture. Critical Care Medicine 1982; **10**:406.
42. Withington PS, Carter JA. Hazards in multiple cannulation of a single vein. Anaesthesia 1985; **40**:700.
43. Powell H, Beechey APG. A reply (to Punt). Anaesthesia 1991; **45**:1087.
44. Punt CD. Route for major vein cannulation. Anaesthesia 1991; **45**:1086.
45. Rao TLK, Wong AY, Salem MR. A new approach to percutaneous catheterization of the internal jugular vein. Anesthesiology 1977; **46**:362.
46. Sulek CA, Gravenstein N. Head rotation during internal jugular vein cannulation and the risk of carotid artery puncture. In response. Anesthesia and Analgesia 1996; **83**:660.
47. Yee LL, Despotis GJ. Increased venous hemoglobin saturation during percutaneous right internal jugular vein cannulation in a patient with a mature right forearm arteriovenous hemodialysis fistula. Anesthesiology 1990; **73**:184.
48. McEnany MT, Austen WG. Life threatening haemorrhage from inadvertent cervical arteriotomy. Annals of Thoracic Surgery 1977; **24**:233.
49. Morgan RNW, Morell DF. Internal jugular catheterisation: a review of a potentially lethal hazard. Anaesthesia 1981; **36**:512.
50. Jobes DR, Schwartz AJ, Greenhow DE, Stephenson LW, Ellison N. Safer jugular vein cannulation: Recognition of arterial puncture and preferential use of the external jugular route. Anesthesiology 1983; **59**:353.
51. Troianos CA, Jobes DR, Ellison N. Ultrasound-guided cannulation of the internal jugular vein. A prospective randomized study. Anesthesia and Analgesia 1991; **72**:823.
52. Peterson GA. Does systemic anticoagulation increase the risk of internal jugular vein cannulation? Anesthesiology 1991; **75**:1124.
53. Boulanger M, Delva E, Maillèet JG, Paiment, B. Une nouvelle voie d'abord de la veine jugulaire interne. Canadian Anaesthetists Society Journal 1976; **23**:609.
54. Mostert JW, Kenny GM, Murphy GP. Safe placement of central venous catheter into internal jugular veins. Archives of Surgery 1970; **101**:431.
55. Belani KG, Buckley JJ, Gordon JR, Castaneda W. Percutaneous cervical central venous line placement: a comparison of the internal and external jugular vein routes. Anesthesia and Analgesia 1980; **59**:40.
56. Brinkman AJ, Costley DO. Internal jugular venipuncture. Journal of the American Medical Association 1973; **223**:182.
57. Jernigan WR, Gardener WC, Mahr MM, Milburn JL. Use of the internal jugular vein for placement of central venous catheter. Surgery, Gynecology and Obstetrics 1970; **130**:520.
58. Daily PO, Griepp RB, Shunway NE. Percutaneous internal jugular vein cannulation. Archives of Surgery 1970; **101**:534.
59. Vaughan RW, Weygandt GR. Reliable percutaneous central venous pressure measurement. Anesthesia and Analgesia 1973; **52**:709.
60. Prince SR, Sullivan RL, Hackel A. Percutaneous catheterization of the internal jugular vein in infants and children. Anesthesiology 1976; **44**:170.
61. Hall DMB, Geefhuysen J. Percutaneous catheterization of the internal jugular vein in infants and children. Journal of Pediatric Surgery 1977; **12**:719.
62. Civetta JM, Gabel JC, Gemer M. Internal-jugular vein puncture with a margin of safety. Anesthesiology 1972; **36**:622.
63. Latto IP, Hughes JA, Falconer RJ. An assessment of an alternative method of internal jugular vein catheterisation. Anaesthesia 1992; **47**:1047.
64. Messahel FM, Al-Mazroa AA. Cannulation of the internal jugular vein. The very high approach. Anaesthesia 1992; **47**:842.
65. Oshima E, Arai T, Urabe N. New anatomic landmarks for percutaneous catheterization of the internal jugular vein. Anesthesiology 1991; **74**:1164.
66. Willeford KL, Reitan JA. Neutral head position for placement of internal jugular vein catheters. Anaesthesia 1994; **49**:202.
67. Hermosura B, Vanags L, Dickey MW. Measurement of pressure during intravenous therapy. Journal of the American Medical Association 1960; **195**:321.
68. Macdonald DJF. Locating the internal jugular vein. British Journal of Anaesthesia 1984; **56**:1447.
69. Cotè CJ, Jobes DR, Schwartz AJ, Ellison N. Two approaches to cannulation of a child's internal jugular vein. Anesthesiology 1979; **50**:371.
70. Korshin J, Klauber PV, Christensen V, Skovsted P. Percutaneous catheterization of the internal jugular vein. Acta Anaesthesiologica Scandinavica 1978; **67**:27.
71. Johnson FE. Internal jugular vein catheterization. New York State Journal of Medicine 1978; **78**:2168.
72. McConnell RY, Fox RT. Experience with percutaneous internal jugular-innominate vein catheterization. California Medicine 1972; **117**:1.

73. Baker JD, Wallace CT. Internal jugular central venous pressure monitoring. A panacea? Anesthesiology Review 1976; **15**.
74. Defalque RJ. Percutaneous catheterization of the internal jugular vein. Anesthesia and Analgesia 1974; **53**:116.
75. Stevens JC, Hamit HF. A simple method for percutaneous cannulation of the internal jugular vein. American Journal of Surgery 1978; **135**:722.
76. Masud KZ, Forster KJ. Percutaneous internal jugular vein catheterization. Michigan Medicine 1973; **72**:699.
77. Petty C. An alternative method for internal jugular venipuncture for monitoring central venous pressure. Anesthesia and Analgesia 1975; **54**:157.
78. Blitt CD, Wright WA, Petty WC, Webster TA. Central venous catheterization via the external jugular vein. A technique employing the J-wire. Journal of the American Medical Association 1974; **229**:817.
79. Stoelting RK, Haselby KA. Evaluation of a catheter with two side holes for external jugular vein catheterization. Anesthesia and Analgesia 1974; **53**:628.
80. Shield CF, Richardson JD, Buckley CF, Hagood CO. Pseudoaneurysm of the brachiocephalic arteries: a complication of percutaneous internal jugular vein catheterization. Surgery 1975; **78**:190.
81. Blitt CD, Wright WA. An unusual complication of percutaneous internal jugular vein cannulation puncture of an endotracheal tube cuff. Anesthesiology 1974; **40**:306.
82. Lingenfelter AL, Guskiewicz RA, Munson ES. Displacement of right atrial and endotracheal catheters with neck flexion. Anesthesia and Analgesia 1978; **57**:371.
83. Khalil KG, Parker FB, Mukherjee N, Webb WR. Thoracic duct injury. A complication of jugular vein catheterization. Journal of the American Medical Association 1972; **221**:908.
84. Majek M, Malatinsky J, Kadlic T. Inadvertent thoracic duct catheterization during trans-jugular central venous cannulation. A case report. Acta Anaesthesiologica Scandinavica 1977; **21**:320.
85. Arnold S, Feathers RS, Gibbs E. Bilateral pneumothoraces and subcutaneous emphysema: a complication of internal jugular venepuncture. British Medical Journal 1973; **1**:211.
86. Cook TL, Dueker CW. Tension pneumothorax following internal jugular cannulation and general anesthesia. Anesthesiology 1976; **45**:554.
87. Koch MJ. Bilateral 'I. V. hydrothorax'. New England Journal of Medicine 1972; **286**:218.
88. Carvell JE, Pearce DJ. Bilateral hydrothorax following internal jugular catheterization. British Journal of Surgery 1976; **63**:381.
89. Ayalon A, Anner H, Berlatzky Y, Schiller MA. A life-threatening complication of the infusion pump. Lancet 1978; **1**:853.
90. Wisheart JD, Hassan MA, Jackson JW. A complication of percutaneous cannulation of the internal jugular vein. Thorax 1972; **27**:496.
91. Butsch JL, Butsch WL, Da Rosa JFT. Bilateral vocal cord paralysis. A complication of percutaneous cannulation of the internal jugular veins. Archives of Surgery 1976; **111**:828.
92. Briscoe CE, Bushman JA, McDonald WI. Extensive neurological damage after cannulation of internal jugular vein. British Medical Journal 1974; **1**:314.
93. Parikh RK. Horner's syndrome. A complication of percutaneous catheterisation of internal jugular vein. Anaesthesia 1972; **27**:327.
94. Ross SM, Freedman PS, Farman JV. Air embolism after accidental removal of intravenous catheter. British Medical Journal 1979; **1**:987.
95. Brown CS, Wallace CT. Chronic hematoma – a complication of percutaneous catheterization of the internal jugular vein. Anesthesiology 1976; **45**:368.
96. Knoblanche GE. Respiratory obstruction due to haematoma following internal jugular vein cannulation. Anesthesia and Intensive Care 1979; **7**:286.
97. Schuster W, Vennebusch H, Doetsch N, Taube HD. Vena cava superior thrombosis following placement of internal jugular vein catheter. Anaesthetist 1978; **27**:546.
98. Nottage WM. Iatrogenic superior vena cava syndrome. A complication of internal jugular venous catheters. Chest 1976; **70**:566.
99. Schwartz AJ. Percutaneous aortic catheterisation a hazard of supraclavicular internal jugular vein catheterization. Anesthesiology 1977; **46**:77.
100. McDaniel MM, Grossman M. Aortic dissection complicating percutaneous jugular-vein catheterisation. Anesthesiology 1978; **49**:213.
101. Ohlgisser M, Kaufman TS, Taitelman U, Burzstein S, Birkhan JH. Cardiac arrest following a complication of internal jugular cannulation. Anaesthesia 1979; **34**:1035.
102. Sprigge JS, Oakley GDG. Carotid artery palpation during internal jugular vein cannulation and subsequent ventricular fibrillation. British Journal of Anaesthesia 1979; **51**:801.
103. Greenall MJ, Blewitt RW, McMahon MJ. Cardiac tamponade and central venous catheters. British Medical Journal 1975; **2**:595.
104. Defalque RJ, Campbell C. Cardiac tamponade from central venous catheters. Anesthesiology 1979; **50**:249.
105. Malatinskÿ J, Kadlic T, Màjek M, Sàmel M. Misplacement and loop formation of central venous catheters. Acta Anaesthesiologica Scandinavica 1976; **20**:237.
106. Kuramota T, Sakabe T. Comparison of success in jugular versus basilic vein technics for central venous pressure catheter position. Anaesthesia and Analgesia 1975; **54**:696.
107. Fischer J, Lundstrom J, Ottander HG. Central venous cannulation: a radiological determination of catheter positions and immediate intrathoracic complications. Acta Anaesthesiologica Scandinavica 1977; **21**:245.
108. Schwartz AJ, Jobes DR, Greenhow E, Stephenson LW, Ellison N. Carotid artery puncture with internal jugular cannulation using the Seldinger technique: incidence, recognition, treatment and prevention. Anesthesiology 1979; **51**:S160.

109. Ellison N, Schwartz AJ, Jobes DR, Greenhow DE, Stephenson LW. Avoidance of carotid artery puncture sequelae during internal jugular cannulation. Anesthesia and Analgesia 1982; **61**:181.
110. Shah KB, Tafikonda LK, Rao MD, Laughlin S, El-Etr A. A review of pulmonary artery catheterization in 6245 patients. Anesthesiology 1984; **61**:271.
111. Peters J, Steinhoff H, Sandmann W. Carotid aneurysm after jugular vein catheterization. Anaesthetist 1984; **33**:330.
112. Aoki H, Mizobe T, Nozuchi S, Hatanaka T, Tanaka Y. Vertebral artery pseudoaneurysm: a rare complication of internal jugular vein catheterisation. Anesthesia and Analgesia 1992; **75**:296.
113. MacGillivray RG. Transverse cervical artery pseudoaneurysm: a complication of internal jugular vein catheterisation. Anesthesia and Analgesia 1995; **81**:1114.
114. Burri C, Ahnefeld FW. The Caval Catheter, p. 45. Berlin: Springer.
115. Verrieres D, Bernard C, Dacheux J. Cervical arteriovenous fistulas following internal jugular catheterisation. Anesthesia Reanimation 1986; **5**:162.
116. Ellison N, Jobes DR, Schwartz AJ. Cannulation of the internal jugular vein: a cautionary note. Anesthesiology 1981; **55**:336.
117. Tyden H. Cannulation of the internal jugular vein – 500 cases. Acta Anaesthesiologica Scandinavica 1982; **26**:485.
118. Powell H. Safety first with triple lumen catheters. Murmurs 1988; **5**:4.
119. Reeves ST, Baliga P, Conroy JM, Cleaver TL. Avulsion of the right facial vein during double cannulation of the internal jugular vein. Journal of Cardiothoracic and Vascular Anaesthesia 1995; **9**:429.
120. Goldfarb G, Lebrec D. Percutaneous cannulation of the internal jugular vein in patients with coagulopathies: an experience based on 1000 attempts. Anesthesiology 1982; **56**:321.
121. Sheep RE, Guiney WB. Fatal cardiac tamponade. Occurrence with other complications after left internal jugular vein catheterisation. Journal of the American Medical Association 1982; **248**:1632.
122. Tovi F, Fliss DM, Noyek AM. Septic internal jugular vein thrombosis. Journal of Otolaryngology 1993; **22**:415.
123. Sagor G, Mitchelmere P, Layfield J, Prentice P, Kirk RM. Prolonged access to the venous system using the Hickman right atrial catheter. Annals of the Royal College of Surgeons of England 1983; **65**:47.
124. Chastre J, Cornud F, Bouchama A, Viau F, Benacerraf R, Gibert C. Thrombosis as a complication of pulmonary-artery catheterization via the internal jugular vein. New England Journal of Medicine 1982; **306**:278.
125. Elinger JH, Bedford RF, Buschi AJ. Do pulmonary artery catheters cause jugular vein thrombosis? Anesthesiology 1981; **57**:A118.
126. Perkins NAK, Bedford RF, Buschi AJ, Cail WS. Internal jugular vein function after Swan-Ganz catheterization studied by venography and ultrasound. Anesthesiology 1983; **59**:A145.
127. Perkins NAK, Cail WS, Bedford RF, Elinger LH, Butschi AJ. Internal jugular vein function after Swan-Ganz catheterization. Anesthesiology 1984; **61**:456.
128. Agraharkar M, Isaacson S, Mendelssohn D, *et al.* Percutaneously inserted silastic jugular haemodialysis catheters seldom cause jugular vein thrombosis. ASAIO Journal 1995; **41**:169.
129. De Bruijn NR, Stadt HH. Bilateral thrombosis of internal jugular veins after multiple percutaneous cannulations. Anaesthesia and Analgesia 1981; **60**:448.
130. Ducatman BS, McMichan JC, Edwards WD. Catheter induced lesions of the right side of the heart. Journal of the American Medical Association 1985; **253**:791.
131. Crowell RH, Adams GS, Koilpillai CJ, McNutt EJ, Montague TJ. In vivo right heart thrombus: precursor of life-threatening pulmonary embolism. Chest 1988; **94**:1236.
132. Joshi P, Bullingham A, Soni N. Septic atrial thrombus: a complication of central venous catheterisation. Anaesthesia 1991; **46**:1030.
133. Gilston A. Internal jugular vein catheterisation. A right sided pleural effusion. Anaesthesia 1982; **37**:221.
134. Bara DP, Dru M, Freffe B. Late venous perforation due to percutaneous central venous cannulation. Canadian Anaesthetists Society Journal 1986; **33**:225.
135. Pina J, Morujao N, Castro-Tavares J. Internal jugular catheterisation. Blood reflux is not a reliable sign in patients with thoracic trauma. Anaesthesia 1992; **47**:30.
136. Punt CD, Swen J, Bovill JG, Obermann WR. Delayed perforations of intrathoracic veins: a comparison between right- and left-sided internal jugular cannulation. European Journal of Anaesthesiology 1990; **7**:25.
137. Forestene JE. Ipsilateral mydriasis following carotid-artery puncture during attempted cannulation of the internal jugular vein. Anesthesiology 1980; **52**:438.
138. Vest JV, Pereira MB, Senior RM. Phrenic nerve injury associated with venipuncture of the internal jugular vein. Chest 1980; **78**:777.
139. Stock MC, Downs JB. Transient phrenic nerve blockade during internal jugular vein cannulation using the anterolateral approach. Anesthesiology 1982; **57**:230.
140. Lange LS, Rees A. Preventing early neurological complications of coronary artery bypass surgery. British Medical Journal 1986; **292**:27.
141. Frasquet FJ, Belda FJ. Permanent paralysis of C5 after cannulation of the internal jugular vein. Anesthesiology 1981; **54**:528.
142. Whittet HB, Boscoe MJ. Isolated palsy of the hypoglossal nerve after central venous catheterisation. British Medical Journal 1984; **41**:288.
143. Nakayama M, Fujita S, Kawamata M, Namiki A, Mayumi T. Traumatic aneurysm of the internal jugular vein causing vagal nerve palsy: a rare complication of percutaneous catheterisation. Anesthesia and Analgesia 1994; **78**:598.

144. Feldman H, Seetzen-Kanaan G. Lesion of vagus nerve: a complication following cannulation of internal jugular vein? Anaesthetist 1984; **33**:322.
145. Burns S, Herbison GJ. Spinal accessory nerve injury as a complication of internal jugular vein cannulation. Annals of Internal Medicine 1996; **125**:700.
146. Zaidi NA, Khan M, Naqvi HI, Kamal RS. Cerebral infarct following central venous cannulation. Anaesthesia 1998; **53**:186.
147. Anagnou J. Cerebrovascular accident during percutaneous cannulation of internal jugular vein. Lancet 1982; **2**:377.
148. Bastulli JA, Orlowski JP. Stroke as a complication of carotid sinus massage. Critical Care Medicine 1985;13/ **10**:867.
149. Brown CQ. Inadvertent prolonged cannulation of the carotid artery. Anesthesia and Analgesia 1982; **61**:150.
150. Sloan MA, Mueller JD, Adelman LS, Caplan LR. Fatal brainstem stroke following internal jugular vein catheterisation. Neurology 1991; **41**:1092.
151. Stephens PH, Lennox G, Hirsch N, Miller D. Superior sagittal sinus thrombosis after internal jugular vein cannulation. British Journal of Anaesthesia 1995; **67**:76.
152. Larkey D, Williams CR, Fanning J, Hilgers RD, Graham DR. Fatal superior sagittal sinus thrombosis associated with internal jugular vein catheterisation. American Journal of Obstetrics and Gynecology 1993; **169**:1612.
153. Stewart RW, Hardjasudarma M, Nall L, Matthews G, Davis R. Fatal outcome of jugular vein cannulation. Southern Medical Journal 1995; **88**:1159.
154. Cozanitits DA. Earache following caval catheterization. Anaesthetist 1981; **30**:150.
155. Gilner LI. The 'ear-gurgling' sign [Letter]. New England Journal of Medicine 1977; **296**:1301.
156. Polglase A. Malpositioned central venous cannulae and the internal jugular vein. Medical Journal of Australia 1976; **2**:714.
157. Klein HO, Di Segni E, Kaplinski E. Unsuspected cerebral perfusion: a complication of the use of a central venous pressure catheter. Chest 1978; **74**:109.
158. Souter RG, Mitchell A. Spreading cortical venous thrombosis due to infusion of hyperosmolar solution into the internal jugular vein. British Medical Journal 1982; **285**:935.
159. Saxena VK, Heilpern J, Murphy SF. Pseudotumour cerebri. A complication of parenteral hyperalimentation. Journal of the American Medical Association 1976; **235**:2124.
160. Stewart DR, Johnson DG, Myers GG. Hydrocephalus as a complication of jugular catheterization during total parenteral nutrition. Journal of Pediatric Surgery 1975; **10**:771.
161. Nagai K, Kemmotsu O. An inadvertent insertion of a Swan-Ganz catheter into the intrathecal space. Anesthesiology 1985; **62**:48.
162. Berlatzjy Y, Freund H, Schiller M. Percutaneous internal jugular vein cannulation in children. Zeitschrift fur Kinderchirurgie 1976; **18**:237.
163. Damen J. Positive bacterial cultures and related risk factor associated with percutaneous internal jugular vein catheterization in pediatric cardiac patients. Anesthesiology 1987; **66**:558.
164. Konichezky S, Saguib S, Soroker D. Tracheal puncture. A complication of percutaneous jugular vein cannulation. Anaesthesia 1983; **38**:572.
165. Levin H, Bursztein S, Heifetz M. Prestenotic dilatation of the oesophagus: a hazard of internal jugular vein cannulation. Anesthesia and Analgesia 1986; **65**:901.
166. Lowe D, Pagel PS. A complication of internal jugular vein double cannulation. Anesthesia and Analgesia 1995; **81**:206.
167. Fielden JM, Monk CR. Caution during double cannulation of the internal jugular vein. Anaesthesia 1996; **51**:794.
168. Randalls B, Toomey PJ. Laryngeal oedema from a neck haematoma. A complication of internal jugular vein cannulation. Anaesthesia 1990; **45**:850.
169. Scott DHT. 'In the country of the blind the one-eyed man is king'. Erasmus (1466–1536). British Journal of Anaesthesia 1999; **82**:820.
170. Hatfield A, Bodenham A. Portable ultrasound for difficult central venous access. British Journal of Anaesthesia 1999; **82**:822.
171. Latto IP. No evidence for seeker needles: a reply. Anaesthesia 1999; **54**:1014.

8 • The External Jugular Vein

PETER LATTO

Cannulation of the external jugular vein for central venous pressure monitoring and fluid infusion was first described by Rams and his colleagues in 1966.[1] They used a surgical cut-down technique. A percutaneous variation of this technique was later described to avoid the disadvantages of a surgical cut-down.[2] Subsequent authors described percutaneous techniques for external jugular vein cannulation both in adults[3–6] and in children.[7–9] The route however remained relatively unpopular for at least another 8 years because of the difficulty in successfully threading catheters past the sharply angulated junction of the external jugular and subclavian veins.

In 1974 Blitt and his colleagues described the value of a J wire in improving the incidence of successful central placement of catheters when using the external jugular route.[10] They achieved a previously unattainable incidence of central placement of 96%. Their four failures were attributed to the presence of a venous plexus formed by the external jugular vein above the clavicle.

In the last few years the J wire kit has become a freely available and affordable item for the British anaesthetist. A number of authors[11–13] have suggested that the external jugular vein route should be more widely adopted because of its low incidence of serious complications. Indeed, there does appear to be a trend towards an increasing use of the external jugular vein in anaesthetic practice.

This change in clinical practice is due to the appreciation of the low risk of complications during insertion, and to the increasing availability of J wires and thus an improved success rate in satisfactory central placement; it has also been shown that valid venous pressure measurements can be made from catheters whose tips are placed just above the junction of the external jugular and subclavian veins.[14]

Pressure Monitoring

Although measurements of central venous pressure can be made with short cannulae in the external jugular vein in anaesthetised patients,[15,16] they may be unreliable since they may be affected by changes in the position of the head as the patient moves around. Improved results are obtained using a catheter with two side holes near its distal end.[17] Reliable measurements cannot be obtained with short cannulae after the chest has been opened.[15] A later study has shown that accurate pressure measurements can be obtained with the catheter tip just above the junction of the external jugular and subclavian veins.[14] Measurements were unaffected by head position or the side of catheterisation. A round-tipped catheter with two side holes was used. This means that by using such a catheter satisfactory pressure measurements can be obtained in 100% of cases if external jugular venous catheterisation is possible.

Clinical Uses of the External Jugular Vein

Since the external jugular vein lies superficially in the neck, the traumatic complications associated with blind venepuncture of deep veins are avoided. This vein, therefore, may be specifically indicated as an alternative to arm veins, particularly if expertise in internal jugular and subclavian vein cannulation is lacking. A short venous catheter can usually be readily inserted into the external jugular vein for intraoperative infusion of drugs or volume replacement. Such a catheter provides a convenient intraoperative access site. The tip of such a short catheter is near the external jugular subclavian junction and thus approximates to a 'halfway' catheter.[18] Such a catheter should be removed immediately at the end of the period of anaesthesia because of the risk of air embolus in the sitting position if a disconnection occurs. This technique may be particularly useful in cardiac arrest patients for 'central' infusion of drugs if a central venous catheter is not immediately available. It should also be recognised that attempts to insert central venous catheters by house officers during a cardiac arrest have a low success rate and a high complication rate.[19]

The vein can also be used for the insertion of one or more single-lumen central venous catheters, a double- or triple-lumen catheter, a haemodialysis catheter, a pacemaker or a Swan–Ganz catheter.

The external jugular vein can be used as a route for long-term (9–50 days) parenteral nutrition in adults.[20] The vein has also been used for inserting Hickman catheters by a surgical cut-down technique in children requiring bone marrow transplant.[21] The catheters were left *in situ* from 1 month to $3\frac{1}{2}$ months. The procedure was done under fluoroscopic control and the catheter tip advanced to the mid-atrial position.

The external jugular vein was the preferred route for percutaneous insertion of flexible, soft Silastic central venous catheters in 15 newborn infants.[22] The fine-bore flexible catheters passed without difficulty into the right atrium and were left *in situ* for a mean of 24.8 days. They were used for administration of total parenteral nutrition. No thrombophlebitis, infection or caval thrombosis was detected.

Some patients do not have a visible or palpable vein on either side. In other patients the vein is visible on one side only. It has been claimed that about 90% of people have a single prominent external jugular vein running down from the angle of the jaw across the sternomastoid muscle to the subclavian vein.[13] There is no difference in the success of central placement between the veins on the right or left side and therefore the most prominent vein should be selected.

In practice the right side of the neck is commonly draped for the more frequently used internal jugular route. The patient should be carefully examined before this procedure to assess the size of external jugular vein. If cannulation of the internal jugular vein is difficult and the attempt abandoned, then the external jugular vein can be used.

Clinical Experience

When external jugular veins are used by junior staff in an emergency the results are worse than for experienced staff under elective circumstances. A success rate of only 53% (18/34) was achieved by house officers on an intensive care unit.[23] It was stressed that operator inexperience was a most important factor and that considerable manipulation of the J wire was often required. In another study inexperienced house officers attempted central venous cannulation.[19] Their success rate with the external jugular vein was 61% (51/84). Surprisingly, failure was attributed most commonly to inability to thread the catheter into the vein. Their success rate was lower than that for internal jugular and subclavian routes.

Practical Points

Various authors have made recommendations to facilitate puncture of the external jugular vein and to advance a guide-wire or catheter centrally. These recommendations appear arbitrary and their validity has not been confirmed by clinical evaluation.

Patient preparation and examination

Place the patient in the Trendelenburg position and examine the neck to determine the degree of venous prominence. If necessary a stethoscope or a finger may be used to distend the vein further by obstructing venous return. In some patients the vein is prominent with the patient in the horizontal position and therefore the Trendelenburg position is not required.

A conscious patient can be asked to perform a Valsalva manoeuvre both before venepuncture and while the J wire is being threaded centrally. In an anaesthetised patient the lungs can be momentarily held in inflation to distend the vein, both during venous catheterisation and while the J wire is threaded centrally. Although the vein is only loosely fixed in the subcutaneous tissues it is not always easy to distend.[13]

Some cardiac patients are unable to tolerate either a Trendelenburg or even a flat position. The external jugular veins may however be dilated in these patients even in the sitting position. In the absence of a suitable arm vein the external jugular vein can be catheterised in the sitting position but great care must be taken to avoid the risk of air embolus. Turning the head fully on to one side can stretch the skin over the vein on the side to be cannulated and make the vein less visible. Bringing the head back towards the mid-line will in some patients make the vein more easily visible.

In some patients the vein is much bigger on one side than the other. Clearly it is sensible to select the bigger vein because it is likely to be easier to cannulate. In one study after insertion of a cannula into the vein a higher successful central placement of a J wire was reported on the left side than that on the right side.[24] Others have not been able to demonstrate a difference in successful central placement between the two sides.[25] It is certainly not usually obvious why the wire passes centrally with the greatest of ease in one patient but extreme difficulty is encountered in another patient. If difficulty is encountered on one side and the external jugular vein is the vein of choice then an attempt can be made on the other side.

Getting into the vein

Use a catheter-over-needle for venepuncture. A steel needle is more likely to cause vein wall puncture and haematoma.[12] Advance the catheter only a few centimetres into the vein to prevent the catheter tip entering a small tributary.[12] Enter the vein from the side rather than the top to minimise transfixion and haematoma formation.[13]

Threading wire or catheter centrally

Repeated insertion of guide-wires is required in a third of all cases.[12] If the wire cannot be threaded centrally retract it fully before making another attempt.[12] If the wire sticks it can be withdrawn and rotated through 180° before a further attemptis made.[13] Alternatively the J wire can be advanced or withdrawn while it is being gently rotated.[26] Avoid prolonged or forceful manipulation of wires and make a skin incision to facilitate easy insertion of the catheter or vein dilator over the guide-wire.

Turning the head to the side being catheterised and medial traction on the skin of the neck will make the angle between the external jugular and subclavian veins less acute.[13,26,27] In addition external manipulation by finger-tip pressure may be helpful; saline can be injected to distend the veins locally. If the arm is raised and pulled to the same side the angle between the subclavian and external jugular veins is made less acute.

Do not advance the catheter with any force past points of obstruction as it may become angulated and stuck, and difficult to remove.[28] Such catheters may require surgical intervention to facilitate removal.

In one study successful central placement of a J wire was achieved in 10 out of 25 (40%) cases by manipulating the shoulder when the wire could not be threaded centrally.[25] The shoulder was first pushed anteriorly by an assistant and if the attempt was still unsuccessful the shoulder was manipulated in the other direction. Blitt[29] recommended that the arm should be rotated internally and upward pressure be applied to the scapula. This raises the clavicle and should help the wire to pass centrally. No information was given on how successful the manoeuvre was in achieving successful central wire placement.

Choice of equipment

A number of studies using different catheters and wires are summarised in Table 8.1. Early studies compared the use of catheter-through-cannula and catheter-through-needle devices.[27,30] In both studies round-ended rather than open-ended catheters gave a higher incidence of successful central placement. The use of catheter-through-cannula rather than through-needle devices will prevent shearing of catheters and the potential for catheter embolisation.

The use of J wires improves the success rate of central placement. Berthelsen *et al.* in 1986[12] concluded that it was nearly always possible to insert a central venous catheter past the external jugular subclavian junction if the vein could be cannulated. More and more authors are recommending the external jugular vein as the route of first choice.

Comparisons have been made between J wires of different radii. It has been suggested by Humphrey and Blitt[31] that a radius of 1.5 mm may increase the incidence of successful central placement in children: the standard radius used is 3 mm. A curved J wire has been shown to result in a higher incidence of successful central placement than a straight Seldinger wire.[32]

Often clinicians may be limited in their choice of equipment. If a J wire kit is available this should be used in preference to simple catheter through cannula devices. If a J wire is not available the use of a round-ended catheter with side holes is preferable to the use of an open-ended catheter.[30,31]

Anatomy

The external jugular vein is formed by the junction of the posterior division of the posterior facial vein and the posterior auricular vein. It receives blood from the deep parts of the face and the surface of the cranium, and runs down the neck from the angle of the mandible, crosses the sternomastoid muscle obliquely, and terminates behind the middle of the clavicle on joining with the subclavian vein. The vein is variable in size and possesses valves 4 cm above the clavicle and just before its junction with the subclavian vein. Natural variations and disease states are responsible for the wide range in the degree of prominence of the external jugular vein.

The vein penetrates the deep fascia of the subclavian triangle. It then passes posterior to the clavicle and enters the subclavian vein at an acute angle. Obstruction to the central passage of a wire could theoretically occur at any acute angle. Possible points of obstruction include the angle as the vein passes through the fascia, at a point behind the clavicle, at the valve in the vein and lastly at the acute angle as the vein joins the subclavian vein. Most clinicians consider the last of these to be the most important but all four could be important and contribute to different degrees of difficulty in different patients. There is an inverse correlation between the sizes of the internal and external jugular veins.[33] Thus if the external jugular vein is very small the chances of successful catheterisation of the internal jugular vein should be increased. Conversely the internal jugular vein may be small if the external jugular vein is large (7 mm or more in external diameter). Stickle and McFarlane recommended the routine measurement of external jugular vein diameter as a screen for small internal jugular vein diameter.[33] If difficulty is encountered in internal jugular cannulation in a patient with a large-diameter external jugular vein then cannulation of the ipsilateral external jugular vein should be considered. There was no correlation between the diameter of the external jugular vein and patient weight, neck circumference or body mass index.

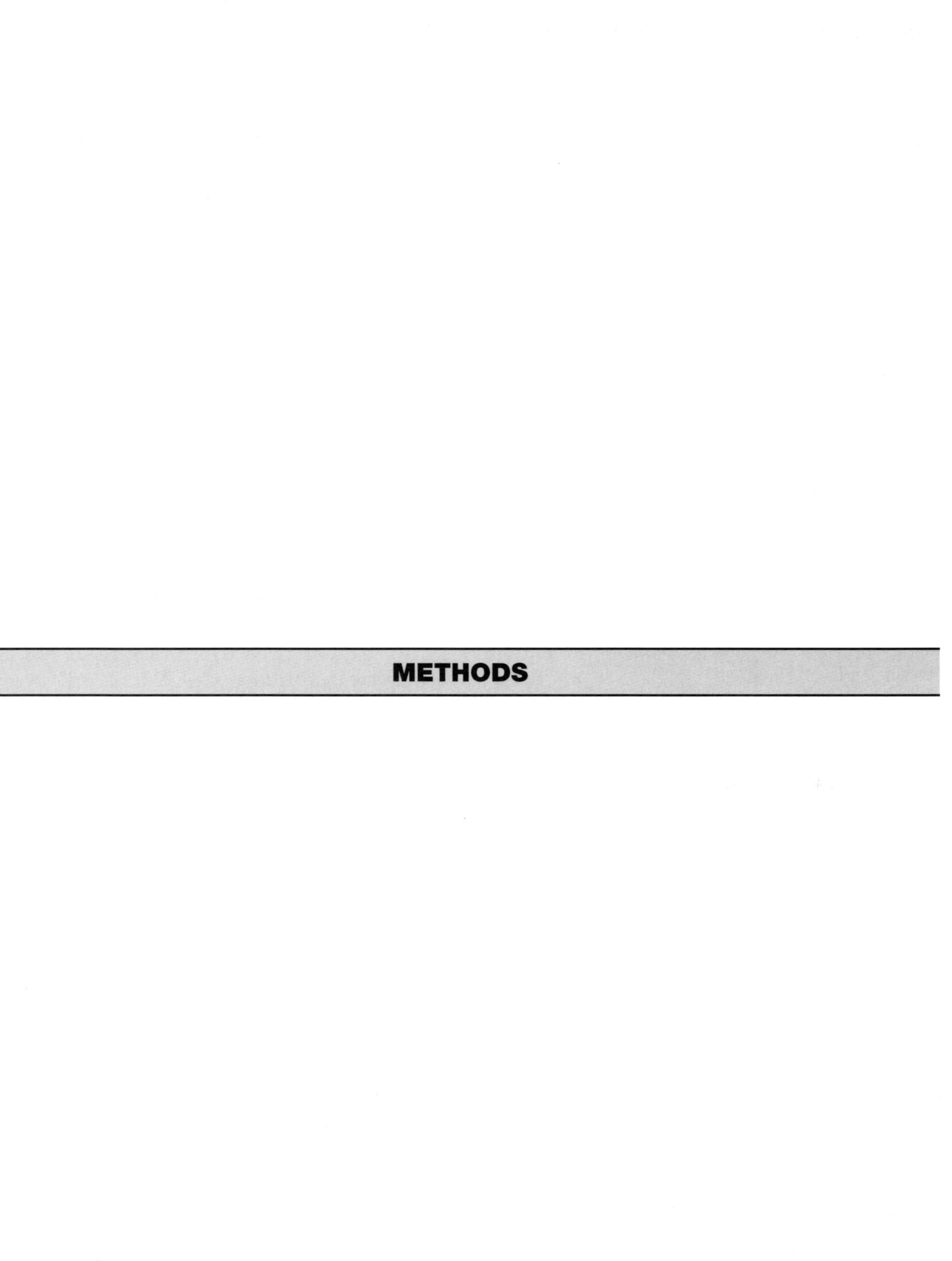

METHODS

EXTERNAL JUGULAR VEIN APPROACH if J wire is unavailable

Authors' method

Patient category

Adults and children.

Advantages and disadvantages

The only contraindication to using the external jugular vein is local sepsis. When catheters or cannulae are used without J wires there is a substantially lower incidence of central placement than when J wires are used. The only reason for using catheters alone therefore is if J wires are unavailable. However, round-ended catheters placed approximately 1 cm above the clavicle will give accurate central venous pressure readings.[14] Such catheters have their tips close to the lateral region of the first rib, and therefore function in a similar way to the 'halfway' catheters described by Gustavsson *et al.* in 1985.[18] The frequency of use of J wires in the developed world is likely to increase. However, in other countries catheters alone will still be frequently required.

Preferred side

Either side may be used.

Position of patient

Place the table in a 25° head-down position. Turn the patient's head away from the side of puncture and place both arms by the sides (Figure 8.1a)

Position of operator

Stand at the head of the patient (Figure 8.1a).

Equipment used

Catheter-through-cannula.

Anatomical landmarks

The landmarks are the external jugular vein and sternomastoid muscle (Figure 8.1b). The external jugular vein is not always palpable or visible; if this is the case, cathererisation should not be attempted.

Preparation

Perform the puncture under sterile conditions using local anaesthesia if indicated.

Precautions and recommendations

Distend the vein if necessary by holding the lungs in inflation for a short time if the patient is anaesthetised, or by asking the patient to perform a Valsalva manoeuvre if awake. Place a finger on the lower portion of the vein to impede venous drainage so as to distend the vein.

Point of insertion of needle

Insert the needle in the line of the vein where it is most easily seen (Figure 8.1b). Cannulate well above the clavicle to avoid the risk of pneumothorax.

Direction of needle and procedure

Attach the needle to a saline-filled syringe. Place the point of the needle on the skin entry site and point the needle caudally (A in Figure 8.1c). Swing the needle and syringe to point the needle in the axis of the vein (A to B). Elevate the syringe just above the skin (B to C, Figure 8.1d, e). Advance the needle and syringe maintaining a slight negative pressure in the syringe. When the vein is entered, remove the needle from the cannula and thread the catheter centrally. Fix the catheter securely. If resistance is encountered when threading the catheter centrally, inject fluid into the catheter as it is advanced, rotate the catheter, and press on the skin just above the clavicle. If central placement proves impossible, leave the catheter at the position reached as this will frequently be satisfactory during anaesthesia for making measurements of central venous pressure and for taking blood samples.

Success rate

A rate of 72% central placement was achieved in 50 patients.[30]

Complications

None.

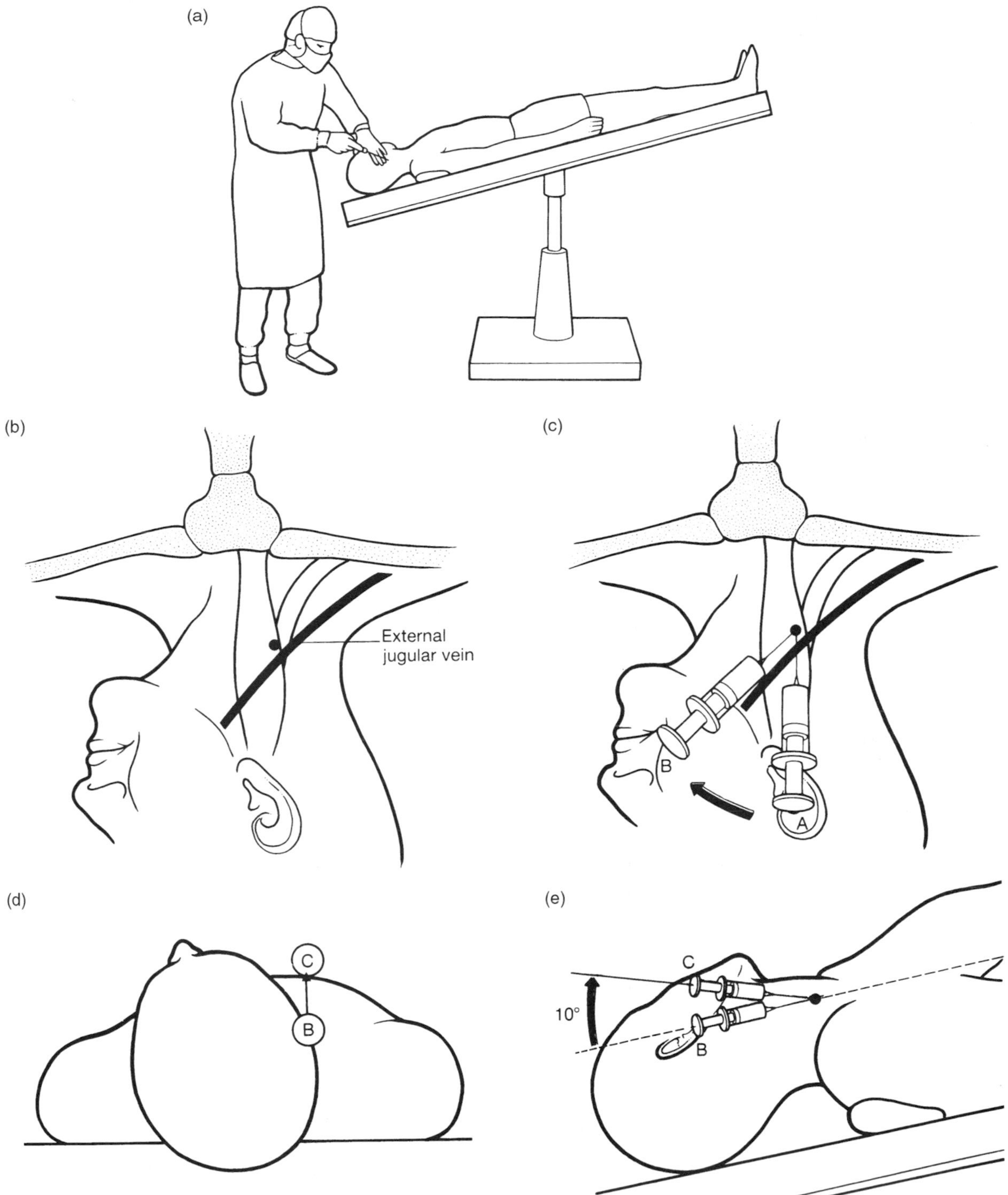

Figure 8.1 Technique of catheterisation: authors' method.

EXTERNAL JUGULAR VEIN APPROACH: J wire technique

Blitt et al. *(1974)*[10]

Patient category

Adults and children.

Advantages and disadvantages

This technique greatly increases the rate of central placement.

Preferred side

Either side may be used. The choice may be influenced by the prominence of the external jugular vein.

Position of patient

Place the table in a 30° head-down position. Turn the patient's head away from the side of puncture and place both arms by the sides (see Figure 8.1a).

Position of operator

Stand at head of patient (see Figure 8.1a).

Equipment used in original description

A 14 gauge or 16 gauge 14 cm Teflon catheter-over-needle; 35 cm long, 0.089 cm diameter, flexible wire catheter guide with a distal radius of curvature of 3 mm (the J wire). This equipment is supplied complete with instructions in a single pack (Figure 8.2).

Advice on current equipment

Use a small needle, a J wire and a soft, flexible non-thrombogenic catheter.

Anatomical landmarks

The external jugular vein and the sternomastoid muscle.

Preparation

Perform the puncture under sterile conditions using local anaesthesia if indicated.

Precautions and recommendations

Distend the vein if necessary by holding the lungs in inflation for a short time if the patient is anaesthetised, or by asking the patient to perform a Valsalva manoeuvre if awake. Place a finger on the lower portion of the vein to impede venous drainage and so distend the vein.

Point of insertion of needle

Insert the needle in the line of the vein where it is easily seen. The point of insertion should be well above the clavicle to avoid the risk of pneumothorax (see Figure 8.1b).

Direction of needle and procedure

Attach the needle to a saline-filled syringe. Place the point of the needle on the skin entry site and point the needle caudally (A in Figure 8.1c). Swing the needle and syringe to point the needle in the axis of the vein (A to B). Elevate the syringe just above the skin (B to C, see Figure 8.1d, e). Advance the needle and syringe maintaining a slight negative pressure in the syringe. When the vein is entered, advance the needle assembly approximately 2.5 cm into the vein. Straighten the J tip of the wire by sliding the plastic insertion sleeve to its end. Remove the needle from the catheter and place the tip of the plastic sleeve into the hub of the catheter. This allows the J wire to be pushed through the catheter and then into the vein. When the wire emerges from the end of the catheter its tip reverts to the original J shape. Advance the wire into the intrathoracic vein, rotating it if obstruction is encountered. Once the wire is in an intrathoracic vein, advance the catheter over the wire. Remove the wire and connect the catheter to the infusion system. Fix the catheter securely and check its position with a chest radiograph.

Success rate

Central placement was achieved in 96 of 100 attempts. In 5 of the 96 cases, measurement of central venous pressure was initially unsatisfactory and alteration of the position of the catheter was needed.

Complications

No complications were reported.

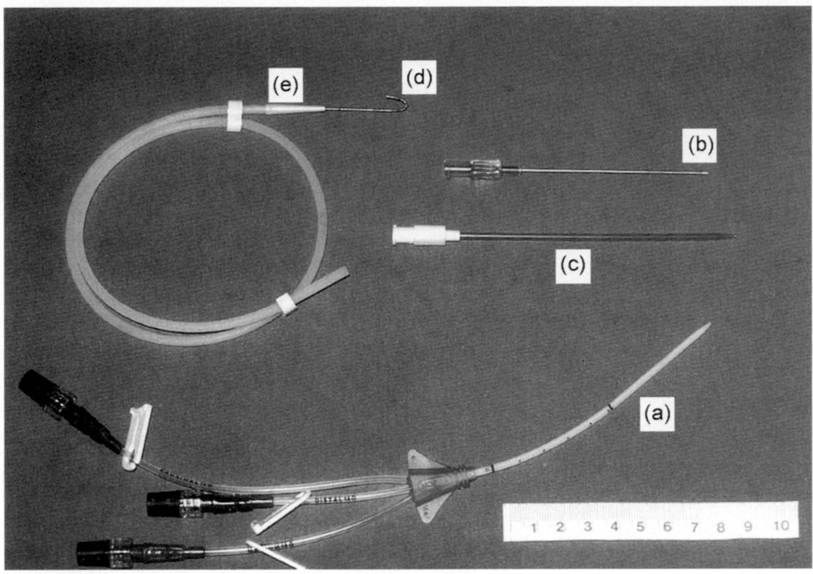

Figure 8.2 The J-wire technique: Blitt *et al.* (1974).[10] (a) Soft flexible triple-lumen catheter; (b) needle; (c) vein dilator; (d) J wire; (e) plastic device to straighten J wire.

Table 8.1 Comparison of results obtained using different types of equipment.

Author and year	Equipment used or cannulation attempts	No. of patients	Successful central placements No. (%)	Comments
Cannulae				
Riddell *et al.* (1982)[30]	Catheter-through-cannula (closed tip)	114 patients with 100 venous cannulations	36/50 (72) (closed tip)	Choice of catheter may influence the success rate
	Catheter-through-needle (open-ended)		30/50 (60) (open-ended)	
Schaps *et al.* (1988)[27]	Closed-tip catheter 60 Open-ended catheter 65	125	51/60 (85) (closed tip) 44/65 (67.7) (open-ended)	Central catheter placement was helped by: 1. Finger-tip pressure at external jugular subclavian junction 2. Injection of saline through the catheterto expand the vein 3. Pulling the arm to the side to improve the angle between external jugular and subclavian veins 4. Turning the head to the side of catheterized vein
Paediatric Seldinger Wire				
Giesy (1972)[6]	Soft, pliable silicone elastomer catheter	112	101/112 (90)	
Humphrey and Blitt (1982)[31]	J wire with 3 mm radius of curvature	20 children with 17 venous cannulations (mean age 56 mo, mean wt 18.9 kg)	10/17 (59)	They suggested that the use of a J wire with a 1.5 mm radius of curvature wire might improve the success rate in children
Nicolson *et al.* (1985)[34]	Seldinger wires	117 patients for EJV study (an investigation in children comparing the IJV and EJV routes)	*Age* — *Attempt* — *Success* <1 mo — 1 — 1 (100) 1 mo –1 yr — 17 — 6 (35) 1–5 yr — 22 — 13 (59) >5 yr — 77 — 56 (73) Total — 117 — 76 (65) 14% of successful cannulations had catheter tips incorrectly positioned	No difference between right and left external jugular vein. They preferred the IJV to the EJV route in children (the IJV route gave an 86% incidence of successful cannulations and a 99.9% incidence of central placement of the catheter tip)
Adult Seldinger Wire				
Blitt *et al.* (1974)[10]	J wire with 3 mm radius of curvature	100	96/100 (96)	The first reported use of the J wire in the external jugular vein. The technique is easy to teach to residents and free of complications. The 4 failures occurred in patients with a venous plexus above the clavicle
Abadair *et al.* (1979)[26]	J wire 0.035 in (0.089 cm) diameter	108	99/108 (91.6) 96 first attempt 3 on opposite side *Failures* 3 failed both EJV 5 no visible EJV 1 advanced to basilic vein	The external jugular vein is suitable for Swan–Ganz catheters

<table>
<tr><td>Belani et al. (1980)[35]</td><td>J wire
0.089 cm OD</td><td>42</td><td>32/42 (76)

30 intrathoracic catheter tips
2 malpositioned tips</td><td>Lower success rate than Blitt et al., possibly due to less vigorous attempts to get the J wire past venous obstructions. This study also compared external and internal jugular routes. The external route was safe but had a lower incidence of central catheter placements</td></tr>
<tr><td>Blyth (1985)[36]</td><td>J wire 0.089 cm OD</td><td>100</td><td>90/100 (90)

Cannulation of vein unsuccessful in 3 cases
Unable to pass wire centrally in 7 cases</td><td>Most important advantage is the absence of major complications. If cannulation of EJV is unsuccessful IJV cannulation can be performed without the need to redrape</td></tr>
<tr><td>Nordstrom and Fletcher (1983)[37]</td><td>Patients randomised to J wire of either 6 mm diameter or 3 mm diameter
If allocated J wire could not be passed then other wire was tried</td><td>138</td><td colspan="2"><table><tr><th>Number</th><th>J wire used first</th><th>Success</th><th>J wire used second</th><th>Success</th></tr><tr><td>77</td><td>6 mm</td><td>54/77 (70%)</td><td>3 mm</td><td>13/23 (56%)</td></tr><tr><td>61</td><td>3 mm</td><td>55/61(88%)</td><td>6 mm</td><td>0/6(0%)</td></tr></table>Difference between two wires was statistically significant ($P < 0.05$)</td></tr>
<tr><td>Schwartz et al. (1982)[11]</td><td>(a) Straight wire – straight central venous catheter</td><td>163</td><td>(a) 19/31 (61)</td><td>The J wire is not necessary for PA catheterisation</td></tr>
<tr><td></td><td>(b) J wire – straight central venous catheter</td><td></td><td>(b) 25/29 (86)</td><td>J wire more successful than straight wire ($P< 0.05$)</td></tr>
<tr><td></td><td>(c) Straight wire – PA catheter with curved tip</td><td></td><td>(c) 91/103 (88)
Total 135/163 (83)</td><td>PA catheter with curved tip sufficient. This technique was recommended as the initial approach in all patients with an appropriate EJV</td></tr>
<tr><td>Blitt et al. 1982)[32]</td><td>(a) Straight wire (0.035 in diameter) was first passed if possible
(b) If this failed a J wire (3 mm radius) was used (successful in all remaining cases)</td><td>36</td><td>(a) 16/36 (44)

(b) 20/20 (100)</td><td>Study to compare straight wires with J wires. The J wire was thought to ‘bounce off’ or ‘roll through’ angles and bends in the vein</td></tr>
<tr><td>Berthelson et al. (1986)[12]</td><td>First attempt – straight wire
Second attempt – J-modified wire (end of straight wire angulated)
Third attempt – J wire</td><td>115 bilateral attempts in 35 patients</td><td>Wire past SC–EJV junction in 148/150 attempts (98.6%)
Successful central placements in 146/150 attempts (97%)</td><td>They concluded that it is nearly always possible to insert a central venous catheter in an adult if the EJV can be cannulated. No difference was found between right and left sides</td></tr>
<tr><td>Sparks et al. (1991)[25]</td><td>J wire (0.9 mm) First 3 tries with head on mattress; if unsuccessful, shoulder was pushed anteriorly (and if necessary then backwards)</td><td>102 (not attempted on 13 patients)</td><td>60/102 (58.8) without shoulder manipulation 10/102 (9.8) with shoulder manipulation</td><td>In 25 patients the wire could not be passed centrally with the shoulder in the neutral position. In 10 of these (40%) shoulder manipulation enabled central placement to be achieved. The technique should therefore be used if difficulty is encountered</td></tr>
</table>

EJV, external jugular vein; IJV, internal jugular vein; OD, outer diameter; PA, pulmonary atery; SC, subclavian vein.

Table 8.2 Complications of external jugular vein cannulation.

Reference	Complication	Comments
Ghani and Berry (1983)[38]	Right hydrothorax secondary to left EJV cannulation in 4 patients	The superior vena cava was eroded by the tip of the catheter 24–48 h after insertion and fluid infusion resulted in hypotension. They recommended using 8 in (20 cm) rather than 6 in (15 cm) catheters. It is particularly important to avoid using stiff catheters on the left side
Eichold and Berryman (1985)[39]	Right hydrothorax secondary to left EJV cannulation in 1 patient	The catheter probably eroded the vein and entered the right pleura. Acute dyspnoea and chest pain developed 4 days after catheter insertion. The clinician should check for lack of venous return and inspect the chest X-ray for evidence of pleural effusion
Ho and Lui (1994)[40]	Bilateral hydrothorax	This complication can be bilateral
Molinari *et al.* (1984)[41]	Right pleural effusion in 3 patients Hyperalimentation fluid in right lung in 1 patient, which was coughed up Left-sided venous cannulation	Use of stiff 6 in (15 cm) PTFE catheters should be avoided on the left side. Perforation of vein wall can occur with insecure catheter fixation and head, neck or cardiopulmonary movement resulting in movement of the tip of the catheter
Fischer and Scherz (1973)[42]	Haemopericardium and death occurred on the fourth postoperative day in a 12-month-old boy. A right-sided EJV cannulation had been performed using a 2 in (5 cm) rigid catheter	This complication might have resulted from catheter tip movement or trauma at the time of insertion. An autopsy study showed that extreme neck movement could result in 2–3 cm movement of the catheter tip and that venous or atrial perforation occurred 60% of the time
Lingenfelter *et al.* (1978)[43]	Catheter tip movement occurred during neck flexion and extension	With jugular catheters the catheter tip may advance into the ventricle during neck flexion
Burri and Krischak (1976)[44]	In 1573 cannulations of the EJV the incidence of venous thrombosis and phlebitis were 1.74% and 2.2% respectively	The incidence of relatively minor complications such as phlebitis and thrombosis should be less with the better-designed, thinner and less thrombogenic catheters available today
Moore *et al.* (1985)[45]	Clinically silent venous thrombosis in paediatric cardiac surgery patients. Teflon non-heparin-bonded catheters were used	This complication was diagnosed by dye wash-out at catheter removal. Thrombosis occurred in 27% of patients (4 out of 15). No significant differences were found between patients with and without silent thrombosis. Thrombosis was more likely to occur if the catheter tip was outside the thoracic cavity. Such catheters should be removed as soon as possible
Jobes *et al.* (1983)[46]	Occasional small subcutaneous haematoma at failed insertion sites	A comparison was made between internal and external jugular routes. The lower success rate and lack of arterial complications with the EJV route must be balanced against the higher success rate and incidence of arterial complications of the IJV route
Berry and Ghani (1982)[47]	Venous occlusion of the left EJV occurred after central venous cannulation. The vein of a jejunal graft was anastomosed to the EJV. The graft became engorged, was not viable and had to be replaced	This case demonstrated the need to understand the surgical procedure thoroughly before inserting cannulae
Stewart *et al.* (1975)[7]	Hydrocephalus. This was reported in a child aged 9 mo in whom catheters had been inserted first into the right EJV and later into the left EJV for parenteral nutrition	Hydrocephalus was thought to have resulted from jugular venous thrombosis and impaired cerebral venous return
Monitoring and removal complications		
McKenzie and Latto (1981)[28]	Difficult removal of soft, pliable central venous catheters occurred in 2 patients; in one case the catheter needed to be surgically removed	Accurate radiographic assessment of the catheter deformity may be helpful. No force should be used if resistance to insertion of the catheter occurs. Non-central placement of round-ended catheter tips is usually satisfactory for pressure monitoring

Finley (1988)[48]	Problem with removal of a 0.018 in (0.45 mm) diameter J wire used to insert a double-lumen catheter	Clinicians should exercise caution when using thin, flexible guide-wires. If difficulties with removal occur the wire and catheter should be removed together
Lawson and Kushins (1985)[49]	Difficulty in removal of a PA catheter inserted via the right external jugular vein. The catheter and introducer wire were then withdrawn at the same time	Multi-purpose pacing PA catheters should be used with caution if there is an acute angle between the external jugular and subclavian veins (probably best avoided in the external jugular vein)
Bromley and Moorthy (1983)[50]	*Intraoperative problems:* Pulmonary artery pressure trace damping Resistance to injection of cold fluid for cardiac outputs Difficulty in advancing or withdrawing the catheter	Acute catheter angulation at the subclavian–EJV junction can lead to kinking of the catheter and monitoring problems

EJV, external jugular vein; IJV, internal jugular vein; PA, pulmonary artery; PTFE, polytetrafluoroethylene.

Complications

As with any technique a haematoma can cause localised swelling. The incidence of major complications with J wire techniques is very low and most serious complications can be avoided by using soft, non-thrombogenic catheters. A summary of the complications reported is given in Table 8.2.

KEY POINTS

- The external jugular vein provides safe and convenient access to the central circulation.
- The most important disadvantage is the difficulty in a significant percentage of patients in threading the catheter centrally after venous cannulation.
- The introduction of the J wire has substantially increased the incidence of successful central placement.
- It can be confidently predicted that this route will be used more frequently in the future.

References

1. Rams JJ, Daicoff GR, Moulder PV. A simple method for central venous pressure measurements. Archives of Surgery 1996; **92**:886.
2. Craig RG, Jones RA, Sproul GJ, Kinyon GE. Alternative methods of central venous system catheterization. American Surgeon 1968; **34**:131.
3. Jernigan WR, Gardner WC, Mahr MM, Milburn JL. Use of the internal jugular vein for placement of central venous catheters. Surgery, Gynecology and Obstetrics 1970; **130**:520.
4. Malatinsky J, Kadlic M, Majek M, Samel M. Misplacement and loop formation of central venous catheters. Acta Anaesthesiologica Scandinavica 1976; **20**:237.
5. Deitel M, McIntyre JA. Radiographic confirmation of site of central venous pressure catheters. Canadian Journal of Surgery 1971; **14**:42.
6. Giesy J. External jugular vein access to central venous system Journal of the American Medical Association 1972; **219**:1216.
7. Stewart DR, Johnson DG, Myers GG. Hydrocephalus as a complication of jugular catheterization during total parenteral nutrition. Journal of Pediatric Surgery 1975; **10**:771.
8. Prince SR, Sullivan RL, Hackel A. Percutaneous catheterization of the internal jugular vein in infants and children. Anesthesiology 1976; **44**:170.
9. Cockington RA. Silicone elastomer for nasojejunal intubation and central venous cannulation in neonates. Anaesthesia and Intensive Care 1979; **7**:248.
10. Blitt CD, Wright WA, Petty WC, Webster TA. Central venous catheterisation via the external jugular vein. A technique employing the J-wire. Journal of the American Medical Association 1974; **229**:817.
11. Schwartz AJ, Jobes DR, Levy WJ, Palermo L, Ellison N. Intrathoracic vascular catherisation via the external jugular vein. Anesthesiology 1982; **56**:400.
12. Berthelsen P, Hansen B, Howardy-Hansen P, Moller J. Central venous access via the external jugular vein in cardiovascular surgery. Acta Anaesthesiologica Scandinavica 1986; **30**:470.
13. Dailey RH. External jugular vein cannulation and its use for CVP monitoring. Journal of Emergency Medicine 1988; **6**:133.

14. Shah M, Swai EA, Latto IP. Comparison between pressures from the proximal external jugular vein and a central vein. British Journal of Anaesthesia 1986; **58**:1384.
15. Briscoe CE. A comparison of jugular and central venous pressure measurements during anaesthesia. British Journal of Anaesthesia 1973; **45**:173.
16. Stoelting RK. Evaluation of external jugular venous pressure as a reflection of right atrial pressure. Anesthesiology 1973; **38**:29.
17. Stoelting RK, Haselby KA. Evaluation of a catheter with two side holes for external jugular vein catheterization. Anesthesia and Analgesia 1974; **53**:628.
18. Gustavsson B, Linder LE, Hultman E, Curelaru I. 'Half-way' venous catheters. I. Theoretical premises and aims. Acta Anaesthesiologica Scandinavica (suppl.) 1985; **80**:30.
19. Bo-Linn GW, Anderson DJ, Anderson KC *et al.* Percutaneous central venous catheterization performed by medical house officers: a prospective study. Catheterization and Cardiovascular Diagnosis 1982; **8**:23.
20. Wilmore DW, Dudrick SJ. Safe long-term venous catheterization. Archives of Surgery 1969; **98**:256.
21. El-Gohary MA. The external jugular vein – a simple access to the central venous system. British Journal of Parenteral Therapy 1985; **4**:154.
22. Dolcourt JL, Bose CL. Percutaneous insertion of silastic venous catheters in newborn infants. Pediatrics 1982; **70**:484.
23. Sessler CN, Glauser FL. Central venous cannulation done by house officers in the intensive care unit: a prospective study. Southern Medical Journal 1987; **80**:1239.
24. Peres PW. Positioning central venous catheters – a prospective survey. Anaesthesia and Intensive Care 1990; **18**:536.
25. Sparks CJ, McSkimming I, George L. Shoulder manipulation to facilitate central vein catheterisation from the external jugular vein. Anaesthesia and Intensive Care 1991; **19**:567.
26. Abadair AR, Kwong AU, Chandry R. Evaluation of external jugular vein for Swan-Ganz catheter insertion. Anesthesiology 1979; **51**:S159.
27. Schaps D, Aiman A, Mehler D, Dransmann NF. External jugular vein catheterisation: a comparison of two different catheter types. Care of the Critically Ill 1988; **4**:21.
28. McKenzie BJ, Latto IP. Difficult removal of external jugular vein catheters. Anaesthesia and Intensive Care 1981; **9**:158.
29. Blitt CD. Monitoring in Anaesthesia and Critical Care Medicine, p. 192. Edinburgh: Churchill Livingstone 1985.
30. Riddell GS, Latto IP, Ng WS. External jugular vein access to the central venous system – a trial of two types of catheter. British Journal of Anaesthesia 1982; **54**:535.
31. Humphrey MJ, Blitt CD. Central venous access in children via the external jugular vein. Anesthesiology 1982; **57**:50.
32. Blitt CD, Carlson GL, Wright WA, Otto C. J-wire versus straight wire for central venous system cannulation via the external jugular vein. Anesthesia and Analgesia 1982; **61**:536.
33. Stickle BR, McFarlane H. Prediction of a small internal jugular vein by external jugular vein diameter. Anaesthesia 1997; **52**:220.
34. Nicolson SC, Sweeney MF, Moore RA, Jobes DR. Comparison of internal and external jugular cannulation of the central circulation in the pediatric patient. Critical Care Medicine 1985; **13**:747.
35. Belani KG, Buckley JJ, Gordon JR, Castaneda W. Percutaneous cervical central venous line placement: a comparison of the internal and external jugular vein routes. Anesthesia and Analgesia 1980; **59**:40.
36. Blyth PL. Evaluation of the technique of central venous catheterisation via the external jugular vein using the J-wire. Anaesthesia and Intensive Care 1985; **13**:131.
37. Nordstrom L, Fletcher R. Comparison of two different J-wires for central venous cannulation via the external jugular vein. Anesthesia and Analgesia 1983; **62**:365.
38. Ghani GA, Berry AJ. Right hydrothorax after left bilateral jugular vein catheterisation. Anesthesiology 1983; **58**:93.
39. Eichold BH, Berryman CR. Contralateral hydrothorax: an unusual complication of central venous catheter placement. Anesthesiology 1985; **62**:673.
40. Ho CM, Lui PW. Bilateral hydrothorax caused by left external jugular venous perforation. Journal of Clinical Anaesthesia 1994; **6**:243.
41. Molinari PS, Belani KG, Buckley JJ. Delayed hydrothorax following percutaneous central venous cannulation. Acta Anaesthesiologica Scandinavica 1984; **15**:107.
42. Fischer GW, Scherz RG. Neck vein catheters and pericardial temponade. Pediatrics 1973; **52**:868.
43. Lingenfelter AL, Guskiewicz RA, Munson ES. Displacement of right atrial and endotracheal catheters with neck flexion. Anesthesia and Analgesia 1978; **57**:371.
44. Burri C, Krischak G. Techniques and complications of the administration of total parenteral nutrition. In: Manni C, Magalini SI, Scrasia J et al., (eds) Total ParenteralAlimentation, 1976. pp. 306–15. Amsterdam: Excerpta Medica.
45. Moore RA, McNicholas KW, Naidech H, Flicker S, Gallagher JD. Clinically silent venous thrombosis following internal and external jugular central venous cannulation in pediatric cardiac patients. Anesthesiology 1985; **62**:640.
46. Jobes DR, Schwartz AJ, Greenhow DE, Stephenson LV, Ellison N. Safer jugular vein cannulation: recognition of arterial puncture and preferential use of the external jugular route. Anesthesiology 1983; **59**:353.
47. Berry AJ, Ghani GA. An unusual complication following cannulation of an external jugular vein. Anesthesiology 1982; **56**:411.
48. Finley GA. A complication of external jugular vein catheterization in children. Canadian Anaesthesia Society Journal 1988; **35**:536.
49. Lawson D, Kushins LG. A complication of multipurpose pacing pulmonary artery catheterization via the external jugular vein approach. Anesthesiology 1985; **62**:377.
50. Bromley JL, Moorthy SS. Acute angulation of a pulmonary artery catheter. Anesthesiology 1983; **59**:367.

9 • The Femoral Vein

SHANG NG

Introduction

The technique of introducing a catheter into the inferior vena cava through a percutaneous puncture of the femoral vein, introduced by Duffy[1] in 1949, was once popular. It was used when patients required long-term intravenous therapy or when markedly hypertonic sugar solutions were being administered to patients in acute renal failure. Peripheral veins quickly became thrombosed by these solutions, but it was found that treatment could be maintained for long periods by catheters introduced into the inferior vena cava through the femoral vein.[2–5] Some authors reported that percutaneous catheterisation of the femoral vein was relatively free from immediate complications or serious late complications.[1,4,6,7] Others recorded an incidence of serious venous thrombosis, thromboembolism and thrombophlebitis.[8,9] The technique received severe criticism from Bansmer and his colleagues,[10] although they did believe that inferior caval catheterisation represented an advance in clinical treatment. Among 24 of their patients in whom an inferior vena caval catheter had been inserted through the femoral vein, 11 suffered serious complications, with 3 subsequent deaths.

However, because of adverse reports and the practical difficulty of keeping the site of skin puncture free from infection, the technique of placing central venous catheters through the femoral vein was largely superseded by the introduction of subclavian venous catheterisation by Wilson in 1962.[11] One of the alleged advantages of subclavian catheters was the reduced risk of venous thrombosis and pulmonary embolism. Femoral vein catheterisation is still occasionally performed in adults when other routes cannot be used. Nevertheless, the femoral vein remains an important alternative to the subclavian and internal jugular routes, especially in cases of emergency and cardiac surgery.[12]

The femoral vein route is still favoured in paediatric practice because of the relatively straightforward nature of femoral venepuncture in such small patients. The anatomy is constant and the femoral arterial pulse provides a reliable landmark. Should accidental arterial trauma occur, it becomes obvious at an early stage and management is facilitated by its relatively superficial position. During resuscitation involving cardiac massage and intubation in these small patients, the femoral vein is conveniently out of the way so it is an eminently suitable route for inserting a venous line if needed. The femoral vein has been used with success and low morbidity by paediatric house staff,[13] and is the site of choice for inserting cardiac catheters in infants and older children.[14]

A study involving cannulation during cardiopulmonary resuscitation in adults, however, showed that the femoral vein was rather less successfully catheterised compared with cannulation through the subclavian vein.[15]

In a prospective study involving a large number of children receiving intensive care, the femoral vein route compared very favourably with catheters placed through the jugular veins, subclavian vein and arm veins.[16] All catheters were introduced with a guide-wire technique; tunnelling was not employed. No difference was found in any of the complication rates including that of infection. Importantly, none of the femoral vein catheterisations was complicated by Gram-negative enteric infections. It appears that provided adequate attention is paid to perineal hygiene then stool contamination is not an important factor in the development of femoral vein catheter-related infection.

It is probable that more recent developments in catheter materials and techniques could decrease the incidence of infection complicating the use of the femoral vein route. Hohn and Lambert[17] introduced Teflon catheters through the femoral vein in 8 children, and left the catheters *in situ* for 2–6 weeks without complications. In one careful study, Silastic catheters were inserted in the femoral vein and led out through a subcutaneous tunnel remote from the groin.[18] The lines were all inserted by surgical cut-down so the results are not necessarily applicable to lines inserted percutaneously. A high standard of management of the lines (all long-term) was maintained with the result that only a small number of complications arose: one case each of infection in the subcutaneous tunnel and the catheter and two cases of thrombosis of the inferior vena cava. The use of Silastic catheters could result in even further improvement. It might also be useful in longer-term infusions to consider subcutaneous tunnelling so as to move the catheter entry site to a point further from the perineum.

A study by Trottier *et al.* compared the incidence of central venous catheter-induced thrombosis in intensive care patients randomised to receive either upper (subclavian or internal jugular vein) or lower (femoral vein) catheterisation.[19] Lower-extremity duplex ultrasound examinations were performed before and after catheterisation up to 7 days after removal of the line. There were no abnormal findings in the upper group but 54% of the femoral vein group developed abnormal ultrasonographic changes and of these 25% developed lower-extremity deep vein thrombosis. Whilst the femoral vein remains an important central venous access route, the danger of thrombosis remains significant.

Other studies show more favourable results. In 123 critically ill patients, only minor complications were reported. Arterial puncture occurred in 9.3% of patients, local bleeding in 10% and local inflammation in 4.7%.[20]

There are times when subclavian or jugular percutaneous access is not available or is contraindicated. This was the case in 465 cancer patients in whom catheterisation of the femoral vein and attachment to an injection port situated in the lower abdomen was performed. Venous access was to be long-term with an average duration of 241 days (range 65–445 days). Late morbidity causing the removal of the implanted port was comparable to the incidence found in patients who had subclavian vein systems in place – 4.9% and 5.9% in the femoral and subclavian routes respectively.[21]

Sato and colleagues demonstrated a successful catheterisation of the distal femoral vein using ultrasound guidance.[22] It is claimed that the puncture of the distal femoral vein is safer than the more proximal site of needle insertion. It is possible that infection problems could be less, as the point of insertion is more distant from the perineal area.

Anatomy

Venous drainage of the leg takes place through a superficial and a deep system of veins. The superficial veins are situated immediately beneath the skin whilst the deep veins accompany the main arteries. The great (long) saphenous vein together with its tributaries provides the main superficial venous drainage: the vein originates in the foot and runs upwards and to the medial side of the thigh, passes through the saphenous opening, and ends in the femoral vein. The femoral vein – the main deep vein – accompanies the femoral artery in the thigh and ends at the level of the inguinal ligament, where it becomes the external iliac vein.

In the femoral triangle (Figure 9.1) the femoral vein is medial to the artery. Here it occupies the middle compartment of the femoral sheath, lying between the femoral artery and the femoral canal. It receives the great saphenous vein on its anterior aspect just below the inguinal ligament. Several smaller superficial veins also enter the femoral vein as it lies in the femoral triangle. The femoral nerve lies lateral to the femoral artery. Thefemoral vein is separated from the skin by superficial and deep fasciae: these layers contain lymph nodes, various superficial nerves, superficial branches of the femoral artery, and the upper part of the saphenous vein before it joins the femoral vein.

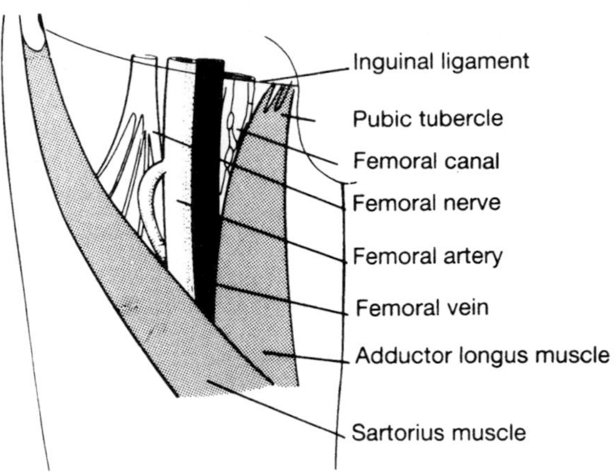

Figure 9.1 Anatomy of the femoral vein.

METHODS

FEMORAL VEIN APPROACH

Duffy (1949)[1]

Patient category

Adults and infants.

Advantages and disadvantages

The femoral route is associated with a high incidence of serious complications (see Table 9.1); therefore it should be used only when venous catheterisation is not possible through other veins.

Preferred side

Either side may be used.

Position of patient

Place the patient in a supine position (Figure 9.2a). Put a pillow under the patient's buttocks to thrust the groin upwards. Abduct and externally rotate the thigh slightly.

Position of operator

Stand on the same side as the puncture site, facing the patient's head (Figure 9.2a). For a right-handed operator, cannulation of the left vein may be more comfortably performed from the patient's right.

Equipment used in original description

Polyethylene catheter through 14 gauge outside diameter (OD) needle (in adults).

Advice on current equipment

Adults: 14 gauge OD needle or introducer, length 40 mm (minimum); catheter length 600 mm (minimum).
Neonates: 20 gauge or 18 gauge OD needle or introducer, length 20 mm (minimum); catheter length 200 mm (minimum).

Anatomical landmarks

Identify the femoral artery below the inguinal ligament by palpation (Figure 9.2b). The vein is medial to the artery.

Preparation

Perform the puncture under sterile conditions using local anaesthesia if indicated.

Precautions and recommendations

Perform the venepuncture with care to avoid puncturing the femoral artery, thereby causing haemorrhage or arterial spasm.

Point of insertion of needle

Adults: about 1 cm medial to the artery just below the inguinal ligament (Figure 9.2b).
Neonates and infants: Immediately medial to the artery just below the inguinal ligament.

Direction of needle and procedure

Adults: place the point of the needle at the entry site on the skin (A in Figure 9.2c) and point the needle cephalad; swing the needle and syringe slightly laterally (A to B). Elevate the needle and syringe above the skin (20–30° to the skin surface, B to C) and advance the needle (Figure 9.2d). Maintain a negative pressure in the syringe as the needle is advanced. The vein is usually entered at a depth of between 2 cm and 4 cm. Insert the catheter to the required distance.
Infants: as above, but elevate the needle and syringe to less of an angle to the skin (10–15° to the skin surface), as the vein is more superficial.

Success rate

The success rate was 100% (28 cases).

Complications

None.

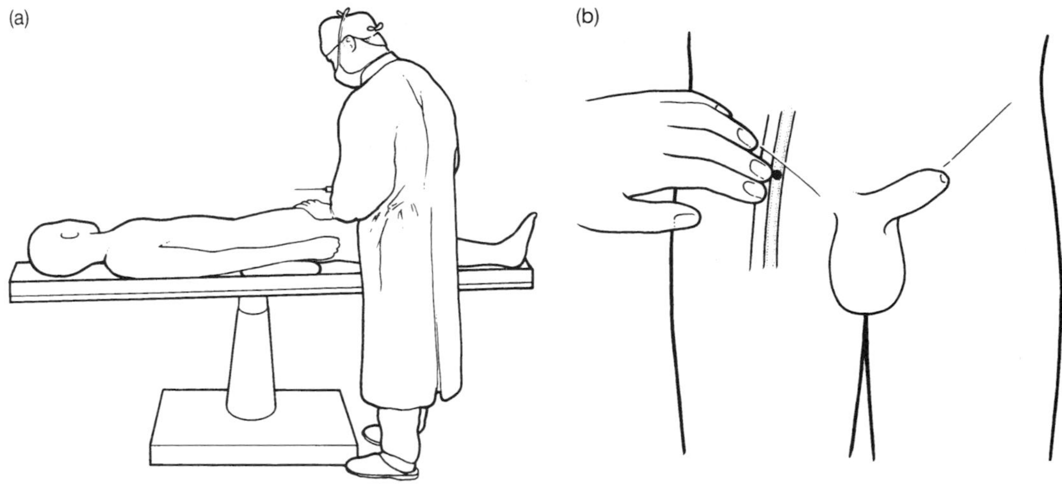

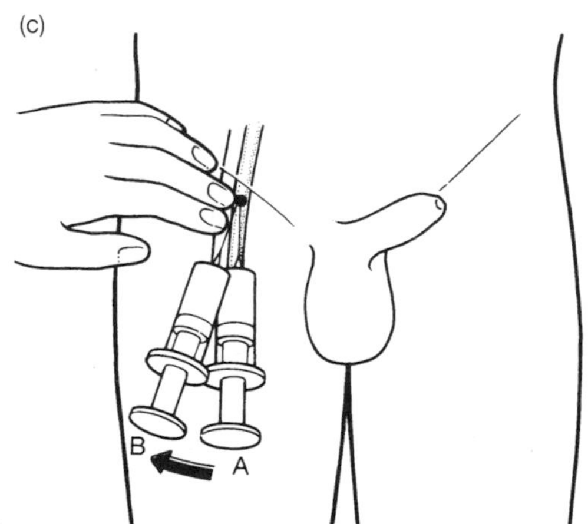

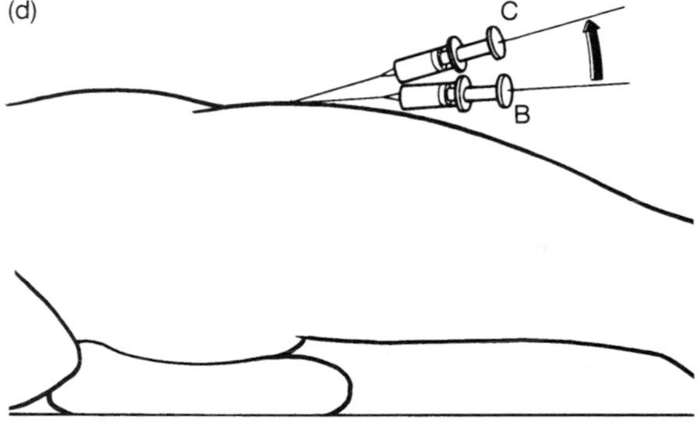

Figure 9.2 Technique of catheterisation: Duffy (1949).[1]

FEMORAL VEIN APPROACH: GUIDE-WIRE TECHNIQUE

Hohn and Lambert (1966)[17]

Patient category

Children over 3 years of age.

Advantages and disadvantages

This technique employs a modified guide-wire (Seldinger) technique. No infant weighing less than 10 kg was included in the original series.

Preferred side

Either side may be used.

Position of patient

Place the patient in the supine position. Put a pillow under the patient's buttocks to make the groin prominent (Figure 9.3a). Abduct and externally rotate the thigh slightly.

Position of operator

Stand on the same side as the puncture site, facing the patient's head (Figure 9.3b).

Equipment used in original description

A 19 gauge OD needle, length 40 mm; nylon filament (continuous nylon, monofilament, 40 lb test fishing line); 19 gauge or 17 gauge OD Teflon catheter, length 500 mm.

Advice on current equipment

A 20 gauge or 18 gauge OD needle or introducing cannula in infants; 200–300 mm catheter or longer in larger children; guide-wire or nylon filament.

Anatomical landmarks

Identify the femoral artery below the inguinal ligament by palpation. The vein lies immediately medial to the artery (Figure 9.3c).

Precautions and recommendations

Perform the puncture under sterile conditions using local anaesthesia if indicated.

Point of insertion of needle

The needle is inserted immediately medial to the femoral artery (Figure 9.3c), below the inguinal ligament (about 2 cm in a 7-year-old child).

Direction of the needle and procedure

Place the point of the needle at the entry site on the skin (A in Figure 9.3d) and point the needle cephalad; then swing the needle and syringe slightly laterally (A to B). Elevate the needle and syringe above the skin (10–15° to the skin surface, B to C in Figure 9.3e) and advance the needle. Maintain a negative pressure in the syringe as the needle is advanced until the vein is entered. Pass the nylon filament (or guide-wire) into the vein through the needle. Enlarge the skin puncture 1–2 mm on each side of the needle with a scalpel blade to help the catheter to pass easily through the skin. Remove the needle. Thread the catheter over the nylon filament (or guide-wire) and advance both into the vein to the required distance. Withdraw the filament (or guide-wire). Confirm the position of the catheter with a chest X-ray.

Success rate

The technique was successful in 8 patients (3–15 years). The rate of successful cannulation was not stated. Catheters were left in for an average of 28 days (range 15–43 days).

Complications

None.

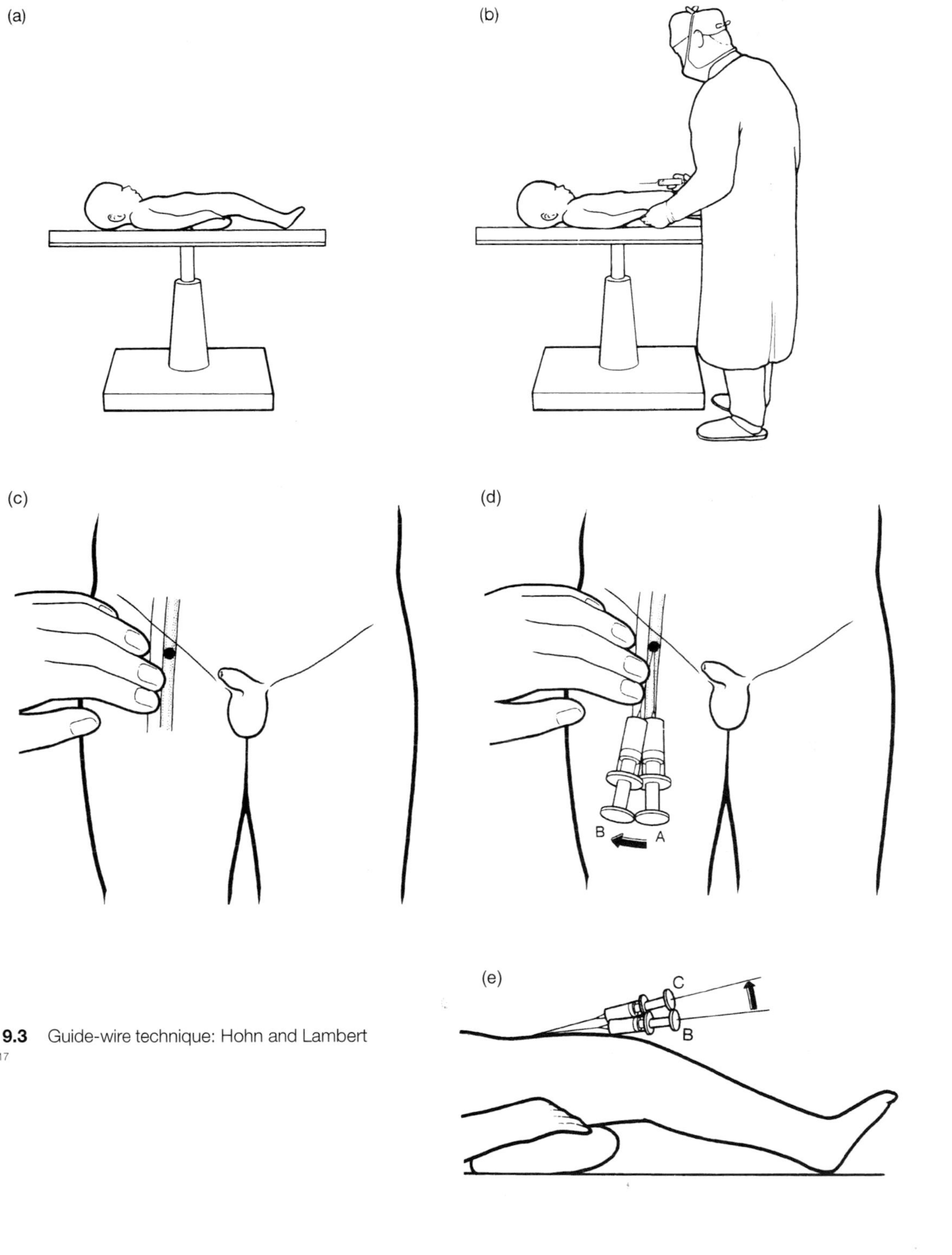

(a)

(b)

(c)

(d)

B A

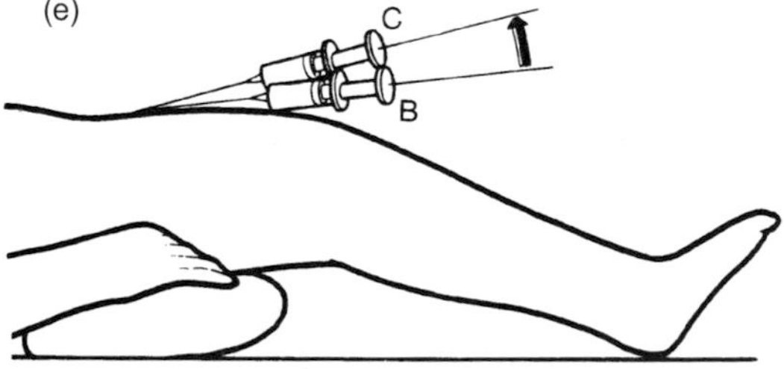

Figure 9.3 Guide-wire technique: Hohn and Lambert (1966).[17]

DISTAL FEMORAL VEIN APPROACH WITH ULTRASOUND GUIDANCE

Sato et al. *(1998)*[22]

Patient category

Adults.

Advantages and disadvantages

The distal femoral vein approach has not been previously described; it is a useful alternative when central venous access is not possible or is undesirable through the more commonly used veins. It is claimed that puncture of the distal femoral vein is safer than the more proximal site of needle insertion. It is possible that infection problems could be less, as the point of insertion is more distant from the perineal area.

Equipment used in original description

Colour Doppler ultrasound unit with a 7.5 MHz probe (Aloka Co. Ltd, Tokyo, Japan).

Adults: 14 gauge cannula-over-needle with catheter inserted through the cannula when in place.

Anatomical landmarks

With the aid of the Doppler probe, the line of the femoral artery and vein travelling longitudinally was marked (line A in Figure 9.4.) A transverse line was marked where the probe showed the cross-sections of artery and vein to best favour advancing the needle (line B).

Point of insertion of the needle

The needle insertion point lies 2 cm lateral to line A (d_1) and 2 cm distal to line B (d_2).

Procedure

After preparing the marked area, wrap the ultrasound probe in a sterile cover containing ultrasound conductive medium. Image the femoral vessels as cross-sections in the short axis. While observing the femoral vein with the probe in the left hand, elevate the syringe 30–40° above the skin and advance the needle, maintaining a slight negative pressure. It may not be possible to see the needle tip on the display but its position can be estimated by observing the stretching movements of the subcutaneous tissue as the tip advances. Entry into the vein is confirmed by easy aspiration of blood. Insert the catheter in the usual way. Take a chest X-ray to confirm satisfactory positioning.

Success rate

The success rate in a group of 20 patients was 100%. The first catheterisation took 15 minutes; the average time for the last 10 cases was 67 seconds to insertion.

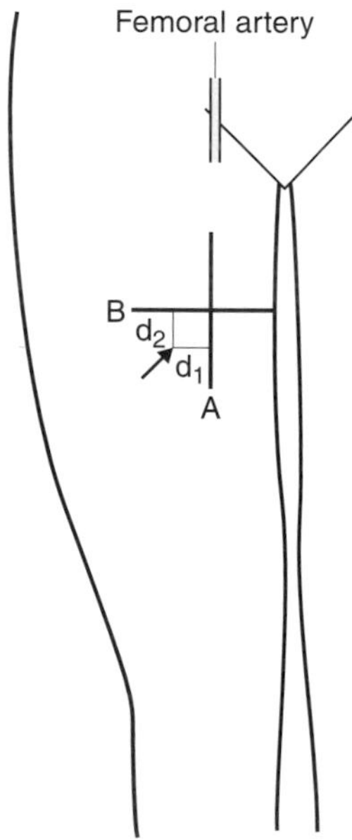

Figure 9.4 Insertion point for the distal femoral vein: landmarks. With kind permission of Sato *et al.* (1998).[22]

Case reports of complications following femoral vein catheterisation

The following complications have been reported:

- ischaemic leg in an infant[23]
- accidental femoral arterial puncture and periarterial haematoma[12]
- retroperitoneal haematoma following perforation of the iliac vein[24]
- transient arteriovenous fistula[24]
- delayed (7 months) arteriovenous fistula[25]
- peritonitis from dislodged catheter[26]
- knot formation when resistance encountered during catheterisation.[27]

KEY POINTS

- The femoral vein is an effective route to the central veins.
- An alternative to catheterisation through the deep veins of the neck.
- Less skill needed and probably safer than cannulating the subclavian and jugular veins.
- Useful in emergency situations.
- May be the only route in patients who have suffered multiple trauma to the head and thorax.
- Main disadvantage is the high incidence of thrombophlebitis.

Table 9.1 Femoral vein catheterisation – results and complications.

Author and year	Success rate (%)	No. of cases	Complications		Comments
			Type	No. (%)	
Duffy (1949)[1]	100	28	Thrombophlebitis	3 (10.7)	Patients mainly postoperative. Catheters used for fluid and electrolyte therapy
Ladd and Schreiner (1951)[6]	Not stated	25	Transient peripheral artery spasm	1 (4)	Catheters used for intravenous alimentation
Bonner (1951)[8]	Not stated	41	Thrombosis of distal leg vein Septic thrombosis leading to septic pulmonary embolus; contamination by faecal fistula	2 (4.8) 1 (2.4)	Duration 1–130 days
Chambers and Smith (1957)[4]	Not stated	9	Deep vein thrombosis of leg	1 (11.1)	Anuric patient treated with hypertonic intravenous infusions
Shaw (1959)[7]	Not stated	13	None. Autopsy in 5 revealed no damage to the inferior vena cava	0	Anuric patients. Heparin added to hypertonic infusions
Bansmer *et al.* (1958)[10]	Not stated	24	Femoral and iliac vein thrombosis Thrombosis of inferior vena cava Thrombophlebitis with suppuration and/or septicaemia	6 (25) 2 (8.3) 5 (20.8)	All patients were severely ill and probably their pathological state contributed to the incidence and severity of complications
Lurie *et al.* (1963)[28]	Not stated	2	None	0	Ages of patients 2 years and 9 years. Guide-wire technique used
Hohn and Lambert (1966)[17]	Not stated	8	None	0	Age of patients 3–15 years Guide-wire technique with Teflon catheter and heparinisation of infusate
Lynn and Maling (1977)[29]		1	Pulmonary embolism from thrombus at puncture site		Patient taking oral contraceptives thought to be a contributory factor
Burri and Ahnefeld (1978)[30]		658	Thrombosis Embolism Phlebitis Sepsis Death	(16.5) (1.8) (4.1) (2.8) (4.1)	Review of complications in 658 cases (16 authors)
Stenzel *et al.* (1989)[16]	41	395	Overall non-infectious Sepsis possibly related to catheter	(2.5) (3.7)	Prospective study Percutaneous technique in all cases Critically ill paediatric cases
Curtas *et al.* (1989)[18]	100	20	Catheter sepsis Infected subcutaneous track Thrombosis IVC	1 (5) 1 (5) 2 (10)	Aseptic cut-down. Silastic catheter tunnelled away from groin. Long-term use (mean 111 days)
DISTAL FEMORAL VEIN					
Sato *et al* (1998)[22]	100	20	None	0	Author only (experienced) Ultrasound guidance

IVC, inferior vena cava.

References

1. Duffy BJ. The clinical use of polyethylene tubing for intravenous therapy. Annals of Surgery 1949; **130**:929.
2. Bull GM. Discussion on the treatment of anuria. Proceedings of the Royal Society of Medicine 1952; **45**:848.
3. Chalmers JA, Fawns HT. Prolonged anuria treated by infusion into the vena cava. Lancet 1955; **i**:79.
4. Chambers JW, Smith G. The use of caval catheterisation in cases of severe oliguria and anuria. British Journal of Surgery 1957; **45**:160.
5. Taylor WH. Management of acute renal failure following surgical operation and head injury. Lancet 1957; **ii**:703.
6. Ladd M, Schreiner GE. Plastic tubing for intravenous alimentation. Journal of the American Medical Association 1951; **145**:642.
7. Shaw G. Acute renal insufficiency treated by caval infusion of dextrose solutions of high concentration. Lancet 1959; **i**:15.
8. Bonner CD. Experience with plastic tubing in prolonged intravenous therapy. New England Journal of Medicine 1951; **245**:97.
9. Page OC, Stephens JW. Prolonged intravenous alimentation: use of polyethylene tubing in inferior vena cava or common iliac veins. Northwest Medicine 1954; **53**:596.
10. Bansmer G, Keith D, Tesluk H. Complications following use of indwelling catheters of inferior vena cava. Journal of the American Medical Association 1958; **167**:1606.
11. Wilson JN, Grow JB, Demong CV et al. Central venous pressure in optimal blood volume maintenance. Archives of Surgery 1962; **85**:563.
12. Gilston A. Cannulation of the femoral vessels. British Journal of Anaesthesia 1976; **48**:500.
13. Kantner RK, Zimmerman JJ, Strauss RH, Stoeckel KA. Central venous catheter insertion by femoral vein: safety and effectiveness for the pediatric patient. Pediatrics 1986; **77**:842.
14. Carter GA, Girod DA, Hurwit RA. Percutaneous cardiac catheterization of the neonate. Pediatrics 1975; **55**:662.
15. Emerman CL, Bellon EM, Lukens TW, May TE, Effron D. A prospective study of femoral versus subclavian vein catheterisation during cardiac arrest. Annals of Emergency Medicine 1990; **19**:26.
16. Stenzel JP, Green TP, Furhman BP, Carlson PE, Marchessault RP. Percutaneous femoral venous catheterizations: a prospective study of complications. Journal of Pediatrics 1989; **114**:411.
17. Hohn AR, Lambert EC. Continuous venous catheterization in children. Journal of the American Medical Association 1966; **197**:658.
18. Curtas S, Bonaventura M, Meguid MM. Cannulation of the inferior vena cava for long term central venous access. Surgery, Gynecology and Obstetrics 1989; **168**:121.
19. Trottier SJ, Veremakis C, O'Brien J. Femoral deep vein thrombosis associated with central venous catheterization: results from a prospective, randomized trial. Critical Care Medicine 1995; **23**:52.
20. Williams JF, Seneff MG, Friedman BC, *et al*. Use of femoral venous catheters in critically ill adults: a prospective study. Critical Care Medicine 1991; **19**:550.
21. Bertoglio S, DiSomma C, Meszaros P, Gipponi M, Cafiero F, Percivale P. Long term femoral vein central venous access in cancer patients. European Journal of Surgical Oncology 1996; **22**:162.
22. Sato S, Ueno E, Toyooka H. Central venous access via the distal femoral vein using ultrasound guidance [letter]. Anesthesiology 1998; **88**:838.
23. Nabseth DC, Jones JE. Gangrene of the lower extremity of infants after femoral venipuncture. New English Journal of Medicine 1962; **268**:1003.
24. Fuller TJ, Mahoney JJ, Juncos LI, Hawkins RF. Arteriovenous fistula after femoral vein catheterization. Journal of the American Medical Association 1976; **236**:2943.
25. Agresti JV, Schwartz AB, Chinitz JL, Krevolin LE, Wilson AR. Delayed traumatic arteriovenous fistula following hemodialysis vascular catheterization. Nephron 1987; **46**:350.
26. Bonadio WA, Losek JD, Melzer-Lange M. An unusual complication from a femoral venous catheter. Pediatric Emergency Care 1988; **4**:27.
27. Hirabayashi Y, Saitoh K, Fukuda H, Hotta K, Mitsuhata H. and Shimizu R. A knotty problem of a central venous catheter. Journal of Anesthesia 1995; **9**:85.
28. Lurie PR, Armer RM, Klatte EC. Percutaneous guidewire catheterisation – diagnosis and therapy. American Journal of Diseases of Children 1963; **106**:189.
29. Lynn KL, Maling TMJ. Case reports. A major pulmonary embolus as a complication of femoral vein catheterisation. British Journal of Radiology 1977; **50**:667.
30. Burri C, Ahnefeld FW. The Caval Catheter. Berlin: Springer, 1978.

Part 2

Central Venous Catheterisation: Paediatric and neonatal procedures

10 • Reasons for Seeking Central Venous Access

PETER JONES

The demands for blood sampling, short-term infusion and long-term intermittent access for corrosive or nutritive fluid therapy are facilitated by the availability of central venous access. Developments in materials and the ingenuity of recently developed devices now enable central venous access to be reliably attained in the smallest of infants.

Nevertheless, compared with the use of peripheral veins, the central venous route may involve substantially greater risk in children. Clinicians differ in the readiness with which they embark upon the central venous route. Both the incidence and severity of complications, measured against the number of catheters inserted, are greater with the central route. However, when the need for intravenous therapy is prolonged, central catheters produce fewer problems than peripheral lines,[1,2] have greater longevity, and are less likely to be associated with poor flow when compared with peripheral lines.

Long-term, continuous central venous access for parenteral nutrition has been, hitherto, largely the domain of surgical cut-down procedures for implanting Hickman or Broviac silicone elastomer catheters. These can now be inserted by percutaneous techniques both in children and adults[3,4]. The Groshong catheter (Bard Ltd, Crawley, UK) is a modification of the Hickman catheter designed for easier percutaneous insertion and reduced need for flushing, and it is available with an antimicrobial-impregnated cuff. It has been shown to survive for extended periods in children receiving antitumour chemotherapy.[5]

In neonatal units, there has been a marked increase in the use of fine silicone elastomer catheters (Silastic, Dow Corning, Reading, UK), the tips of which are delivered to central venous locations from a variety of peripheral venous puncture sites.[6–8] The silicone catheters, some as small as 27 gauge, are introduced through needles, cannulae or splittable introducers. Polyurethane catheters are also used for this application[6,9] and some (22 gauge) are introduced over Seldinger wires.[10]

Periodic, repetitive access to a central vein, as may be required for children who need repeated intermittent courses of antibiotic or cytotoxic medication, is best served by the surgical introduction of an implantable infusion port device connected to a central vein by a silicone elastomer catheter.[11–13] These devices offer the best long-term reliability, combined with low complication rates and minimal maintenance (see Chapter 3). They have the added advantage that the child is able to live a more normal life and maintain a better self-image. The use of an implanted port in preference to a catheter device should be seriously considered if the child's family owns a dog or other boisterous pet!

Flow directed balloon-tipped pulmonary artery catheters can be used for haemodynamic measurements in infants and children.[14] Their relatively large size makes a multi-stage vein dilatation technique obligatory. Extracorporeal venovenous life support in infants weighing 2–5 kg[15] has now been achieved with a percutaneous cannulation technique using a 12 French scale (F) double-lumen cannula introduced through the internal jugular vein. The cannula was introduced over a guide-wire.

References

1. Ziegler M, Jakobowski D, Hoelzer D, Eichenberger M, Koop CE. Route of pediatric parenteral nutrition: proposed criteria revision. Journal of Pediatric Surgery 1980; **15**:472.
2. Newman BM, Jewett TCJ, Karp MP, Cooney DR. Percutaneous central venous catheterisation in children: first line choice for venous access. Journal of Pediatric Surgery 1986; **21**:685.
3. Mirro J, Rao BN, Kumar M *et al.* A comparison of placement techniques and complications of externalized catheters and implantable parts used in children with cancer. Journal of Pediatric Surgery 1990; **25**:120.
4. Dudrick SJ, O'Donnell JJ, Englert GM *et al.* 100 patient-years of ambulatory home total parenteral nutrition. Annals of Surgery 1984; **199**:770.
5. Hull JE, Hunter CS, Luiken GA. The Groshong catheter: initial experience and early results of imaging-guided placement. Radiology 1992; **185(3)**:803.
6. Rudin C, Nars PW. A comparative study of two different percutaneous venous catheters in newborn infants. European Journal of Pediatrics 1990; **150(2)**:119.
7. Soong WJ, Jeng MJ, Hwang B. The evaluation of percutaneous central venous catheters&em;a convenient technique in pediatric patients. Intensive Care Medicine 1995; **21(9)**:759.
8. Sterniste W, Vavrik K, Lischka A, Sacher M. Effectiveness and complications of percutaneous central venous catheters in neonatal intensive care. Klinische Padiatrie 1994; **206(1)**:18.
9. Nakamura KT, Sato Y, Erenberg A. Evaluation of a percutaneously placed 27-gauge central venous catheter in neonates weighing less than 1200 grams. Journal of Parenteral and Enteral Nutrition 1990; **14(3)**:295.
10. Valk WJ, Liem KD, Geven WB. Seldinger technique as an alternative approach for percutaneous insertion of hydrophilic polyurethane central venous catheters in newborns. Journal of Parenteral and Enteral Nutrition 1995; **19(2)**:151.
11. Wallace J, Zeltzer PM. Benefits, complications and care of implantable infusion devices in 31 children with cancer. Journal of Pediatric Surgery 1987; **22**:833.
12. Wesley JR. Permanent central venous access devices. Seminars in Pediatric Surgery 1992; **1(3)**:188.
13. Sola JE, Stone MM, Wise B, Colombani PM. Atypical thrombotic and septic complications of totally implantable venous access devices in patients with cystic fibrosis. Pediatric Pulmonology 1992; **14(4)**:239.
14. Damen J. Positive bacterial cultures and related risk factors associated with the percutaneous internal jugular vein catheterization in pediatric cardiac patients. Anesthesiology 1987; **66**:558.
15. Reickert CA, Schreiner RJ, Bartlett RH, Hirschl RB. Percutaneous access for venovenous extracorporeal life support in neonates. Journal of Pediatric Surgery 1998; **33(2)**:365.

11 • Choosing the Vein

PETER JONES

Anatomical Considerations

The smaller dimensions of blood vessels in infancy and the relatively extreme contours of their routes make it more difficult to advance a catheter that has been successfully introduced into the vein.

Peripheral Veins

As in adults, the advantage of peripheral veins is that they can be seen – or at least palpated. The veins of the head, the arm (basilic, cephalic) and the leg (femoral, long saphenous) have been advocated as entry points for central venous catheterisation in infants and children. In neonates, the median basilic vein can be difficult to cannulate. The proximal basilic vein is often not visible or palpable in infants even when distended by axillary compression.[1] The majority of available catheters tend to fill the vein completely, although 27 gauge catheters are now available, suffering only the disadvantage that they will not reliably deliver packed red blood cells.[2] If the vein goes into a state of spasm during insertion, advancement of the catheter is impeded and time must be allowed for the vessel to relax. The cephalic vein carries the disadvantage of tortuosity at the clavipectoral fascia. Nevertheless, fine silicone catheters can be advanced successfully from a variety of peripheral veins,[3] including the long saphenous vein at the ankle[4] and the femoral vein.[5] The technique is established as an effective method of securing venous access in very low-birthweight infants.[6] These limitations disappear as children become larger and approximate the adult anatomy. One multicentre review of the use of central venous access in paediatric oncology identified the frequency of use of the cephalic vein as 7% and the saphenous vein as 3% of all insertions.[7]

Axillary Vein

The axillary vein is accessible to catheterisation from its origin as the basilic vein passes over the inferior border of the teres major muscle to the point at which it becomes obscured by the pectoralis major. Throughout its course it is closely related to the axillary artery and the branches of the brachial plexus within a neurovascular bundle. It is therefore desirable to identify the axillary or proximal basilic vein either visually or by palpation before making any attempt at puncturing the vein in order to minimise accidental arterial puncture or nerve injury.[8] Identification of the vein is much more difficult in infants and small children, but if the dangers are borne in mind, the method is an alternative to using other peripheral and deep veins. It is particularly useful when a tracheostomy threatens to contaminate points of venous access on the neck and chest wall.[9] The route is probably unsuitable for operators with limited experience, especially when dealing with infants.

External Jugular Vein

The external jugular vein offers the advantage of being visible and palpable. Serious traumatic complications are therefore unusual. Unfortunately, the course of the vein is tortuous (Figure 11.1), which makes the passage of stiff catheters into acentral vein almost impossible. Nevertheless, highly flexible catheters can traverse the vein. It is a favoured vein for inserting a flexible silicone elastomer catheter through a metal winged needle.[10] The vein is usually of an adequate calibre, and external jugular venous catheterisation bears little risk of iatrogenic complications. The several valves in the lower portion of the external jugular vein frequently offer obstruction to the easy passage of a catheter, but once past these, a catheter inserted through the right external vein runs a straight course to the right atrium. From the left side, the catheter traverses the left innominate vein to meet the right innominate vein at an angle which encourages its passage into the right atrium.

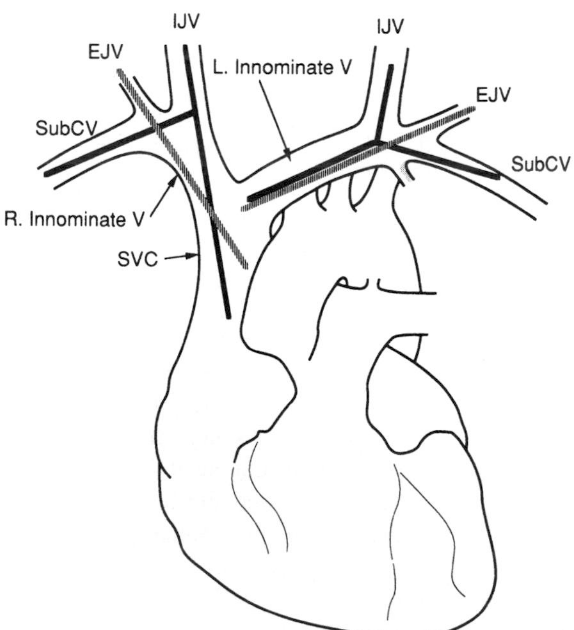

Figure 11.1 The axes of the various venous approaches to the superior vena cava in infants. Modified from Cobb *et al.* (1987).[14] EJV, external jugular vein; IJV, internal jugular vein; SubCV, subclavian vein; SVC, superior vena cava.

Internal Jugular Vein

The internal jugular vein is intimately related to the carotid artery throughout its course. Throughout its length it lies deep to the sternomastoid muscle, presenting to the outer margin of the triangle formed by the sternal and clavicular heads of that muscle. When the head is turned towards the opposite side, the vein tends to be just covered by the medial margin of the clavicular head of the muscle. A catheter inserted through the right internal jugular vein runs an almost straight course through the right innominate vein and superior vena cava into the right atrium. In contrast, the left internal jugular vein joins the left innominate vein which has an almost horizontal course to the point at which it meets the confluence of the right innominate vein and the superior vena cava at virtually a right angle. For this reason, cannulation of the right side is preferred for central venous catheterisation through the internal jugular veins.[11]

Cannulation of the left internal jugular vein carries the risk of damaging the thoracic duct. This is a serious problem because a punctured duct tends to be slow to heal, risking a prolonged and attenuating chylothorax.

The tortuous course from the left internal jugular vein precludes the safe introduction of the more rigid paraphernalia of the renal dialysis suite. In fact, the risks of immediate and delayed puncture arising from use of semirigid haemodialysis catheters are such that one should seriously doubt the wisdom of inserting one into the right internal jugular vein now that more flexible polyurethane and silicone devices are available.

Cannulation of the internal jugular vein is often considered to be facilitated by some degree of neck extension combined with rotation of the head away from the side of cannulation. In infants and young children, the relatively large size of the head makes it necessary to lift the chest by means of a pad under the shoulders or extension of the head over the edge of the mattress. It should be remembered that extreme lateral rotation of the head tends to make the sternomastoid muscle move further over the vein and compress it. If the child is anaesthetised, the sternomastoid muscle can be relaxed, reducing the tendency for the vein to be compressed, whilst positive pressure ventilation can increase the venous pressure, making the vein more prominent. Sustained positive pressure applied to the airway, though, produces a Valsalva effect which tends to move the apex of the lung further through the thoracic inlet making injury to the lung from an exploring needle more likely. It should be noted that 18% of children have been reported to have anomalous internal jugular venous anatomy.[12]

Subclavian Vein

The subclavian vein tends to arch higher into the neck in infants than in adults. This is more pronounced on the right side, causing the right subclavian vein to join the innominate vein at a right angle. Because of this, guide-wires and catheters inserted through this vein tend to be directed up into the neck rather than into the superior vena cava (see Figure 11.1) and right-sided subclavian puncture is less likely to result in satisfactory location of the catheter tip than when the left side is cannulated.[13] Beyond the age of 1 year, as in adults, both right and left subclavian veins have an almost horizontal course.[14]

The subclavian vein route is more hazardous than the internal or external jugular techniques because of the proximity of the adjacent artery (which cannot be palpated) and the close relation of the pleura. Furthermore, if severe bleeding is accidentally produced, haemostasis by the application of pressure to the vessel is virtually impossible because of the overlying clavicle. Although this approach has been successfully used in children suffering from haemophilia,[15] it would seem prudent to seek an alternative route in an infant with coagulopathy.

Cannulation of the infraclavicular portion of the subclavian vein carries yet another hazard – that of

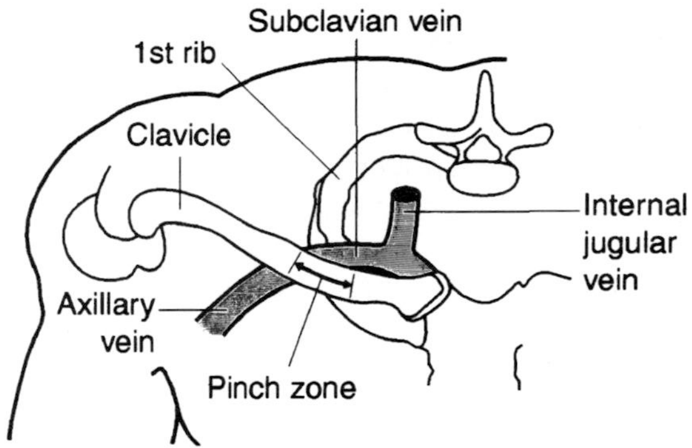

Figure 11.2 The relations of the subclavian vein.

the 'pinch' effect whereby the catheter can become occluded by compression of the apposing surfaces of the clavicle and the first rib. It is important to avoid approaching the vessel from a point medial to the midpoint of the clavicle. The junction of the middle and lateral thirds of the lower margin of the clavicle represents a suitable point of entry for the exploring needle if this problem is to be avoided (Figure 11.2). A cannula introduced in the axis of the clavipectoral groove is appropriately lateral.

Femoral Vein

The femoral vein is usually medial to the femoral artery although it can sometimes lie directly behind the artery.[16] Ultrasound imaging can be helpful in identifying the position and patency of the femoral vein relative to the palpable adjacent artery.[17] Ultrasound imaging reveals a close correlation between femoral artery diameter and the patient's weight. The femoral vein is often larger than the artery, particularly in infants, and is subject to great variation in size with the respiratory cycle. The vein expands to double its 'resting' size when a Valsalva manoeuvre is induced.

Because the vein is relatively remote from the thorax, radiological confirmation of the position of the catheter tip is essential.[18]

The risk of infection through the cannulation site is always a concern when this route is used because of the proximity of the perineum, though modern wound dressing systems minimise the problem. The presence of a femoral hernia would be a contraindication to the use of this site.

Other Vessels

Infants and children requiring long-term central venous access for parenteral nutrition may develop occlusion of the conventional vessels as well as the cavae because of thrombus organisation. In these circumstances, it has been necessary to surgically insert catheters directly into the azygos vein or the right atrium at open thoracotomy or under thoracoscopic guidance.[19]

Percutaneous access to the inferior vena cava of young children has also been achieved using ultrasound-guided needles and a Seldinger technique to deliver tunnelled catheters into the right atrium. The catheters have been delivered by transhepatic and translumbar routes[20–22] and haemostasis has been achieved after inserting sheaths of 5–12 F into the liver by injecting Gelfoam (Pharmacia and Upjohn Co., Upjohn Co., Kalamazoo, Mi, USA) into the sheath track.[23]

KEY POINTS

- Peripheral vein access to central veins has the advantage that venepuncture is relatively safe and easy though the delivery of the catheter tip to the right atrium is uncertain, relatively time consuming and may require significant x-ray exposure.
- The axillary vein is suitable access when head and neck access is limited or inappropriate, e.g. tracheostomy.
- The internal jugular veins can be safely cannulated with controlled ventilation. The right internal jugular vein (IJV) offers the shortest and most certain access to the right atrium. Access via left IJV risks thoracic duct damage, malposition of the catheter tip and venous trauma.
- The subclavian vein is best avoided for central venous access because of technical uncertainty and its potential for relatively sinister immediate complications.
- The femoral vein offers reasonably safe access for veno-venous haemodialysis catheters because of its relatively straight course to the inferior vena cava. It is unsuitable for access in active childre.
- Trans-lumbar and trans-hepatic routes to the IVC carry high risk and should be contemplated only when no other option is available.

References

1. Ayim EN. Percutaneous catheterisation of the axillary vein and proximal basilic vein. Anaesthesia 1977; **32**:753.
2. Nakamura KT, Sato Y, Erenberg A. Evaluation of a percutaneously placed 27-gauge central venous catheter in neonates weighing less than 1200 grams. Journal of Parenteral and Enteral Nutrition 1990; **14(3)**:295.
3. Durand M, Ramanathan, R, Martinelli B, Tollentino M. Prospective evaluation of percutaneous central venous silastic catheters in newborn infants with birth weights of 510 to 3920g. Pediatrics 1986; **78**:245.
4. Ohki Y, Nako Y, Morikawa A, Maruyama K, Koizumi T. Percutaneous central venous catheterization via the great saphenous vein in neonates. Acta Paediatrica Japonica 1997; **39(3)**:312.
5. Serrao PR, Jean-Louis J, Godoy J, Prado A. Inferior vena cava catheterization in the neonate by the percutaneous femoral vein method. Journal of Perinatology 1996; **16**(2 Pt 1):129.
6. Cairns PA, Wilson DC, McClure BG, Halliday HL, McReid M. Percutaneous central venous catheter use in the very low birth weight neonate. European Journal of Pediatrics 1995; **154**(2):145.
7. Wiener ES, McGuire P, Stolar CJ *et al.* The CCSG prospective study of venous access devices: an analysis of insertions and causes for removal. Journal of Pediatric Surgery 1992; **27(2)**:155; discussion 63.
8. Metz RI, Lucking SE, Chaten FC, Williams TM. Percutaneous catheterization of the axillary vein in infants and children. Pediatrics 1990; **85**:531.
9. Jourdan C, Convert J, Terrier A, Chiara Y, Lamy B, Charlot M, Artru F. A prospective study of 180 percutaneous catheterizations of the axillary vein during resuscitation. Cahiers d'Anesthesiologie 1991; **39(7)**:469.
10. Dolcourt JL, Bose CL. Percutaneous insertion of silastic central venous catheters in newborn infants. Pediatrics 1982; **70**:484.
11. English ICW, Frew RM, Piggott JF. Percutaneous catheterisation of the internal jugular vein. Anaesthesia 1969; **24**:521.
12. Alderson PJ, Burrows FA, Stemp LI, Holtby HM. Use of ultrasound to evaluate internal jugular vein anatomy and to facilitate central venous cannulation in paediatric patients. British Journal of Anaesthesia 1993; **70(2)**:145.

13. Casado-Flores J, Valdivielso-Serna A, Perez-Jurado L, *et al.* Subclavian vein catheterization in critically ill children: analysis of 322 cannulations. Intensive Care Medicine 1991; **17(6)**:350.
14. Cobb LM, Vinocur CD, Wagner CW, Weintraub WH. The central venous anatomy in infants. Surgery, Gynecology and Obstetrics 1987; **165**:230.
15. Fontes B, Ferreira Filho AA, Carelli CR, Fontes W, Birolini D, Bevilacqua RJ. Percutaneous catheterization of the subclavian vein in hemophiliac patients: report of 47 cases. International Surgery 1992; **77(2)**:118.
16. Bosch GT, Kengeter JP, Beling CA. Femoral venepuncture. American Journal of Surgery 1950; **79**:722.
17. Sahn DJ, Goldberg SJ, Allen HD, Valdez-Cruz LM, Canale JM, Lange L, Friedman MJ. A new technique for non-invasive evaluation of femoral artery and venous anatomy before and after percutaneous cardiac catheterisation in children and infants. American Journal of Cardiology 1982; **49**:349.
18. Kelley MA, Finer NN, Dunbar LG. Fatal neurologic complication of parenteral feeding through a central vein catheter. American Journal of Diseases of Children 1984; **138**:352.
19. Bax NM, van der Zee DC. Thoracoscopic guided percutaneous cannulation of the azygos vein in children [letter]. Surgical Endoscopy 1996; **10(8)**:863.
20. Azizkhan RG, Taylor LA, Jaques PF, Mauro MA, Lacey SR. Percutaneous translumbar and transhepatic inferior vena caval catheters for prolonged vascular access in children. Journal of Pediatric Surgery 1992; **27(2)**:165.
21. Robertson LJ, Jaques PF, Mauro MA, Azizkhan RG, Robards J. Percutaneous inferior vena cava placement of tunneled silastic catheters for prolonged vascular access in infants. Journal of Pediatric Surgery 1990; **25(6)**:596.
22. Malmgren N, Cwikiel W, Hochbergs P, Sandstrom S, Mikaelsson C, Westbacke G. Percutaneous translumbar central venous catheter in infants and small children. Pediatric Radiology 1995; **25(1)**:28.
23. Johnson JL, Fellows KE, Murphy JD. Transhepatic central venous access for cardiac catheterization and radiologic intervention. Catheterization and Cardiovascular Diagnosis 1995; **35(2)**:168.

12 • Choosing the Equipment

PETER JONES

There are two important considerations in choosing equipment for central venous catheterisation in very small patients. The first consideration is an immediate one: how best to successfully puncture the chosen vein and advance a catheter whilst minimising traumatic complications. Equipment must be scaled down to accommodate the smaller dimensions and thinner walls of the infant vein. The catheter must be capable of negotiating, without kinking, curves of a much tighter radius than in adults. The second consideration is how to reduce the longer-term complications of catheterisation. In this respect, the importance of catheter materials is highlighted.

Dimensional Considerations

It is useful to consider the implications of scaling. If it is assumed that the neonate is essentially a miniature adult, the full-term neonate (3 kg), who is approximately one third of the adult length, will have 1/3 × 1/3 = 1/9 of the surface area and 1/3 × 1/3 × 1/3 = 1/27 of the weight of the 70 kg adult. All linear dimensions will be similarly reduced. A 12 mm diameter internal jugular vein in the adult will be 4 mm in a neonate. A 14 gauge cannula (2.1 mm outside diameter; OD) is considered large in an adult; its equivalent in a neonate would be 22 gauge (0.71 mm OD). However, catheters as large as 1.6 mm OD (5 French) have been passed percutaneously into the pulmonary artery in infants.[1] Such catheters must virtually fill the cannulated vein. Notwithstanding these 'first principle' calculations, it must be recognised that the real child has a, proportionately, much larger head and shorter limbs than the adult, and that the venous architecture is more variable than that of the arteries. Furthermore, any fibrous scarring that occurs in the growing vessel as a result of previous cannulation will impede growth and leave the vessel strictured, occluded or significantly distorted,[2] so that the success and safety of cannulation may be seriously compromised.

A perhaps more important consideration is the need, in infants, for catheters to negotiate curves of much smaller radius than in adults and to do so without exerting excessive pressure on the infant vein wall or kinking. Applying the scaling concept, a catheter inserted into an infant must have an elastic recoil much smaller than that acceptable in adults in order to avoid excessive and damaging pressure on the intima of the vein as the catheter negotiates a curve. The narrower catheter applies its force on a smaller area of intima, resulting in greater pressure on the tissue. It should also be remembered that the lower blood pressure of the infant results in reduced capillary pressure and a proportionately minimised ability to withstand sustained distortion or pressure before ischaemia results in tissue necrosis.

It is not surprising that the incidence of catheter-related damage is higher in infants. The catheter material must provide great flexibility with little force. At body temperature, a catheter that describes a tortuous course must be something of a 'wet noodle'.

Catheter Materials

Silicone elastomer

Silicone elastomer is a natural choice for central venous catheters. It is a chemically and biologically inert material which has the facility to readily recover its shape after being deformed when the deforming force is removed. Catheters made of this material tolerate repeated bending and kinking without any tendency to kink at the same point. Radio-opaque marker material renders silicone elastomer an opaque white and results in some stiffening. Fluid, particulate matter and gas bubbles within the tubing cannot therefore be observed. The disadvantages of silicone elastomer are that it is difficult to fashion into a tapered point and it tends not to thread easily over a guide-wire. Therefore, catheters of this material are inserted either surgically or through a needle or cannula previously inserted into the vein. If the introducer is to be removed completely, the catheter cannot be provided with a connector bonded to the proximal end of the catheter. At one time, it was common practice to provide a makeshift connector by pushing the catheter over the tip of a winged needle. Such a technique was sure to produce an incidence of accidental shearing of the catheter with subsequent migration of the catheter into the heart and beyond. This danger could be reduced by deliberately blunting the needle tip before attaching the catheter.[3] The Tuohy Borst adaptor is unsuitable as a connector because it compresses and occludes a silicone rubber catheter without achieving a secure grip. If a Tuohy-Borst adaptor is to be used it is necessary to feed the catheter over some form of stiffener tube before applying compression. These problems have been overcome by the introduction of the 'peel away' introducer. Once the catheter with its bonded connector has been successfully placed, the introducer cannula can be split lengthways and removed completely.[4,5]

Polyvinyl chloride

Polyvinyl chloride (PVC) materials are made more flexible by the addition of plasticisers. These additives tend to leach out of the material with the passage of time so that such catheters become harder. They are therefore unsuitable for long-term use (i.e. several weeks or months). The tendency for PVC to soften when warm makes it possible to formulate a material that is sufficiently stiff to be readily inserted over a guide-wire but softens effectively at body temperature.

Polyethylene and PTFE

Polyethylene and polytetrafluoroethylene (PTFE) are relatively stiff and are readily tapered to conform over guide-wires. Suitably lubricated, they are easily advanced into a vein. These catheters have a tendency to kink repeatedly at the same site and eventually to weaken and fracture. They are therefore usually unsuitable for use in infants unless the chosen vein has a straight course.

Polyurethane copolymers

Polyurethane copolymers represent a significant advance. They can be formulated to produce material characteristics ranging from a rubbery elastomer to the near-rigid vein dilator devices, whilst retaining the ease with which tip contours can be constructed for easy insertion and minimum tip trauma. They can be chemically bonded, making complex assemblies feasible. The material tends to soften considerably when warmed from room to body temperature. The outstanding feature of this class of material is its low elastic memory. For this reason, polyurethane behaves more like rubber than other synthetic plastics materials. Tubing made of polyurethane recovers completely from having been kinked, showing no tendency to be weakened by the extreme distortion.

Surface Characteristics

The ideal surface characteristic of an indwelling catheter is that it should be biologically inert and'invisible' to platelets. Failing this it should be so 'slippery' that platelets, having aggregated, cannot organise a firm thrombus sheath around the material.

The plastics materials of which catheters are made greatly influence their surface characteristics. With silicone elastomer, polyethylene and PTFE, a fibrin sheath forms after about 24 hours use. Some polyurethane formulations appear to have the best surface characteristics.

The formation of a fibrin sheath can be minimised by coating the catheter with heparin.6 The value of heparin coating diminishes as the heparin is lost from the catheter, although some recent techniques of heparin bonding can extend the period of protection from the present limit of about 7 days to 9–10 days.

An alternative to heparin bonding is to coat the catheter with a hydrophilic substance (one that attracts water molecules to its surface). Platelets encounter nothing foreign to cause them to initiate the clotting mechanism, and the reduced tendency for clot formation results in a reduced incidence of infection.[7] The Viggo Hydrocath (Viggo-Spectramed, Swindon, UK) is coated with Hydromer (biocompatiable hydrophilic material). These catheters become very slippery when wetted because of their hydrophilic characteristic. The Hydromer coating is delicate when wetted andeasily damaged by handling during catheter insertion.

Needles, Catheters and Guidewires

The introducing needle and cannula

It is commonly believed that the use of an introducing needle for a Seldinger wire is less traumatic than using an introducing cannula because of its thinner wall. It should be remembered that the needle which has a lumen just sufficient for thepassage of the wire will create a track through the superficial tissues and through the vessel wall which is smaller than the external diameter of the catheter. The catheter may then be difficult to pass into the lumen of the vessel. This is particularly true of multilumen catheters and is the reason why these devices require the intermediate step of introducing a vein dilator. If a cannula-over-needle device is used for the introduction of the guidewire, the needle diameter needs to be no larger than the wire itself, minimising exploratory trauma, whilst the cannula, doubling as a vein dilator, provides a better track through which the catheter may be introduced. The introducing cannula, once safely introduced into the vessel with the needle removed, forms a secure access for the insertion of the wire. Being flexible, it assumes the axis of the vessel, easing the passage of the wire into the vessel lumen and having no tendency to cut out of the vessel. The greatest danger of using needle introducers is their tendency to cut through the wire guide or catheter if any attempt is made to withdraw them. This disadvantage should be sufficient incentive to cause the elimination of most needle introducers from catheter introducer packs. They can only be justified if the vein is too tortuous and flexible to permit the relatively higher friction of the cannula-over-needle device to be readily admitted to its lumen. This situation applies almost exclusively to low-birthweight infants.

J Wire

The success of central venous cannulation through the external jugular vein is greatly enhanced by the use of a J-ended Seldinger wire which assists in negotiating the tortuous pathway of the vein as it joins the subclavian vein.[8] It has been suggested that the relatively poor success of the external jugular vein approach to the central veins in infants and children is related to the excessive radius of the curve of the tip of the J wire. This is consistent with the finding that the technique is less successful in smaller children and infants.[9]

Manufacturers should consider revising the designs of J wire provided for cannulation in infants. Currently available J contours are often too large to be safely deployed in the peripheral veins of infants and many small children. Consequently, straight wires are often of more use in these groups.

Length of catheter

The head grows very quickly in early life, reaching very nearly its final dimensions by the age of 3 years. This largely explains the disproportionate rate of increase of the full and sitting heights with increasing age. Height is a reasonably linear predictor of intravenous catheter length. Figure 12.1 has been drawn on the assumption that there is a perfect direct relationship between standing height and catheter lengths. Clearly, the disproportionate rate of head growth would make this assumption untrue for fine-bore flotation catheters introduced to a central vein from a scalp vein, but for catheters approaching a central vein from elsewhere, the prediction is useful.

Figure 12.2 relates catheter length to the weight of the child.[10] The graph can be used as a guide for ordering purposes, but is not an alternative to direct surface measurement and radiological confirmation in determining the correct catheter length in an individual patient.

Table 12.1 shows the relationship which exists between the various measurement units used for needle and catheter size. The Charièrre or French scale represents the circumference of a tubular instrument. Thus, the circumference of a catheter of 2 mm outside diameter is 2 π (GK_{pi}) mm = 2 × 3.14 mm = 6.3 F.

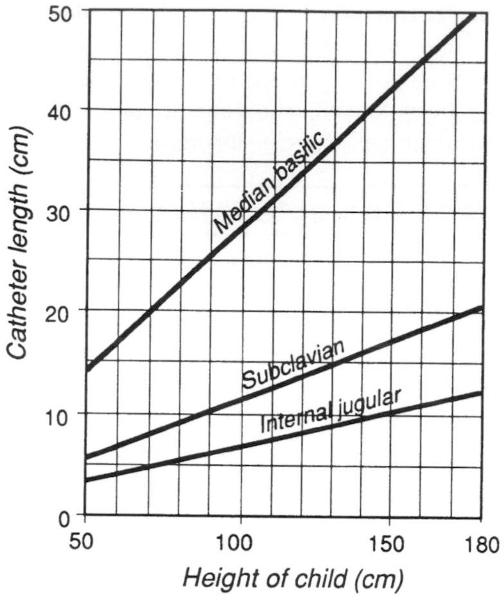

Figure 12.1 Predicted catheter length plotted against height of the child.

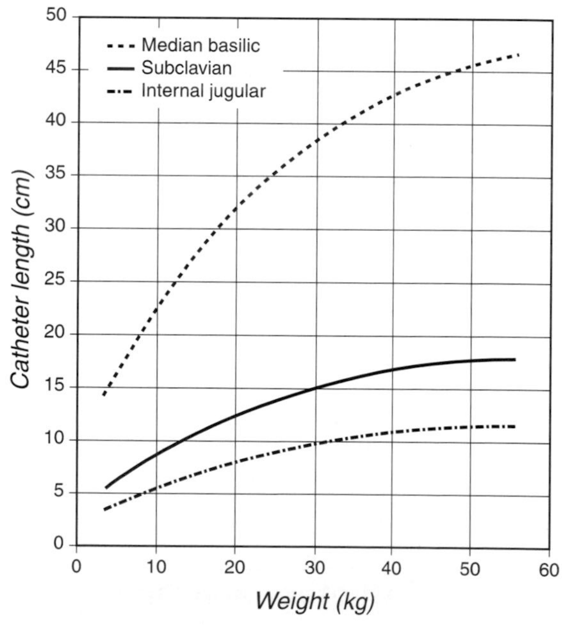

Figure 12.2 Catheter length predicted for weight of child. Central venous catheter length plotted against the weight of the child. Data from Figure 12.1 has been translated for predicted weight by combining male and female data from charts published by the Child Growth Foundation 1996/1, derived from multiple British data sources.

Implantable catheters

Implantable, cuffed silicone elastomer catheters were introduced in 1973 by Broviac[11] for the prolonged administration of total parenteral nutrition solutions. The catheter bears a Dacron felt cuff which is embedded within a subcutaneous tunnel. As time passes, the material becomes infiltrated by fibroblasts and is incorporated into the fibrous lining of the tissue conduit which forms around the

Table 12.1 Equivalent values of various catheter size units.

Standard Wire Gauge	Diameter (mm)	French or Charrière scale
30	0.31	0.99
29	0.34	1.08
28	0.38	1.18
27	0.42	1.31
26	0.46	1.43
25	0.51	1.59
24	0.56	1.75
23	0.61	1.91
22	0.71	2.23
21	0.81	2.55
20	0.91	2.87
19	1.02	3.20
18	1.22	3.83
17	1.42	4.46
16	1.63	5.12
15	1.83	5.75
14	2.02	3.20
13	2.34	7.35
12	2.64	8.29
11	2.95	9.26
10	3.25	10.20

catheter. The cuff forms an obstruction to fluid passing along the outside of the catheter and anchors the device, making skin anchorage unnecessary. These devices have tended to be inserted by surgical cut-down because of concern about the difficulty in controlling haemorrhage, particularly in patients with malignancy and thrombocytopenia However, satisfactory results can be obtained by percutaneous insertion. In one series in which Broviac catheters were inserted percutaneously into 37 patients with thrombocytopenia (including 5 children with ages ranging from 1 month to 16 years) a 10% incidence of relatively trivial complications resulted. There were three arterial punctures (without sequelae) and one cervical haematoma.[12] These results compare favourably with some studies where catheters inserted by surgical cut-down have produced a 20% incidence of subcutaneous tunnel haematomas in one series[13] and a 6% incidence of significant postoperative bleeding in another.[14]

The terms 'Hickman' and 'Broviac' are widely regarded by clinicians as representing generic design configurations and can be applied to appropriate products of any manufacture. The manufacturer Bard Ltd (Crawley, UK) has registered the names Hickman, Broviac and Leonard in the company's range of long-term, silicone elastomer, cuffed, tunnelled central venous catheters and has also registered the SureCuff tissue in-growth cuff design and the antimicrobial-impregnated VitaCuff. All these catheters are available as open lumen devices which requires that they be clamped and capped when not in use and frequently flushed with heparin–saline solution – a process that risks introducing contaminating organisms into the blood stream. The company has also developed a three-way valve device which is incorporated in the round-ended catheter tip. The valve is normally closed but can be opened for injection, infusion or aspiration by applying an adequate pressure gradient in either direction. This device has the registered name of Groshong and has the advantage that the isolation of the catheter lumen prevents it from becoming contaminated with the patient's blood. As a result it needs to be flushed only with saline and at weekly intervals. It is available on a variety of Bard silicone elastomeric devices including implanted ports, long-term catheters[15] and (non-cuffed) peripherally inserted central catheters. The design offers the potential benefits of reduced maintenance and incidence of infection compared with open catheters, particularly when combined with the VitaCuff. Initial studies suggest that the product has satisfactory long-term survival but is more prone to technical failure than the simpler alternatives.[16–18] All of these devices (termed 'chronic', 'long-term' or 'permanent') are available in kits that facilitate percutaneous introduction, and some include the CathTrack facility, an accessory device that permits the location and direction of the catheter tip to be predicted during insertion. These products are available in sizes suitable for paediatric use (4.2 F or 1.34 mm).

Multiple-lumen catheters

Multiple-lumen catheters in sizes that are sufficiently small to be introduced into infants are now available. They tend to be rather less flexible than single-lumen devices and are therefore more likely to become associated with vein trauma. Nevertheless, their use greatly facilitates the simultaneous administration of incompatible solutions and blood sampling. The percutaneous route may also be used for inserting haemodialysis catheters in small infants, though the device may require extensive modification.[19]

Haemodialysis catheters

Haemodialysis catheters are multilumen catheters designed for the simultaneous delivery and withdrawal of blood. As such, they require minimised flow resistance; they therefore tend to be manufactured of relatively stiff, thin-walled plastics material which constitutes a major hazard with regard to delayed vessel rupture and the consequences of cardiac tamponade, haemothorax and exsanguination. Wherever lower flow rates are acceptable, a compromise design composed of softer, thicker-walled materials such as polyurethane and silicone elastomer should be used. Haemodialysis catheters are designed to minimise recirculation between their two terminal ports by separating them as proximal and distal ports. This complicates the contour of the device and, combined with an optional cuff on devices that are designed for longer-term use, makes insertion something of a bloodbath in the hands of the novice. The company Bard Ltd (Crawley, UK) manufacture the VasCath range of haemodialysis catheters, a name that is believed by many to be a generic description and wrongly appears in reports relating to catheters produced by other manufacturers.

KEY POINTS

- The linear dimensions (diameter, length) of vascular catheters used in children can be predicted by reducing them in proportion to the ratio of the height of the child and that of a 'standard' adult.
- Softer catheter materials such as silicone elastomer and certain polyurethane materials can follow the tighter vessel contours of infants and children while applying reduced forces to tissues.
- Surface coatings and treatments such as heparin bonding and hydrophilic polymer coatings are particularly indicated in infants and small children.
- Cannula-over-needle introducers for guide-wire insertion are safer than needle introducers.
- J-ended guide wires must have appropriately tight contours to avoid vessel damage when deployed in small vessels.
- Imperial Standard Wire Gauge or Stubs Wire Gauge (both referred to as SWG or sometimes G or g) are nearly identical measures used for identifying the external dimension of a needle or obturator.
- French Gauge (Fg. or F and occasionally Ch. (Charriere)) indicates the external circumference of a catheter in millimetres. It is suitable for gauging flexible catheter materials and can be converted readily to diameter (mm) by dividing its value by Pi (π) or, for most purposes, by three (3).
- The internal and external diameters are more useful in predicting the suitability of associated needles and catheters.
- The terms 'Hickman' and 'Broviac', widely used to represent generic designs of vascular catheter have now been patented by C.R. Bard Ltd as trade marks for a range of products.
- High-flow haemodialysis catheters which have been manufactured of exceptionally inflexible materials in order to facilitate their haemodynamic performance are unsuitable for introduction into tortuous vessels. This restricts the routes by which they may be safely inserted.

References

1. Pollack MM, Reed TP, Holbrook PR, Fields AI. Bedside pulmonary artery catheterization in pediatrics. Journal of Pediatrics 1980; **96**:274.

2. Alderson PJ, Burrows FA, Stemp LI, Holtby HM. Use of ultrasound to evaluate internal jugular vein anatomy and to facilitate central venous cannulation in paediatric patients [see comments]. British Journal of Anaesthesia 1993; **70(2)**:145.
3. Cockington RA. Silicone elastomer for naso jejunal intubation and central venous cannulation in neonates. Anaesthesia and Intensive Care 1979; **7**:248.
4. Kirkemo A, Johnstone MR. Percutaneous subclavian vein placement of the Hickman catheter. Surgery 1982; **91**:349.
5. Dudrick SJ, O'Donnell JJ, Englert GM et al. 100 patient-years of ambulatory home total parenteral nutrition. Annals of Surgery 1984; **199**:770.
6. Curnow A, Idowu J, Behrens E et al. Urokinase therapy for Silastic catheter-induced intravascular thrombi in infants and children. Archives of Surgery 1985; **120**:1237.
7. Valk WJ, Liem KD, Geven WB. Seldinger technique as an alternative approach for percutaneous insertion of hydrophilic polyurethane central venous catheters in newborns. Journal of Parenteral and Enteral Nutrition 1995; **19(2)**:151.
8. Blitt CD. Central venous catheterization via the external jugular vein: a technique employing the 'J' wire. Journal of the American Medical Association 1974; **229**:817.
9. Nicolson SC, Sweeney MF, Moore RA, Jobes DR. Comparison of internal and external jugular cannulation of the central circulation in the pediatric patient. Critical Care Medicine 1985; **13**:747.
10. United Kingdom cross-sectional reference data: 1996/1, Child Growth Foundation (Publishers), 2 May Field Ave., London W4 1PW.
11. Broviac JW, Cole JJ, Scribner BH. A silicone rubber atrial catheter for prolonged parenteral alimentation. Surgery, Gynecology and Obstetrics 1973; **136**:602.
12. Stellato TA, Gauderer MW, Lazarus HM, Herzig RH. Percutaneous silastic catheter insertion in patients with thrombocytopenia. Cancer 1985; **56**:2691.
13. Adami GF, Bacigulupo A, Bonalumi U. Use of Hickman right atrial catheter for vascular access in marrow transplant recipients [letter]. Archives of Surgery 1981; **116**:1099.
14. Reed WP, Newman KA, de Jongh C et al. Prolonged venous access for radiotherapy by means of the Hickman catheter. Cancer 1983; **52**:185.
15. Hull JE, Hunter CS, Luiken GA. The Groshong catheter: initial experience and early results of imaging-guided placement. Radiology 1992; **185(3)**:803.
16. Lang W, Schweiger H, Richter U, Richter R, Beck JD, Krasa M, Luthin D. Hickman catheter for long-term parenteral therapy. A prospective interdisciplinary study. Medizinische Klinik 1992; **87(8)**:412.
17. Cogliati AA, Dell'Utri D, Picardi A, Testi AM, Micozzi A, Pasotti E, Rosa G. Central venous catheterization in pediatric patients affected by hematological malignancies. Haematologica 1995; **80(5)**:448.
18. Warner BW, Haygood MM, Davies SL, Hennies GA. A randomized, prospective trial of standard Hickman compared with Groshong central venous catheters in pediatric oncology patients. Journal of the American College of Surgeons 1996; **183(2)**:140.
19. Weiss M, Sutherland DE. Percutaneous subclavian vein catheterisation for haemodialysis in small children. Surgery 1984; **95**:353.

13 • Practical Aspects of Technique

PETER JONES

The reader is directed to Chapter 3 where many additional practical considerations in the insertion and maintenance of central venous lines are discussed.

Sedation and Anaesthesia

The lack of cooperation of many small patients during attempts at venous access can result in a thoroughly unpleasant experience for both patient and attendant. Several approaches have been employed to overcome this problem.

Pin-down techniques

The literature on securing venous access in small children not infrequently refers to restraint, splinting of the head to the table with adhesive tape, and similar undesirable stratagems.

Sedation

'Sedation' when administered to a child who is to be subjected to a painful experience is generally ineffective unless carried to a point at which it is virtually identical to general anaesthesia. Unfortunately, appropriate personnel and facilities which are the prerequisites of safe anaesthetic practice may not be present when sedation is carried to such lengths.

Local anaesthesia

The development of effective local anaesthetic skin creams represents a major advance for gaining venous access in children. Emla cream 5% (Astra Pharmaceuticals Ltd; King's Langley, UK) is an eutectic mixture of lignocaine and prilocaine in an emulsion base. It is applied for 1–5 hours before attempting to obtain venous access. A liberal coating of the cream is isolated under an occlusive dressing and a further outer absorbent bandage is applied.[1] Ametop (Smith & Nephew Healthcare Ltd, Hull, UK) is a gel containing 4% amethocaine. It is applied in a similar manner to Emla cream but must be removed after 45 minutes to avoid excessive absorption of the drug.

The widespread use of these creams is producing a generation of children who do not associate attempted venepuncture with pain. Neither product is recommended by the manufacturers for use in infants, though Emla has been successfully used and has been found to be both effective and safe for infants[2] (dose 1–1.25 g) and small children.[3]

General anaesthesia

General anaesthesia is appropriate in a number of circumstances. Its value in facilitating successful and safe cannulation of deep neck veins such as the internal jugular vein is obvious when compared with attempts at venepuncture in a child who is struggling, crying and straining. The anaesthetised child is still, the neck muscles are relaxed, and a Valsalva effect to increase venous pressure in the neck and so distend the vein can easily be induced by positive pressure applied to the airway.

Positioning the Child for Central Venous Catheterisation

The size of the child has an important influence upon the optimal positioning for central venous catheterisation. When neck veins are being cannulated in adults it is customary to place the patient in a head-down position by tilting the couch or operating table in order to increase the venous pressure in the neck to above atmospheric pressure. This has three benefits: (a) it makes the vein more obtrusive; (b) it becomes easier to enter the vein rather than transfix it with the needle; and (c) there is less likelihood of air being aspirated during the respiratory cycle.

A 15° head-down tilt in an adult may elevate the venous pressure in the neck 10–15 mmHg above atmospheric pressure. The same tilt in an infant, one-third the length of an adult, is likely to have one-third of the effect in raising the venous pressure, achieving a rise of only 3–5 mmHg. Furthermore, the relatively large head (Figure 13.1a) requires that the shoulders and chest are raised to permit the necessary extension of the neck to provide access for venepuncture. The result of these manoeuvres is actually a reverse Trendelenburg tilt (Figure 13.1b) which must then be corrected by exaggerating the tilt head-down to 25° or more (Figure 13.1c,d).

Achieving this posture in an awake, uncooperative child is not always easy. The use of general anaesthesia may well offer the best solution in these cases.

Radiological Assistance

The use of X-ray imaging can reveal the position of a catheter against the background of the bony skeleton and other radiologically identifiable structures. Blood vessels are not revealed unless radio-opaque contrast is injected. The tendency of naive operators to employ long screening times when confronted with these limitations renders the technique potentially injurious and of little use for catheter guidance. The most useful benefit of radiology is in providing a permanent record of the final location of the catheter and in identifying complications such as pneumothorax, haemothorax, haemopericardium and the location of dislodged fragments. The encouraging reports proclaiming the virtues of fluoroscopy[4–6] in placing conventional central venous catheters should be regarded in the light of these facts. The limitations of many radiology departments in providing adequate environmental conditions for sick, preterm infants should also be considered.

Ultrasound Guidance

Two-dimensional, real-time ultrasound imaging provides a sectional image where vessels are highlighted as echo-free cavities. Their location and diameter can be accurately estimated with a suitable probe[7] and the state of the vessel fullness in

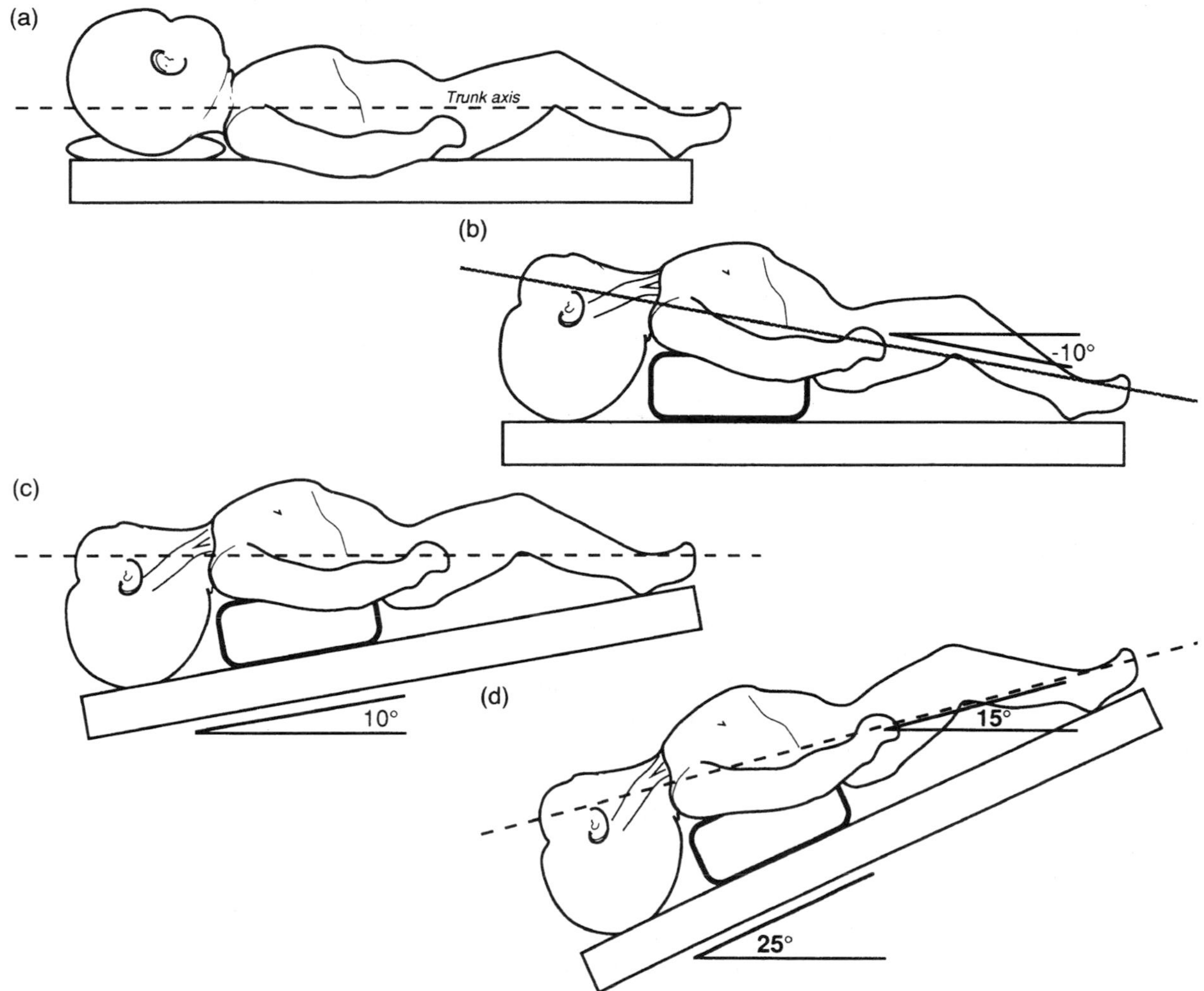

Figure 13.1 (a) The trunk axis is horizontal. An infant lying with a small pillow under the head presents no access to the neck for cannulation; (b) placing a large pad under an infant's shoulders and bak achieves full extension of the head. Note that the long axis of the trunk is now 10° head-down even though the table mattress remains horizontal; (c) as in (b) but note how 10° of head-down table tilt has been necessary to regain a horizontal axis for the trunk; (d) as in (b) but note how 25° of head-down table tilt has been necessay to achieve 15° head-down axis for the trunk.

response to positional manoeuvres is readily determined. Although the introducer needle may not be clearly visible, the image of its effect on the vessel as it approaches and then punctures the vessel graphically confirms successful cannulation.[8] Arteries are distinguishable from veins by their relative resistance to deformation when the probe pressure is increased. Two-dimensional ultrasound guidance, therefore, offers unique advantages in accessing otherwise unidentifiable vessels, although it offers no assistance in monitoring the progress and direction of the advancing catheter. The portable equipment can be taken to the preferred location for the procedure, eliminating the hazards of relocating a sick infant. The position of the catheter can be identified indirectly if cold saline is injected, as some machines will register the cloud of microbubbles released into the circulation. Tamponade can be diagnosed by ultrasound.[9]

Determining the Correct Length for the Catheter

It is important that the catheter tip is optimally located. It must be sufficiently advanced to ensure that corrosive fluids are delivered to a central location for adequate mixing to avoid vessel damage. The tip should not pass into the heart because excessive catheter movement induced by cardiac action can encourage material fatigue and premature failure of the catheter with an increased risk of tip embolisation. The Food and Drug Administration in the USA has recommended that the catheter tip should not be permitted to lie within the heart.[10]

The difficulty of determining the correct inserted length of catheters introduced from peripheral veins can be alleviated by using predictive formulae[5,11] or observing the electrocardiographic (ECG) signal obtained from the saline-filled catheter as it is advanced.[12] The ECG technique, as reported by Neubauer,[12] involves reconnecting the chest electrode lead to a conductive connector (Alphacard Syringe, electrical conductive, cat. no. 18040112, Sterimed Saarbrücken, Hennef/Sieg, Germany) which is applied to the hub of the hypertonic saline-filled (NaCl 5.85%) catheter as it is advanced (Figure 13.2). The P wave becomes greatly enlarged as the catheter tip approaches the sinoatrial node (Figure 13.2, A to C). The catheter is then withdrawn slowly until the P wave becomes smaller (Figure 13.2 B) and then fixed in that position.[12] This method can be used with a variety of long catheter techniques. It is essential that only an ECG monitor with a type CF applied part circuit should be used for this application.[13] Neubauer[12] developed a nomogram for calculating the appropriate length of catheter from the data he obtained using the ECG technique. Formulae derived from the published nomogram are:

Length (in cm) of indwelling catheter (from *left* elbow) = (patient length in cm × 0.288) + 0.71

Length (in cm) of indwelling catheter (from *right* elbow) = (patient length in cm × 0.265) + 0.87

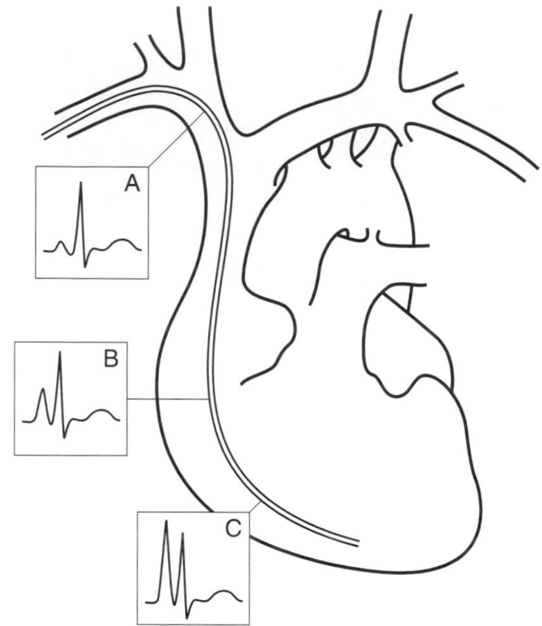

Figure 13.2 Electrocardiographic method of determining catheter position.

Care of Infusion Systems

Fixing catheters in place

Simple catheters (no cuff)

If the catheter emerges from the skin through a wound that is a tight, dry fit around the catheter, such as might be the case when a catheter has been inserted over a guide-wire using a vein dilator, then the primary dressing might be a single layer of a vapour-permeable, transparent adhesive film dressing (e.g. Tegaderm, 3M Health Care Ltd, Loughborough, UK). If the catheter has been tethered to the skin with sutures, local pressure should be applied until all bleeding stops before the adhesive film dressing is applied. If there is any residual bleeding, as might be the case if the catheter was inserted through a needle or introducer, an absorbent dressing needs to be applied until the wound is dry before re-dressing the wound with a vapour-permeable, transparent adhesive film dressing.[14] In small infants, a suture tether may be inappropriate. In such cases, a substantial strain relief adhesive tab must be fashioned and applied so that it is separated from the wound dressing. This should enable the wound dressing to be replaced when soiled or loose with a minimal risk of the catheter being accidentally withdrawn.

Catheters with Dacron cuffs

The Dacron cuff applied to Hickman, Broviac, Groshong and similar catheters is intended to be located in a subcutaneous tunnel where it eventually becomes inextricably involved in scar tissue, thereby acting as a secure anchor for the catheter and an interruption to the passage of infectious organisms along the track from the skin surface. It has recently been shown that, for the fixation to be properly effective, the cuff should be more than 2 cm distant from the skin emergence site and that this partly accounts for the greater likelihood of accidental dislodgement in smaller children.[15] The dressing of a Hickman catheter immediately after its insertion must provide absorption for minor bleeding from the two incisions while retaining an uncontaminated field. Because the catheter itself provides a means by which organisms can track under the dressing, a microporous dressing without an absorbent pad is likely to become partly loosened by blood and exudate in the first 24 hours, presenting a sodden track for the ingress of organisms alongside the route of the catheter as it lies on the skin.

At the time of insertion and for the next 5–10 days, the catheter remains vulnerable to being accidentally pulled out. It must therefore be supported in much the same way as a non-cuffed catheter until the scar tissue forms. Thereafter, it remains only necessary to dress the exit point of the catheter aseptically, possibly using an antibacterial cream such as one containing povidone and a vapour-permeable, transparent adhesive film dressing. The Luer connectors are capped off until required after flushing with saline and the external portion of the catheter needs to be protected from being snagged or gnawed by pets.

Blockage of catheters

Preventing blockage by blood clot

The loss of a possibly vital central line as a result of blockage of its lumen with clot is a frustrating experience.

Simple gravity infusion is insufficiently precise for use with central venous catheters because the flow is easily reversed by thrombus in the vein, Valsalva manoeuvre, external compression and similar incidents. Reversal of the fluid flow permits reflux of blood into the catheter lumen where it may clot, causing an obstruction. Ladd and Schreiner[16] found that as many as 44% of venous catheters failed because of such problems. Intermittent flushing with heparin solution followed by capping of the catheter was a more reliable method of keeping long-term central venous catheters patent than a continuous fluid infusion. The use of a volumetric pump, or at least a one-way valve, would seem to be prudent in these circumstances. An institution that provides central venous access for monitoring or fluid infusion in infants and children should always be able to ensure that reversal of flow cannot occur in the line and that there is no opportunity for toxic concentrations of drugs or electrolytes to be delivered. These requirements preclude the use of burette administration sets for drug addition and necessitate the provision of volumetric infusion pumps, syringe pumps and (while gravity delivery is unavoidable) non-return valves. The 'primary' infusion set (e.g. Flo-Gard Continu-Flo, Baxter Healthcare Ltd, Thetford, UK), which incorporates such a valve, is a suitable device, capable of gravity delivery as well as inclusion in a dedicated volumetric infusion pump. The transportation of children, for example from ward to operating theatre, is frequently associated with failure of a precious central (or even peripheral) line unless care is exercised. The practice of clamping the infusion line and then removing it from the infusion pump for transport may cause a substantial quantity of blood to be aspirated into the line because of release of the compression pumping device. If the line is not then immediately flushed, the blood will clot, blocking the catheter. If possible, the pump should remain connected to the catheter and the fluid flow maintained during transport.

Thrombolytic therapy

Thrombolytic therapy using urokinase has been employed successfully to salvage catheters occluded with thrombus in children.[17,18] Long-term catheters used for total parenteral nutrition are liable to blockage with crystalline deposits of calcium phosphate.[19,20] These incidents can be minimised by carefully selecting the relative concentrations of the two ions in solutions or by arranging to prescribe calcium and phosphate sequentially. Theoretically, the occurrence can be eliminated by using a multilumen catheter, with one lumen reserved for each of the supplements. Repeated irrigation with hydrochloric acid and heparin solution to dissolve catheters blocked by calcium phosphate crystals has been recommended.[19] This solution is prepared by mixing 0.1 N HCl (1 ml/kg) with 10 ml of heparin–saline (10 IU/ml), and 0.2 ml aliquots are used to irrigate the catheter using a 'to-and-fro' action from a 1 ml tuberculin syringe. The process is repeated hourly, as necessary.

Detachment of catheter fragments

The most common cause for embolisation of catheter fragments used to be the severing of the catheter by the cutting edge of the introducing needle. Improved techniques for insertion of catheters, including Seldinger technique devices and introducer sheaths, have minimised this complication. Accidental cutting of the catheter while removing retaining sutures was implicated in 6 out of 8 reported cases of catheter embolisation.[21] Techniques in which the catheter is secured by a suture which is wrapped around it at the point of its entry through the skin, or within a tunnel track,[22] are particularly likely to be associated with accidental severance of the catheter and the subsequent loss of its distal portion into the circulation.

When catheter embolisation occurs, removal of the detached component must be attempted since the mortality associated with retention of the fragment has been estimated at 37%.[22] There have been numerous reports of successful removal of catheter fragments from preterm infants as well as from older children using percutaneous techniques involving catheter-guided snares[23–34] as well as surgical means.[35,36]

Prevention of Infection

Systemic infection is a serious limiting factor in the long-term usefulness of central venous catheters in infants and children. Catheter-induced sepsis resulting in endocarditis and subsequent mortality has been reported[37] and associated with intracardiac thrombi following central venous catheterisation.[38] The incidence of catheter contamination as evidenced by positive catheter tip culture is related to the duration of use.

There is a widespread practice of providing antibiotic prophylaxis for infants and children undergoing cardiothoracic surgery by giving a second-generation cephalosporin for 2 days or until transthoracic devices are removed.[39] However, no equivalent consensus exists for similar prophylaxis following insertion of central venous catheters. Harms *et al.*,[40] in a retrospective study of 497 catheters introduced into high-risk preterm infants, recorded an incidence of septicaemia of 1.9%, though 22% of all catheters, on removal after an average of 11 days use, showed evidence of tip infection. The same authors[41] later conducted an elective, randomised study of the use of prophylactic amoxycillin (100 mg/kg per day) for the insertion of 75 of 148 central venous catheters. The control group had 2 cases of septicaemia compared with none in the amoxycillin group, though positive blood cultures were discovered in 6 and 3 subjects in each group, respectively. The apparent benefit of antibiotic prophylaxis was not statistically significant.

It is generally believed that the colonisation of the catheter tip is the result of bacteria becoming attached to and growing on the fibrin sheath which forms around most catheters. These organisms may arise from any number of unrelated sources, being dispersed by the circulation and infecting the catheter in much the same way as is thought to occur with other prosthetic devices such as cardiac valves. This would explain the delay which often occurs between catheter insertion and the onset of clinical symptoms. Catheter surfaces which are treated to minimise platelet adhesion and fibrin deposition should therefore be less readily involved in septicaemia incidents. Nevertheless, the nature of the organisms encountered suggests that skin-borne organisms migrate through the lumen or through the track of the catheter. Needles and catheters that are introduced over needles or guide-wires are likely to be contaminated with skin pathogens on insertion. Venepuncture and catheter insertion may inoculate deeper layers of the track, facilitating the passage of organisms to the fibrin sheath. This view is supported by the finding of suppurative arthritis of the hip joint in association with femoral venepuncture.[42] The argument for tunnelling catheters is that it lengthens this path.[43] The Dacron felt cuff incorporated into the tunnelled portion of long-term silicone catheters interrupts the continuity of the track for migrating organisms while serving also to anchor the catheter in a fibrous scar. This logic is borne out in clinical practice where tunnelled, Dacron-cuffed catheter lines have been demonstrated to survive five times longer than conventionally inserted catheters, to be associated with half the septicaemia rate, and to be less prone to accidental removal.[44]

Staphylococcus epidermidis, once considered to be a non-pathogenic skin contaminant, has emerged as a serious pathogen in hospitalised, immunosuppressed, premature and malnourished paediatric patients. In these infants, the presence of an indwelling venous catheter greatly enhances the likelihood of infection. In one series of such patients, central venous catheters were identified as the source of 23 out of 56 cases of *Staphylococcus epidermidis* sepsis infestation.[45]

Full sterile precautions must be taken when inserting a central venous catheter, particularly when it is intended for long-term use. Skin preparation should include a recognised antibacterial agent, though it must be emphasised that excess fluid should be wiped away. Both alcohol and iodine have been shown to be absorbed after extended exposure to a neonate's skin. Disturbance of thyroid function has been demonstrated in very low-birthweight infants after the use of povidone–iodine as a skin preparation.[46]

Recommendations have been made for arbitrary removal or replacement of catheters in children after 3–7 days in order to reduce the incidence of catheter-related sepsis.[37,47,48] Such policies are totally unacceptable for patients requiring long-term central venous access for chemotherapy. In these instances, there is justification for retaining the catheter for as long as it is clinically necessary, and treating any infectious incident by administering antibiotics down the catheter before considering its removal.[49] This applies whether or not the infection is proved to be catheter-related. By this means, it has proved possible to retain suitable catheters for a year or more.

There is a widespread practice of incorporating a terminal bacterial filter between an infusion set and the central venous catheter. These devices may include a hydrophobic section which eliminates air. A study designed to evaluate the performance of these devices in neonates failed to demonstrate their effectiveness in reducing complications.[50]

There is good evidence that percutaneously introduced Hickman and Broviac silicone elastomer catheters are less likely to be associated with subsequent obstructive or infectious complications than catheters introduced by surgical cut-down.[51]

Infants undergoing cardiac surgery in whom an internal jugular vein catheter had been introduced were more susceptible to catheter-related infection in spite of prophylactic antibiotic cover than older children. The evidence suggested that it would be safe to leave catheters *in situ* for 3 days in infants and 6 days in older children.[52] *Staphylococcus epidermidis*, an organism capable of causing endocarditis, was the organism most commonly found on the catheter tips in this series. Opsonins, necessary to coat the organisms to make phagocytosis possible, are much depleted in infants compared with adults,[53] and the levels are further reduced by anaesthesia and surgery[54] and by cardiopulmonary bypass.[55]

There appears to be no consistent relationship between positive tip cultures and the duration of insertion of the catheter. There is some evidence that catheters introduced through the basilic vein become less frequently infected than those introduced through the internal or external jugular veins.[56]

Femoral venepuncture has been implicated in several incidents of suppurative arthritis of the hip joint in infants.[57,58] This is hardly surprising when one recommended technique includes advancing the needle until the bone is felt before aspirating gently on withdrawal. Clavicular periostitis has also been reported as a complication of central venous cannulation.[59]

In summary, there can be no doubt that central venous cannulae intended for long-term use should be introduced under optimum conditions to minimise bacterial contamination, vessel injury and haematoma formation. In children, this will require full surgical precautions in an operating theatre with the patient under general anaesthesia and correctly positioned. Ultrasound and image intensifier assistance should be used whenever necessary. Attempts to introduce catheters in less favourable environments[60] inevitably increase the risk of contamination, technical failure and accident.

KEY POINTS

- Local anaesthetic creams greatly reduce pain and stress in conscious children undergoing venepuncture.
- Sedation offers uncertain cooperation for central venous access procedures in children and may risk air embolism.
- General anaesthesia offers optimum conditions for central venous catheterisation techniques in children and minimises the risks of technical accidents.
- Correct positioning greatly facilitates the success of a procedure.
- Radiological screening is generally necessary whenever a long catheter is 'floated' to a central vein and all intra-thoracic catheters should be radiologically checked to confirm position and to exclude evidence of complications.
- Ultrasound guidance to secure safe venepuncture should be considered to be mandatory when available.
- Catheters which are intended to be used for long-term access should be suitably designed and may include special materials, coatings and accessories to reduce infection, blockage and accidental extraction.
- The care of an in-dwelling central venous catheter requires meticulous and fastidious procedures and management.

References

1. Norman J, Jones PL. Complications of the use of EMLA [letter]. British Journal of Anaesthesia 1990; **64(3)**:403.
2. Garcia OC, Reichberg S, Brion LP, Schulman M. Topical anesthesia for line insertion in very low birth weight infants. Journal of Perinatology 1997; **17(6)**:477.
3. Miser AW, Goh TS, Dose AM *et al.* Trial of a topically administered local anesthetic (EMLA cream) for pain relief during central venous port accesses in children with cancer. Journal of Pain and Symptom Management 1994; **9(4)**:259.
4. Bonventre EV, Lally KP, Chwals WJ, Hardin WD, Atkinson JB. Percutaneous insertion of subclavian venous catheters in infants and children. Surgery, Gynecology and Obstetrics 1989; **169(3)**:203.
5. Lein BC, Vinocur CD, Reyes C, Geissler G, Billmire DF, Weintraub WH, Dunn SP. Simple technique for determination of the correct length of percutaneous tunnelled catheters in neonates and children. Journal of Pediatric Surgery 1993; **28(2)**:162.
6. Nosher JL, Shami MM, Siegel RL, DeCandia M, Bodner LJ. Tunneled central venous access catheter placement in the pediatric population: comparison of radiologic and surgical results. Radiology 1994; **192(1)**:265.
7. Alderson PJ, Burrows FA, Stemp LI, Holtby HM. Use of ultrasound to evaluate internal jugular vein anatomy and to facilitate central venous cannulation in paediatric patients. British Journal of Anaesthesia 1993; **70(2)**:145.
8. Randolph AG, Cook DJ, Gonzalez CA, Pribble CG. Ultrasound guidance for placement of central venous catheters: a meta-analysis of the literature. Critical Care Medicine 1996; **24**:2053.
9. Chatel-Meijer MP, Roques-Gineste M, Fries F, Bloom MC, Laborie S, Lelong-Tissier MC, Regnier C. Cardiac tamponade secondary to umbilical venous catheterization accident in a premature infant. Archives Francaises de Pediatrie 1992; **49(4)**:373.
10. Report TF. Precautions necessary with central venous catheters. FDA Drug Bulletin 1989; **19**:15.
11. Ohki Y, Nako Y, Morikawa A, Maruyama K, Koizumi T. Percutaneous central venous catheterization via the great

saphenous vein in neonates. Acta Paediatrica Japonica 1997; **39(3)**:312.

12. Neubauer AP. Percutaneous central i.v. access in the neonate: experience with 535 silastic catheters. Acta Paediatrica 1995; **84(7)**:756.
13. 601-1 DN. Safety of Medical Electrical Equipment, Part 1: General Requirements: International Electrotechnical Commission (IEC), 1979.
14. Trotter CW. A national survey of percutaneous central venous catheter practices in neonates. Neonatal Network 1998; **17(6)**:31.
15. Wiener ES, McGuire P, Stolar CJ *et al.* The CCSG prospective study of venous access devices: an analysis of insertions and causes for removal. Journal of Pediatric Surgery 1992; **27(2)**:155; discussion 63.
16. Ladd M, Schreiner GE. Plastic tubing for intravenous alimentation. Journal of the American Medical Association 1951; **145**:642.
17. Winthrop AL, Wesson DE. Urokinase in the treatment of central venous catheters in children. Journal of Pediatric Surgery 1984; **19**:536.
18. Curnow A, Idowu J, Behrens E *et al.* Urokinase therapy for Silastic catheter-induced intravascular thrombi in infants and children. Archives of Surgery 1985; **120**:1237.
19. Breux C, Duke D, Georgeson KE, Mestre JR. Calcium phosphate occlusion of central venous catheters used for total parenteral nutrition in infants and children: prevention and treatment. Journal of Pediatric Surgery 1987; **22**:829.
20. Eggert LD, Rusho WJ, MacKay M *et al.* Calcium compatibility in parenteral nutrition solutions for neonates.American Journal of Hospital Pharmacy 1982; **39**:49.
21. Grabenwoeger F, Bardach G, Dock W, Pinterits P. Percutaneous extraction of centrally embolised foreign bodies: a report of 16 cases. British Journal of Radiology 1989; **61**:1014.
22. Alfieris GM, Wing GW, Hoy GR. Securing Broviac catheters in children. Journal of Pediatric Surgery 1987; **22**:825.
23. Moncada R, Demos TC. Iatrogenic cardiovascular foreign bodies. Revista Interamericana de Radiologica 1977; **2**:205.
24. Fisher RG, Mattox KL. Percutaneous extraction of an embolised hyperalimentation catheter fragment. Southern Medical Journal 1978; **71**:1438.
25. Millan VG. Retrieval of intravascular foreign bodies using a modified bronchoscopic forceps. Radiology 1978; **129**:587.
26. Chung KJ, Chernoff HL, Leape LL, Kreidberg MB. Transfemoral snaring of broken catheters from the right heart in small infants. Catheterization and Cardiovascular Diagnosis 1980; **6**:331.
27. Weber J, Sartor K. Percutaneous removal of intravascular fragments from infusion, angiographic, and CSF drainage catheters with the loop-snare technic. Chirurgie 1980; **51**:711.
28. Endrys J, Rubacek M, Podrabski P. Percutaneous retrieval of foreign bodies from the cardiovascular system. Cor Vasa 1985; **27**:36.
29. Uflacker R, Lima S, Melichar AC. Intravascular foreign bodies: percutaneous retrieval. Radiology 1986; **160**:731.
30. Alzen G, Mertens R, Gunther R. Percutaneous catheter extraction of a ruptured Portacath in a small child. Klinische Pediatrie 1987; **199**:296.
31. Gross DM, Cox MA, Denson SB, Ferguson L. Unique use of a tip-deflecting guide wire in removing a catheter embolus from an infant. Pediatric Cardiology 1987; **8**:117.
32. Engelhardt W, Muhler E, Lang D, von Bernuth G. Percutaneous removal of embolised catheters from pulmonary arteries or the right heart in children. Klinische Pediatrie 1989; **200**:444.
33. Ochikubo CG, O'Brien LA, Kanakriyeh M, Waffarn F. Silicone-rubber catheter fracture and embolization in a very low birth weight infant. Journal of Perinatology 1996; **16(1)**:50.
34. Hwang B, Hsieng JH, Lee BC, Lu JH, Soong WJ, Chen SJ, Meng CC. Percutaneous removal of a nonopaque silastic catheter from the pulmonary artery in two premature infants. Cardiovascular and Interventional Radiology 1997; **20(4)**:319.
35. Abbruzzese PA, Chiappa E, Murru P, Stefanini L, Longo S, Balagna R. Surgical retrieval of an embolized central venous catheter in a premature baby. Annals of Thoracic Surgery 1998; **66(3)**:938.
36. Khilnani P, Toce S, Reddy R. Mechanical complications from very small percutaneous central venous Silastic catheters. Critical Care Medicine 1990; **18(12)**:1477.
37. Stanton BF, Baltimore RS, Clemens JD. Changing spectrum of endocarditis in children. An analysis of 26 cases, 1970–1979. American Journal of Diseases of Children 1984; **138**:720.
38. Mecrow IK, Ladusans EJ. Infective endocarditis in newborn infants with structurally normal hearts. Acta Paediatrica 1994; **83(1)**:35.
39. Lee KR, Ring JC, Leggiadro RJ. Prophylactic antibiotic use in pediatric cardiovascular surgery: a survey of current practice. Pediatric Infectious Disease Journal 1995; **14(4)**:267.
40. Harms K, Herting E, Kruger T, Compagnone D, Speer CP. Percutaneous Silastic catheters in newborn and premature infants. A report of experiences with 497 catheters in 5 years. Monatsschrift Kinderheilkunde 1992; **140(8)**:464.
41. Harms K, Herting E, Kron M, Schiffmann H, Schulz-Ehlbeck H. Randomized, controlled trial of amoxicillin prophylaxis for prevention of catheter-related infections in newborn infants with central venous silicone elastomer catheters. Journal of Pediatrics 1995; **127(4)**:615.
42. Asnes RS, Arendar GM. Septic arthritis of the hip: a complication of femoral venepuncture. Pediatrics 1966; **38**:837.
43. Dudrick SJ, Groff DB, Wilmore DW. Long term venous catheterisation in infants. Surgery, Gynecology and Obstetrics 1969; **129**:805.
44. Henneberg SW, Jungersen D, Hole P. Durability of central venous catheters. A randomized trial in children with

malignant diseases. Paediatric Anaesthesia 1996; **6(6)**:449.

45. Scherer LR, West KW, Weber TR, Teiman M, Grosfeld JL. *Staphylococcus epidermidis* in pediatric patients: clinical and therapeutic considerations. Journal of Pediatric Surgery 1984; **19**:358.
46. Jeng MJ, Lin CY, Soong WJ, Hsiao KJ, Hwang B, Chiang SH. The effect of povidone-iodine on thyroid function of neonates with different birth sizes. Chung-Hua Min Kuo Hsiao Erh Ko i Hsueh Hui Tsa Chih 1998; **39(6)**:371.
47. Rao TL, Wong AY, Salem MR. A new approach to the percutaneous catheterisation of the internal jugular vein. Anesthesiology 1977; **46**:362.
48. Notterman DA. Invasive Haemodynamic Monitoring. Philadelphia:WB Saunders, 1985.
49. Klein JF, Shahrivar F. Use of percutaneous silastic central venous catheters in neonates and the management of infectious complications. American Journal of Perinatology 1992; **9(4)**:261.
50. Ginies JL, Joseph MG, Champion G, Bouderlique C. A prospective study of the efficacy of bacterial filters in preventing complications of central parenteral nutrition in the newborn infant. Agressologie 1990; **31(8)**:495.
51. Mirro J, Rao BN, Kumar M *et al.* A comparison of placement techniques and complications of externalized catheters and implantable parts used in children with cancer. Journal of Pediatric Surgery 1990; **25**:120.
52. Damen J. Positive bacterial cultures and related risk factors associated with the percutaneous internal jugular vein catheterization in pediatric cardiac patients. Anesthesiology 1987; **66**:558.
53. Fleer A, Gerards LJ, Aerts P, Westerdaal NAC, Senders RC, Van Dijk H, J Venning. Opsonic defence to *Staphylococcus epidermidis* in the premature neonate. Journal of Infectious Disease 1985; **152**:930.
54. Perttila J, Lilius EM, Salo M. Effects of anaesthesia on serum opsonic capacity. Acta Anaesthesiologica Scandinavica 1986; **30**:173.
55. Jones HM, Matthews N, Vaughan RS, Stark JM. Cardiopulmonary bypass and complement activation. Anaesthesia 1982; **37**:629.
56. Gertner J, Herman B, Pescio MD, Wolff MA. Risk of infection in prolonged central venous catheterization. Surgery, Gynecology and Obstetrics 1979; **149**:798.
57. Samilson RL, Bersani FA, Watkins MG. Acute suppurative arthritis in infants and children. Pediatrics 1958; **21**:798.
58. Baitch A. Recent observations of acute suppurative arthritis. Clinical Orthopaedics 1962; **22**:157.
59. Marty F, Truong P. Clavicular periostitis: an unusual complication of percutaneous subclavian venous catheterization. Radiology 1983; **64**:139.
60. Slavc I, Urban C. Percutaneous insertion of Broviac catheters by pediatricians on the oncology ward [letter]. Pediatric Hematology and Oncology 1992; **9(2)**:191.

14 • Choice of Technique

PETER JONES

Introduction

The many factors to be taken into account when choosing a particular route for central venous catheterisation are discussed in Chapter 1.

Some reviews of published data concerning intravenous alimentation in children have concluded that the jugular veins offer the best means of access in infants, with the catheter tunnelled subcutaneously to an exit point behind and above the right ear. The subclavian route is more appropriate in larger children. It has been argued that the femoral vein is best avoided because of the increased infection risk.[1]

Ultrasound Imaging as a Guide to Central Venous Access

The use of real-time two-dimensional ultrasound imaging provides useful information about the suitability of veins for puncture, improving the ease and success of cannulation and minimising the incidence of complications during superior vena caval cannulation.[2] It has been predicted that the use of ultrasound imaging for central venous access will become medicolegally mandatory in the near future.[3]

This author routinely uses ultrasound imaging (Dymax Site-Rite, Dymax Corporation, Pittsburgh, Pa, USA) as a real-time guide for placement of central venous catheters via the internal jugular route for neonates (some weighing less than 1 kg) and children, using the 9 megahertz probe. The benefits are such that the view is now held that ultrasound imaging is highly desirable if not yet mandatory in this age group. The only indication for proceeding without such imaging is the acceptance of increased risk of failure and iatrogenic injury in the absence of appropriate imaging equipment. An alternative technique for using the device is included in the internal jugular vein section, though it is also valuable in assessing other large vessels.

PERIPHERAL VEINS

Flexible silicone catheters, inserted through thin-walled needles, are usually employed to gain central venous access through peripheral veins. Their bore is necessarily fine and therefore susceptible to blockage by clot and calcium phosphate crystals from parenteral nutrition solutions.[4,5] These catheters can accommodate a maximum flow rate of 50 ml/h.[6] Several studies in infants show conclusively that percutaneous central venous catheterisation compares favourably with insertion of Silastic catheters (sometimes of a large diameter) by surgical cut-down on deeper veins.[6–11]

INSERTION OF A FINE-BORE SILICONE CENTRAL VENOUS CATHETER THROUGH A WINGED INTRODUCING NEEDLE INTO ANY SUITABLE PERIPHERAL VEIN

Durand et al. *(1986)*[12]

Patient category

Infants weighing between 0.51 kg and 3.92 kg.

Advantages and disadvantages

Any convenient peripheral vein can be used. There is no risk of causing raised intracranial pressure with head movement as is the case with internal jugular cannulation.[13,14]

Equipment used in original description

A winged needle from which the flexible tubing and plastic hub had been detached, a 25 gauge blunted needle, and a length of Silastic silicone rubber tubing (Dow Corning, Reading, UK) of 0.025 inch (0.635 mm) outside diameter (OD) and 0.012 inch (0.305 mm) internal diameter (ID).

Advice on current equipment

Examples of suitable kits are as follows.

Infant < 1 kg

The Premicath 27 gauge kit (Vygon UK Ltd, Cirencester, UK) includes a 27 gauge polyurethane radio-opaque catheter which is permanently bonded to a winged suture flange and has a short, flexible, clear plastic extension and a Luer connector. It is introduced through either a 24 gauge needle which may be split longitudinally to separate it from the inserted catheter after successful venepuncture (code 1261.21) or through a slightly larger peel-apart cannula (code 1261.22).

Infant > 1 kg

The Epicutaneo Cave or ECC kit (Vygon UK Ltd, Cirencester, UK). The 23 gauge silicone catheter, graduated at 5 cm, 10 cm, 15 cm and 20 cm, connects to a short extension tube via a compression hub after the winged 19 gauge introducer needle has been removed.

Anatomical landmarks

Visualise and identify the vein directly.

Preparation

Perform the procedure under sterile conditions using local anaesthesia as indicated.

Precautions and recommendations

Suitable sites for venepuncture include the antecubital fossa, forearm, leg and scalp veins (preferably anterior to the ear).

Procedure

Puncture the vein and insert the catheter for a distance that has been pre-measured so that the catheter tip will lie in a suitable central position. Withdraw and discard the needle. Attach a blunt cannula to the external end of the catheter, securing it with a suture. Confirm the catheter tip position by X-ray. Clean the insertion site again with povidone–iodine solution and fix the catheter to the skin using Steristrip skin closures before covering the site with a vapour-permeable self-adhesive membrane such as OpSite (Smith & Nephew Medical Ltd, Hull, UK). Change the dressing only when necessary but change the infusates and infusion sets daily under sterile conditions. Add 1 IU/ ml heparin to all infusion fluids.

Success rate

Fifty successful cannulations were achieved in the first 55 attempts. The mean duration that the catheter remained in position was 25.4 ± 16. 7 days. There were 4 cases (6.7%) of bacteraemia. Mechanical complications occurred in 26.4% of cases, mostly blockage of catheter due to calcium phosphate precipitation.

Modification of the Durand Technique *Puntis (1986)*[6]

The technique is essentially the same as the Durand *et al.* procedure described above. An Abbott Butterfly (Abbott Laboratories, Abbott House, Norden Road, Maidenhead, Berks, SL6 4XE) 25 gauge needle whose cutting edge is first blunted using the ridged surface of a needle holder or similar surface is used as an improvised connector for the silicone rubber tubing.

1. Introduce a Silastic feeding line (0.64 mm OD) through a 19 gauge winged needle from which the tubing has been removed (Figure 14.1a).
2. Remove and discard the winged needle (Figure 14.1b).
3. Thread Silastic tube over a 25 gauge winged needle which has been prepared as above. With the needle guard in place, the whole assembly is sandwiched between two small squares of elastic adhesive bandage (Figure 14.1c).

The catheter recommended for insertion into the vein is a Silastic feeding line (cat. no. 602.105, Dow Corning, Reading, UK)[15] which is a silicone elastomer tube of 0.64 mm OD, 0.3 mm ID. The catheter can be inserted into the scalp vein, antecubital fossa vein or long saphenous vein. Where possible, antecubital fossa veins are reserved for candidates for parenteral nutrition.

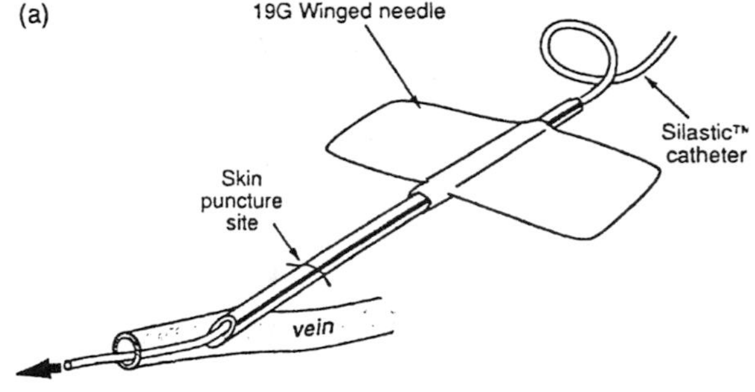

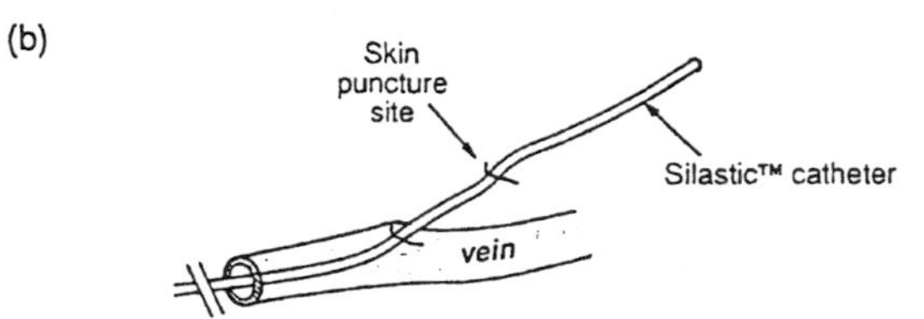

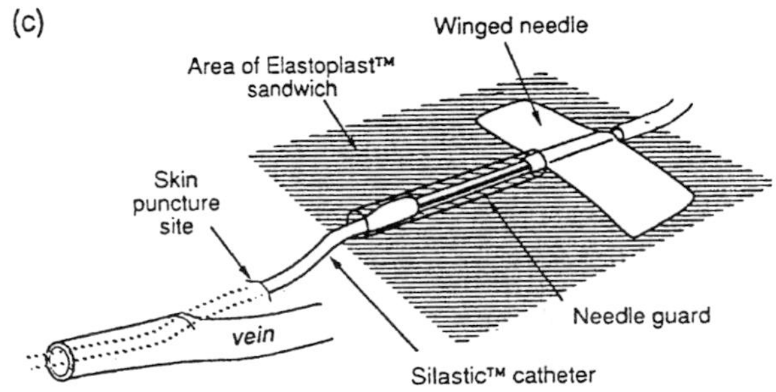

Figure 14.1 Technique described for Durand *et al.* 1986.[12]

AXILLARY VEIN

Central venous catheterisation through the axillary vein avoids the potentially serious complications associated with catheterisation of the deep neck veins.[16,17] The shorter catheter needed for the axillary vein route is easier to pass centrally, in comparison with catheters inserted through more peripheral veins. The axillary route is well suited to long-term fluid and nutritional therapy, blood transfusion and concurrent venous pressure monitoring.

Two techniques are detailed below. The technique described by Oriot and Defawe[18] seeks to identify the vein directly, whilst that of Metz *et al.*[19] identifies the axillary artery and defines its relation to the vein. The advantages of the latter method are its application to children with an impalpable vein and the reduced risk of arterial puncture. A third technique (described by Nickalls in 1987 and Taylor and Yellowlees in 1990 for use in adults and infants, see Chapter 5) seeks to access the middle part of the axillary artery by using indirect landmarks. Of the three methods, it is probably the least appropriate for infants.

INSERTING A SILICONE CATHETER THROUGH AN INTRODUCING NEEDLE INTO AN AXILLARY VEIN

Oriot and Defawe (1988)[18]

Patient category

Low-birthweight neonates.

Advantages and disadvantages

Facility and comparatively low incidence of complications.

Preferred side

None.

Position of patient

Supine with arm abducted to 120° (Figure 14.2a). The humerus is maximally externally rotated.

Position of operator

Not stated.

Equipment used in original description

A 19 gauge thin-walled needle (Vygon UK Ltd, Cirencester, UK); 30 cm, 24 gauge silicone elastomer microcatheter (Vygon).

Anatomical landmarks

With the arm abducted away from the side of the body, palpate the axillary artery (Figure 14.2a). This lies between the medial side of the head of the humerus and the small tuberosity of the humerus. The axillary vein lies medial (i.e.on the chest side) to the axillary artery. In low-birthweight neonates the vein is frequently visible.

Preparation

Perform the puncture under sterile conditions using local anaesthesia as indicated.

Precautions and recommendations

Infusions should contain 1 IU/ml heparin, up to 100 IU per day.

Point of insertion of needle

Insert the needle subcutaneously, 1 cm below the lesser tuberosity of the humerus (Figure 14.2b).

Direction of the needle and procedure

Slowly advance the needle in a line parallel to the axis of the humerus, aspirating gently until flashback of blood signals entry into the vein (Figure 14.2b,c). With fine forceps, insert the catheter into the needle shaft and advance it to a predetermined length such that the tip lies in the superior vena cava. Withdraw the needle from the vein. Immobilise the arm with a small board acting as a splint.

Attach the catheter to an appropriate infusion system and fix the portion of the catheter outside the skin entry site to the arm. Confirm the correct positioning of the catheter tip by X-ray, having first filled the catheter with radio-opaque dye.

Success rate

There were 217 successful catheterisations with 226 attempts (96%), 187 neonates had a birthweight less than 1.5 kg.

Complications

There were 3 cases of catheter-related sepsis with positive blood and catheter-tip cultures, and 8 cases of shoulder oedema which subsided when the catheter was removed. Examination after 6 months revealed no vascular or limb abnormalities.

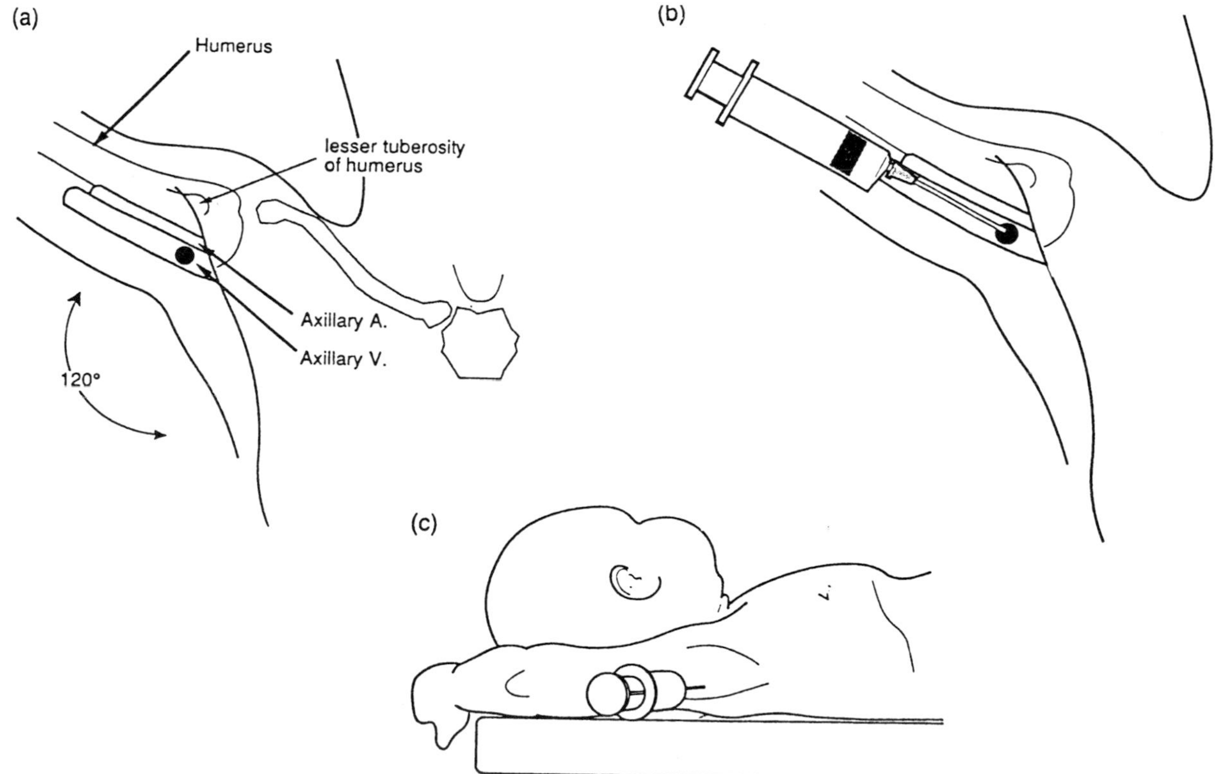

Figure 14.2 Inserting a silicone catheter through an introducing needle into the axillary vein (Oriot and Defawe, 1988).[18]

CENTRAL VENOUS CANNULATION VIA THE AXILLARY VEIN, USING THE AXILLARY ARTERY AS A LANDMARK

Metz et al. *(1990)*[19]

This technique is similar to that described by Nickalls (1987)[20] for adults (see Chapter 5).

Patient category

Age range 4 days to 12 years (3–59 kg), median age 0.9 years (median weight 7 kg).

Advantages and disadvantages

Favourable complication rate.

Preferred side

Not stated.

Position of patient

The Trendelenburg position was preferred, with the arm abducted 100–130° and rotated externally (Figure 14.3a,b).

Position of operator

Not stated.

Equipment used in original description

A 22 gauge short (2.5 cm) cannula-over-needle device or a thin-walled needle for insertion of a Seldinger wire introducer for a suitable single- or multiple-lumen catheter device.

Advice on current equipment

Use a flexible catheter introduced over a Seldinger wire. Estimate the length to be inserted by measuring from axilla to sternal notch.

Anatomical landmarks

Palpate the axillary artery (Figure 14.3c).

Preparation

Perform the procedure under sterile conditions using local anaesthesia as indicated.

Point of insertion of needle

The needle is inserted in the axilla, parallel and inferior (i.e. on the chest wall side) to the axillary artery (Figure 14.3c).

Direction of needle and procedure

Palpate the axillary artery (Figure 14.3d,e). Insert the needle into the vein by assuming it lies immediately medial (i.e. on the chest side) to the artery. Confirm entry into the vein by aspirating blood. Thread the catheter or guide-wire centrally.

Success rate

The success rate was 79% – 41 out of 52 attempts: 33% of catheter tips were located in the superior vena cava; 61% reached the subclavian vein; 5.6% terminated in the axillary/subclavian junction. Duration of catheterisation was 2–22 days (median 8 days).

Complications

Catheters became dislodged with subsequent tissue infiltration in 10%, and were accidentally removed in a further 4 cases. Catheter occlusion occurred in 7% and there were solitary instances of venous thrombosis, venous stasis and suspected sepsis. There was one pneumothorax, and one axillary haematoma due to accidental axillary artery puncture.

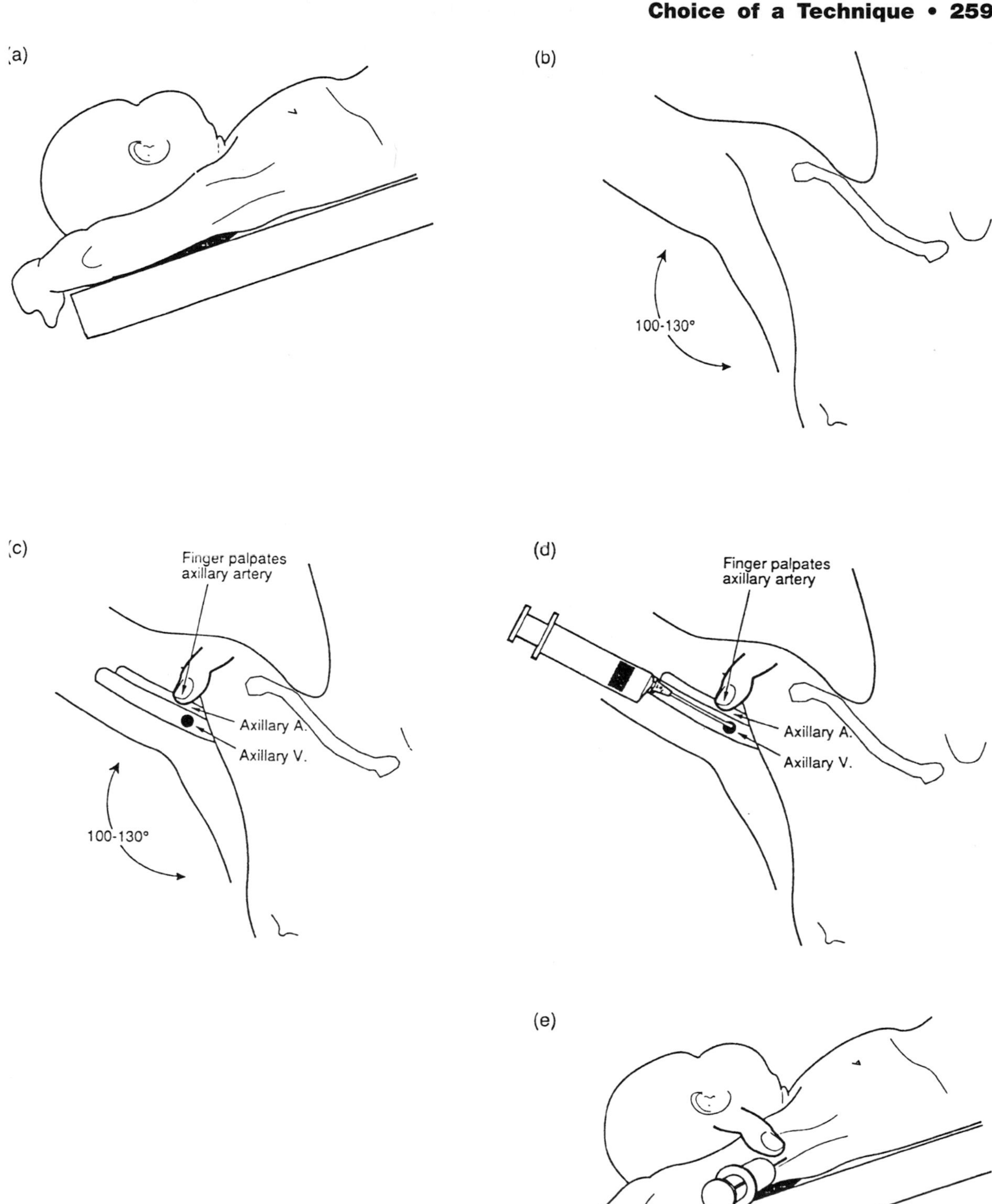

Figure 14.3 Central venous cannulation via the axillary vein, using the axillary artery as a landmark (Metz *et al.*, 1990).[19]

SUBCLAVIAN VEIN

Reports of central venous catheterisation through the subclavian vein in infants are confined to the infraclavicular approach, presumably because of fear of inflicting serious trauma to the lung and other vital structures.

Some workers warn against the subclavian route in infants weighing less than 4.5 kg.[16,19,21] Other reports, however, describe the method in very small children weighing between 0.6 kg and 5 kg.[17,22] Nevertheless, the reported incidence of serious complications cannot be overlooked. Careful consideration should therefore be exercised before choosing the subclavian vein route in very small patients. The subclavian approach should not be attempted by the inexperienced without appropriate supervision.

Puncture of the subclavian vein is necessarily a 'blind' procedure. In most techniques the needle is inserted below the midpoint of the clavicle and identifies the direction in which the needle is advanced by aiming for a target in the suprasternal notch.[16,17] Both Filston and Grant[22] and Eichelberger *et al.*[23] recommend the deltopectoral groove as an additional landmark.

Holland and Ford[24] have recommended the infraclavicular approach to the subclavian vein, using fluroscopic guidance and assisting the passage of the vein dilator and its peel-away sheath by lifting the ipsilateral shoulder of the child in a shrugging manoeuvre.

CENTRAL VENOUS ACCESS VIA THE INFRACLAVICULAR PORTION OF THE SUBCLAVIAN VEIN

Dudrick et al. *(1969)*[21]

Patient category

Adults, and infants over 4.5 kg.

Advantages and disadvantages

Catheter exit site is easy to manage.

Preferred side

Not stated.

Position of patient

Place the patient in a 25° head-down position (Figure 14.4 a,b). Throw the child's shoulders back maximally or hyperextend over a roll placed beneath the vertebral column. Rotate the head to the opposite side.

Position of operator

Not stated.

Equipment used in original description

Longdwel (Becton Dickinson, Swindon, UK) PTFE catheter (size not specified for infants); Deseret Angiocath (Bard, Crawley, UK).

Advice on current equipment

Any catheter-through-needle, catheter-through-cannula or catheter-over-wire device of suitable size.

Anatomical landmarks

Midpoint of inferior border of clavicle; suprasternal notch (Figure 14.4c).

Preparation

Perform the procedure under sterile conditions using local anaesthesia as indicated.

Point of insertion of needle

The point of insertion lies immediately below the midpoint of the inferior border of the clavicle (Figure 14.4c,d).

Direction of needle and procedure

Place the point of the needle on the entry site and

swing the syringe and needle laterally so that the needle is directed towards a finger-tip pressed firmly in the suprasternal notch (A to B) (Figure 14.4d,e). Advance the tip of the needle maintaining gentle aspiration all the time and keeping the syringe and needle parallel to the coronal plane of the patient. A flashback signals entry into the vein; advance the needle 2–3 mm more to ensure complete entry of the tip into the vein. Remove the needle and introduce the catheter to the required distance. Ensure that blood can be freely aspirated from the catheter before it is connected to an appropriate infusion system. Secure and apply a suitable sterile dressing. Take a chest X-ray to confirm the position of the catheter tip and to exclude a pneumothorax.

Success rate

Not stated, but authors advise that infants below 4.5 kg are better catheterised by a cut-down technique, using the internal or external jugular vein.

Complications

Not stated.

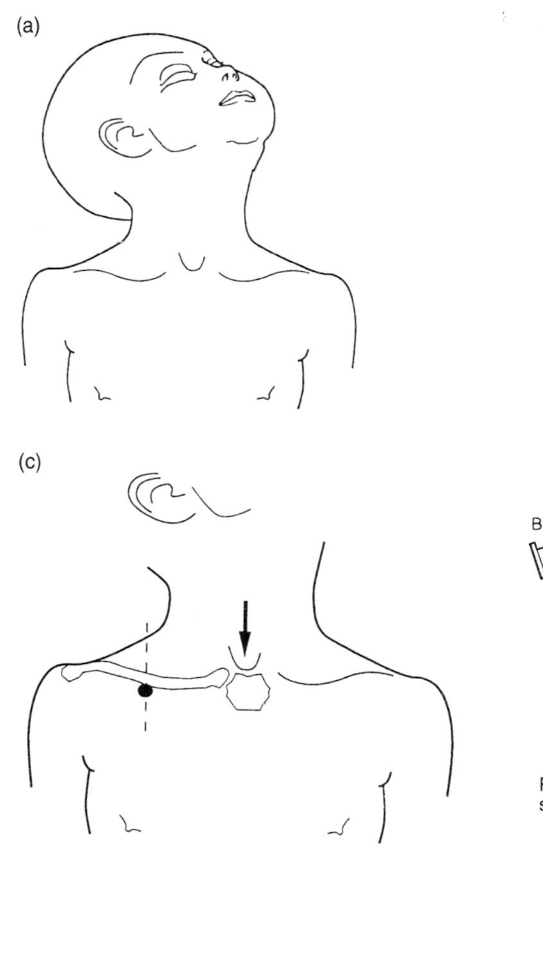

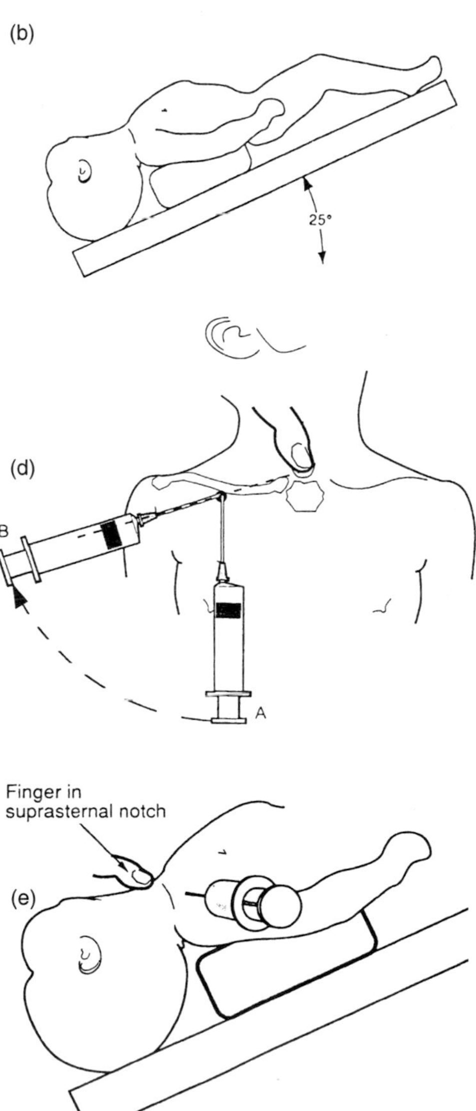

Figure 14.4 (a, b) Position with head hyperextended and rotated; (c) midpoint of clavicle and suprasternal notch; (d, e) axis of needle insertion (Dudrick *et al.,* 1969).[21]

CENTRAL VENOUS ACCESS VIA THE INFRACLAVICULAR PORTION OF THE SUBCLAVIAN VEIN: AN EXTENSION OF THE TECHNIQUE DESCRIBED BY DUDRICK *et al.*

Groff and Ahmed (1974)[17]

Groff and Ahmed used the technique described by Dudrick *et al.*[21] but added a number of salient points. This description should be read in conjunction with Figures 14.4 (a–e).

Patient category

Patients under 2 years old.

Preferred side

Not stated.

Position of patient (Figure 14.5a,b)

Carefully restrain the patient if conscious. Turn the head away from the side of the procedure. The head-down position is optional (Figure 14.5a and b).

Equipment used in original description

A 19 gauge thin-walled, 1.5 inch (3.75 cm) needle with Bardic or Deseret type catheters (the use of a 14 gauge needle for this purpose has been reported in infants).[17] A syringe attached to the needle hub is advised to prevent air embolism.

Advice on current equipment

Catheter-through-needle device with a removable catheter so that the syringe can be attached directly.

Point of insertion of needle

The point of insertion lies at the midpoint of the lower border of the clavicle (Figure 14.5c,d).

Direction of needle and procedure

The needle *must* be inserted and withdrawn in a straight line because searching for the vein beneath the clavicle is dangerous. As many as six or seven insertions can be made in this way.

Place the point of the needle on the entry site and swing the syringe and needle laterally (A to B) so that the needle is directed towards a finger-tip pressed firmly in the suprasternal notch (Figure 14.5d,e). Advance the tip of the needle maintaining gentle aspiration all the time and keeping the syringe and needle parallel to the coronal plane of the patient. A 'flashback' signals entry into the vein; advance the needle 2–3 mm more to ensure complete entry of the tip into the vein. Remove the needle and introduce the catheter to the required distance. Ensure that blood can be freely aspirated from the catheter before it is connected to an appropriate infusion system. Secure and apply a suitable sterile dressing. Take a chest X-ray to confirm the position of the catheter tip and to exclude a pneumothorax.

It is often necessary to manipulate the catheter to make it pass from the subclavian vein to the superior vena cava. This is in contrast to adults where the catheter is almost always easily inserted after the needle is positioned in the vein. If the catheter binds on the needle, the catheter and needle are withdrawn together to avoid severing the catheter on the sharp needle bevel.

Success rate

Each catheter insertion required, on average, 3 needle insertions (range 1–8).

Complications

One pneumothorax, 2 hydrothoraces (1 died), 1 haemothorax, 6 catheter sepsis, 1 uncontrolled bleeding (died).

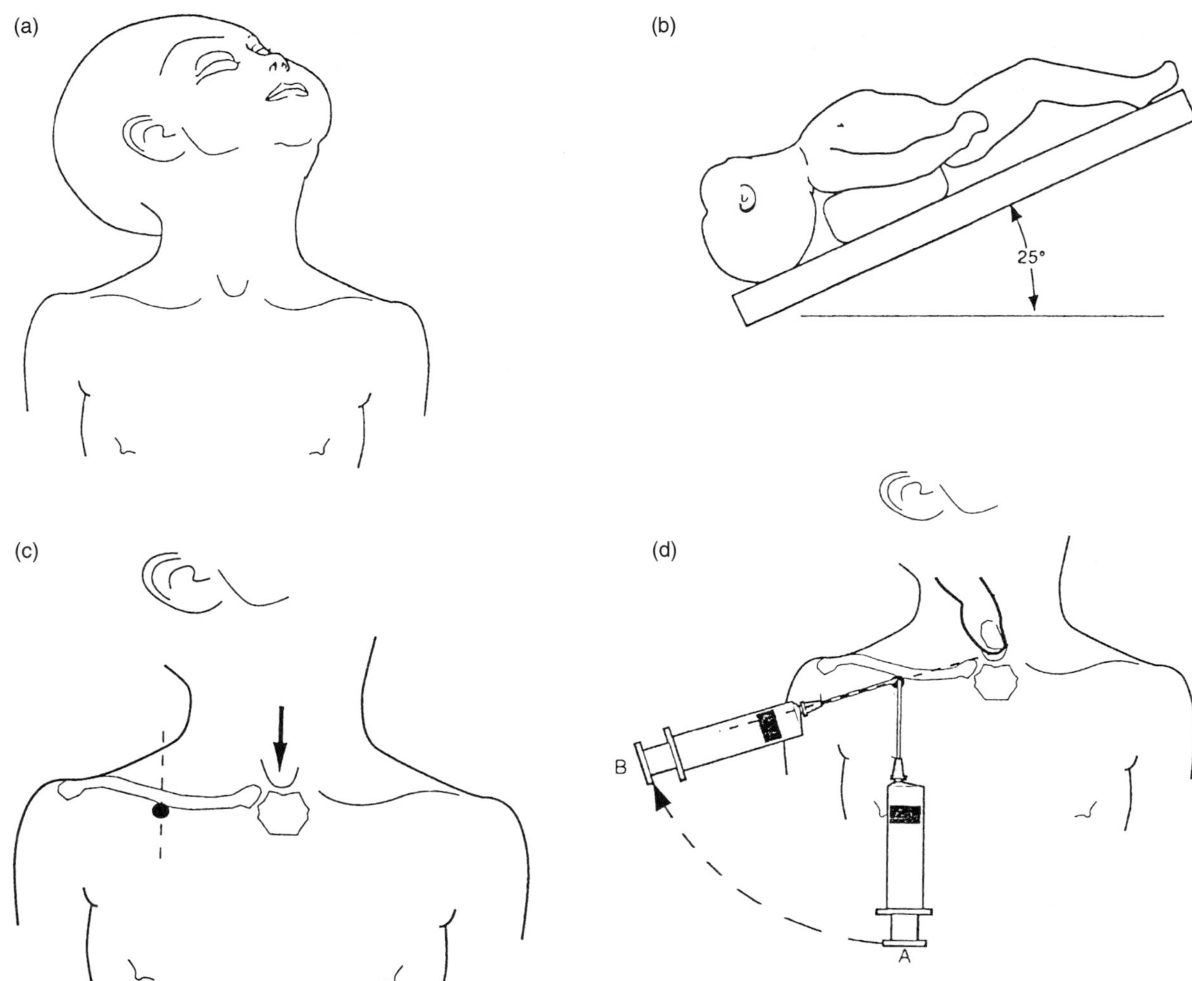

Figure 14.5 (a,b) Position with head hyperextended and rotated; (c) Midpoint of clavicle and suprasternal notch; (d,e) axis of needle insertion (Groff and Ahmed, 1974).[17]

INFRACLAVICULAR APPROACH TO THE SUBCLAVIAN VEIN USING THE DELTOPECTORAL GROOVE AS A LANDMARK

Filston and Grant (1979)[22]

Patient category

Age from 1 day to 6 months; weight 690–5270 g.

Advantages and disadvantages

The deltopectoral groove is usually easily identified.

Preferred side

Left side preferred. In this series 7% required cannulation on the right side after failure on the left.

Position of patient

Tie down hands and feet (conscious patient) and tape the head so that it faces forward with the neck extended (Figure 14.6a,b). Tilt the table head-down.

Position of operator

Not stated.

Equipment used in original description

Catheter-through-cannula device (Argyl Intramedicut Catheter, Sherwood Medical Industries Tyco Healthcare, Gosport, Hants, UK).

Advice on current equipment

Catheter-through-cannula device or guide-wire technique.

Anatomical landmarks

Midpoint of lower border of clavicle; deltopectoral groove; suprasternal notch (Figure 14.6c).

Preparation

Perform the procedure under sterile conditions using local anaesthesia as indicated.

Point of insertion of needle

The needle is inserted infraclavicularly, just lateral to the midpoint of the clavicle (Figure 14.6c,d).

Direction of needle and procedure

Place the needle point on the site of insertion and swing needle and syringe laterally (A to B) until they lie along the line that aims the tip of the needle towards a point 1–1.5 cm above the suprasternal notch (Figure 14.6d,e). The syringe and needle should now lie along the deltopectoral groove.

Elevate the needle and syringe 45° above the coronal plane (Figure 14.6e) at first. This enables the needle to pass under the clavicle. This angle is then reduced to 15–20° above the coronal plane (Figure 14.6f). If the patient has a prominent pectoral region, the needle is flattened against the chest wall. Advance the needle into the vein.

When blood is aspirated, withdraw 0.5 ml blood and inject it forcefully, advancing the needle a few millimetres further into the vein.

Success rate

The success rate was 95% in 80 patients.

Complications

Malpositioned catheter 4%, arterial puncture 2%, hydrothorax 1%, pneumothorax 1%, pneumomediastinum 1%, haemorrhage 1%, hydrothorax due to catheter migration 1%, arm swelling 1%, catheter fault – broken hub 1%, septicaemia due to line 2.5%.

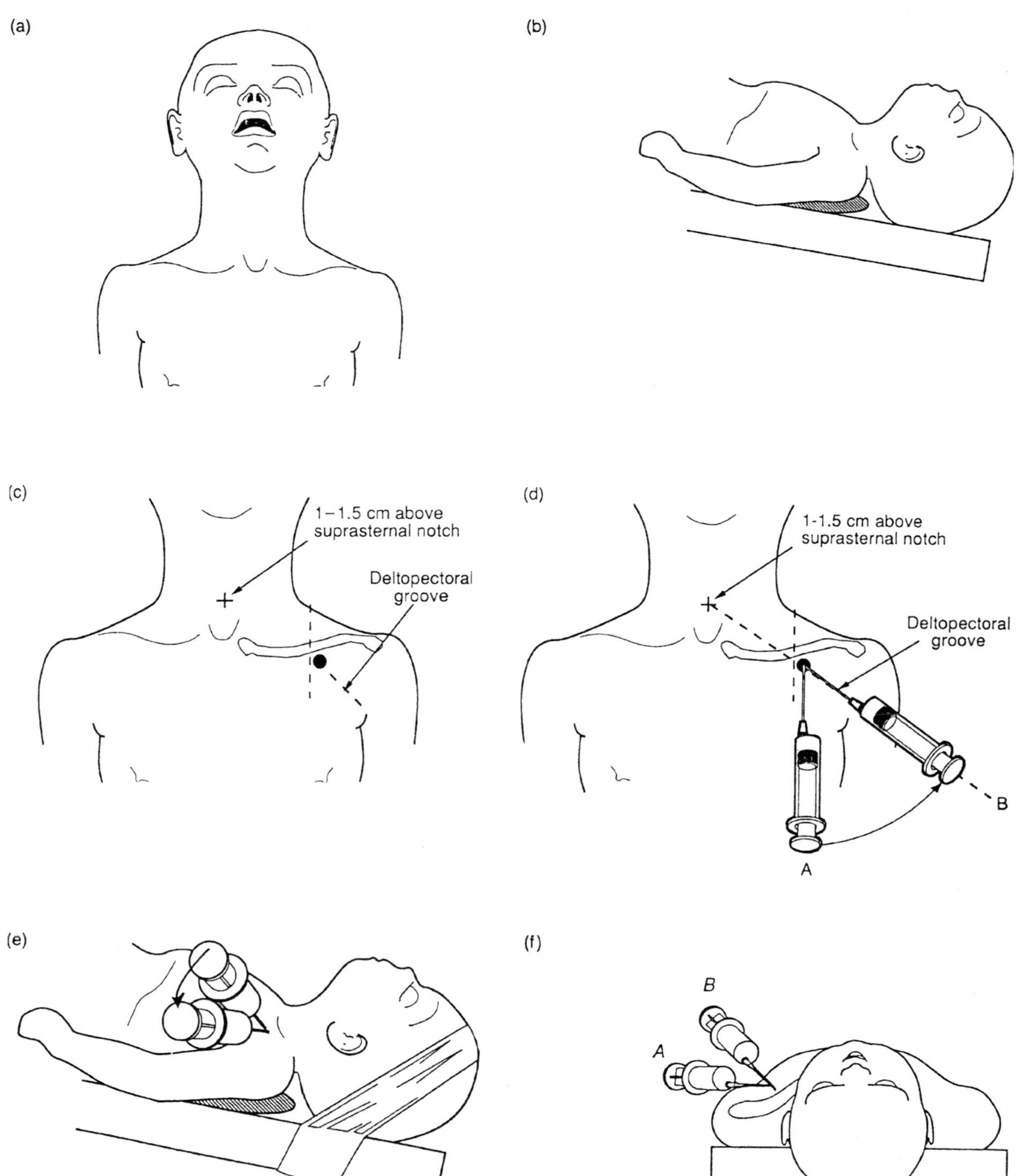

Figure 14.6 (a,b) Position with head extended; (c) midpoint of sternum, deltopectoral groove and suprasternal notch; (d) axis of needle insertion; (e,f) syringe is angled for needle to pass under clavicle, then lowered (Filston and Grant, 1979).[22]

INFRACLAVICULAR APPROACH TO THE SUBCLAVIAN VEIN USING THE DELTOPECTORAL GROOVE AS A LANDMARK

Eichelberger et al. *(1981)*[3]

This technique represents a modification of that described by Filston and Grant. (see above).

Patient category

Infants and small children.

Advantages and disadvantages

The puncture site is easy to manage. No major complications reported.

Preferred side

None stated.

Position of patient

Supine (with restraint if conscious). Place a cylindrical roll of 10 cm ×10 cm gauze longitudinally in the interscapular region to enhance the backward lie of the shoulders (Figure 14.7a,b). Keep the head facing forwards by means of adhesive tape strapped across the forehead. Tilt the table head-down.

Position of operator

Not stated.

Equipment used in original description

An 18 gauge or 20 gauge PVC catheter-through-cannula (Argyl Intramedicut).

Advice on current equipment

Silicone elastomer or similarly flexible catheter, introduced through a cannula.

Anatomical landmarks

Deltopectoral groove; lower border of clavicle; suprasternal notch (Figure 14.7c).

Preparation

Perform the procedure under sterile conditions using local anaesthesia as indicated.

Precautions and recommendations

Use a fenestrated, translucent self-adhesive drape so that the child can be easily seen through it.

Point of insertion of needle

Insert the needle in the deltopectoral groove, 2 cm from the lower margin of the clavicle (Figure 14.7d,e).

Direction of the needle and procedure

Identify the palpable deltopectoral groove where the clavicle crosses the first rib and insert the needle at the point of insertion. Swing the syringe and needle laterally to lie in the deltopectoral groove (A to B), keeping the needle in the coronal plane (Figure 14.7d). Advance the needle tip, bevel down, until aspiration of blood confirms entry into the subclavian vein as the latter passes between the clavicle and first rib.

Immediately redirect the syringe so that the needle is aimed at a point above the suprasternal notch (B to C) (Figure 14.7e,f). This point should be 1 cm above the notch, but in children older than 1 year the distance should be less than 1 cm.

Advance the needle a few millimetres into the vein and if a cannula-over-needle is being used, advance the cannula into the vein and remove the needle. The catheter is introduced through the cannula and advanced to the superior vena cava. The cannula is then withdrawn along the catheter. This is important, because if the cannula were to remain in the vein, accidental extraction of the catheter would leave the cannula open to the atmosphere with the attendant grave risk of air embolism or haemorrhage.

Success rate

A total of 191 catheters were inserted into 135 patients. Of these insertions, 34.6% were on neonates, another 34.6% were on infants 1–12 months old and the remainder (30.8%) were on patients 1–18 years old. Mean duration of catheter usage was 23.7 days. Failed catheter insertions are not identified.

Complications

There were no incidents of pneumothorax, haemopneumothorax, haemorrhage, superior vena cava obstruction or facial oedema. Sixty cases (31.4%) suffered catheter-related sepsis though the catheter was considered to be the primary cause in 3.4% of children over 12 months of age and in 6.8% of younger children. Routine blood cultures are essential to monitor for infection and all catheter tips should be sent for culture. There were 3 cases (1.6%) of pleural effusion, 2 instances (1%) of subclavian vein thrombosis and 9 lines (4.7%) became blocked. The line or its hub cracked in 14 cases (7.3%).

(a)

(b)

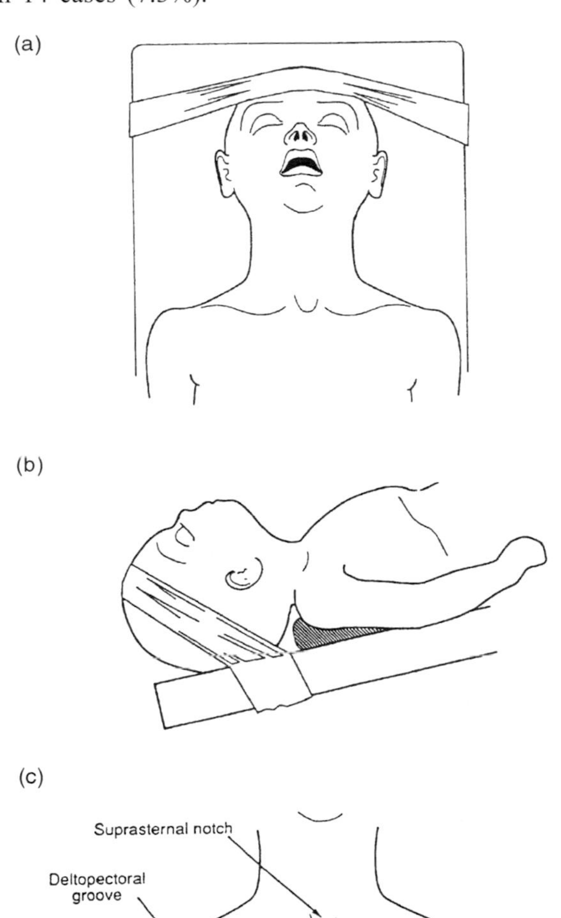

(c)

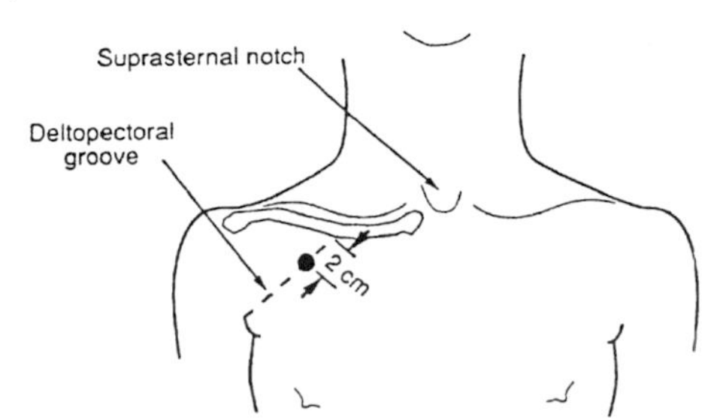

d)

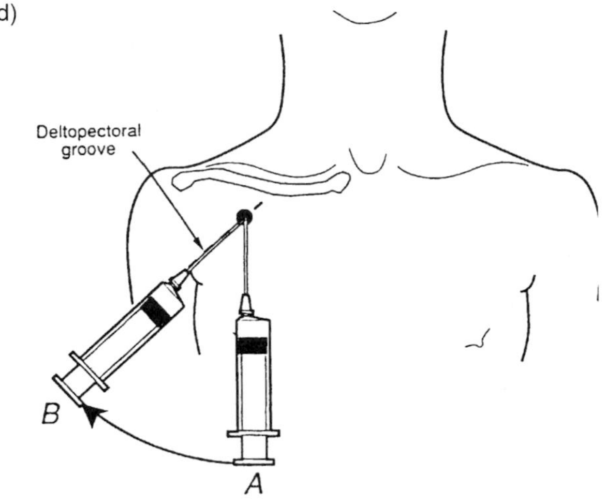

e)

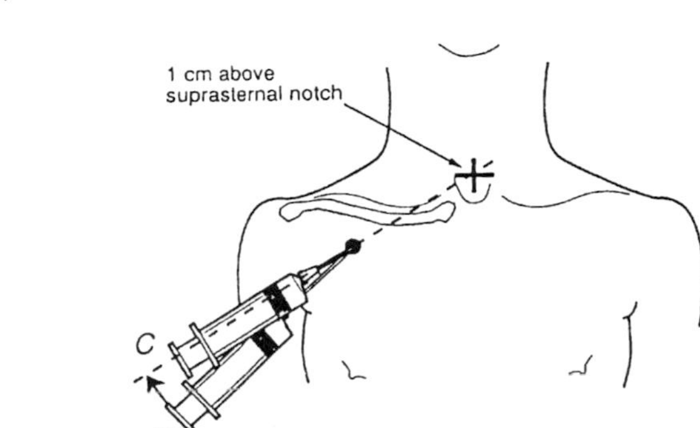

f)

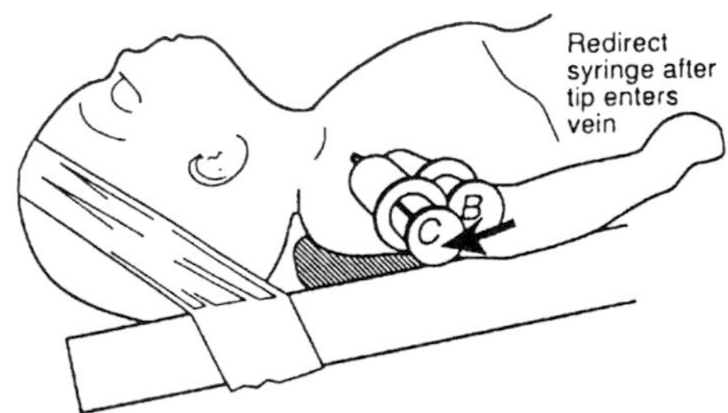

Figure 14.7 (a) Position with head restrained and extended; (b) head-down tilt; (c) deltopectoral groove, lower border of clavicle, suprasternal notch; (d) swing syringe to align with deltopectoral groove; (e,f) redirect needle towards suprasternal notch after achieving venepuntcture.

INTERNAL JUGULAR VEIN

English *et al.*[25] described two alternative techniques for central venous cannulation via the internal jugular vein and reported the results of 500 attempted cannulations which included 85 children and infants. Their 'elective' technique is unique in that it demands that the internal jugular vein is positively identified by palpation. For patients – particularly small children and infants – in whom this is not possible, the authors described an 'alternative' technique, using the clavicular head of the sternomastoid as the sole identifier of the location of the internal jugular vein.

Long-term cannulation of the internal jugular vein for parenteral nutrition in infants and children was first described by Dudrick *et al.*[21] They and several other groups of workers advocated tunnelling the catheter to a point behind the ear as a means of limiting infection problems. Although a Broviac catheter with its Dacron wool cuff can be used in full-term infants and children, premature babies requiring nutrition have insufficiently large veins for the use of this device. Pereyra *et al.*[26] described a novel technique in which a plain silicone central venous catheter is introduced surgically into the internal jugular vein and then tunnelled to the preferred position on the chest wall, where it is fixed by cementing silicone sheet material to the catheter material and sewing this to the skin. This technique could be used to enhance the fixation of percutaneously introduced silicone catheters.

The internal jugular vein can be approached at one of three levels. English *et al.*[25] seek to identify the vein by palpation (high approach), whilst three groups (English *et al.*, Hall and Geefhuysen[257] and Korshin *et al.*[258] exploit the relationship of the vein with the triangle formed by the two heads of the sternomastoid muscle and the clavicle (low approach). Korshin *et al.* also describe a method of identifying the carotid artery and deflecting it medially in order to minimise accidental arterial puncture (high approach). This technique is described below. Rao *et al.*[2514] favour identifying a 'notch' on the upper border of the clavicle (very low approach). Most of these authors recommend a steep angle between the needle and the skin in order to minimise the risk of traumatising the adjacent apex of the lung. Korshin *et al.* do not subscribe to this precaution. Two techniques (Krausz *et al.*[259] and Hall and Geefhysen[256] approach the vein at an extreme angle from behind the lateral margin of the sternomastoid muscle, minimising lung trauma at the expense of inheriting some inevitable difficulty in causing the wire or catheter to advance into a central vein.

Most of the recommendations on adult internal jugular vein catheterisation (Chapter 7), which seek to maximise the success rate and minimise complications, are as pertinent to children as they are to adults. High techniques are preferable to low approaches. The number of stabs at a given vein should be limited. The large head and short neck in the infant and very small child can make access to the neck difficult. A high priority should therefore be given to careful positioning of the patient before attempting venepuncture. Equipment of appropriate design and scaled-down dimensions can influence the success and complication rates. Central venous catheterisation in infants and very small children should ideally be carried out only by those whose work regularly involves performing these techniques in children.

Techniques that can be used in children are described in detail in Chapter 7 which deals with the internal jugular vein route in depth. Two methods not included in Chapter 7 are described below. In this section, techniques for percutaneous introduction of tunnelled Hickman (and Broviac) catheters and pulmonary artery balloon catheters are included because they are most appropriately and safely introduced through the internal jugular vein because of its straight course to the right atrium and the relative safety of catheter introduction.

CENTRAL VENOUS CATHETERISATION VIA THE INTERNAL JUGULAR VEIN (HIGH TECHNIQUE): MEDIAL APPROACH, CAROTID ARTERY METHOD

Korshin et al. *(1978)*[28]

Patient category

Ages from 4 months to 81 years.

Advantages and disadvantages

Positively identifies the carotid artery and seeks to avoid it.

Preferred side

The right side.

Position of patient

Place the table with a 10–15° head-down tilt. Hyperextend the head and turn it towards the contralateral side (Figure 14.8a,b).

Position of operator

Not stated.

Equipment used in original description

Bardic Intracath (a catheter-through-needle device); 16 gauge, 12 inch (30 cm) catheter with 14 gauge needle for larger children; 19 gauge, 12 inch (30 cm) catheter with 17 gauge needle for infants and children.

Advice on current equipment

Any suitable guide-wire device.

Anatomical landmarks

Mid-neck technique: palpate the common carotid artery at the level of the cricoid cartilage (Figure 14.8c).

Preparation

Perform the puncture under sterile conditions using local anaesthesia as indicated.

Precautions and recommendations

If the patient is breathing spontaneously, whether anaesthetised or awake, advance the needle only during expiration.

Point of insertion of needle

The needle is inserted immediately lateral to the carotid artery and medial to the border of the sternomastoid muscle at the level of the cricoid cartilage (Figure 14.8d).

Direction of needle and procedure

Palpate the carotid artery with the left hand and retract the artery slightly medially (Figure 14.8d). Place the point of the needle on the skin and point the syringe caudally (A). Swing the syringe and needle so that it points 'slightly laterally' (A to B). Elevate the syringe 10–15° above the skin surface (B to C). Point the needle towards the junction of the first and middle thirds of the ipsilateral clavicle, which usually positions the needle pointing more or less towards the ipsilateral nipple. Advance the needle into the vein. Confirm correct positioning of the catheter tip by chest X-ray.

Success rate

The results of the carotid artery technique are presented together with an alternative method using the triangle formed by the two heads of the sternomastoid muscle and clavicle as a guide (see below). A total of 162 patients were involved of whom 54 were infants and children (median age 5 years). The overall success rate was 86.4%. Four catheters (7.4%) were found to be malpositioned.

Complications

One puncture of right pleural dome. Accidental carotid puncture also occurred.

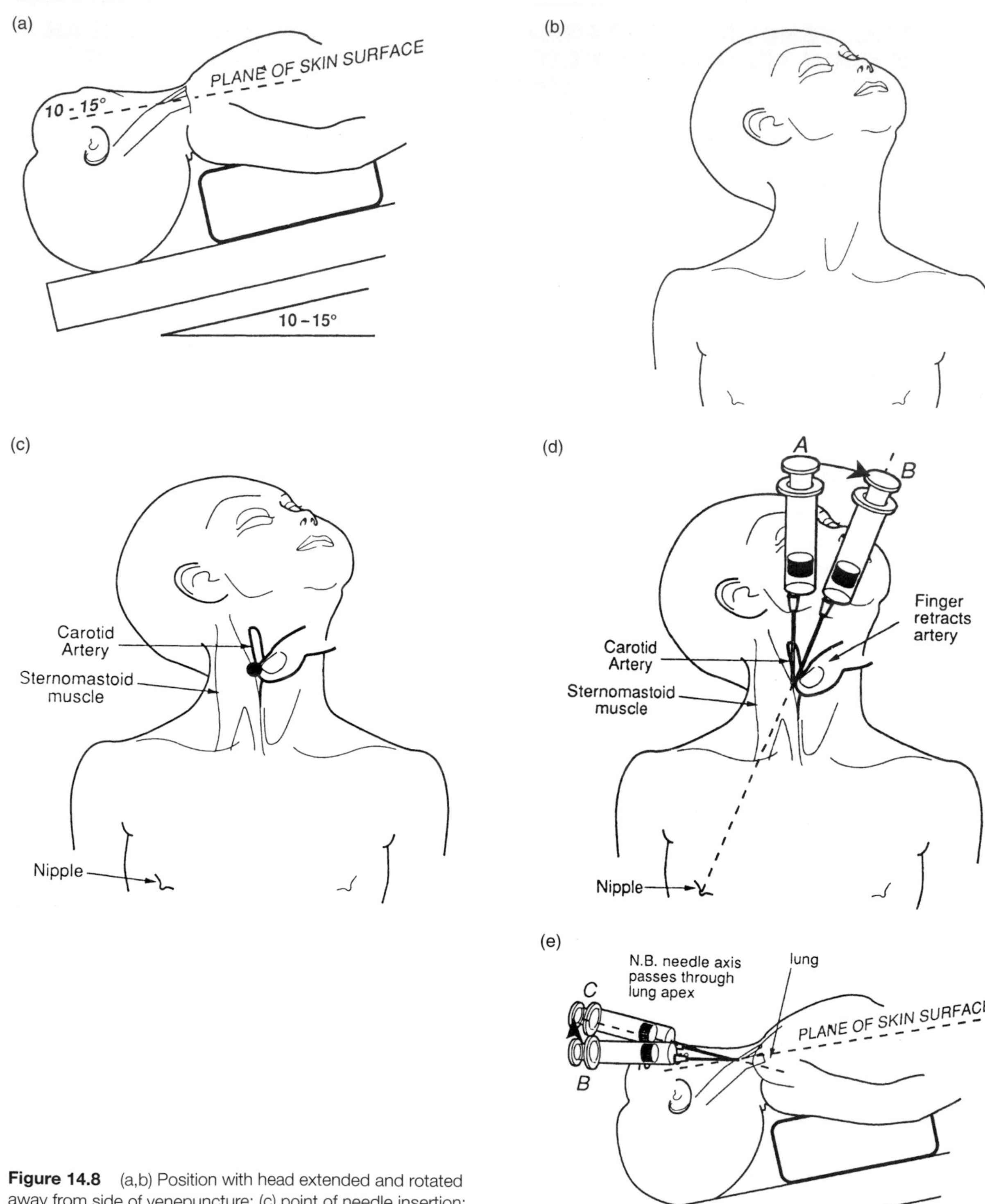

Figure 14.8 (a,b) Position with head extended and rotated away from side of venepuncture; (c) point of needle insertion; (d) palpating the carotid artery, and sighting the ipsilateral nipple; (e) the needle is roated into a plane which includes the ipsilateral (Korshin et al. 1978).[28]

CENTRAL VENOUS CATHETERISATION VIA THE INTERNAL JUGULAR VEIN (HIGH TECHNIQUE): CENTRAL APPROACH, ALTERNATIVE (TRIANGLE) METHOD

Korshin et al. *(1978)*[28]

Patient category

All ages.

Advantages and disadvantages

The triangle formed by the two heads of the sternomastoid muscle is not always easy to demonstrate.

Preferred side

The right side.

Position of patient

Place the table with a 10–15° head-down tilt. Hyperextend the head and turn it towards the contralateral side (Figure 14.9a)

Position of operator

Not stated.

Equipment used in original description

Bardic Intracath (a catheter-through-needle device); 16 gauge, 12 inch (30 cm) catheter with 14 gauge needle for larger children; 19 gauge, 12 inch (30 cm) catheter with 17 gauge needle for infants and children.

Advice on current equipment

Any suitable guide-wire device.

Anatomical landmarks

Identify both sternal and clavicular heads of the sternomastoid muscle and the medial head of the clavicle (Figure 14.9b).

Preparation

Perform the puncture under sterile conditions using local anaesthesia as indicated.

Precautions and recommendations

If the patient is breathing spontaneously, whether anaesthetised or awake, advance the needle only during expiration.

Point of insertion of needle

Insert the needle at the apex of the triangle formed by the two heads of the sternomastoid muscle (Figure 14.9c).

Direction of needle and procedure

Palpate the carotid artery with the left hand and retract the artery slightly medially. Place the point of the needle on the skin and point the syringe caudally (A) (Figure 14.9d). Swing the syringe and needle so that it points 'slightly laterally' (A to B). Elevate the syringe 10–15° above the skin surface (B to C) (Figure 14.9e,f). Point the needle towards the junction of the first and middle thirds of the ipsilateral clavicle, which usually positions the needle pointing more or less towards the ipsilateral nipple. Advance the needle into the vein. Confirm correct positioning of the catheter tip by chest X-ray.

Success and complication rates

See under 'carotid' method above.

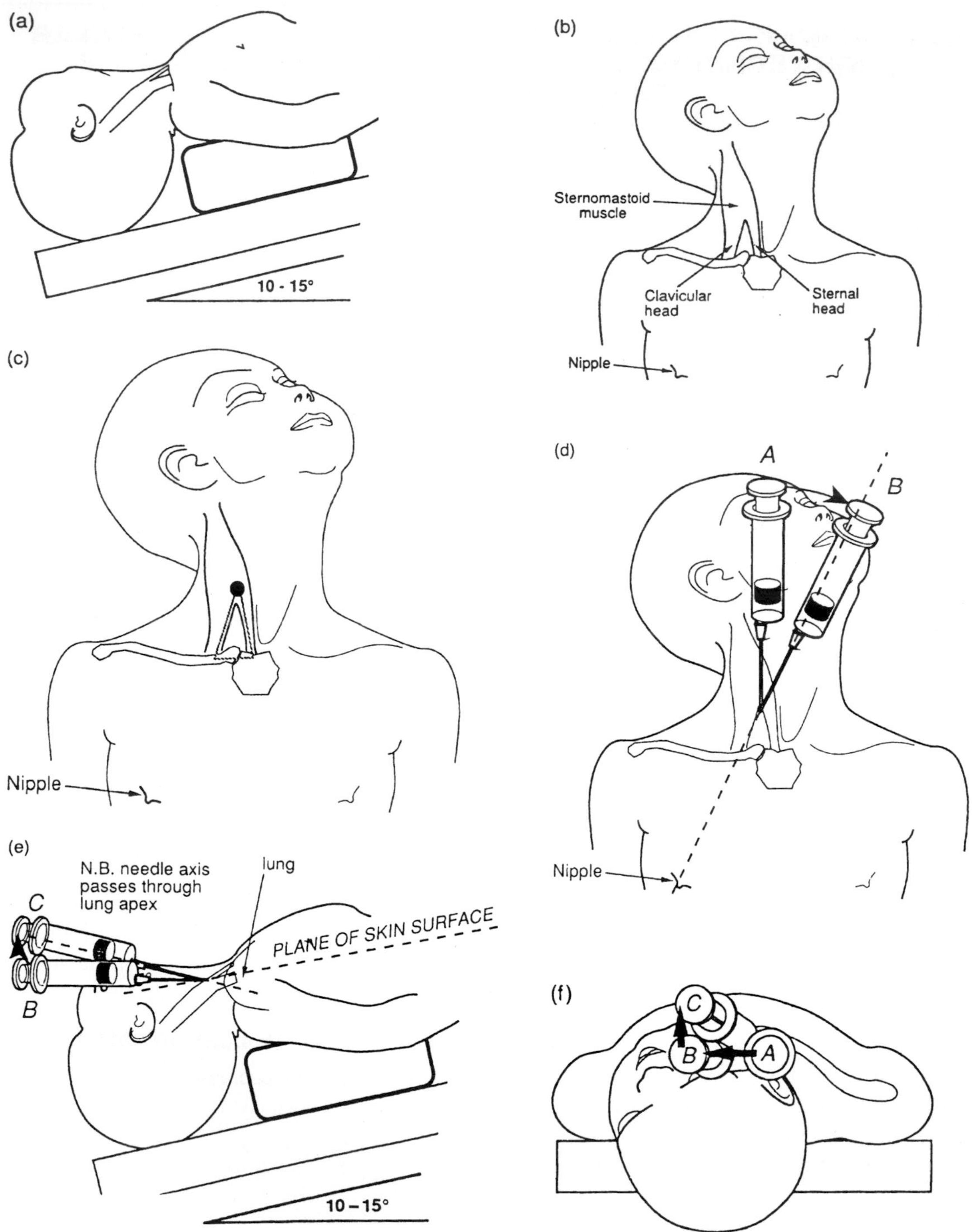

Figure 14.9 Alternative (triangle) method. (a) Position with head extended and rotated away from the side of venepuncture; (b) the two heads of sternomastoid; (c) sternal and clavicular heads of sternomastoid with needle insertion point at apex of triangle formed between them; (d) introduce the needle and swing it into place, pointing more or less towards the ipsilateral nipple; (e) raise the barrel of the syringe to form a 15° angle with skin; (f) top view (Korshin *et al.,* 1978).[28]

CENTRAL VENOUS ACCESS VIA THE INTERNAL JUGULAR VEIN USING TWO-DIMENSIONAL ULTRASOUND IMAGING

Author's method

Patient category

All ages.

Advantages and disadvantages

This method avoids the need for surgical cut-down, and clearly identifies the location, size and course of the target vessel and the adjacent artery. It virtually eliminates failure to cannulate patent vein and minimises complications.

Equipment used in original description

Twenty gauge and 22 gauge Hydromer-coated polyurethane catheters (Viggo Hydrocath, Becton Dickinson, Swindon, UK); 22 gauge PTFE cannula (Abbocath, Abbott Laboratories, Maidenhead, UK) (optional); portable two-dimensional ultrasound imager (Dymax Site-Rite, Dymax Corporation, Pittsburgh, Pa, USA).

Advice on current equipment

Any product requiring percutaneous introduction.

Anatomical landmarks

Supraclavicular area, preferably right side.

Preparation

Perform the procedure with the patient under light general anaesthesia with tracheal intubation or laryngeal mask airway, with a facility for controlling lung ventilation. Raise the shoulders and extend the head moderately over a neck pad. Plastic bubble wrap can easily be fashioned into a suitable size and shape of pad. Rotate the head 15–20° away from the side proposed for examination and puncture.

Procedure

1. Prepare the skin area widely using an alcoholic solution of chlorhexidine. Let the first application dry before spraying a second time. This wetting of the skin acts as the ultrasound transmitting medium.
2. Drape the face and head using sterile drapes or swabs.
3. Switch on the Dymax Site-Rite with its depth graticule active and apply the 9 MHz probe gently to the skin of the neck, ensuring that the face of the probe is lying flat on the patient's skin.
4. Explore the vein by sliding the probe over the wetted skin of the neck and determine the optimum point for vein puncture. If the vein appears insubstantial or blocked, move to the other side of the neck.
5. Hand the probe to an assistant, with instructions to keep the vein image in the centre of the screen and to continue to identify it by gently ballotting the neck with the probe. The vein will 'wink' whereas the artery will not be distorted by gentle downward pressure. It may be necessary to reapply the alcoholic chlorhexidine solution to maintain the quality of the image.
6. Don sterile gloves and introduce the supplied switched cannula or the 22 gauge alternative cannula (with 5 ml syringe attached) into the skin approximately 1 cm craniad to the centre of the probe tip (Figure 14.10).
7. Advance the cannula, pointing it in the direction of the vein (usually slightly) medially and at 45° to the skin surface with the objective of making the needle tip coincide with the long axis of the probe at approximately 1 cm below the skin surface (the vein lies rather less than 1 cm deep in infants).
8. Aspirate gently on the syringe and advance intermittently in short increments. The screen image will reveal the extent to which anatomy is deformed by the frictional drag of the cannula, possibly causing the vein to become completely collapsed. It may be necessary to transfix the vein in this case.

9. When flashback is obtained or the vein is thought to have been transfixed, withdraw the needle from the cannula, apply the syringe to the cannula and withdraw until flashback is once more obtained and blood aspirates freely. Gently advance the cannula as far as possible into the vein. This is necessary to ensure that the coil of the J wire deploys only in a large central vein. Alternatively, choose a straight guide-wire.
10. Introduce the guide-wire and advance it until only enough remains outside the patient to allow the catheter to be passed over it.
11. Withdraw the introducer cannula, insert the vein dilator then exchange it for the catheter. Introduce enough catheter to ensure that the tip lies at the junction between the right atrium and the superior vena cava. In term neonates, this will be no more than 6 cm.
12. Remove the guide-wire and attach a syringe filled with heparin–saline. Check for free bi-directional flow and flush the catheter. If aspiration is intermittent, adjust the inserted length of catheter until flow is free. Connect the catheter to a flushing line or appropriate closure device (the kit includes an on-off switch).
13. Clean the skin and secure the catheter according to the appropriate policy. This may include the use of a suture tether. Ensure that a secondary strain-relieving tether is applied so that the catheter dressing can be changed at intervals with a minimised risk of the catheter 'falling' out.

Success rate

The success rate is 100% for veins that are not blocked or seriously distorted.

Complications

There have been very occasional arterial punctures but only when the vein overlies the artery. The ultrasound display reveals the intimate relationship of the vein to the artery and identifies the impossibility of effectively deflecting the artery medially since any attempt to do so almost invariably causes the vein to be deformed and occluded. The manoeuvre actually invites complications.

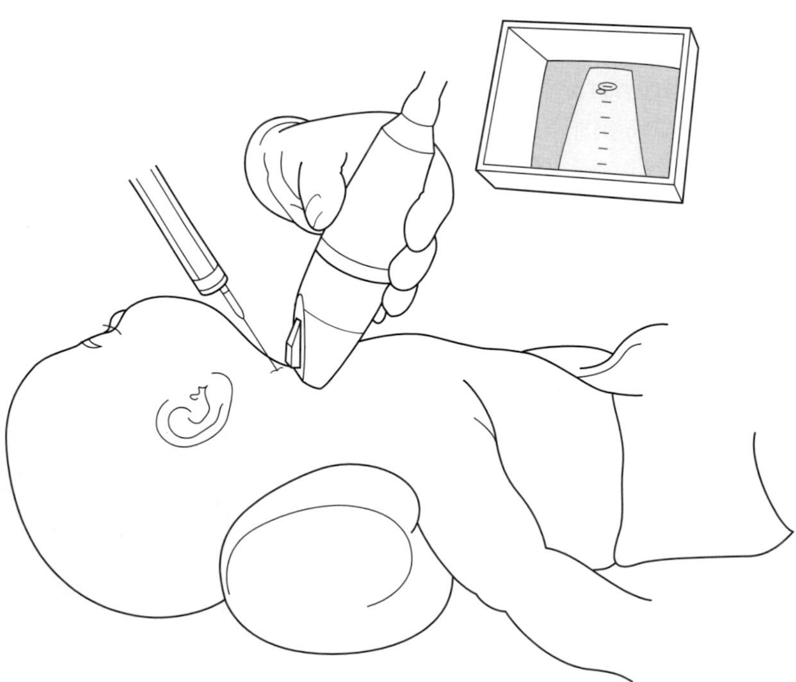

Figure 14.10 Applying the ultrasound probe to locate the target vessel (head drape removed for clarity).

PERCUTANEOUS INSERTION OF A SUBCUTANEOUSLY TUNNELLED HICKMAN CATHETER

Dudrick et al. *(1984)*[30]

Patient category

All ages.

Advantages and disadvantages

Avoids the need for surgical cut-down, minimising damage to the vein.

Equipment used in original description

An introducer system originally designed for the placement of transvenous cardiac pacemaker leads. The kit comprised: 18 gauge needle, 9 cm long; J wire, 47 cm long; syringe; linearly splittable (peel-away) winged introducer cannula of an internal diameter sufficient to pass the selected Hickman catheter; vein dilator of sufficient length and diameter to act as an obturator for the introducer.

Advice on current equipment

Any product containing these components.

Anatomical landmarks

As appropriate for the chosen technique – preferably an infraclavicular subclavian cannulation technique.

Preparation

Perform the puncture under sterile conditions using local anaesthesia as indicated.

Procedure

1. Introduce the needle into the chosen vein and check its position by aspiration.
2. Advance the J wire through the needle until its tip lies several centimetres beyond the needle tip. Ideally, the position of the J wire tip in the superior vena cava should be confirmed by radiological screening (Figure 14.11a).
3. Remove the needle.
4. Make a 1 cm incision in the skin to include the wire insertion site (Figure 14.11b).
5. Make a second, similar incision at the selected point of exit of the catheter. This site should provide easy access for the patient and attendants for routine wound cleaning and dressing procedures (Figure 14.11c).
6. Create a tunnel between the two incisions with a suitable blunt shunt-passing device (Figure 14.11d).
7. Widen the distal end of the tunnel using arteryforceps (haemostat) to permit entry of the Dacron cuff of the catheter (Figure 14.11e).
8. Thread the catheter through the tunnel by attaching it to the shunt-passing device and drawing it through the tunnel until the cuff is located in its final chosen position, several centimetres within the tunnel (Figure 14.11f).
9. Cut the catheter to the correct length by laying it over its proposed course and cutting it at the level of the second intercostal space adjacent to the angle of Louis.
10. Fill the catheter with heparinised saline and apply an obturator with a latex injection site to the Luer connector.
11. Thread the vein dilator over the J wire and dilate the track into the lumen of the vein.
12. Having removed the dilator, pass it through the splittable introducer sheath and thread both (i.e. dilator and splittable introducer), assembled, over the J wire.
13. Remove the J wire and the vein dilator, staunching the flow of blood from the introducer with the finger of a gloved hand.
14. Introduce the cut end of the catheter through the introducer (Figure 14.11g).
15. Carefully remove the introducer by separating its wings and splitting it as it is withdrawn, taking care to prevent the catheter from being delivered with it (Figure 14.11h).
16. Close both wounds with a skin suture or an adhesive dressing (Figure 14.11i).
17. Apply rigorous antiseptic/aseptic dressing technique.

Success rate

Suitable for parenteral feeding over an extended period.

Complications

As apply to the route employed.

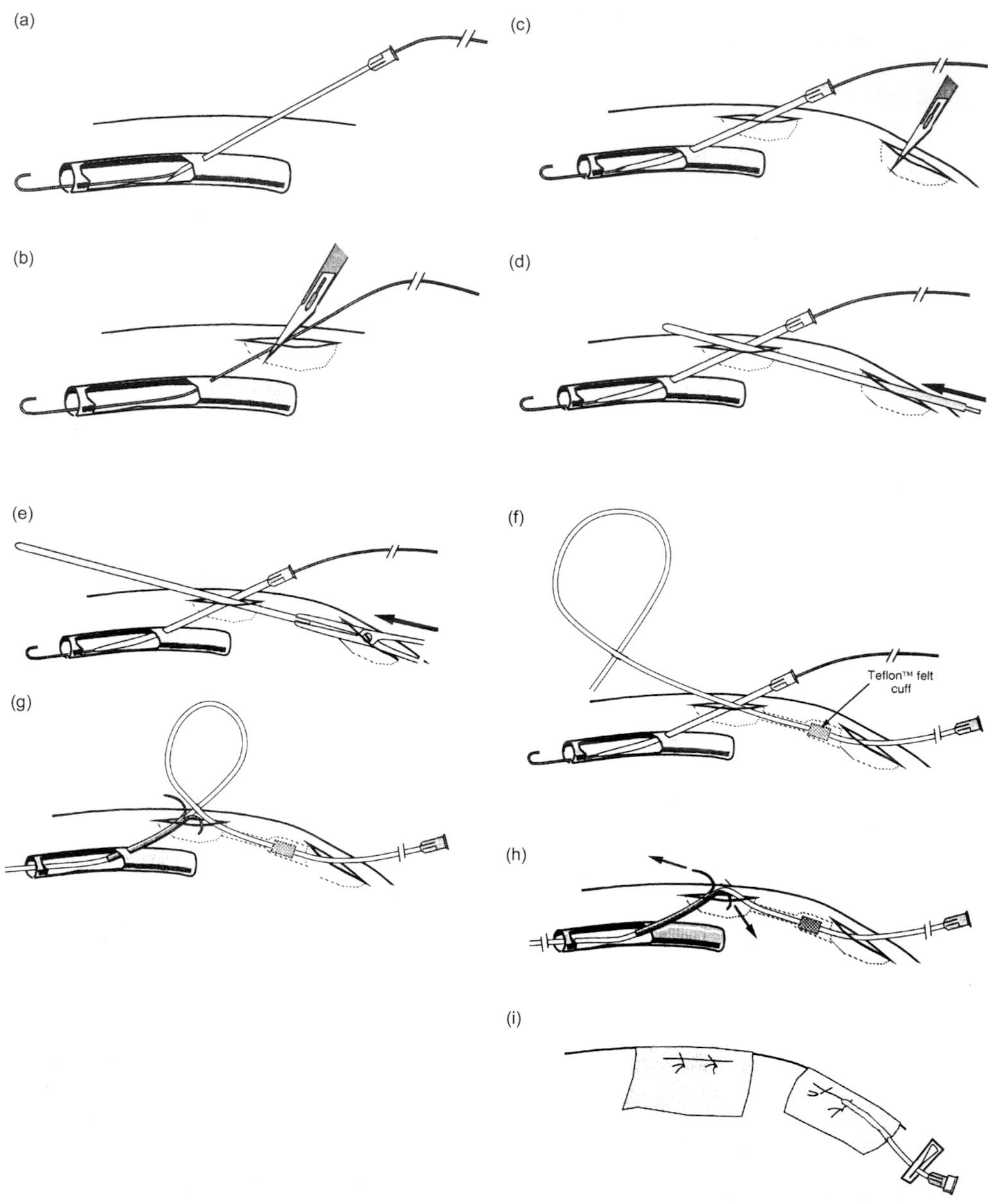

Figure 14.11 Percutaneous insertion of a Hickman line. (a) Introduce the J wire after confirming position of needle in vein by aspiration; (b) make first skin incision to include J-wire point of emergence from skin; (c) insertion of vein dilator over J wire and second skin incision for proposed site of emergence of Hickman line; (d) creation of a tunnel between the two incisions using a blunt catheter insertion device; (e) widening the tunnel at the distal end by introducing a haemostat; (f) the catheter is drawn through the tunnel using the catheter insertion device; (g) the twin dilator is removed, leaving the J wire in place; a splittable catheter sleeve is placed over the vein dilator and the assembly reinserted into the vein. The vein dilator is again removed leaving the sleeve in position. The catheter is cut to the correct length and advanced through this sleeve; (h) the splittable introducer is removed by pulling the two split ends apart, and the catheter is advanced until it lies entirely beneath the skin level; (i) close both wounds and apply an adhesive dressing (Dudrick *et al*., 1974).[30]

PRECUTANEOUS INSERTION OF A BALLOON-TIPPED PULMONARY ARTERY FLOTATION CATHETER THROUGH THE INTERNAL JUGULAR VEIN IN CHILDREN

Damen and Wever (1987)[31]

Patient category

Children up to 5 years old.

Preferred side

The right side.

Equipment used in original description

Children weighing less than 20 kg: 5 F Swan–Ganz catheter (Edwards Company, Santa Ana, Calif, USA) with 6 F introducer. Balloon volume 0.5 ml. *Children weighing more than 20 kg*: 7 F or 7.5 F Swan–Ganz catheter with 8 F introducer. Balloon volume 1.5 ml.

Introducers by Cordis Corporation, Miami, Fla, USA.

Advice on current equipment

Any equivalent product.

Preparation

Perform the puncture under sterile conditions using local anaesthesia as indicated.

Precautions and recommendations

Locate the right internal jugular vein using a seeker needle of 25 gauge or 23 gauge.

Point of insertion of needle

As appropriate for technique chosen.

Procedure

1. Having located the right internal jugular vein with the seeking needle, puncture the vessel with a 20 gauge or 18 gauge needle and introduce a guide-wire through it.
2. Advance an 18 gauge or 16 gauge catheter over the guide-wire. Replace the guide-wire with a thicker one.
3. Replace the catheter with a 6 F or 8 F introducer over the larger guide-wire.
4. In small babies, it may be necessary to shorten the introducer to the appropriate length before insertion.
5. Test the catheter balloon and fill the catheter lumina with heparinised saline.
6. When the catheter is being inserted for the purpose of managing a child undergoing corrective heart surgery, introduction of the balloon catheter into the pulmonary artery may be deferred until it is anatomically possible, either during or after corrective surgery. Place a sterile sleeve over the catheter and advance it into the introducer, using the pressure trace derived from the terminal lumen as a guide to progress and an ECG to monitor possible cardiac arrhythmias.
7. Inflate the balloon to its full diameter when the catheter passes beyond the tip of the introducer and after an acceptable right atrial pressure trace has been obtained. Advance the catheter until it can be demonstrated to have wedged in the pulmonary artery.
8. Deflate the balloon until the next estimation of pulmonary artery wedge pressure is made.

Success rate

The success rate was 100%. There were 57 out of 59 successful insertions of the introducer into the right internal jugular vein; 2 out of 59 were located successfully through the left internal jugular vein.

Complications

Accidental carotid artery punctures by the seeker needle – 6 in 59 (10%); no serious haematoma or bleeding problems. The catheter could not be wedged in only 3 instances (5%). Balloon inflation affected the systemic pressure in 5 instances.

EXTERNAL JUGULAR VEIN

The superficial nature of the external jugular vein has made it a favoured site for surgical access for the insertion of long-term silicone elastomer catheters since these are sufficiently pliable to follow the tortuous route by which this vein reaches the subclavian vein. Its use for percutaneous central venous access in children is limited by the unsuitability of the narrower veins to the introduction and manipulation of a J wire[325] which is so effective in adults in assisting in the navigation of the tortuous course of the vein in the region of the clavipectoral fascia.

FEMORAL VEIN

Of the routes available for central venous catheterisation, the femoral vein tends to be avoided on the basis of a small number of reported serious complications[33,34] which have included two instances of gangrene of the extremities after femoral venepuncture. There is a high incidence of catheter-related thrombus formation (20–46% in adults) found at autopsy in patients who had central venous catheters inserted through the femoral vein[35,36] However, this incidence still compares favourably with an incidence of 67% with pulmonary artery catheters inserted via the internal jugular vein[37] and with 61% for umbilical artery catheters.[38]

A prospective analysis has shown that central venous catheterisation through the femoral vein for the purpose of haemodynamic monitoring is safe and effective and a reasonable method to teach to paediatric trainees.[33] When attempting femoral venepuncture, there is a risk of entering the capsule of the hip joint and striking the femoral head with the possibility of producing a subsequent suppurative arthritis. This risk is increased in infants and in very small children.[39]

CENTRAL VENOUS CANNULATION VIA THE FEMORAL VEIN

Kanter et al. *(1986)*[33]

Patient category

All children requiring haemodynamic monitoring.

Advantages and disadvantages

This is a safe and effective technique which can be effectively taught to all trainees.

Preferred side

Not stated.

Position of patient

Supine and immobilised (Figure 14.12a).

Position of operator

Not stated.

Equipment used in original description

Seldinger guide-wire technique using a 19 gauge needle, 0.025 inch (0.635 mm) wire and a PVC or polyethylene 19 gauge pulmonary artery catheter.

Advice on current equipment

Any flexible catheter introduced over a Seldinger wire. A J wire may be unsuitable in infants because the radius of the curved tip could be too great in such a small vessel.

Anatomical landmarks

Identify the inguinal ligament. Palpate the femoral artery; the vein lies immediately medial to the artery (Figure 14.12b).

Preparation

Perform the puncture under sterile conditions using local anaesthesia as indicated.

Point of insertion of needle

Insert the needle just medial to the palpated femoral artery, 2–3 cm inferior to the inguinal ligament (Figure 14.12b).

Direction of needle and procedure

Place the point of the needle at the entry site (A). Swing the needle slightly laterally (A to B in Figure 14.12c). Elevate the syringe above the skin surface 15–30° (B to C in Figure 14.12d); this helps to avoid the risk of puncturing the capsule of the hip joint. Advance the needle while aspirating gently on the attached syringe. If the vein is not immediately entered, withdraw the needle tip to the skin surface before redirecting it in order to minimise the risk of lacerating the vein. In infants and very small children, advance the needle very slowly and to a depth of 0.5–0.75 cm only to avoid entering the hip joint. Advance the tip a further 1 mm into the vein after withdrawing blood. Introduce the guide-wire and advance it 5–10 mm into the vein before removing the needle. Insert the catheter over the wire. In the event of inadvertent arterial puncture, withdraw the needle and apply firm pressure for 5 minutes. Advance sufficient length of catheter so that its tip lies in the intrathoracic portion of the inferior vena cava and not in the right atrium. Confirm correct positioning of the tip by X-ray.

Success rate

Successful cannulation was achieved in 25 of 29 (86%) patients. Ten of the patients weighed less than 10 kg and 14 were 'in shock' at the time of cannulation. Trainees were successful in cannulating 17 of 25 patients presented (68%).

Complications

Inadvertent femoral artery puncture occurred in 4 of the 29 patients (14%) and 4 patients (14%) experienced leg swelling which resolved when the catheter was removed. A catheter thrombus was found in one child at autopsy. There had been no associated signs in this case.

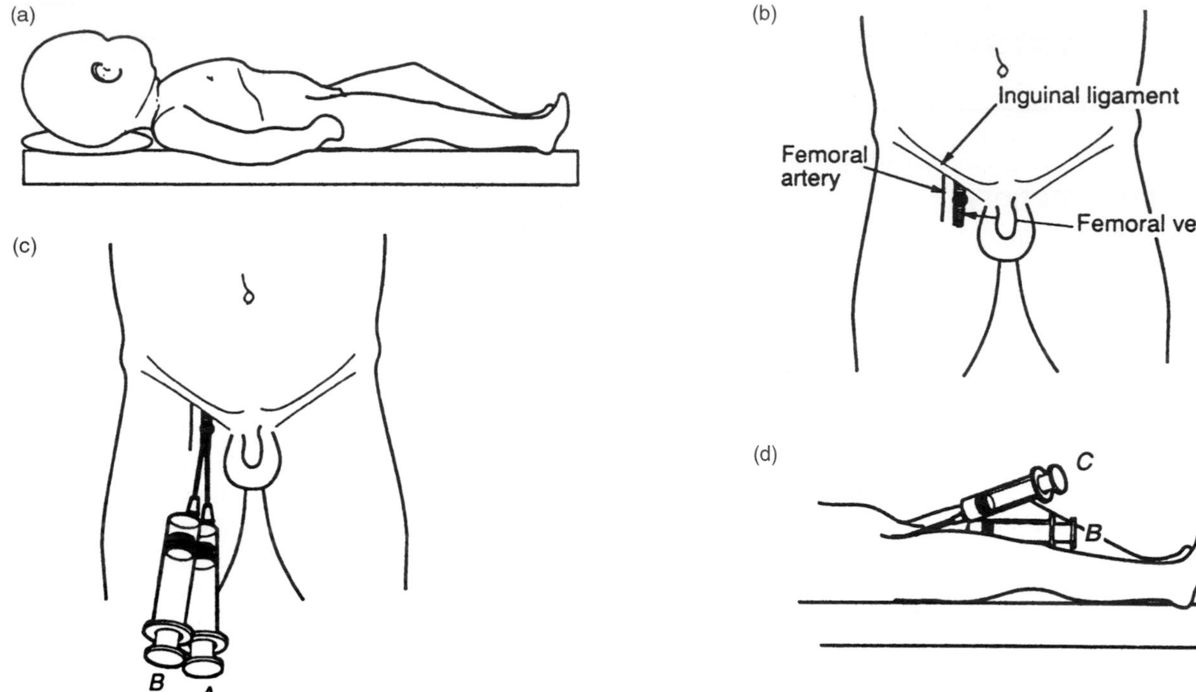

Figure 14.12 Central venous cannulation via the femoral vein (Kanter *et al.*, 1986).[33]

References

1. Heird WC, Driscoll JM, Schullinger JN, Grebin B, Winters RW. Intravenous alimentation in pediatric patients. Journal of Pediatrics 1972; **80**:351.
2. Randolph AG, Cook DJ, Gonzalez CA, Pribble CG. Ultrasound guidance for placement of central venous catheters: a meta-analysis of the literature. Critical Care Medicine 1996; **24**:2053.
3. Scott DHT. Editorial II. British Journal of Anaesthesia 1999; **82**:820.
4. Eggert LD, Rusho WJ, MacKay M, et al. Calcium compatibility in parenteral nutrition solutions for neonates. American Journal of Hospital Pharmacy 1982; **39**:49.
5. Breux C, Duke D, Georgeson KE, Mestre JR. Calcium phosphate occlusion of central venous catheters used for total parenteral nutrition in infants and children: prevention and treatment. Journal of Pediatric Surgery 1987; **22**:829.
6. Puntis JW. Percutaneous insertion of central venous feeding catheters. Archives of Disease in Childhood 1986; **6**:1138.
7. Dolcourt JL, Bose CL. Percutaneous insertion of silastic central venous catheters in newborn infants. Pediatrics 1982; **70**:484.
8. Shulman RJ, Pokorny WJ, Martin CG, Petitt R, Baldaia L, Roney D. Comparison of percutaneous and surgical placement of central venous catheters in neonates. Journal of Pediatric Surgery 1986; **21**:348.
9. Evans JR, Allen AC, Stinson DA. Percutaneous insertion of central venous catheters [letter]. Pediatrics 1983; **71**:668.
10. Carrera G, Liberatore A. Percutaneous silicone catheters in the newborn infant. Pediatrie 1985; **40**:285.
11. Carrera G, Coccia C, Coppalini B, Liberatore A, Minoli I. Percutaneous central venous silastic catheters in newborn infants [letter]. Pediatrics 1987; **79**:837.
12. Durand M, Ramanathan R, Martinelli B, Tollentino M. Prospective evaluation of percutaneous central venous silastic catheters in newborn infants with birth weights of 510 to 3920g. Pediatrics 1986; **78**:245.
13. Scherer LR, West KW, Weber TR, Teiman M, Grosfeld JL. *Staphylococcus epidermidis* in pediatric patients: clinical and therapeutic considerations. Journal of Pediatric Surgery 1984; **19**:358.
14. Rao TL, Wong AY, Salem MR. A new approach to the percutaneous catheterisation of the internal jugular vein. Anesthesiology 1977; **46**:362.
15. Perttila J, Lilius EM, Salo M. Effects of anaesthesia on serum opsonic capacity. Acta Anaesthesiologica Scandinavica 1986; **30**:173.

16. Dudrick, SI. Groff DB Wilmore DW. Long term venous catheterisation in infants. Surgery, Gynecology and Obstetrics 1969; **129**:805.
17. Groff BD, Ahmed NO. Subclavian vein catheterisation in the infant. Journal of Pediatric Surgery 1974; **9**:171.
18. Oriot D, Defawe G. Percutaneous catheterisation of the axillary vein in neonates. Critical Care Medicine 1988; **16**:285.
19. Metz RI, Lucking SE, Chaten FC, Williams TM. Percutaneous catheterization of the axillary vein in infants and children. Pediatrics 1990; **85**:531.
20. Nickalls, RWD. A new percutaneous infraclavicular approach to the axillary vein. Anaesthesia 1987; **42**:151
21. Dudrick SJD, Wilmore DW, Vars HM, Rhoads JE. Can intravenous feeding as the sole means of nutrition support growth in the child and restore weight loss in the adult? Annals of Surgery 1969; **169**:974.
22. Filston HC, Grant JP. A safer system for percutaneous subclavian venous catheterisation in newborn infants. Journal of Pediatric Surgery 1979; **14**:564.
23. Eichelberger MR, Rous PG, Hoelzer DJ, Garcia VF, Koop CE. Percutaneous, subclavian venous catheters in neonates and children. Journal of Pediatric Surgery 1981; **16** (suppl. 1): 547.
24. Holland AJ, Ford WD. Improved percutaneous insertion of long-term central venous catheters in children: the 'shrug' manoeuvre. Australian and New Zealand Journal of Surgery 1999; **69(3)**:231
25. English ICW, Frew RM, Piggott JF. Percutaneous catheterisation of the internal jugular vein. Anaesthesia 1969; **24**:521.
26. Pereyra R, Andrassy RJ, Mahour GH. Central venous cannulation in neonates. Surgery, Gynecology and Obstetrics 1980; **151**:253.
27. Hall DM, Geefhuysen J. Percutaneous catheterisation of the internal jugular vein in infants and children. Journal of Pediatric Surgery 1977; **12**:719.
28. Korshin J, Klauber PV, Christensen V, Skovsted P. Percutaneous catheterisation of the internal jugular vein. Acta Anaesthesiologica Scandinavica 1978; (suppl.): 27.
29. Krausz MM, Berlatzky Y, Ayalon A, Freund H, Schiller M. Percutaneous cannulation of the internal jugular vein in infants and children. Surgery, Gynecology and Obstetrics 1979; **148**:591.
30. Damen J, Wever JEAT. The use of balloon-tipped pulmonary artery catheters in children undergoing cardiac surgery. Intensive Care Medicine 1987; **13**:266.
31. Damen J, Wever JEAT. The use of balloon-tipped pulmonary artery catheters in children undergoing cardiac surgery. Intensive Care Medicine 1987; **13**:266.
32. Blitt CD. Central venous catheterization via the external jugular vein: a technique employing the 'J' wire. Journal of the American Medical Association 1974; **229**:817.
33. Kanter RK, Zimmerman JJ, Strauss RH, Stoeckel KA. Central venous catheter insertion by femoral vein: safety and effectiveness for the pediatric patient. Pediatrics 1986; **77**:842.
34. Nabseth DC, Jones JE. Gangrene of the lower extremities of infants after femoral venepuncture. New England Journal of Medicine 1963; 268:1003.
35. Moncrief JA. Femoral catheters. Annals of Surgery 1958; **147**:166.
36. Bansmer G, Keith D, Tesluk H. Journal of the American Medical Association 1958; **167**:1606.
37. Chastre J, Cornud F, Bouchama A. Thrombus as a complication of pulmonary artery catheterization via the internal jugular vein. New England Journal of Medicine 1982; **306**:278.
38. Symansky MR, Fox HA. Umbilical vessel catheterization. Journal of Pediatrics 1972; **80**:820.
39. Asnes RS, Arendar GM. Septic arthritis of the hip: a complication of femoral venepuncture. Pediatrics 1966; **38**:837.

15 • Results and Complications

PETER JONES

Introduction

The wide range of successful cannulation rates and reported complications occurring in both adults and children are described in detail in the relevant adult chapters as well as in Table 15.1 which concentrates on those particularly related to paediatric practice.

The complications of central venous catheterisation can be divided into two groups: (a) complications that are encountered at the time of cannulation and consist of trauma to surrounding vital structures (the incidence and severity of injuries are much higher when 'blind' puncture of deep neck veins is attempted, compared with cannulation of visible and palpable peripheral veins or when an ultrasonic imaging device is used); and (b) complications that become manifest at some later stage and are the consequence of thrombus formation, intravascular accidents and catheter-related infection.

Congenital abnormalities

Most complications are applicable to both adult and paediatric practice. Nevertheless, some problems are peculiar to infants and small children. Particular care must be exercised when attempting to cannulate veins in children with suspected or known cardiovascular abnormalities. For instance, the absence of a right superior vena cava, with the persistence of a left superior vena cava, occurs in 0.2% of the population. This congenital anomaly has been responsible for failure to cannulate the right internal jugular vein.[1] The catheter, which was introduced into the right subclavian vein, crossed the midline to terminate in the left superior vena cava. In another incident, multiple attempts to cannulate the right internal jugular vein resulted in the puncture of a 6 cm Gore-tex shunt between the right subclavian artery and the right pulmonary artery.[2] Both patients had Fallot's tetralogy.

Specific vessels

Peripheral veins

Not surprisingly, complications are rarely encountered at the catheterisation sites of peripheral veins. Generally, the catheters float with the venous flow towards the heart, though aberrant destinations are recorded, including the ascending lumbar vein when the saphenous vein was used for insertion of the catheter.[3] Malpositioned narrow-bore catheters tend to correct themselves in time; in one trial, every one of 7 out of 187 catheters (4%) which wereinitially malpositioned assumed the correct location within 24 hours. Knowledge of this phenomenon can avoid the trauma of extended attempts to achieve primary accuracy with catheter positioning. Despite the extremely flexible and yielding nature of narrow-gauge silicone catheter material, there have been a number of reported instances of tamponade arising from vessel perforation by the catheter tip[4–9] and migration into the heart wall,[8] causing cardiac arrest,[10] often after several days or weeks of use. Similar incidents have been reported from the use of an umbilical vein catheter.[11,12] A review of more than 500 peripherally inserted central venous catheters in neonates identified sepsis to be more than twice as common in infants weighing less than 1 kg than in heavier infants; phlebitis being most prevalent in saphenous vein cannulations and least in basilic cannulations.[8] Retention of the catheters as a result of tethering within the vein has also been reported in association with infection[13–15] and low-dose urokinase infusion has assisted in their release.

Pulmonary oedema arising from the insertion of excessive lengths of silicone peripherally inserted central catheters has been reported.[16] The tips of all the catheters were discovered to be located in the pulmonary artery or its branches. The symptoms and signs improved when the catheter tips were withdrawn into the right atrium.

Although the majority of published evidence applies to silicone catheters, polyurethane catheters have been used and evaluated. They appear to enjoy a somewhat shorter duration of use, failing for a number of minor mechanical reasons,[17–19] but are immune to the fracture and embolisation disasters which occasionally beset silicone catheters in this application.[20]

Axillary veins

The reports of experience with techniques utilising the axillary vein are few. Clearly, the method requires more skill than venepuncture of visible or palpable arm veins.

Jugular veins

Catheterisation through the external jugular vein is safer than through the internal jugular vein but successful cannulation is less predictable.[21,22] In contrast to the internal jugular vein approach, where the age of the child appears to play no part, attempts to insert a J wire into the external jugular vein in children become more successful with advancing age. The poorer performance in small children has been attributed to the inappropriately large radius of curvature of the J-tipped wire.[21]

Success rates with the internal jugular vein route are consistently good. Comparing complications arising with techniques using the high approach, the clinical significance of sequelae associated with the low approach would tend to caution against its use.[23]

Subclavian veins

Good results with few complications have been reported with this technique in infants and small children[24] but more recent literature confirms that subclavian venepuncture should be undertaken only when there is a specific indication. The technique has tended to be abandoned in favour of safer approaches[25] as it carries an inevitable risk of accidental serious incident (pneumothorax, hydrothorax, haemothorax) requiring immediate resuscitation. The incidence of these disasters has been reported variously as 0–3% of all attempted insertions.[26,27] Thrombosis of the subclavian vein[28] is another complication almost unique to this approach to the right atrium. The left-sided approach is more likely to result in satisfactory tip position.[26] Clavicular periostitis has been reported complicating subclavian cannulation.[29] Supervision of the inexperienced attempting this technique in the paediatric patient is essential.

Femoral veins

Fear of infectious complications has been a deterrent in the use of the femoral vein for central venous catheterisation. However, the femoral vein has been recommended as a safe route for central venous catheterisation in the infant and small child[27] because there was no great risk of sepsis and the approach did not expose the patient to intrathoracic complications. This conclusion is echoed by Serrao *et al.*[30] There were no significant differences in infectious or other sequelae when compared with those of catheterisation through other routes.[31]

Other approaches

It is hardly surprising that attempts to access the central veins in children who have lost all conventional routes should be associated with complications. Acute Budd–Chiari syndrome has been reported following transhepatic placement of a percutaneous inferior vena caval catheter.[32]

Table 15.1 Venous cannulation in paediatric practice: summary of results and complications.

Authors and year	Vein	Technique, insertion point	Side	Distance between skin and vein (mm)	Age range	Successes/ patients (%)	Complications		Personnel	Comments
							Type	Incidence		
Oriot and Defawe (1988)[33]	AxV	Axilla	Either	10	Neonates	217/226 (94)	Shoulder oedema Catheter sepsis	3.5% 1.3%	?	
Metz *et al.* (1990)[34]	AxV	Medial to AxA Seldinger technique via needle or cannula			4 d–12 yr	41/52 (79)	AxA haematoma Pneumothorax Tissue infiltration Venous thrombosis	1/41 1/41 4/41 1/41	Mostly consultants plus 5 trainees	
Taylor & Yellowlees 1990)[35]	AxV	Percutaneous, Seldinger			Mostly adult	98/102 (96)	Malposition Arterial puncture Transient paraesthesia Pneumothorax	6.0% 5.0% 2.0% 1.0%	Consultants and trainees	
Wirrell *et al.* 1993)[7]	AxV	Percutaneous	R		740 g	1 case report	Cardiac tamponade			Day 38, Silastic catheter
Nicolson *et al.* (1985)[21]	EJV	Visualise and cannulate vessel using Seldinger technique with J wire	R then L		<1 mo 1 mo–1 yr 1–5 yrs 5 yr	1/1 (100) 6/17 (35) 13/22 (59) 56/77 (73)	Failed CephV access	14.5%	Trainees and consultants	15–20° Trend., head extended away from puncture side
Krul *et al.* (1986)[36]	EJV	Surgical cut-down of implantable closed system – Abbott Portacath	R side preferred		0–16 yr	33/42	Innominate v. placement Wound dehiscence Haematoma Catheter disconnection Catheter occlusion Catheter-related sepsis	21% 2.4% 2.4% 4.8% 9.5% 4.8%	?Authors	Authors conclude that this is the preferred method for long-term venous access
Khilnani *et al.* (1990)[37]	EJV	Percutaneous	R		Preterm	2 case reports	Cardiac tamponade Catheter embolisation	1 case 1 case		
Hohn & Lambert (1966)[38]	FV	PTFE catheter over nylon monofilament (modified Seldinger technique)			3–15 yr	8/8 (100)	Clot within tube	25.0%	?	IVC access
Kanter *et al.* (1986)[39]	FV	Percutaneous, Seldinger training programme			Paediatric	25/29 (86)	Arterial puncture Leg swelling	14.0% 14.0%	Mostly trainees	Technique easy to teach
Talbott *et al.* (1995)[40]	FV	Percutaneous observed post-insertion by Doppler US			Infants and children	20	Thrombus formation	7/20		Failure to aspirate and leg swelling related to thrombi
Serrao *et al.* (1996)[30]	FV	Percutaneous			Neonates	44/44 (100)	None			Recommended femoral vein route is safe

English *et al.* (1969)[41]	IJV	Two techniques: (a) palpate IJV; if failure, (b) blind 500 cases incl. 85 children	R	–	1–15 yr	0–1 yr, 11/12 1–5 yr, 23/27 5–15 yr, 43/46	Pneumothorax Arterial puncture Misplaced tip	0.2 0.6 0.2	Consultants and trainees	Complication rate for all cases
Prince *et al.* (1976)[42]	IJV	Skin puncture at apex of triangle formed by 2 heads of sternomastoid and clavicle. Needle at 45°to skin towards nipple	R then L	1–2	6/52–14 yr	40/52 on R side (77)	Carotid puncture Horner's syndrome Haematoma	23.0 3.8 5.8	Trainees	15–20° Trend., head extended away from puncture side
Hall & Geefhuysen (1977)[43]	IJV	(a) Enter at apex of 'sternomastoid triangle' Advance at 30° to skin slightly laterally *or* (b) posterior edge of sternomastoid	Either	–	2 wk–9 yr	>90/100 (>90)	None serious Arterial puncture Troublesome bleeding	 ?3		Head extended over edge of bed & away from site
Rao *et al.* (1977)[44]	IJV	Needle in palpable notch 0.25–1 cm from sternal end of clavicle parallel to sagittal plane and at 30–40° to coronal plane	Mostly R	–	0–11 yr	180/192 (94) on 1st attempt 97% at 2nd on same side	2/23 on L side punctured thoracic duct Carotid A. puncture	9.0 0.8	Trainees and consultants	25°Trend., head extended slightly away from puncture side
Korshin *et al.* (1978)[45]	IJV	(a) Lateral to carotid (b) Apex of triangle	mostly R	–	0–14 yr	86.4% in 54 cases 54 cases	Punctured lung apex Carotid A. puncture	1.8 ?	Consultants (naive)	Carotid a. puncture rate not stated
Coté *et al.* (1979)[46] IJV		Rao (low)R Needle at 30–45°	R	28	0–19 yr	38/51 (74)	Haematoma Pneumothorax	3.9 2.0	Authors	
		Prince (high) Needle at 30–45°	R	22	0–19 yr	59/71 (83)	Haematoma Carotid a. puncture	4.2 8.5	Authors	
Krausz *et al.* (1979)[47]	IJV	Posterior edge of sternomastoid muscle	Either	10–20	0–12 yr	201/206 (97.6)	Mediastinal extravasation SVC obstruction Pneumothorax Tracheal puncture R hydrothorax Catheter sepsis	1.5 1 0.5 0.5 0.5 10.6	Authors	Intracath used Extreme head-down tilt with legs elevated vertically
Nicolson *et al.* (1985)[21]	IJV	Confluence of two heads of sternomastoid m., towards nipple and at 30–45° to skin Seldinger technique	R then L	–	1 mo 1 mo–1 yr 1–5 yr 5 yr	4/5 (80) 32/38 (84) 24/28 (86) 49/57 (86)	Failed CV access Carotid a. puncture	0.9 8.0	Trainees and consultants	15–20° Trend., head extended away from puncture side
Damen & Wever (1987)[48]	IJV	Balloon-tipped PA catheters, 6 & 8 F introducers	R	–	24 1 yr 34 1 yr	58/58 (100)	Carotid puncture Catheter sepsis	10 4.0	Consultant	Wedge success 92%
Reickert *et al.* (1998)[49]	IJV	Percutaneous insertion of 12–15 gauge double-lumen venovenous ECLS catheter	R	–	Infants	14/20 (70)	Surgically assisted Pneumothorax Blockage	6/20 1/20 1/20		Catheters for venovenous ECLS

Table 15.1 *Continued*

Authors and year	Vein	Technique, insertion point	Side	Distance between skin and vein (mm)	Age range	Successes/ patients (%)	Complications: Type	Complications: Incidence	Personnel	Comments
Evans *et al.* (1983)[50]	PV	Silicone catheter through needle			Infants	18/20 (90)	Septicaemia	11	Authors	EJV, BasV, AxV, superficial Temp V used
Durand *et al.* (1986)[51]	PV	Percutaneous, scalp or limb vein access with floated silicone catheter through needle			Newborn 0.51–3.9 kg	50/55 (91) (1st attempt)	Sepsis Occlusion Dislodgement Fluid extravasation	7.0 15.0 8.0 4.0	–	Indwelling for 25 (2–80) days
Puntis *et al.* (1986)[52]	PV	Percutaneous, scalp or limb vein access with floated silicone catheter			1–7 kg	41/57 (72)	Sepsis Blockage Limb swelling	10 17 10	Consultant	Indwelling for 17 days average 'Scalp, long', Saph V and ACV
Carrera *et al.* (1987)[53]	PV	Fine-bore silicone catheters, various veins			Neonates	555 (?100)	Infection Dislodgement Extravasation Occlusion Thrombosis Pulm. oedema	0.2 18 16 10 0.7 0.5	?	Electively used for mean of 16 days
Klein & Shahrivar (1992)[54]	PV	Percutaneous			Approx. 1000 g	34/35	Bacteraemia (MRSA)	12		2/4 cases cured without catheter removal
Neubauer (1995)[8]	PV	Catheter-through-needle	Both		Neonates	340/535 (1st attempt)	Sepsis (1 kg) Sepsis (1 kg) Thrombosis Myocardial perforation	6.9 3.1 1.0 0.4		ECG guidance for 273 cases, very effective
Soong *et al.* (1995)[55]	PV	Percutaneous			Neonates	1218/1318	Probable catheter sepsis	2.7		Small, medium and large catheters equally successful
Valk *et al.* (1995)[19]	PV	Percutaneous, Seldinger BasV CephV AxV SaphV Scalp	Mostly R		'Newborns'	130/138 78/81 25/28 9/9 16/17 2/3	Obstruction Thrombophlebitis Thrombosis Perforation Catheter related sepsis	3.8 20 0.8 1.5 0.8	? Authors	Viggo Hydrocath 22 gauge, 10 cm or 20 gauge, 20 cm via 24 gauge Insyte BD cannula 8 days average usage
Ochikubo *et al.* (1996)[20]	PV	Percutaneous			28 wk	1 case report	Embolised catheter fragment (5.5 cm)			Removed by transvenous technique
Luyt *et al.* (1996)[27]	PV	Percutaneous			12 yr	241/273	Minor bleeding Pneumothorax	23 1.24		All serious complications were in

						Tachyarrhythmia	0.83		subclavian route group
						Major bleed	0.83		
						Catheter tip infection	51		Femoral route safest
						Septicaemia	5.7		
Rastogi *et al.* (1998)[56]	PV	Percutaneous PICC		Infants	186/187	Malpositioned tip	3.7		All self-corrected in time
Lussky *et al.* (1997)[3]	SaphV	Percutaneous		Neonates	2 case reports	Tips in ascending lumbar vein	2	cases	
Ohki *et al.* (1997)[57]	SaphV	Percutaneous		Neonates	46/46	Blockage	37		Catheter tip moves with leg flexion
						Oedema of leg	6		
						Catheter breakage	4		Best sited between T9 and L3
Eichelberger *et al.* (1981)[58]	SubCV	Infraclavicular using deltopectoral groove	20		191/?	Clotted line	4.7		Success not stated
						SVC thrombus	1		
						Migration & pleural Effusion	1.6		
						Arm swelling	1.6		
						Sepsis	31		
Scherer *et al.* (1981)[59]	SubCV	All cases with ***Staph. epidermidis*** septicaemia		2 wk–15 yr		Infected catheters	35.0		Review for cause of septicaemia
Stellato *et al.* (1985)[60]	SubCV	Percutaneous Broviac for thrombocytopenia		1 mo–16 yr	5/5(100)	Arterial puncture	8.0	?	5 children in series of 199
						Haematoma	2.7		
Pollack *et al.* (1980)[61]	FV (6) IJV (5) ACV (8)	PA balloon catheter at bedside without fluoroscopy		2d–19yr	22/22 (100) (6/22 cut-down)	Pneumothorax (IJV)	4.5	Supervised by consultants	PA, 4-lumen Swan –Ganz catheter 5–7 F
						Bleeding (FV)	4.5		
						BP down at PAWP	4.5		
Ziegler *et al.* (1980)[62]	SubCV IJV EJV	Infraclavicular		Neonates and children	SubCV 118/? IJV, EJV 82/?	Pleural effusion	2.5	Consultants and trainees	Using Filston's technique
						Central v. thrombosis	1		
						Catheter sepsis	10.5		
Dolcourt Bose (1982)[63]	BasiV or EJV	Silicone catheter-through-needle		27–35 wk gestation	15/17	Accidental removal	20	Authors	No infection observed
						$Ca_3 (PO_4)_2$ blockage	7		
Kanter *et al.* (1986)[39]	FV	All percutaneous		Paediatric	44/?	Leg swelling	7.0		Review of 161 catheters indwelling 1–15 days (median 3 days)
						Transient cyanosis	5.0		
						Cellulitis	1.0		
	SCV	Infraclavicular			37/?	Sepsis	3.0		
	IJV				48/?	None/48	0.0		
	EJV				4/?	None/4	0.0		
	ACV	Percutaneous and cut-down			23/?	Arm, neck swelling	9.0		
						Sepsis	4.0		
						Bleeding	4.0		
Newman *et al.* (1986)[64]	IJV SCV FV	XRO polyethylene catheters used in a comparison of central and peripheral venous lines for access		1 d–17 yr	77/83 (93)	Arterial puncture	3.0	Senior staff	Percutaneous technique
						Catheter slippage	5.0		
						Poor flow	3.0		
	PV	PVs all cut-down techniques			40/49 (82)	Poor flow	65.0	Senior staff	Cut-down technique
						Infiltration	37.5		
						Phlebitis	27.5		

Table 15.1 *Continued*

Authors and year	Vein	Technique, insertion point	Side	Distance between skin and vein (mm)	Age range	Successes/ patients (%)	Complications		Personnel	Comments
							Type	Incidence		
Shulman *et al.* (1986)[65]	PV	Floated silicone catheter from ACV			Neonates	29/29 (100)	Displacement	17	? Consultants only	0.635 mm OD 0.305 mm ID float catheter
							Malposition	7		
							Block (clotted)	14		
							Block (precip.)	7		
							Brachial V thrombosis	4		
	JV	Cut-down technique with 4–5 cm tunnel				25/25 (100)	Displacement	12		16 gauge silicone catheter
							Difficult removal	7		
							Blocked (clotted)	4		
							Blocked (precip.)	0		
							SVC syndrome	4		
Wallace & Zeltzer (1987)[66]	CFV JV	Cut-down insertion of implanted ports			5 mo–16 yr	?100%	Positive blood culture	6.5	Surgeon	Catheters survived 163 149 days
							Extravasation	6.5		
							Spontaneous extrusion	3.2		
Stenzel *et al.* (1989)[31]	FV	Percutaneous, Seldinger			<18 mo	92/?	Infectious	5.4	All specialists	
							Thrombosis	2.2		
					1.5–6 yr	48/?	Infectious	2.1		
							Thrombosis and	4.2		
	Non-FV	Various					embolism	0		
					>6 yr	22/?	Infectious	0		
							Non-infectious	8.6		
					<18 mo	116/?	Infectious	0		
							Non-infectious	6.5		
					1.5–6 yr	46/?	Infectious	2.1		
							Perforation	4.3		
							Bleeding	8.7		
					<6 yr	71/?	Infectious	1.4		
							Thrombosis			
Mirro *et al.* (1990)[67]	CV	(a) Percutaneous, Seldinger			'Children'	69/70 (99)	Pneumothorax Migration	1.5	Specialist	Ports best for long term
		(b) Surgical via CephV				195/196 (99)		0.35	"	Catheter:
		(c) Implanted port device				92/93 (99)	–	0	Specialists	percutaneous less problems than surgery
Mecrow & Ladusans (1994)[68]	Various	Percutaneous and surgical	Both		Infants	Case reports	12 cases of vegetations at SVC-RA junction			All had positive blood cultures
Nosher *et al.* (1994)[69]	Mostly SubCV	Percutaneous in X ray dept.	Both	7 mo–14 yr	X-ray: 16/18 (89)	Removed for technical failure or infection		38		Authors claim results
		Percutaneous and cut-down in theatre			Theatre: 27/35 (77)	Removed for technical failure or infection		63		in X-ray 'safe'

Malmgren *et al*. (1995)[70]	Trans. lumbar	Percutaneous	Infants and small children	12/12 (100)	None		Catheters lasted 4.8 (1–10) mo
Morimoto *et al*. (1993)[15]		Percutaneous	Child	2 case reports	Difficulty in removing catheter		Surgery and urokinase required
Sasidharan *et al*. (1996)[10]	–	Percutaneous	<1000 kg	1 case report	Cardiac arrest		Myocardial infiltration with hyperalimentation lipid
Sterniste *et al*. (1994)[71]	Various	Peripheral percutaneous	Neonate	114/114 (100)	Catheter-related infection	3.5	
					Serious complications	0	
Warner *et al*. (1996)[72]	–	Groshong catheters	Children	10/10 (100)	Catheters removed	5/10	Groshong catheters unsuitable for paediatric use
					Catheters needing daily flush	'Several'	
		Hickman catheters			Catheter removed	0/10	
Weiner *et al* (1992)[73]	Various	Cut-down 67% Percutaneous 33%	Children	822	Removal for complications	39	Multi-centre prospective study of Childrens' Cancer Study Group. EJV 33%, IJV 22%, SubCV 35%, Ceph-V 7%, SaphV 3%
					Infection (various centres)	8.5–31	
					Dislodgement (various centres)	2.8–24	
					Occlusion (various centres)	0–13	

ACV, antecubital vein; AxA, axillary artery; AxV, axillary vein; BasV, basilic vein; BP, blood pressure; CephV, cephalic vein; CFV, common facial vein; ECG, electrocardiographic; ECLS, extracorporeal life support; EJV, external jugular vein; FV, femoral vein; ID, inner diameter; IJV, internal jugular vein; IVC, inferior vena cava; JV, jugular vein; L, left; MRSA, methicillin-resistant ***Staphylococcus aureus***; OD, outer diameter; PA, pulmonary artery; PAWP, pulmonary artery wedge pressure; PICC, peripherally inserted central catheter; PTFE, polytetra fluoroethylene (Teflon); PV, peripheral vein; RA, right atrium; SaphV, saphenous vein; SubCV, subclavian vein; SVC, superior vena cava; TempV, temporal vein; Trend., Trendelenburg position; US, ultrasound.

References

1. Mehta Y, Bhavani SS, Sharma KK. A difficult cannulation of the right internal jugular vein [letter]. Anaesthesia 1990; **45**:1087.
2. Watson D, Simpson JC. Yet another hazard of percutaneous central venous cannulation [letter]. Anesthesiology 1984; **60**:524.
3. Lussky RC, Trower N, Fisher D, Engel R, Cifuentes R. Unusual misplacement sites of percutaneous central venous lines in the very low birth weight neonate. American Journal of Perinatology 1997; **14**(2):63.
4. Scharf J, Rey M, Schmiedl N, Stehr K. Pericardial tamponade as a complication of the use of peripheral percutaneous silastic catheters. Klinische Padiatrie 1990; **202**(1):57.
5. Mupanemunda RH, Mackanjee HR. A life-threatening complication of percutaneous central venous catheters in neonates [letter]. American Journal of Diseases of Children 1992; **146**(12):1414.
6. Beattie PG, Kuschel CA, Harding JE. Pericardial effusion complicating a percutaneous central venous line in a neonate. Acta Paediatrica 1993; **82**(1):105.
7. Wirrell EC, Pelausa EO, Allen AC, Stinson DA, Hanna BD. Massive pericardial effusion as a cause for sudden deterioration of a very low birthweight infant. American Journal of Perinatology 1993; **10**(6):419.
8. Neubauer AP. Percutaneous central i.v. access in the neonate: experience with 535 silastic catheters. Acta Paediatrica 1995; **84**(7):756.
9. Fioravanti J, Buzzard CJ, Harris JP. Pericardial effusion and tamponade as a result of percutaneous silastic catheter use. Neonatal Network 1998; **17**(5):39.
10. Sasidharan P, Billman D, Heimler R, Nelin L. Cardiac arrest in an extremely low birth weight infant: complication of percutaneous central venous catheter hyperalimentation. Journal of Perinatology 1996; **16**(2 Pt 1):123.
11. Chatel-Meijer MP, Roques-Gineste M, Fries F, Bloom MC, Laborie S, Lelong-Tissier MC, Regnier C. Cardiac tamponade secondary to umbilical venous catheterization accident in a premature infant. Archives Francaises de Pediatrie 1992; **49**(4):373.
12. Levkoff AH, Macpherson RI. Intrahepatic encystment of umbilical vein catheter infusate. Pediatric Radiology 1990; **20**(5):360.
13. Bautista AB, Ko SH, Sun SC. Retention of percutaneous venous catheter in the newborn: a report of three cases. American Journal of Perinatology 1995; **12**(1):53.
14. Gladman G, Sinha S, Sims DG, Chiswick ML. Staphylococcus epidermidis and retention of neonatal percutaneous central venous catheters. Archives of Disease in Childhood 1990; **65**(2):234.
15. Morimoto T, Hosoya R, Matsufuji H, Tachi M, Yokoyama J, Nishimura K. Difficulty in removing a percutaneous central venous catheter inserted from a peripheral vein. Acta Paediatrica Japonica 1993; **35**(4):352.
16. Carrera G, Liberatore A, Villa G, Riboni G. Pulmonary edema. A rare complication of the percutaneous insertion of silastic central venous catheters. Minerva Pediatrica 1989; **41**(10):521.
17. Nakamura KT, Sato Y, Erenberg A. Evaluation of a percutaneously placed 27-gauge central venous catheter in neonates weighing less than 1200 gram. Journal of Parenteral and Enteral Nutrition 1990; **14**(3):295.
18. Rudin C, Nars PW. A comparative study of two different percutaneous venous catheters in newborn infants. European Journal of Pediatrics 1990; **150**(2):119.
19. Valk WJ, Liem KD, Geven WB. Seldinger technique as an alternative approach for percutaneous insertion of hydrophilic polyurethane central venous catheters in newborns. Journal of Parenteral and Enteral Nutrition 1995; **19**(2):151.
20. Ochikubo CG, O'Brien LA, Kanakriyeh M, Waffarn F. Silicone-rubber catheter fracture and embolization in a very low birth weight infant. Journal of Perinatology 1996; **16**(1):50.
21. Nicolson SC, Sweeney MF, Moore RA, Jobes DR. Comparison of internal and external jugular cannulation of the central circulation in the pediatric patient. Critical Care Medicine 1985; **13**:747.
22. Belani KG, Buckley JJ, Gordon JR, Castaneda W. Percutaneous cervical central vein placement: a comparison of the internal and external jugular vein routes. Anesthesia and Analgesia Current Researches 1980; **5940-4**:40.
23. Cot CJ, Jobes DR, Schwartz AJ, Ellison N. Two approaches to the cannulation of a child's internal jugular vein. Anesthesiology 1979; **50**:371.
24. Morgan WW, Harkins GA. Percutaneous introduction of long-term in dwelling venous catheters in infants. Journal of Pediatric Surgery 1972; **7**:538.
25. Postel JP, Quintard JM, Ricard J, Delaplace R, Bernard F, Canarelli JP. Development of a safe technique for central venous access in pediatrics. Our experience with 700 percutaneous central catheters. Chirurgie Pediatrique 1990; **31**(4–5):219.
26. Casado-Flores J, Valdivielso-Serna A, Perez-Jurado L *et al.* Subclavian vein catheterization in critically ill children: analysis of 322 cannulations. Intensive Care Medicine 1991; **17**(6):350.
27. Luyt DK, Mathivha LR, Litmanovitch M, Dance MD, Brown JM. Confirmation of the safety of central venous catheterisation in critically ill infants and children – the Baragwanath experience. South African Medical Journal 1996; **86**(5 suppl.):603.
28. Chung DH, Ziegler MM. Central venous catheter access. Nutrition 1998; **14**(1):119.
29. Marty F, Truong P. Clavicular periostitis: an unusual complication of percutaneous subclavian venous catheterization. Radiology 1983; **64**:139.
30. Serrao PR, Jean-Louis J, Godoy J, Prado A. Inferior vena cava catheterization in the neonate by the percutaneous femoral vein method. Journal of Perinatology 1996; **16**(2 Pt 1):129.

31. Stenzel JP, Green TP, Fuhrman JB, Carlson PE, Marchessault RP. Percutaneous femoral venous catheterisations: a prospective study of complications. Journal of Pediatrics 1989; **114**:411.
32. Pieters PC, Dittrich J, Prasad U, Berman W. Acute Budd–Chiari syndrome caused by percutaneous placement of a transhepatic inferior vena cava catheter. Journal of Vascular and Interventional Radiology 1997; **8**(4):587.
33. Oriot D, Defawe G. Percutaneous catheterisation of the axillary vein in neonates. Critical Care Medicine 1988; **16**:285.
34. Metz RI, Lucking SE, Chaten FC, Williams TM, Mickell JJ. Percutaneous catheterization of the axillary vein in infants and children. Pediatrics 1990; **85**:531.
35. Taylor BL, Yellowlees I. Central venous cannulation using the infraclavicular axillary vein. Anesthesiology 1990; **72**:55.
36. Krul EJ, van Leeuwen EF, Vos A, Voute PA. Continuous venous access in children for long-term chemotherapy by means of an implantable system. Journal of Pediatric Surgery 1986; **21**:689.
37. Khilnani P, Toce S, Reddy R. Mechanical complications from very small percutaneous central venous Silastic catheters. Critical Care Medicine 1990; **18**(12):1477.
38. Hohn AR, Lambert EC. Continuous venous catheterisation in children. Journal of the American Medical Association 1966; **197**:658.
39. Kanter RK, Zimmerman JJ, Strauss RH, Stoeckel KA. Central venous catheter insertion by femoral vein: safety and effectiveness for the pediatric patient. Pediatrics 1986; **77**:842.
40. Talbott GA, Winters WD, Bratton SL, O'Rourke PP. A prospective study of femoral catheter-related thrombosis in children. Archives of Pediatrics & Adolescent Medicine 1995; **149**(3):288.
41. English ICW, Frew RM, Piggott JF. Percutaneous catheterisation of the internal jugular vein. Anaesthesia 1969; **24**:521.
42. Prince SR, Sullivan RL, Hackel A. Percutaneous catheterisation of the internal jugular vein in infants and children. Anesthesiology 1976; **44**:170.
43. Hall DM, Geefhuysen J. Percutaneous catheterisation of the internal jugular vein in infants and children. Journal of Pediatric Surgery 1977; **12**:719.
44. Rao TL, Wong AY, Salem MR. A new approach to the percutaneous catheterisation of the internal jugular vein. Anesthesiology 1977; **46**:362.
45. Korshin J, Klauber PV, Christensen V, Skorsted P. Percutaneous catheterisation of the internal jugular vein. Acta Anaesthesiologica Scandinavica, Supplementum 1978; **1978**:27.
46. Coté CJ, Jobes DR, Schwartz AJ, Ellison N. Two approaches to the cannulation of a child's internal jugular vein. Anesthesiology 1979; **50**:371.
47. Krausz MM, Berlatzky Y, Ayalon A, Freund H, Schiller M. Percutaneous cannulation of the internal jugular vein in infants and children. Surgery, Gynecology and Obstetrics 1979; **148**:591.
48. Damen J, Wever JEAT. The use of balloon tipped pulmonary artery catheters in children undergoing cardiac surgery. Intensive Care Medicine 1987; **13**:266.
49. Reickert CA, Schreiner RJ, Bartlett RH, Hirschl RB. Percutaneous access for venovenous extracorporeal life support in neonates. Journal of Pediatric Surgery 1998; **33**(2):365.
50. Evans JR, Allen AC, Stinson DA. Percutaneous insertion of central venous catheters (letter). Pediatrics 1983; **71**:668.
51. Durand M, Ramanathan R, Martinelli B, Tollentino M. Prospective evaluation of percutaneous central venous silastic catheters in newborn infants with birth weights of 510 to 3920 g. Pediatrics 1986; **78**:245.
52. Puntis JW. Percutaneous insertion of central venous feeding catheters. Archives of Disease in Childhood 1986; **61**:1138.
53. Carrera G, Coccia C, Coppalini B, Liberatore A, Minoli I. Percutaneous central venous silastic catheters in newborn infants. Pediatrics 1987; **79**:837.
54. Klein JF, Shahrivar F. Use of percutaneous silastic central venous catheters in neonates and the management of infectious complications. American Journal of Perinatology 1992; **9**(4):261.
55. Soong WJ, Jeng MJ, Hwang B. The evaluation of percutaneous central venous catheters – a convenient technique in pediatric patients. Intensive Care Medicine 1995; **21**(9):759.
56. Rastogi S, Bhutada A, Sahni R, Berdon WE, Wung JT. Spontaneous correction of the malpositioned percutaneous central venous line in infants. Pediatric Radiology 1998; **28**(9):694.
57. Ohki Y, Nako Y, Morikawa A, Maruyama K, Koizumi T. Percutaneous central venous catheterization via the great saphenous vein in neonates. Acta Paediatrica Japonica 1997; **39**(3):312.
58. Eichelberger MR, Rous PG, Hoelzer DJ, Garcia VF, Koop CE. Percutaneous, subclavian venous catheters in neonates and children. Journal of Pediatric Surgery (Supplement 1) 1981; **16**:547.
59. Scherer LR, West KW, Weber TR, Teiman M, Grosfeld JL. *Staphylococcus epidermidis* in pediatric patients: clinical and therapeutic considerations. Journal of Pediatric Surgery 1984; **19**:358.
60. Stellato TA, Gauderer MW, Lazarus HM, Herzig RH. Percutaneous silastic catheter insertion in patients with thrombocytopenia. Cancer 1985; **56**:2691.
61. Pollack MM, Reed TP, Holbrook PR, Fields AI. Bedside pulmonary artery catheterization in pediatrics. Journal of Pediatrics 1980; **96**:274.
62. Ziegler M, Jakobowski D, Hoelzer D, Eichenberger M, Koop CE. Route of pediatric parenteral nutrition: proposed criteria revision. Journal of Pediatric Surgery 1980; **15**:472.
63. Dolcourt JL, Bose CL. Percutaneous insertion of silastic central venous catheters in newborn infants. Pediatrics 1982; **70**:484.
64. Newman BM, Jewett TC Jr, Karp MP, Cooney DR. Percutaneous central venous catheterisation in children: first line choice for venous access. Journal of Pediatric Surgery 1986; **21**:685.

65. Schulman RJ, Pokorny WJ, Martin CG, Petitt R, Baldaia L, Roney D. Comparison of percutaneous and surgical placement of central venous catheters in neonates. Journal of Pediatric Surgery 1986; **21**:348.
66. Wallace J, Zelter PM. Benefits, complications and care of implantable diffusion devices in 31 children with cancer. Journal of Pediatric Surgery 1987; **22**:833.
67. Mirro J, Rao BN, Kumar M, Rafferty M, Hancock M, Austin BA, Fairclough D, Lobe TE. A comparison of placement techniques and complications of externalized catheters and implantable parts used in children with cancer. Journal of Pediatric Surgery 1990; **25**:120.
68. Mecrow IK, Ladusans EJ. Infective endocarditis in newborn infants with structurally normal hearts. Acta Paediatrica 1994; **83**(1):35.
69. Nosher JL, Shami MM, Siegel RL, DeCandia M, Bodner LJ. Tunneled central venous access catheter placement in the pediatric population: comparison of radiologic and surgical results. Radiology 1994; **192**(1):265.
70. Malmgren N, Cwikiel W, Hochbergs P, Sandstrom S, Mikaelsson C, Westbacke G. Percutaneous translumbar central venous catheter in infants and small children. Pediatric Radiology 1995; **25**(1):28.
71. Sterniste W, Vavrik K, Lischka A, Sacher M. Effectiveness and complications of percutaneous central venous catheters in neonatal intensive care. Padiatrie 1994; **206**(1):18.
72. Warner BW, Haygood MM, Davies SL, Hennies GA. A randomized, prospective trial of standard Hickman compared with Groshong central venous catheters in pediatric oncology patients. Journal of the American College of Surgeons 1996; **183**(2):140.
73. Wiener ES, McGuire P, Stolar CJ. *et al.* The CCSG prospective study of venous access devices: an analysis of insertions and causes for removal. Journal of Pediatric Surgery 1992; **27**(2):155; discussion 63.

Part 3

Arterial Catheterisation: General considerations and adult procedures

16 • Introduction to Arterial Cannulation

BRIAN JENKINS

Indications

The main indications for arterial cannulation are blood pressure measurement, arterial blood sampling and radiological procedures. Under some circumstances the displayed form of the arterial pressure wave itself may be useful diagnostically, although it is seldom used in isolation. In recent years, improvements in technology have led to the development of continuous intra-arterial blood gas monitors so that near-instantaneous measurement of pH, Pao_2 and $Paco_2$ is now possible.

Arterial cannulation may be associated with complications that could result in severe injury, or even death in some cases. In most circumstances, therefore, informed consent should be obtained from either the patient or a close relative prior to the procedure. However, in many cases, particularly in critical care, arterial cannulation may have to be performed as an urgent procedure when the patient's life is at risk, and there may be no opportunity for formal consent procedures beforehand. Under these circumstances, implied consent is assumed because the procedure is regarded as necessary for the continued well-being of the patient. Arterial cannulation is now a common procedure. It has been estimated that 8 million arterial cannulations for blood pressure measurement are made every year.[1]

Blood pressure measurement

Non-invasive methods of blood pressure rely on a variety of methods to infer blood pressure within an artery. Most have an external cuff that is fitted around the arm in order to occlude the arterial blood flow intermittently. Manual methods involve listening over the artery with a stethoscope for sounds associated with blood flow as the pressure is released in the occluding cuff, or by palpating a distal artery for return of the pulse. At this point, the cuff pressure gives an indication of systolic arterial blood pressure. Diastolic pressures are typically more difficult to measure by indirect methods. Automatic devices commonly measure pressure fluctuations within the cuff as the pressure is released. Because of this reliance on an occluding cuff, measurement may be difficult in obese patients, small children or where the size of the cuff is inappropriate to the size of the arm.

Indirect blood pressure measurement infers arterial pressure from blood flow under the occluding cuff, and may be unable to estimate blood pressure adequately in situations of reduced blood flow to the extremities. Direct pressure monitoring simply measures the pressure in the artery, and is capable of accurately measuring pressure even where there is no flow at all.

Most non-invasive methods of blood pressure measurement are intermittent, while direct methods are capable of beat-to-beat measurement of pressure. Intermittent measurements are adequate in most circumstances, but if rapid changes in blood pressure are anticipated, continuous direct blood pressure measurement will usually be preferable.

Non-invasive methods are prone to error from mechanical interference, which may be a problem in operating theatres where surgeons or other personnel intermittently press on the occluding cuff, producing an error message instead of a blood pressure measurement. In these circumstances, there is a danger of misinterpreting an error message as mechanical interference, when it is actually due to a rapid change in blood pressure or a fall in blood pressure to a level at which it cannot be accurately estimated.

Many of the problems of non-invasive methods are overcome by the use of direct blood pressure monitoring. This is useful in the management of severe hypertension, hypotension and shock, and when vasoactive drugs are being administered. It is also useful in surgical procedures where rapid changes in blood pressure and/or cardiac output occur, especially where deliberate manipulation of these parameters is required. In extremely obese patients, accurate blood pressure measurement may only be possible with direct blood pressure monitoring.

Direct blood pressure monitoring is associated with practical problems that vary according to the method of measurement and display. Accurate measurement of blood pressure depends on the correct assembly of apparatus, which includes saline-filled, non-distensible plastic tubing, connected at one end to the arterial cannula and at the other to a transducer or other pressure measuring device. The pressure measurement device needs to be zeroed and calibrated. If measurements are made for more than a short period, the tubing needs to be continuously flushed and pressurised in order to prevent back-flow of blood and thrombus formation within the cannula. Continuous flushing also has the effect of reducing the incidence of complications associated with intermittent flushing such as embolization of thrombus or air. Most continuous flushing systems use a fixed orifice device and a pressurised bag of fluid to consistently deliver 2–4 ml per hour at a bag pressure at 300 mmHg. The flushing solution is usually normal saline that is heparinised in order to prolong the life of the catheter and to reduce the incidence of thrombosis.[2] The high resistance of the fixed orifice 'isolates' the pressurised solution from the measurement system, thus reducing the likelihood of pressure measurement errors. Errors in pressure measurement associated with these systems are clinically insignificant.[3] In small children, the volume of fluid delivered by fixed orifice systems may be excessive in relation to the body weight. In order to overcome this problem, syringe drivers may be used as an alternative.

The resonance frequency of the manometer tubing is also important in the accurate measurement of blood pressure. It is related to the length and rigidity of the manometer tubing; the shorter and more rigid the tube, the more accurately the pressure wave will be transmitted to the measurement device. However, in some circumstances the pressure wave may hyperresonate, exaggerating the measured systolic blood pressure. In many circumstances, transmission characteristics may be improved by the use of damping devices to modify resonance frequency in a controlled way.[4]

Transducers are the most commonly used pressure measurement devices, but other simpler devices (e.g. aneroid systems) have also been described. However, with the introduction of cheap, high-performance, low-maintenance, portable transducer systems the use of alternative devices has declined.

Transducer systems

Transducer systems consist of the transducer itself, a device that processes and displays the signal, and in most cases another system to intermittently store blood pressure values for retrospective display and analysis. The system may have an internal battery to store information when the mains supply is discontinued. The transducer converts a fluctuating pressure into either an analogue or a digital electrical signal. This signal is then usually processed by a dedicated microprocessor system and the result displayed on a monitor. Calibration is usually automatic, and zeroing the pressure trace is achieved by opening the system to air at the level of the heart and then simply pressing a button.

In recent years, these systems have achieved a high degree of reliability. The transducer unit itself is now commonly disposable and is also available in combined units in order to measure blood pressure, central venous pressure and pulmonary artery pressures simultaneously. Standards adopted by the American National Standards Institute (ANSI) have helped to enable interchangeability of components between manufacturers.

Liquid manometers

Simple liquid manometer systems were first used to measure human blood pressure by Faivre in 1856. They may be useful as a quick and simple method of estimating direct blood pressure during transfer of a patient between intensive care and theatre. Because of the magnitude of blood pressure, an open limb full of liquid is usually impractical, so that one end of the manometer tubing is closed with the other in direct contact with the arterial blood. The blood pressure may then be displayed and measured by the oscillation of a heparinised blood/air interface or a heparinised blood/saline interface against a scale.[5,6] The scale may be calibrated by a transducer system prior to transfer, and discarded when reconnected to a more accurate system.

These types of liquid manometers have limited accuracy, but may be useful when intermittent measurements of non-invasive blood pressure are impractical because of patient movement, or when battery-powered transducer systems are unavailable.

Aneroid manometers

The use of aneroid manometers to continuously measure direct arterial pressure was initially proposed by Severinghaus.[7] They have since been used by many authors for blood pressure measurement during major surgery.[8–10] A column of heparinised saline in contact with the arterial blood may be used to transmit the arterial pressure wave from the arterial blood. Flickering of the needle on the gauge indicates blood pressure changes between systolic and diastolic. With the exception of cardiopulmonary bypass machines, aneroid manometers are now rarely used for direct blood pressure measurement.

Inaccuracies

Inaccuracies that occur during direct blood pressure measurement may be classified into local reasons at the site of cannulation, problems with pressure wave conduction in the saline-filled tubing, and problems with pressure wave measurement.

Local causes

Local causes of inaccuracy include intra-arterial or intracannular thrombus, stenosis or occlusion of the artery proximal to the measurement site, kinking of the cannula, abutment of the cannula against the vessel wall, and changes in vascular tone. These usually result in damping of the transmitted waveform.

Following insertion, the tip of the cannula may abut against the vessel wall or an atheromatous plaque, decreasing the frequency response of the transmitted waveform. If the cannula completely occludes the artery, the pressure wave becomes reflected on the tip of the cannula, changing the appearance of the pressure waveform by augmenting the high-frequency components and artificially elevating the measured blood pressure.

Cannulae that have become kinked may sometimes be salvaged by partial withdrawal and reinsertion, using a guide-wire if necessary, or by rotating the cannula along its axis through 180°. A change in position of the insertion point may also be helpful, especially in distal arterial punctures such as the radial and dorsalis pedis arteries. However, with all these manoeuvres there is the potential for an increased incidence of infection of the cannula site when the dressing is removed and the cannula moved in relation to the skin, risking bacterial migration along the tract of the cannula. Thrombus that has built up on the outside of the cannula may be dislodged.

Intra-arterial and intracannular thrombus can sometimes be removed by aspirating and discarding a small amount of arterial blood via a three-way tap positioned close to the cannula. If this does not work, flushing the cannula or attempting to pass a guide-wire may result in embolisation of thrombus, and should not be attempted. Other problems of this nature are best resolved by removing the cannula and using another artery. Kinking of the cannula can sometimes be corrected by repositioning the cannula in relation to the skin, cleaning the surrounding area and fixing the cannula in a more favourable position. However, in most cases this is only a temporary solution. Once the cannula has become kinked, the lumen is permanently narrowed and is more likely to occlude owing to repeated bending of the cannula at this weak point, or through the accumulation of thrombus.

Pressure wave conduction

If air is present in the manometer tubing or the measurement chamber of the transducer, the pressure waveform detected by the transducer will become severely damped, and if enough air is present, the tubing may not be able to transmit pressure waves at all. As well as causing problems with measurement, the presence of air represents a potentially fatal hazard if it is inadvertently flushed through the cannula into the arterial system and by retrograde flow reaches arteries that perfuse the brain.

If the connecting tubing is not made of a sufficiently rigid material, or if the tubing is excessively long, damping of the waveform may again result. Small leaks in the conduction system also cause damping and a decrease in the quality of the transmitted waveform.

Measurement

Problems in measurement may occur because of miscalibration, failure to establish a satisfactory zero point or changes in patient position following zeroing. Other inaccuracies may occur as a result of problems in the method of measurement, such as changes in the tension of a disposable transducer diaphragm producing artefactual hypotension.[11]

Whatever the cause of inaccuracy, miscalculation of the blood pressure may lead to inappropriate and potentially lethal treatment.[12,13] If the blood pressure measured using an arterial cannula does not correlate with clinical signs or with blood pressure measured by other means, causes of inaccuracy should be sought immediately.

Radial artery pressures, and to a lesser extent brachial artery pressures, are known to overestimate systolic blood pressure compared with direct aortic measurement, but immediately following cardiopulmonary bypass the reverse situation occurs, with peripheral arterial measurement underestimating ‘true’ central aortic pressure by approximately 1–5%. This may be related to a decrease in vascular resistance in the hand following bypass.[14] The relationship between central and peripheral arterial pressures may change with changes in peripheral blood flow and systemic vascular resistance (see later).

Blood sampling

Frequent arterial blood sampling is another indication for arterial cannulation. During surgery and in critical care management, arterial blood can be obtained rapidly without the complications associated with multiple skin punctures. The sampling port may be remote from the puncture site, allowing convenient access even though the cannulation site itself may be inaccessible.

Blood gas sampling is one of the most common tests performed, giving direct measurement of Pao_2 and acid–base status, and being particularly useful in intensive care and thoracic surgery. In recent years, the need for these intermittent measurements has decreased with the greater availability and improved accuracy of continuous, non-invasive devices such as pulse oximeters and capnographs. Technological advances have also resulted in the development of intra-arterial probes capable of continously measuring pH and Pao_2.[15] These are likely to become cheaper and more widely available, and in the future may replace intermittent sampling of blood, at least for some parameters.

Diagnosis

The displayed arterial waveform may in itself be a useful diagnostic tool. Waveforms transmitted from the ascending aorta are thought to be the most useful diagnostically, as they most accurately reflect pressure changes close to the heart. The slope of the upstroke correlates with myocardial contractility, although it may also correlate with an increase in systemic vascular resistance.[16] When the arterial waveform shows large respiratory variation and a narrowed pulse pressure, hypovolaemia may be a cause.[17] If arrhythmias occur, the cardiovascular consequences can be immediately assessed, and appropriate measures taken.

The appearance of the arterial waveform arises from an interaction between the kinetic energy of flowing blood and the vessel walls, and differs according to the size and compliance of the transmitting artery. As the pressure wave is transmitted from the aorta to distal arteries, high-frequency components such as the anacrotic and dicrotic notches are filtered out, causing a change in the appearance of the waveform. Other changes are thought to be due to reflection of the waveform, resonance within distal arteries and changes in compliance between central and peripheral arteries.[18,19] The further away from the aorta, the greater the transmission delay, and the narrower and taller the waveform becomes. As arteries become smaller, the component of the waveform that is due to reflection becomes more prominent. In cases of peripheral vasodilatation, the waveform passes more distally and this component is reduced.

There is also a change in the measured blood pressure; the systolic pressure is increased and the diastolic pressure decreased in peripheral arteries, although the mean blood pressure is unchanged in most circumstances. In the dorsalis pedis artery, measured systolic blood pressure is 10–20 mmHg higher and measured diastolic blood pressure 10–20 mmHg lower than that in the aorta.[20]

The presence of a cannula in a peripheral artery invariably results in some degree of narrowing which is exacerbated by the presence of thrombus, and this in itself may result in an altered waveform and a change in the magnitude of the measured blood pressure.

Radiological procedures

Cannulation of arteries is required for many radiographic diagnostic and therapeutic procedures, including coronary artery angioplasty, arteriography and embolectomy. In most procedures, a relatively large cannula is introduced for a short time.

Choosing an artery

Several factors should be considered in choosing an artery that is most suitable for the purpose intended. Some of the major considerations are listed below.

Dominant hand

In upper limb cannulation, it is common practice to avoid using the dominant hand and arm in order to minimise the risk of disability should serious complications occur.

Difficulty with fixation and patient movement

If an arterial puncture site overlies a joint it may be associated with particular complications due to movement of the cannula and the dressing. Movement at the cannulation site may cause kinking of the cannula, which may in turn result in dampening of the arterial pressure wave and inaccuracies in blood pressure measurement. Withdrawal of blood from the cannula may be difficult, and in some cases complete occlusion of the cannula lumen may occur, necessitating removal. Dressings are subject to shear forces, creating air space under the dressing and encouraging infection, particularly when the cannula is able to move in and out of the puncture site. This is more of a problem during long-term cannulation, such as in critical care, but may also be a problem during short-term cannulation for surgical procedures, especially when positioning the patient prior to surgery.

In critical care, the brachial and femoral sites may cause particular problems. Brachial cannulae are likely to kink during spontaneous patient movement, and enforcing full extension at the elbow by means of a splint is particularly difficult and uncomfortable for the patient over a prolonged period. Femoral arterial lines may be troublesome during periods of weaning from a ventilator, when the patient gradually assumes a more upright position in order to facilitate spontaneous ventilation. Repositioning of the cannula to a more suitable site may then be required.

Particular positions adopted during surgery may limit access to the arterial site or may compress the arterial circulation, resulting in a measured arterial pressure that is not reliable. This may not be a problem if the site is only being used for sampling. If a lateral position is adopted during surgery, either the upper limb should be used or particular care must be taken in order to avoid compression of the axillary and brachial arteries in the cannulated arm.

Adequacy of a collateral circulation

Cannulation sites with a good alternative blood supply are ideal, because if the cannulated artery becomes occluded by thrombus, the collateral circulation should then prevent ischaemic complications ensuing. Of course, this assumes that the collateral circulation is adequate to meet the metabolic needs of the perfused tissue. Wherever possible, the quality of the collateral circulation should be assessed prior to cannulation, and the results of the assessment documented. If it is assessed as inadequate, or if tests are equivocal, then it would be wise to choose an alternative site if possible. In larger arteries such as the femoral, the risk of complete occlusion occurring as a direct result of cannulation may be remote, although embolisation is still a risk. Prior to cannulation of a large artery, the presence of distal pulses should therefore be confirmed and documented.

Presence of local infection

If skin adjacent to the proposed puncture site is inflamed or infected, or if the site itself is thought to be more prone to infection, then another site should be used because of the risk of introducing infection into the artery during cannulation. Other complications related to the presence of infection such as thrombosis are also more likely.

Accuracy of recorded blood pressure

Large arteries are more likely to reflect 'true' arterial blood pressure than are peripheral arteries, although in most circumstances this will not make a difference to patient management. This may be a major consideration when blood pressure in small arteries is significantly different from that recorded in large arteries, as in situations of reduced peripheral circulation in shocked states and following bypass.

Patient pathology

A particular cannulation site may have disadvantages because of pathological abnormalities, or for other reasons connected with the type of surgery.

It is common practice to use two cannulation sites during cardiac surgery, one in the radial artery, one in the femoral. Blood pressure recorded from a large vessel such as the femoral artery may be more accurate than that from the radial artery during and after cardiac bypass, and the former is therefore used for blood pressure measurement. With the radial artery also cannulated, arterial blood may be aspirated without temporarily losing the blood pressure display. The second cannula also acts as a back-up in case of occlusion or displacement of the femoral cannula.

In pathological conditions of the thoracic aorta such as coarctation or dissecting aneurysm there may be large differences in the blood pressure measured in the upper and lower parts of the body, or between the left and right arms, depending on the location of the lesion. Measurement of direct blood pressure from two arteries that arise above and below the lesion gives valuable information about the blood pressure to the brain and lower body prior to and during surgical repair. In cases where the aorta is cross-clamped, blood pressure measurement in the femoral artery gives an indication of the adequacy of flow through a shunt, and may help to prevent postoperative complications because of lower body ischaemia.[21] Before operations of this type, the site of surgery needs to be carefully considered in order to place the arterial cannulae appropriately.

A patent ductus arteriosus may influence the oxygen content in sampled arterial blood. If the cannulated artery is distal to the ductus, the measured oxygen concentration will be lower than in the blood actually perfusing the brain. This may be of particular significance in neonates if the measured oxygen tension is misinterpreted as a safe level with which to perfuse the retinal vessels. Sampling of arterial blood from vessels proximal to the patent ductus would give a better estimate of oxygen tension in the blood perfusing the brain and retinal vessels.

Conditions that affect the patency and reactivity of small arteries such as Buerger's disease and Raynaud's disease are relative contraindications to small artery cannulation. In vascular surgery for complications of these conditions, cannulation of larger arteries may often be required in order to measure blood pressure, although it would seem wise to limit the duration of cannulation in order to minimize the risk from embolisation of thrombus.

Previous surgery

If a potential arterial site has undergone previous surgical treatment, especially if a synthetic graft has been used to repair an artery, this is an absolute contraindication to the use of that site. Arteriovenous fistulae that have been fashioned to facilitate renal dialysis may become thrombosed or infected from arterial cannulae on the same limb, so this is usually contraindicated.

Locating the artery

In most patients location of an artery by direct palpation will be easy, and attempts at subsequent cannulation will have an acceptable success rate. Difficulty with palpation may be experienced where an artery is deep to the skin, where the pulse volume is small, or where the artery itself is of small diameter or in spasm. These situations may coexist in many circumstances, for example in a child in hypovolaemic shock. Where difficulties exist, a technique using a localisation aid may be an alternative to – or an adjunct to – simple palpation of a pulse, and may be associated with higher success rates. Fluoroscopy has been used to guide femoral artery puncture,[22] but the most commonly used localisation aids are Doppler probes in adults and children, and transillumination in neonates and infants.

Doppler probes

Doppler probes are used to locate a point on the skin where auditory signals from the pulsating artery are maximal, corresponding to the midpoint of the artery. This method is useful where an artery is difficult to palpate owing to its depth or small size, and has been used extensively in children.[23,24]

During cannulation, the probe is held over the artery. When the cannula enters the artery, the Doppler tones become high-pitched or may disappear, thus reducing the need to rely on backflow into the needle hub in order to identify the arterial lumen. A statistically significant difference in success rate between use of Doppler location techniques and blind techniques has been noted in infants weighing less than 6 kg.[24] Doppler probes placed on a distal branch of an artery may also facilitate cannulation by detecting sound frequency changes as the needle penetrates the artery, and further changes due to blood-flow turbulence as a guide-wire is introduced. A technique has been described in which the Doppler probe was placed over the dorsalis pedis artery in order to facilitate femoral artery cannulation.[25]

Transillumination

Pearse has described the transillumination technique for radial artery cannulation in newborn babies.[26,27] In this group, profound difficulties may be experienced because of the small size of vessels such as the radial artery. A fibreoptic cold light source is used, with a funnel attachment both to hold the light source at a fixed distance from the skin and to increase the area transilluminated. During radial artery cannulation, the light source is positioned over the dorsal surface of the wrist while the wrist is held in dorsiflexion. The radial artery can then be identified as a pulsatile shadow over a bright background. Reducing the ambient light level prior to attempting cannulation may help visualisation. Pearse reported an 85% success rate for cannulation after some experience with the technique.[27]

Cannula insertion

Types of cannula

Arterial cannulae need to be hard enough to penetrate the skin without being damaged, and should also be made of a substance that is associated with a low incidence of thrombosis. They have been made from a variety of compounds, including polyvinyl chloride, polyethylene, polypropylene and polytetrafluoroethylene (PTFE, Teflon). Polypropylene and polyethylene cannulae have the strength to penetrate the skin without damage to the cannula tip, but are associated with a higher incidence of thrombosis than Teflon cannulae.[28–31] Teflon cannulae tend to be softer and more easily damaged during insertion, particularly with smaller-gauge cannulae, but have low thrombogenic potential when compared with other cannulae.[29,30,32–34]

Heparin bonding to cannulae may reduce the incidence of thrombosis in the short term[35] and may be useful for short procedures such as some radiographic studies, but after a few days in vivo the heparin leaches out and this advantage is lost. Following removal, a slightly longer compression time may be needed than with untreated cannulae. It is presumed that thrombus that has accumulated outside untreated cannulae during their time in the artery is stripped off and helps to plug the hole in the artery when it is removed.

From the perspective of blood pressure measurement, the larger the internal diameter of the cannula, and the larger the diameter and the shorter the length of the conducting tubing, the better. This will ensure that the frequency response of the system will be large enough to measure all components of the pressure waveform. However, as previously discussed, there is a risk of hyperresonance, which would exaggerate the measured blood pressure.

The external diameter of the cannula in relation to the size of the cannulated vessel influences the incidence of thrombosis, with large cannulae in small arteries being associated with the highest risk.[36] When an artery is cannulated for a prolonged period this may be a major consideration, perhaps favouring the use of larger arteries such as the femoral.[37] To optimise the transmitted pressure wave whilst minimising the external diameter of the cannula, non-tapered thin-walled cannulae are most commonly used, although their use may lead to an increased incidence of cannula damage during cannulation attempts. It is known that 20% of 20 gauge cannulae kink within 24 hours of insertion, resulting in deterioration of performance.[36]

There is thus a trade-off between the incidence of thrombotic complications, ease of insertion, and performance. Generally, a 20 gauge cannula is suitable for most adult arteries. If possible, a 22 gauge or smaller cannula should be used in children.

Transcutaneous techniques

Direct cannulation

In the direct cannulation technique, correct positioning of the cannula in the arterial lumen is confirmed by free flow of arterial blood through a needle that is located inside the cannula (Figure 16.1b). When the lumen is identified, the position of the needle is fixed, the cannula railroaded over the needle (Figure 16.1c), and the needle withdrawn (Figure 16.1d). A 20 gauge or smaller intravenous cannula is commonly used in adults, but dedicated arterial cannulae offer some advantages.

One potential problem with this technique is the distance between the needle tip and cannula tip. If this is large, the tip of the cannula may lie outside the arterial lumen even though the needle is correctly positioned. This may make it difficult or impossible for the cannula to follow the needle into the artery, and the cannula may be stripped off the needle with continued attempts.

Transfixion

Transfixion is a variation on the direct cannulation technique (Figure 16.2). The needle is deliberately passed through the posterior wall of the artery, thus transfixing it (Figure 16.2b). The needle is then withdrawn completely from the cannula (Figure 16.2c), and the cannula is slowly withdrawn until arterial blood passes freely into the hub (Figure 16.2d). The cannula is then gently advanced, ensuring that blood continues to flow until the whole length is inserted.

A variation of this technique is to leave the needle partially retracted but still within the cannula while it is being withdrawn in order to facilitate cannulation. Whatever method is used, the needle must never be reintroduced into the cannula once withdrawn because of the risk of damage to the cannula by the cutting edge of the needle. If penetration of the cannula wall by the needle occurs, further attempts at cannulation are likely to result in damage to the arterial wall; also the tip of the cannula may be sheared off, risking embolisation.

Because this technique involves penetration of the anterior and posterior arterial walls, concern has been expressed about possible increased risk of subsequent haematoma and/or occlusion compared with techniques where only one side of the artery is penetrated. However, there does not appear to be any evidence to support this hypothesis.[28,38,39]

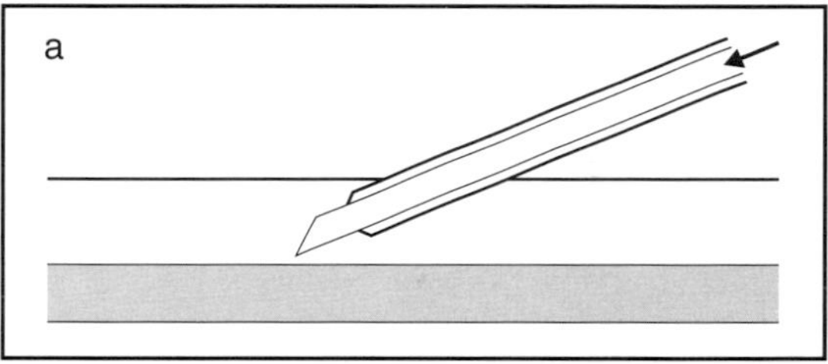

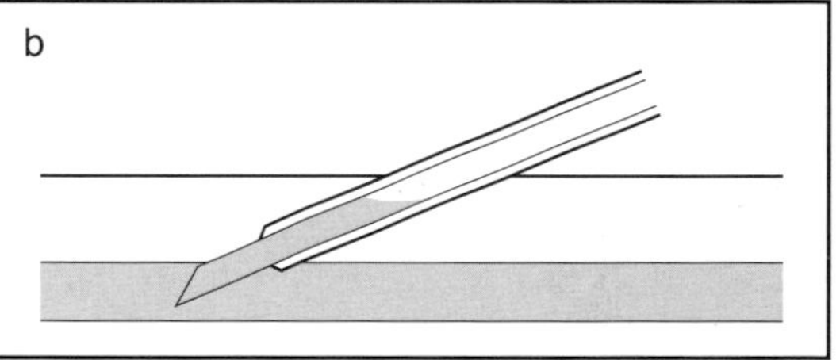

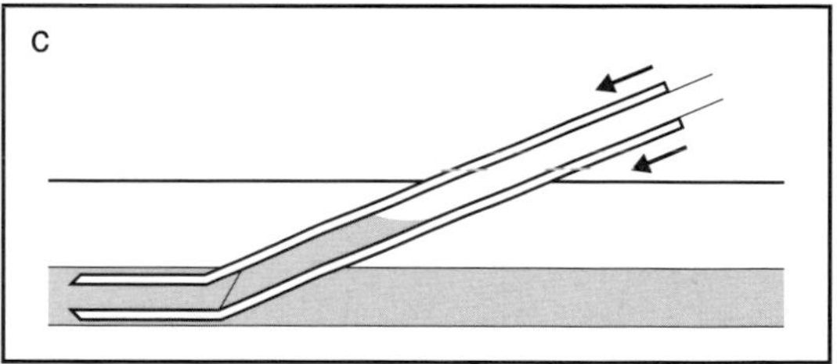

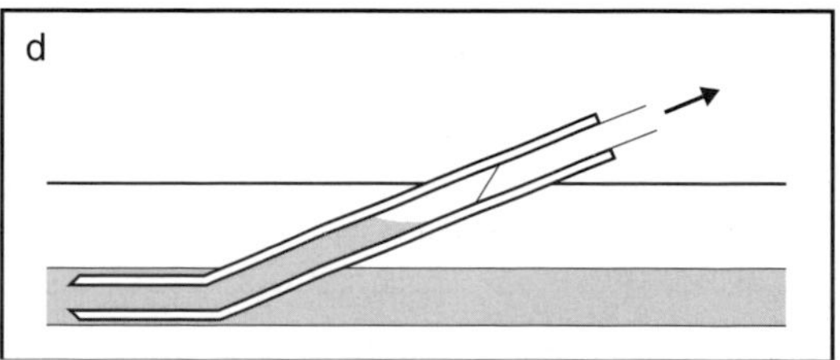

Figure 16.1 Direct cannulation.

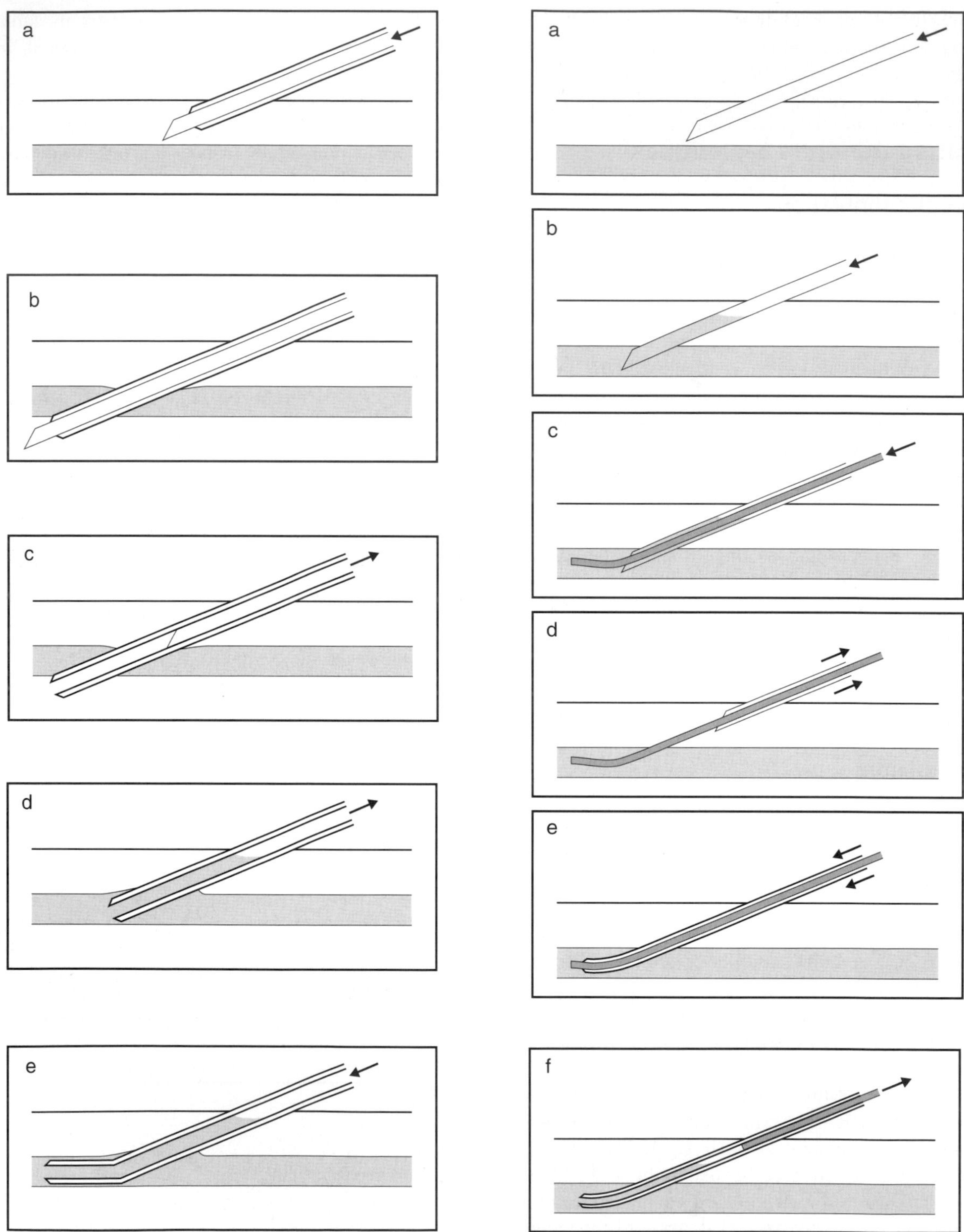

Figure 16.2 Transfixion.

Figure 16.3 Catheter-over-wire technique.

Catheter-over-wire (Seldinger technique)

In the catheter-over-wire technique (Figure 16.3) the artery is located with a needle. A wire is then passed through the needle and left *in situ* as the needle is withdrawn (Figure 16.3d). A cannula is then railroaded over the wire into the arterial lumen (Figure 16.3e) and the wire withdrawn (Figure 16.3f).

If the wire cannot be easily threaded into the artery, it should be entirely withdrawn, the angle of the needle changed in order to reduce the angle between the needle and the arterial lumen, and then reintroduced. If, despite resistance, introduction of the wire continues to be attempted, the wire may be placed outside the artery, through the artery, or may dissect along the intima, and significant damage to the arterial wall and surrounding tissues is likely. It is also possible for the wire to become impacted in the periarterial tissues so that it cannot be advanced or withdrawn. Increasingly desperate attempts to free the wire may result in uncoiling of the wire and further damage to the arterial wall and surrounding tissue. In these cases, open surgical removal is often the safest course of action.

This technique has been shown to have a higher success rate than the direct technique for radial artery cannulation, particularly in patients with small arteries,[40] but is thought to be associated with a higher risk of infection.

Cannula-through-needle

The cannula-through-needle technique is similar to the Seldinger technique, but instead of a wire being passed through the needle into the artery and a cannula then being railroaded over the wire, a smaller cannula is passed directly through the lumen of the needle into the artery (Figure 16.4). One disadvantage of this technique is that the hole in the arterial wall made by the passage of the needle is necessarily larger than the cannula, so that leakage of blood around the cannula following insertion may be a problem, especially in patients with prolonged clotting times or thrombocytopenia. The cannulae used with this technique tend to be long with a narrow lumen, which may dampen the pressure wave and limit the accuracy of the blood pressure measurement. There is also a risk of the cannula shearing on the cutting edge of the needle if cannula withdrawal is attempted. This means hat if, after locating the arterial lumen with the needle, the cannula is difficult to thread into the lumen, the needle and the cannula must be removed from the artery, necessitating another skin puncture. Because of these problems, this technique is now rarely used.

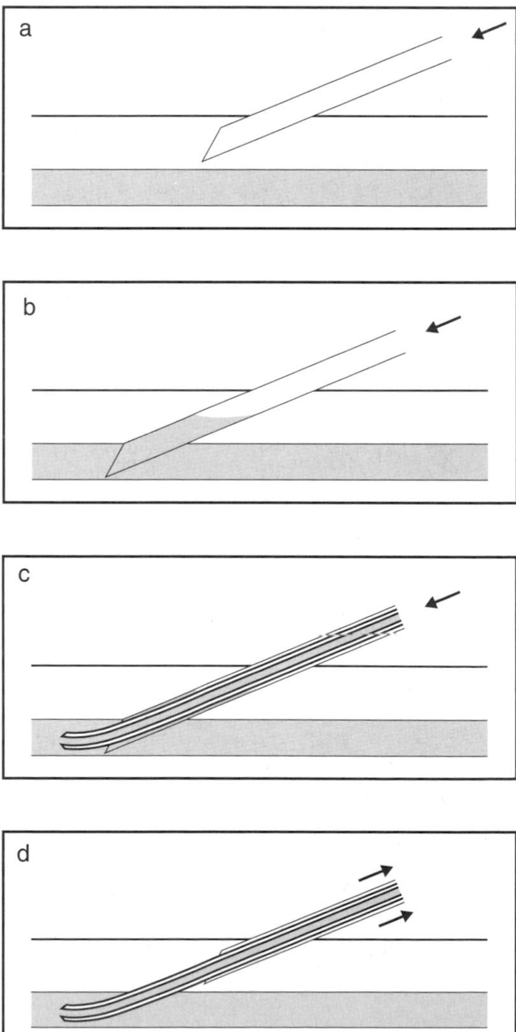

Figure 16.4 Cannula-through-needle technique.

Surgical techniques

Surgical cut-down (Figure 16.5) may occasionally be useful when cannulation is difficult or impossible using percutaneous techniques. Under most circumstances percutaneous techniques are a better choice, and are associated with a lower incidence of complications than open surgical cannulation. Surgical cut-down is easier and safer to perform in superficial arteries, such as the radial, brachial, temporal and dorsalis pedis arteries. However, identification of the artery may be difficult in shocked patients, and it is wise to attempt to improve peripheral arterial flow prior to cannulation, rather than to attempt it under difficult circumstances and risk damage to adjacent structures such as nerves.

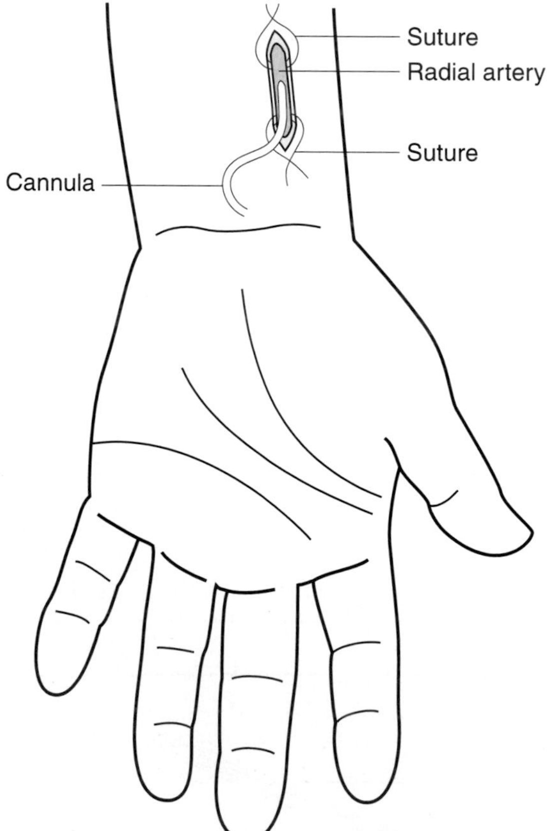

Figure 16.5 Surgical cut-down, left hand. Radial artery dissected out and held by retaining sutures. Cannula introduced into the artery after longitudinal incision.

Surgical cut-down should only be performed using fully aseptic techniques. A suitable artery is chosen prior to a full surgical scrub. The skin is cleaned using antiseptic solutions and isolated with sterile drapes. The skin overlying the artery is then infiltrated with a suitable volume of local anaesthetic solution (2–3 ml 1% lignocaine) and a small longitudinal incision is made in the skin overlying the artery. The artery is then identified and mobilised so that forceps can be passed beneath the artery. Ligatures are threaded under the proximal and distal ends of the exposed artery and are used to ensure adequate control and stabilisation of the artery during cannula insertion. The cannula is inserted into the artery over a needle, or through a small longitudinal incision made in the arterial wall.

Management of cannulation

Preparation

It is essential to have all required equipment near to hand. This includes facilities to flush the cannula immediately following cannulation, so that the cannula does not become obstructed with thrombus. Minimum equipment requirements are:

- antiseptic fluids for skin preparation
- local anaesthetic solution (0.5–1% lignocaine, plain)
- sterile gloves and drapes
- syringes for aspiration of blood
- a syringe containing heparinised saline
- a continuous flush system, irrigated with heparinised saline and all air bubbles eliminated
- a needle and suture (if required)
- a transparent sterile dressing

In addition to these items, a sterile guide-wire of a diameter and type suitable to assist cannulation should be available. This may be used to replace a damaged wire during a Seldinger technique, or may help to cannulate the artery where difficulty is experienced using other techniques.

Cannulation

Correct positioning of the site is essential for consistently successful cannulation. Sufficient time should be taken to correctly position the subject *before* scrubbing.

If the pulse is not readily palpable it may be located by one of the other techniques previously described. The use of location aids may also help to prevent problems with insertion of the cannula. If the lumen of the artery is more easily identified, insertion problems due to penetration of the side wall of the artery and consequent difficulty with threading the cannula should be less likely to occur. Other complications associated with inaccurate arterial puncture such as haemorrhage and pseudoaneurysm formation may also be reduced.

Local anaesthesia is commonly used when the patient is conscious. Giving 1–2 ml of 1% lignocaine is usually sufficient to provide good analgesia without imparing palpation of the pulse; the injection should be made over the point of maximal pulsation.

The cannula should be inserted under aseptic conditions in order to reduce the incidence of early infection. The skin is cleaned with iodine and alcohol solutions, taking care to avoid erasing skin markings, and the area of cannulation isolated with sterile drapes, ensuring that only the smallest area necessary for cannulation is exposed.

Prior to insertion, it is useful to fixate the artery as much as possible by placing a thumb distal to the insertion point. This limits lateral movement of the artery during cannulation attempts, and may help to distend the arterial lumen.

If the artery is not entered at the first attempt, the needle is withdrawn, and another attempt may be made. If a cannula-over-needle technique if being used, the cannula should be inspected for damage prior to any further attempts, and discarded if there is any damage to the tip or kinking of the cannula.

Difficulty with threading the cannula into the artery may be an indication of the presence of atheromatous plaques within the artery, dissection of the intima or other damage to the arterial wall. In Seldinger techniques the guide-wire may be threaded through the cannula to ensure that it is still in the lumen of the artery, but in cannula-over-needle techniques no attempt should ever be made to reintroduce the needle through the cannula. If difficulty is encountered using a cannula-over-needle technique, it is usually the best policy to withdraw the cannula slowly until blood flows freely from the cannula hub, and then attempt to reintroduce the cannula into the artery. If this fails, the arterial lumen can sometimes be relocated using a guide-wire introduced through the cannula, but in most cases cannulation of another artery will be a better option.

Identification of arterial puncture is usually easy, as rapid back-flow of arterial blood confirms the location of the needle within the vessel lumen. Unfortunately, this does not always occur. Coring of the skin may occur when the needle is introduced through the skin, which then blocks the needle lumen and prevents back-flow of blood, even when the lumen is entered. If this has occurred, a new cannula may be used in a more proximal position. Inserting the cannula tip through the hole left by the local anaesthetic injection or using a small incision in the skin may help to reduce this complication, and may also reduce damage to the cannula tip during skin penetration, particularly if a Teflon cannula is being used. In circumstances where penetration of the artery is not detected, it is likely that the posterior wall of the artery will be punctured, perhaps increasing the incidence of localised haematoma.

Filling the needle with saline and allowing a bubble in the hub has been described as an aid to identification of arterial puncture.[41] Pulsation of the bubble allows identification of initial entry of the cannula into the artery, maximum pulsation occurring when the needle lies fully within the lumen, and a damping of oscillations as the posterior wall is approached. Some devices have been designed to allow visualisation of the pulsation of blood as it enters the arterial lumen as an aid to cannulation.[42] Another method involves removal of the stopper from the needle so that maximum flow of blood out of the needle identifies the point when the needle bevel lies within the lumen. This presents a hazard of blood contamination to staff; either appropriate precautions should be used to reduce its incidence, or the technique should not be used at all.

Once the arterial lumen is located, the needle must be fixed at the skin in order to avoid displacement while introducing the cannula or a wire. Failure to do this may result in the needle leaving the arterial lumen and making cannulation impossible. In many cases, aspiration of blood is still possible owing to blood accumulating around the artery as a haematoma.

Difficulty with threading the cannula into the arterial lumen is a common problem. This may simply be due to the small size of the artery in relation to the size of the cannula, but may also be due to the presence of arterial spasm, arteriosclerotic plaques or misalignment between the direction of the artery and the angulation of the cannula. The situation can sometimes be rescued by withdrawing the cannula until free flow of arterial blood is obtained, but frequently the cannula tip is damaged at the first attempt, so that subsequent attempts will be unsuccessful.

Good technique can reduce the incidence of threading difficulty, which may occur even with an experienced operator. It seems to be less common with the catheter-over-wire technique, and failure with other insertion methods may be an indication for the use of this technique. Attaching a fluid infusion to the cannula prior to withdrawing it, then using back-flow of blood to recognize the intraluminal position of the cannula, may also help, as may noting the pulsation of air bubbles in the infusion fluid.[41] Another technique is described as using a 'liquid stylet', where a 10 ml syringe filled with 0.9% sodium chloride is attached to the cannula hub and the cannula withdrawn until free flow of blood is obtained. The cannula is then inserted while injecting saline to distend the arterial lumen.[43]

When the cannula has been threaded into the arterial lumen to a length of at least 1 cm, the cannula is aspirated to ensure good arterial blood flow and to remove air bubbles which may be present in the cannula. A small amount of heparinised saline should be injected prior to connection to the flush tubing. Finally, the cannula is fixed to the skin with adhesive tape, and sterile transparent film stretched over the cannula and the injection site so that the skin above the cannula entry point can be inspected without removing the dressing. A suture may be used to secure the cannula to the skin and prevent inadvertent decannulation, but may also act as a focus for infection. If the cannulated artery overlies a joint, it may be held in the correct position by means of a splint to avoid kinking of the cannula at the skin entry point.

Whichever technique is used to locate the artery, the success rate associated with cannulation depends on the integrity of the arterial wall and patency of the arterial lumen. Failed cannulation attempts tend to result in arterial spasm, making further attempts futile. In these circumstances, waiting 30 minutes for the arterial spasm to diminish may resolve the problem, provided that haematoma has not obscured the site. A previously cannulated artery with a damaged wall or a thrombosed and narrowed lumen may be difficult to cannulate successfully, even if the arterial lumen is located with a high degree of accuracy.[40]

Post-insertion management

When the cannula is inserted and fixed securely tothe skin, the cannula and all injection ports should be clearly labelled 'ARTERIAL LINE', preferably with a large, red indelible marker. The tissues supplied by the cannulated artery should be inspected for signs of decreased perfusion, both immediately after cannulation and at frequent intervals subsequently. A sudden blanching of the skin may signify arterial spasm due to the flushing of cold saline, inadvertent arterial injection, or the embolisation of thrombus. If perfusion does not improve rapidly, an urgent referral to a vascular surgeon may be necessary. If the most likely diagnosis is inadvertent injection of a drug, the cannula may need to be left *in situ* in order to administer vasodilators and other drugs into the artery in order to provide analgesia, reduce spasm and prevent clot formation. If it is associated with severe and prolonged arterial spasm, sympathetic blockade of the limb may also be indicated.

When long-term cannulation is carried out, the insertion site should be inspected on a regular basis for signs of inflammation, infection and displacement of the cannula. After every 24 hours the dressing should be discarded, the site of insertion disinfected and a new dressing applied under sterile conditions.

KEY POINTS

- The main indications for arterial cannulation are blood pressure measurement, arterial blood sampling, and radiological procedures requiring access to the arterial system.
- Direct, continuous blood pressure monitoring has significant advantages over intermittent non-invasive monitoring in conditions of hypotension and hypertension, reduced peripheral circulation, in circumstances where blood pressure changes rapidly, or during infusion of vasoactive drugs.
- Successful measurement of blood pressure depends on a suitable system consisting of a cannula, transmitting tubing filled with saline, and a system for measuring and displaying blood pressure.
- Successful cannulation depends upon technique, attention to detail and a knowledge of the associated potential problems.
- Localisation aids may help to increase the success rate and to prevent problems arising from inaccurate cannulation attempts.
- The safety of arterial cannulation depends upon a system of post-cannulation monitoring and a knowledge of acute treatment options should complications occur.

References

1. Gardner RM. Direct arterial blood pressure monitoring. Current Anaesthesia and Critical Care 1990; **1**:239.
2. Bedford RF, O'Brien TE. Comparison of bovine lung and porcine intestinal heparin for arterial thrombosis in man. American Journal of Hospital Pharmacy 1977; **34**:936.
3. Gardner RM, Bond EL, Clark JS. Safety and efficacy of continuous flush systems for arterial and pulmonary artery catheters. Annals of Thoracic Surgery 1977; **23**:534.
4. Abrams JH, Olson ML, Marino JA, Cerra FB. Use of a needle valve variable resistor to improve invasive blood pressure monitoring. Critical Care Medicine 1984; **12**:978.
5. Blackburn JP. A disposable monitor for arterial blood pressure. Anaesthesia 1966; **21**:109.
6. Cooperman LH, Mann PEG. A simple method for direct arterial pressure measurement. Anesthesiology 1966; **27**:93.
7. Severinghaus J. Aneroid manometer for arterial blood pressure. Anesthesiology 1957; **18**:906.
8. Hale DE. Arterial and venous pressure readings during open-heart operations; apparatus and technic. Cleveland Clinic Quarterly 1964; **31**:45.
9. Aarons BJ. Simple apparatus for the simultaneous monitoring of central venous and mean arterial pressures in the ward. Thorax 1965; **20**:382.
10. Zorab JSM. Continuous display of the arterial pressure. A simple manometric technique. Anaesthesia 1969; **24**:431.
11. Sisko F, Hagerdal M, Neufeld GR. Artifactual hypotension without damping, a hazard of disposable diaphragm domes. Anesthesiology 1979; **51**:263.
12. Saka D, Liu TY, Oka Y. An unusual cause of false radial artery blood pressure readings during cardiopulmonary bypass. Anesthesiology 1975; **43**:487.
13. Diamant M, Arkin DB. False radial-artery blood-pressure readings. Anesthesiology 1976; **44**:273.
14. Pauca AL, Hudspeth AS, Wallenhaupt SL, Tucker WY, Kon ND, Mills SA, Cordell AR. Radial artery-to-aorta pressure difference after discontinuation of cardiopulmonary bypass. Anesthesiology 1989; **70**:935.
15. Shapiro BA, Cane RD, Chomka CM, Gehrich JL. Evaluation of a new intra-arterial blood gas system in dogs. Critical Care Medicine 1987; **15**:361.
16. Bruner JMR, Krenis LJ, Kunsman JM, Sherman AP. Comparison of direct and indirect methods of measuring arterial blood pressure. Medical Instrumentation 1981; **15**:11.
17. Kaplan JA. Hemodynamic monitoring. In: Kaplan JA, ed. Cardiac Anesthesia, 2nd edn. Philadelphia: WB Saunders, 1987, p183.
18. Remington JW, Wood EH. Formation of the peripheral pulse contour in man. Journal of Applied Physiology 1956; **9**:433.
19. Remington JW. Contour changes of the aortic pulse during propagation. American Journal of Physiology 1960; **199**:331.
20. Husum B, Palm T, Eriksen J. Percutaneous cannulation of the dorsalis pedis artery. A prospective study. British Journal of Anaesthesia 1979; **51**:1055.
21. Kopman EA, Ferguson TB. Intraoperative monitoring of femoral artery pressure during replacement of aneurysm of descending thoracic aorta. Anesthesia and Analgesia 1977; **56**:603.
22. Dotter CT, Rosch J. Fluoroscopic guidance in femoral artery puncture. Radiology 1978; **127**:266.

23. Fukutome T, Kojiro M, Tanigawa K, Sese A. Doppler-guided 'percutaneous' radial artery cannulation in small children. Anesthesiology 1988; **69**:434.
24. Morray JP, Brandford HG, Barnes LF, Oh SM, Furman EB. Doppler-assisted radial artery cannulation in infants and children. Anesthesia and Analgesia 1984; **63**:346.
25. Becker CJ, Towbin RB. Doppler flow monitoring of the dorsal artery of the foot facilitates puncture of the femoral artery in children. American Journal of Roentgenology 1990; **155**:131.
26. Cole FS, Todres ID, Shannon DC. Technique for percutaneous cannulation of the radial artery in the newborn infant. Journal of Pediatrics 1978; **92**:105.
27. Pearse RG. Percutaneous catheterization of the radial artery in newborn babies using transillumination. Archives of Disease in Childhood 1978; **53**:549.
28. Davis FM. Methods of radial artery cannulation and subsequent arterial occlusion [letter]. Anesthesiology 1982; **56**:331.
29. Bedford RF. Percutaneous radial-artery cannulation – increased safety using Teflon catheters. Anesthesiology 1975; **42**:219.
30. Kim JM, Arakawa K, Bliss J. Arterial cannulation: factors in the development of occlusion. Anesthesia and Analgesia 1975; **54**:836.
31. Downs JB, Chapman RL, Hawkins IF Jr. Prolonged radial-artery catheterization. An evaluation of heparinized catheters and continuous irrigation. Archives of Surgery 1974; **108**:671.
32. Downs JB, Rackstein AD, Klein EF Jr, Hawkins IF. Hazards of radial-artery catheterization. Anesthesiology 1973; **38**:283.
33. Davis FM, Stewart JM. Radial artery cannulation: a prospective study in patients undergoing cardiothoracic surgery. British Journal of Anaesthesia 1980; **52**:41.
34. Feeley TW. Re-establishment of radial artery patency for arterial monitoring. Anesthesiology 1977; **46**:73.
35. Eldh P, Jacobssen B. Heparinized vascular catheters: a clinical trial. Radiology 1974; **111**:289.
36. Bedford RF. Wrist circumference predicts the risk of radial-arterial occlusion after cannulation. Anesthesiology 1978; **48**:377.
37. Soderstrom CA, Wasserman DH, Denham CM, Caplan ES, Cowley RA. Superiority of the femoral artery for monitoring: a prospective study. American Journal of Surgery 1982; **144**:309.
38. Cronin KD, Davies MJ, Domaingue CM, Worner MJ, Koumoundouros E. Radial artery cannulation – the influence of method on blood flow after decannulation. Anaesthesia and Intensive Care 1986; **14**:400.
39. Jones RM, Hill AB, Nahrwold ML, Bolles RE. The effect of method of radial artery cannulation on postcannulation blood flow and thrombus formation. Anesthesiology 1981; **55**:76.
40. Mangar D, Thrush DN, Connel GR, Downs JB. Direct or modified Seldinger guide wire-directed technique for arterial catheter insertion. Anesthesia and Analgesia 1993; **76**:714.
41. Edelman JD. An aid in arterial cannulation [letter]. Anesthesiology 1980; **53**:79.
42. Gray RJ, Rundback JH, Dolmatch BL, Horton KM. Ergonomic vascular access needle with blood-containment capability: clinical evaluation during arterial access procedures. Journal of Vascular and Interventional Radiology 1995; **6**:115.
43. Stirt JA. Liquid stylet for percutaneous radial artery cannulation. Canadian Anaesthetists Society Journal 1982; **29**:492.

17 • Arteries

BRIAN JENKINS

Introduction

As discussed in Chapter 16, there are many reasons for choosing a particular artery. When all these factors are considered, the choice is usually also dependent on a large body of experience and a history of safe use. Cannulation of the radial artery has the largest body of research associated with it, and has been used in most medical applications where arterial cannulation is required (Table 17.1).

For invasive radiological procedures, large arteries tend to be required because of the size of cannula used, although smaller arteries such as the radial artery are being increasingly used. Virtually all the arteries discussed in this section have been used in critical care, although experience with ulnar and posterior tibial artery cannulation is limited. Cannulation of the superficial temporal artery and umbilical arteries in neonates and infants has been associated with a high incidence of serious complications, and the use of these arteries is no longer recommended.

Table 17.1 Arteries used by medical specialty

Artery	Anaesthesia	Intensive care (adult)	Intensive care (paediatric)	Radiology
Axillary		√		√
Brachial		√		√
Radial	√	√	√	√
Ulnar		√	√	
Femoral	√	√	√	√
Dorsalis pedis		√	√	
Posterior tibial		√	√	

Arteries

Axillary artery

Because of the large size of the axillary artery, the waveform and measured blood pressure more closely approximate those of the aorta following cannulation than the blood pressure measured in smaller arteries such as the radial artery.[1] It has an extensive collateral blood supply, and ischaemic complications following cannulation are rare, even when the arterial lumen is completely occluded by thrombus.[2,3] The site has been used for perioperative blood pressure monitoring in a patient with Buerger's disease,[4] again without subsequent ischaemic complications.

The axillary artery arises close to the origin of the carotid arteries, so that particular attention should be paid to elimination of air from all lines in order to avoid retrograde embolisation during flushing. Embolisation of thrombus from the axillary cannula to the brain through the carotid artery is also a possible risk, particularly if the length of the cannula is excessive. If the right side is used, the tip of the cannula may lie within the innominate artery, so the left side is usually preferred.[5]

Percutaneous cannulation of the axillary artery has been used for long-term monitoring and arterial sampling in the intensive care unit.[6] In this situation it seems to have an acceptable complication rate[7] and advantages have been claimed over radial artery cannulation, in particular a lower incidence of major ischaemic complications.[2,6] The axillary artery may also be more easily palpable than the radial artery in shocked patients.

The axillary artery has been a popular site for radiographic examinations of the aorta and coronary vessels since the early 1960s,[8–10] being used either when the femoral artery is unavailable or when technical considerations make it the best choice for cannulation. It has been associated with neurological damage to nerves of the brachial plexus, mostly secondary to haematoma formation, although it is argued that long-term sequelae can be prevented by prompt surgical intervention in the majority of cases.[11]

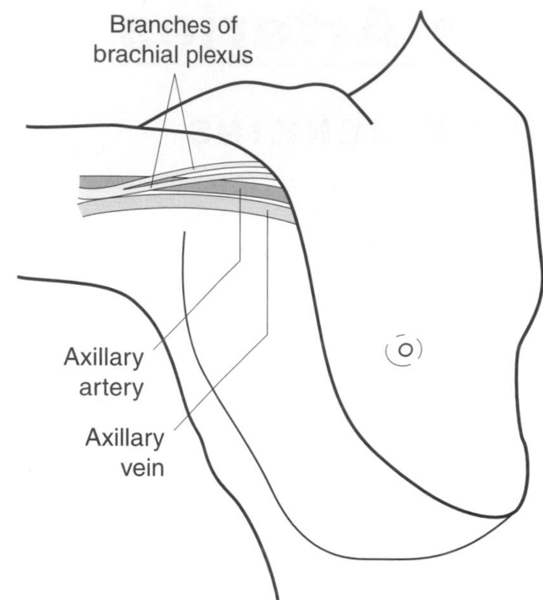

Figure 17.1 Axillary artery.

Anatomy

The axillary artery is the main artery to the arm (Figure 17.1). It is a continuation of the subclavian artery beyond the outer border of the first rib and becomes the brachial artery at the lower border of teres major. It is enclosed in the axillary sheath along with the axillary vein, axillary nerve and branches of the brachial plexus. It is normally cannulated in the first part of its course, where the brachial plexus is posterior to the artery. More distally, the nerves of the brachial plexus surround the artery where they can be more easily damaged.

Technique

The artery is most easily palpated with the arm supinated and extended, with hyperabduction to 135° or as close to this as possible, in a manner similar to that employed when performing a brachial plexus block by the axillary approach. If possible, the patient should lie supine without a pillow, with the head resting on the hand of the side to be used. In this position the artery may be palpated immediately posterior to the pectoral muscles, and may be cannulated at the junction of the deltoid and pectoral muscles.

A transfixion technique has been described for insertion,[2] but as the needle emerges through the posterior wall of the artery, it risks damaging the nerves of the brachial plexus. The Seldinger technique is therefore recommended, and has been reported to be satisfactory.[5,7]

The area to be cannulated is shaved and cleaned in the usual way. Immediately prior to insertion, the axillary artery is identified and pressed against the humerus to fix the artery prior to insertion of the cannula. The cannula is then inserted at 45° to the skin. When blood returns into the hub of the needle, the angulation of the needle and cannula is changed to a more acute angle (approximately 10°) to assist the passage of the wire into the arterial lumen.

During palpation of the artery, subjects commonly experience paraesthesiae due to pressure on the brachial plexus by the palpating finger. They should therefore be warned of the possibility of shooting pains or numbness in their arm. If this occurs during needle insertion, it is likely that the needle is aimed too high and is touching a root of the brachial plexus. It should be withdrawn and redirected to a slightly lower position.

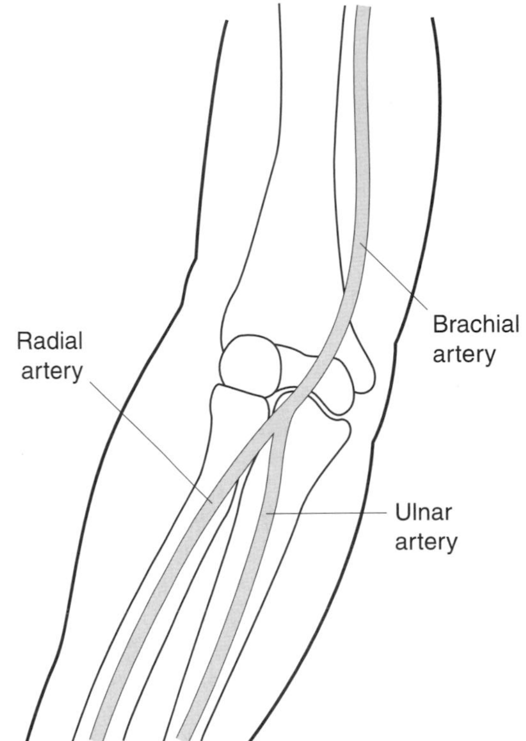

Figure 17.2 Anterior aspect of right arm, showing brachial artery.

Brachial artery

The brachial artery has been used extensively for radiological procedures such as coronary angiography[12] and aortography.[13] It has also been used for blood pressure measurement and arterial blood sampling, usually when a more distal artery such as the radial or dorsalis pedis is either inaccessible or contraindicated. Complications from percutaneous cannulation of the brachial artery for monitoring are known to be less than when the artery is accessed surgically for angiography and cardiac cannulation.[14] However, other studies have suggested a higher complication rate than that for other arteries when used for similar procedures.[15]

Brachial arterial pressures and waveforms approximate to those measured in the femoral artery, and are closer approximations of central arterial pressures than radial artery pressure measurements before and after cardiopulmonary bypass.[16,17] Percutaneous cannulation has an acceptable incidence of complications when used for cardiac surgery,[17] and during critical care.[14] Following cannulation, the collateral circulation is usually adequate to prevent distal ischaemic injury, even with complete occlusion.[18]

The brachial artery is an acceptable site for most purposes, but does necessitate full extension of the arm at the elbow in order to prevent kinking of the cannula. This may well be uncomfortable for the patient and makes routine nursing tasks difficult.

Anatomy

The brachial artery is a continuation of the axillary artery into the middle and lower arm (Figure 17.2). It divides into the radial and ulnar arteries in the cubital fossa, at the level of the neck of the radius. It passes medial to the biceps tendon and lateral to the medial nerve at the elbow. In most subjects, the brachial artery is easily palpated medial to the biceps tendon at the level of the elbow joint in the antecubital fossa. This is the most common site for cannulation.

Technique

The arm is fixed to a board in a supinated position with the arm fully extended at the elbow. The position of the brachial artery is identified by palpation or by a Doppler technique, and the point of maximal pulsation marked on the skin. A Seldinger technique is recommended. If the artery cannot be readily palpated, there is no role for expectant probing with a needle, as the antecubital fossa contains many structures that are easily damaged. Particular care should be taken to avoid damaging the median nerve, which usually passes medial to the brachial artery in the antecubital fossa.

The needle is introduced though the skin at a level just above the antecubital fossa. An entry site below this may result in cannulation of the radial or ulnar arteries. The needle is directed through the skin at an angle of 45° until the lumen of the artery is detected by flashback of blood into the needle hub. The guide-wire may then be introduced, followed by a cannula.

If the subject complains of shooting pains down the arm during attempted cannulation, it is likely that the sheath of the median nerve has been entered. The site should be marked, and the needle repositioned to avoid this area during further attempts. A more distal or proximal approach may be required.

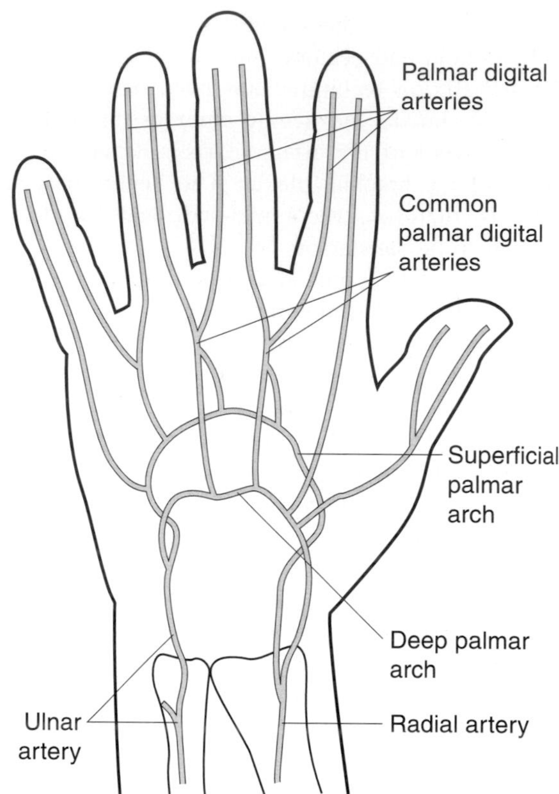

Figure 17.3 The palmar arches (palm, right hand).

Arterial supply to the hand

The palmar arches

The palmar arches form an anastomotic network between the radial and ulnar arteries, which supply arterial blood to the hand and to the fingers (Figure 17.3). The arrangement of the network is such that occlusion of one artery rarely results in ischaemia.

From a study of 650 subjects,[19] three arterial arches which anastomose between the radial and ulnar circulations have been identified, although considerable anatomical variation exists. A superficial arch, formed from a continuation of the ulnar artery, is complete in 86% of subjects; a deep arch, formed from a continuation of the radial artery, is complete in 50%; and a dorsal arch, formed from a continuation of the dorsal radial artery, is complete in 85%. As well as the arterial blood supply from the ulnar and radial arteries, interosseous and carpal networks also feed the palmar arches. The ulnar artery is usually the larger, and supplies most of the blood flow to the hand in the majority of subjects, but in approximately 10% the radial artery supplies most of the flow.[20]

Assessing collateral circulation of the hand

Following radial artery cannulation, collateral blood flow to the hand is almost entirely dependent on the patency of the ulnar artery.[21] Flow through the ulnar artery is usually adequate to maintain perfusion pressure to distal arteries,[22] but many cases have been reported in which cannulation of the radial artery has resulted in ischaemic damage to the hand. In contrast to this, a case has been described in which both the radial and ulnar arteries were completely occluded, and a satisfactory arterial blood supply to the hand was maintained entirely by palmar collaterals.[23]

In 1929, Allen described a simple test to assess the adequacy of collateral blood flow to the hand following complete radial or ulnar artery occlusion,[24] originally in patients with Buerger's disease. The classical test requires good patient cooperation, although a modified technique[25] may be performed in anaesthetised patients by exsanguinating the hand using an Esmarch bandage, and then assessing collateral circulation in the normal way. The basis of the test uses the time in which normal colour returns to an exsanguinated hand after complete radial artery occlusion. If the radial artery is to be cannulated, the ulnar and radial arteries are simultaneously occluded by digital pressure. The pressure on the ulnar artery is then released, and the time taken for normal colour to return to the hand is noted. A time longer than 15 seconds was regarded as signifying an inadequate ulnar collateral circulation. However, it is known that reperfusion may be delayed by factors other than ulnar artery blood flow, such as hyperextension of the fingers resulting in overstretching of the skin.[26] Patients in shock may also have reduced perfusion to the hand despite normal ulnar arteries, so that arterial return and collateral circulation may be difficult to assess in these subjects. The test is inconclusive if return of colour to the hand is delayed for 10–15 seconds.

There are also other problems with the period used to signify adequate circulation. If the original period of 15 seconds is accepted as a cut-off point, there remains a 10% incidence of thumb underperfusion.[27] If a reduced period of 7 seconds is used as a criterion for adequate collateral circulation, 15% of patients have been reported as having significantly reduced perfusion as assessed by Doppler techniques.[28]

Clinical reports have also suggested that Allen's test is not accurate enough as a predictor of post-cannulation complications. In a series of 16 patients, no complications were seen when radial artery cannulation was carried out despite inadequate ulnar blood flow as assessed by Allen's test.[29] In contrast, some cases of ischaemia following radial artery cannulation have been described, despite Allen's test signifying an adequate ulnar circulation.[30,31] In another report, a patient developed ischaemic complications despite adequate flow as assessed by Allen's test, performed as suggested by compressing the radial artery at the level of the radial styloid process.[32] The patient was found to have an aberrant artery that allowed blood to flow to the hand during a standard compression procedure and gave a false estimate of the adequacy of collateral circulation. It was suggested that in order to avoid this complication, the radial artery should be compressed at the level of proposed puncture, rather than at the level of the styloid process of the radius as described in Allen's test.

Because of concerns about the accuracy of Allen's test, alternative methods of estimating collateral circulation have also been described. The ulnar and radial arterial circulations are usually in continuity via the palmar arch, so that the presence of pulsation in the radial artery following proximal digital occlusion may be an indication of both ulnar artery perfusion and palmar arch patency.[33] Doppler techniques,[28,34,35] plethysmography[34] and pulse oximetry[36] have been used to assess the adequacy of collateral arterial flow. They may be used to estimate blood return via ulnar collaterals following radial artery occlusion in a similar manner to Allen's test, or a Doppler probe may be used to directly assess and quantify collateral circulation.

Because of the conflicting data on the usefulness of Allen's test as a means of predicting ischaemic problems following radial artery cannulation, it is difficult to advise its use as the sole means of assessing ulnar collateral blood flow. It seems reasonable to regard it as a means of supplying some information about the adequacy of collateral circulation when radial artery cannulation is required. However, it would seem prudent to also consider other factors such as history of previous cannulation and predisposition to thrombosis, rather than to rely solely on Allen's test as a determinant of whether or not radial artery cannulation can be safely accomplished.

Radial artery

Percutaneous cannulation of the radial artery was first described by Barr in 1961.[37] Since then it has achieved considerable popularity for long-term blood pressure measurement and arterial blood sampling. There are many reasons for this popularity. First of all, the artery is almost always superficial and readily palpable. The usual site for cannulation at the extremity of the upper limb enables easy access under most circumstances, and in long-term cannulation the site can easily be kept clean and accessible. There is usually a good collateral circulation, and when correct procedures are used, there is a low incidence of complications compared with cannulation of other arteries.[15] A great body of experience exists for radial artery cannulation, both in adult and paediatric patients, and the number of reports reflects this.

Blood pressure measurement is probably the most common reason for cannulation, and under most circumstances the radial artery is usually a good choice for this use. However, radial artery pressure may not be a good estimate of central aortic blood pressure in situations where peripheral circulation is reduced, or following cardiopulmonary bypass.[38,39] Previous cannulation of the brachial artery by surgical cut-down may result in a falsely low radial arterial blood pressure being recorded.[21]

Radial artery cannulation has been performed in order to introduce a long cannula in a retrograde direction into the aorta, to measure true aortic blood pressure[40,41] and also to perform coronary artery angioplasty.[42,43] These procedures appear to have a low incidence of complications.

Anatomy

The radial artery is formed near the apex of the cubital fossa from a terminal branch of the brachial artery. It descends deep to brachioradialis through the anterior compartment of the forearm. In the lower forearm it lies subcutaneously and is usually easily palpable for 1–4 cm over the lower end of the radius. Distally, it crosses over the wrist joint in a lateral position and passes deep to the tendons that border the anatomical snuff box (Figure 17.4). It then emerges in a dorsal position to pass between the heads of the first dorsal interosseous muscle to form the deep palmar arch.

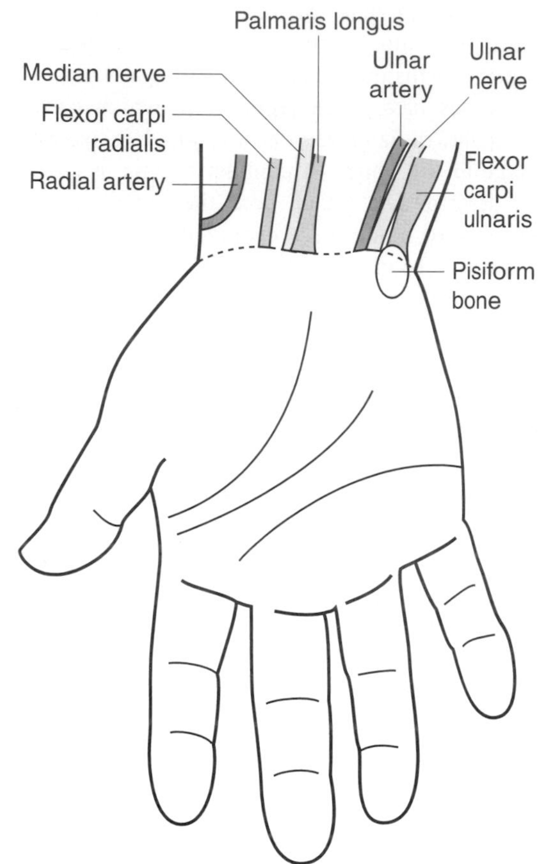

Figure 17.4 Right palm and wrist showing radial and ulnar arteries and their relations.

Technique

The wrist is first dorsiflexed and immobilised over an arm-board. Care should be taken to avoid excessive dorsiflexion, as this may reduce the anteroposterior diameter of the artery and make it difficult to palpate. The wrist may be kept in a relaxed, comfortable position by placing a small sandbag, an unopened bag of intravenous fluid or a roll of general-purpose padding under the back of the wrist. If the radial pulse is difficult to palpate, it is sometimes helpful to mark the location of the artery on the skin between the proposed needle entry point and a point approximately 2 cm proximal, or until the course of the artery can no longer be accurately palpated.

All the techniques described have been used to cannulate the radial artery, but a cannula-over-needle technique is probably most commonly used. The skin is usually penetrated between 1 cm and 4 cm from the wrist joint, where the radial artery is straighter than in more distal positions. The needle is inserted at an angle of 30–45° to the skin surface, towards the marked artery or directly beneath a gloved finger which is continuously palpating the site of maximum pulsation, until the artery is entered, indicated by a rush of blood into the hub of the cannula. The cannula is then threaded into the artery, either directly or over a wire.

Ulnar artery

The ulnar artery has been used extensively for blood pressure measurement and blood sampling, but the more superficial position of the radial artery and the greater body of experience of cannulation associated with it has made cannulation of the ulnar artery second or third choice in most circumstances. The position of the ulnar nerve in relation to the ulnar artery, making it vulnerable to injury by an advancing needle, has also influenced this decision.

Anatomy

The ulnar artery is formed near the apex of the cubital fossa as a terminal branch of the brachial artery and passes deep to the median nerve. It descends over flexor digitorum profundus through the anterior compartment of the forearm accompanied by the ulnar nerve from the middle of the forearm downward. In the lower forearm it lies below flexor carpi ulnaris lateral to the ulnar nerve. At the wrist it passes between the tendons of flexor carpi ulnaris and flexor digitorum profundus, then crosses the flexor retinaculum to end laterally to the pisiform bone. The ulnar pulse is impalpable in 3.4% of normal individuals.[44]

Technique

The ulnar artery may be cannulated at the wrist in a similar manner to the radial artery. It is common to cannulate it percutaneously, but an open surgical technique may also be used. Similar considerations to the radial artery apply with regard to the collateral circulation. The adequacy of the collateral circulation via the radial artery may be checked in a similar manner to that used with Allen's test.

Femoral artery

The femoral artery is commonly used for cannulation in critical care when smaller arteries are not palpable owing to shock or hypovolaemia, or where access via other arteries has been restricted by injury. The large size of the vessel and its constant position make cannulation relatively easy, even when no pulse is palpable.

The location of the artery may make cannula placement difficult in obese patients, where skin folds may obscure the normal anatomical landmarks. If a femoral arterial cannula is required, assistance will be required to retract abdominal skin during the procedure, and even then it may be extremely difficult to perform. The presence of chronic skin infection under skin folds and the difficulty in keeping these areas clean may also lead to cannula-related infection problems in these subjects.

The length of the cannula may prove to be a problem in some patients. Long cannulae have a larger area in which to accumulate thrombus, and may be associated with an increase in the incidence of thrombosis and thromboembolism associated with arterial cannula placement. In the case of the femoral artery there may be an additional problem in that if a long cannula is used, the tip may extend as far as the common iliac artery. In one reported case,[45] clot formation on the cannula was thought to have extended into the contralateral artery. It is advised that only the minimum length of cannula should remain in the femoral artery following placement.

Cannulation of the femoral artery has been reported to have a low complication rate in critical care.[46] It has also been used in the past for haemofiltration and extracorporeal membrane oxygenation techniques, although it is now more common to use a double-lumen venous catheter. The artery is also a common site of puncture for radiological procedures such as selective angiography. It is said to have a lower complication rate than the brachial artery when used for similar radiological procedures.[47]

Indications for cannulation in theatre include cardiac surgery, and thoracic surgery when the blood supply to the lower body may be impaired during the surgical procedure. Other reasons for cannulation may be for a variety of radiological procedures in which a large artery is required.

Blood pressure in the femoral artery is a closer approximation to aortic blood pressure than that measured in the radial artery, and the waveform is also a closer approximation. Long-term cannulation by this route is associated with a high incidence of cannula-related infection, with an incidence of 8–17% when cannulation is longer than 4 days.[6,45,46]

Doppler flow detection devices have been placed over a peripheral foot artery to detect when femoral arteries have been occluded by direct digital pressure.[48] This method of indirect detection of the femoral artery has also been suggested as an aid to insertion.[48]

Common post-cannulation complications, especially when large cannulae are used for radiographic procedures, include the development of pseudoaneurysms and periarterial haematomas. These two conditions may be reliably distinguished by colour Doppler imaging;[49] pseudoaneurysms may require surgical repair, but simple haematomas are usually treated conservatively.

Anatomy

The femoral artery is the main artery of the leg, and originates below the inguinal ligament as a continuation of the external iliac artery (Figure 17.5). It passes below the inguinal ligament in the femoral

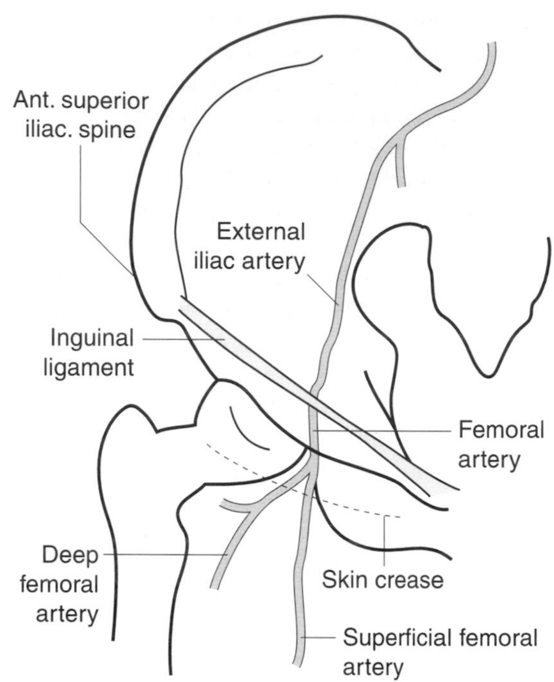

Figure 17.5 Femoral artery.

sheath in a position lateral to the femoral vein and medial to the femoral nerve. It is separated from the hip bone by psoas major. As it emerges from under the femoral ligament, it enters the femoral triangle, and is at this point anterior to the femoral head. It leaves the femoral triangle at its apex, accompanied by the saphenous nerve, the nerve to vastus medialis and the femoral vein. The common femoral artery bifurcates approximately 6.5 cm below the inguinal ligament, dividing into the superficial femoral artery and the profunda femoris.

Technique

Whether the superficial or common femoral artery is punctured during cannulation depends on the technique used. Puncture of the superficial femoral artery has been reported as having a higher incidence of complications such as arteriovenous fistula, pseudoaneurysm and thrombosis compared with puncture of the common femoral artery.[50–52] This may be because the common femoral artery overlies bone (pubic ramus and femoral head) for most of its palpable course and is therefore easier to compress with external pressure compared with the superficial femoral artery. On the other hand, the risk of retroperitoneal haemorrhage is likely to be greater with a 'high' puncture of the common femoral artery.

The most popular single landmark for cannulation of the femoral artery is the inguinal skin crease at the site of maximal femoral pulsation.[53] However, the position of the inguinal skin crease in relation to the underlying artery may be variable, especially in obese patients, and the bifurcation of the common femoral artery is higher than the inguinal skin crease in up to 75% of patients,[54] making superficial femoral artery puncture most likely if the inguinal skin crease is used as the primary landmark.

Prior to cannulation, the subject should be fully supine. A sandbag or other device may be put under the buttock on the side of the artery to be cannulated in order to further open the inguinal skin crease and aid identification of landmarks. The area to be cannulated usually needs to be shaved.

Identification of the point of maximal pulsation may be aided by palpation with both the forefinger and the second finger, with the aim being to obtain maximum pulsation in both fingers when the fingertips are spread 1 cm apart. The artery should then lie between the two palpating fingers. The needle should enter the skin at this point and be directed at an angle of 60° to the skin until the artery is entered, and maximum blood flow obtained from the hub. The needle is then redirected so that it lies at a more acute angle to the skin surface, thus aiding introduction of the cannula.

It may occasionally be difficult to thread the wire or cannula into the arterial lumen despite its large size. Redirecting the needle usually helps. In some circumstances the wire or cannula may dissect along the wall of the artery, and unless care is taken the artery may be damaged. A misplaced wire may become difficult to remove if it has been forcefully inserted against resistance, necessitating surgical removal.

Arterial supply to the foot

Arterial blood is supplied to the foot by the posterior tibial arteries, the dorsalis pedis artery, the peroneal artery and the malleolar network.

The posterior tibial artery terminates as the lateral plantar artery. The plantar artery, which is the main arterial arch of the foot, is supplied by the lateral plantar artery and the dorsalis pedis artery in a manner similar to the arterial supply of the hand. Both main arteries can thus potentially supply arterial blood to any part of the foot. As long as flow is adequate in the complementary artery, complete occlusion of one major artery can occur without necessarily incurring ischaemia.

The arterial network supplying the foot is very variable.[55] Studies using strain gauge plethysmography have suggested almost equal arterial dominance between the dorsalis pedis artery and the posterior tibial artery,[56] but in 16% of patients the dorsalis pedis artery was shown to supply almost the entire arterial blood flow to the toes.[57] In 2% of healthy subjects collateral circulation was judged to be inadequate on the basis of great toe arterial pressure when the dorsalis pedis artery was occluded,[56] but in another, older, population, 21% of the collateral circulation was judged to be inadequate on the same basis.[58]

The dorsalis pedis artery is thought to be absent in 3–12% of cases in anatomical studies,[55] which correlates well with the incidence of absent dorsalis pedis pulse in other studies.[56,59–61] Arterial blood supply to the feet is known not to be symmetrical,[62] so that it is worth checking both feet for the presence of pulses and collateral circulation before deciding on a suitable cannulation site.

Assessing collateral circulation of the foot

Collateral circulation is evaluated by tests that involve compressing the artery to be cannulated and assessing the subsequent circulation in a manner similar to Allen's test. The arterial blood pressure distal to the obstruction may also be measured,[56] or in the case of proposed dorsalis pedis cannulation, the artery is occluded by direct pressure and the collateral circulation assessed by the rapidity of return of colour following blanching by compression of the great toe.[63] However, this test may be affected by factors other than arterial blood flow, such as external temperature.

Return of the circulation within 10 seconds of occlusion of the relevant artery has been suggested as a suitable criterion for inferring the adequacy of the collateral circulation.[56] As with radial artery cannulation, the collateral blood supply may also be assessed by pulse plethysmography or Doppler techniques.[55,64]

Dorsalis pedis artery

Cannulation of the dorsalis pedis artery is useful when the radial artery is inaccessible or unusable because of limitations of surgical access, injuries or damage from previous cannulations. It is ideal for blood pressure measurement during neurosurgical procedures when access to the upper part of the body may be limited. It has many of the advantages of radial artery cannulation, with a subcutaneous straight portion of the artery ideally suited to cannulation.

The blood supply to the big toe is dependent upon dorsalis pedis blood flow in a substantial proportion of subjects.[56] Where the blood supply to this part of the foot is decreased because of shock or other causes, cannulation of the dorsalis pedis is probably best avoided.

When using this artery for blood pressure measurement, the systolic blood pressure is overestimated by about 10 mmHg and the diastolic blood pressure underestimated by 10–15 mmHg compared with aortic pressures.[58,64] Quantitatively, these effects are greater in the dorsalis pedis artery compared with the radial artery, and there is also a longer delay between ventricular contraction and arrival of the pressure wave compared with the radial artery.

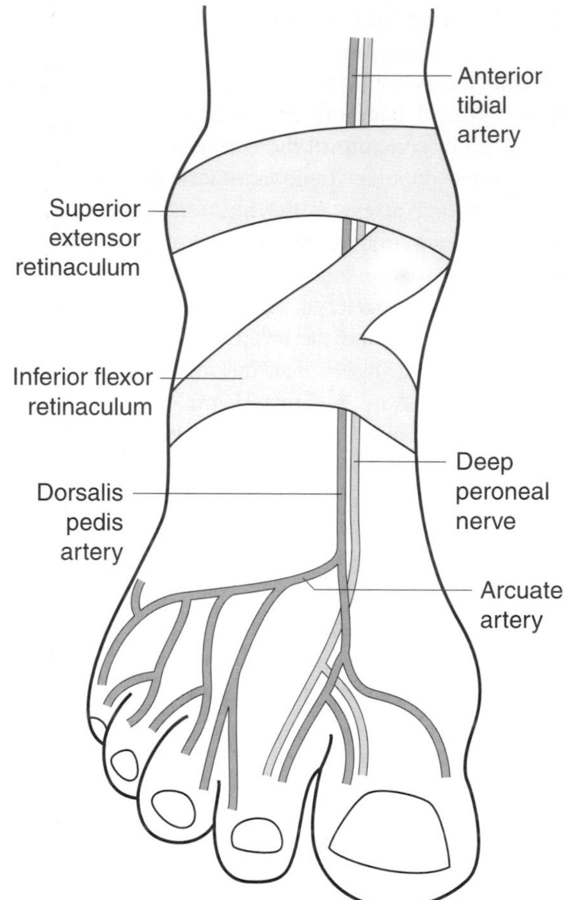

Figure 17.6 Dorsal aspect of foot, showing dorsalis pedis artery.

Anatomy

The dorsalis pedis artery is a continuation of the anterior tibial artery, and arises over the anterior aspect of the ankle joint (Figure 17.6). It passes from the ankle over the tarsus bones to the great toe and lies parallel and lateral to the extensor hallucis longus tendon in a superficial position, making palpation, localisation and cannulation relatively easy. At the proximal end of the first intermetatarsal space it divides into the first dorsal metatarsal artery and the arcuate artery.

Technique

After checking for an adequate collateral circulation as described above, the position of the artery may be identified with a marker pen prior to cleaning the skin. The artery may be cannulated using any of the techniques described. Fixation of the cannula following insertion is usually easy because of the superficial position of the artery. Keeping the site clean is also easier than following femoral artery cannulation.

Posterior tibial artery

When lower limb arterial cannulation is required, the dorsalis pedis will be the artery of choice in the vast majority of subjects. Because of the depth of the posterior tibial artery and its awkward position behind the medial malleolus, it is more difficult to cannulate, but may be used when local infection or other problems make the dorsalis pedis unsuitable. The posterior tibial artery has been successfully cannulated in neonates, with a low incidence of complications.[65] While dorsalis pedis pulses are congenitally absent in 5–12% of normal individuals, absence of a posterior tibial pulse is said to be almost always pathological.[60,61]

Anatomy

The posterior tibial artery is the main artery of the foot, and also supplies blood to the deep muscles of the back of the leg (Figure 17.7). It arises at the lower border of popliteus and descends into the foot behind the medial malleolus accompanied by the tibial nerve, and divides into the medial and lateral plantar arteries in the foot deep to the flexor retinaculum.

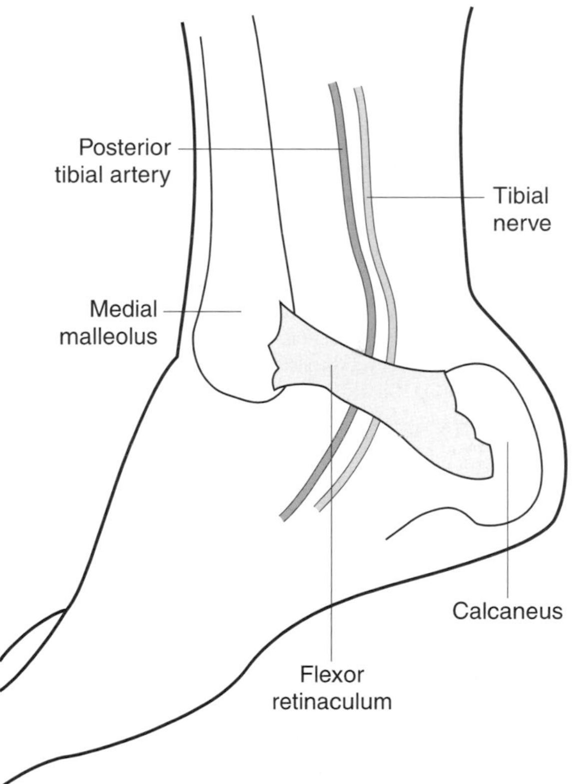

Figure 17.7 Medial aspect of foot, showing posterior tibial artery.

Technique

In adults, the posterior tibial pulse may be palpated approximately one finger's breadth behind the medial malleolus. The collateral circulation via the dorsalis pedis artery should be assessed prior to cannulation in a similar way to that described for the dorsalis pedis. The artery is most easily cannulated with the knee flexed, so that the lower leg lies across the other leg. A pillow can be placed between the legs to stabilize the position prior to cannulation. An assistant then holds the foot in a neutral position during cannulation attempts. Because of the difficulty of matching the angle of the needle to the direction of the artery, a catheter-over-wire technique is recommended.

Other arteries

Umbilical artery

The umbilical arteries rapidly occlude and fibrose soon after birth, so that cannulation is only possible in neonates. The technique is useful in some patients, but because of the well-recognised high incidence of complications compared with other sites such as the radial and femoral arteries the technique has lost popularity. Complications include thrombosis and vascular spasm with or without a reduction in distal organ perfusion.[66,67] A high incidence of infection has also been reported.[68]

The umbilical arteries arise from the internal iliac arteries, crossing the bladder and ureters before emerging from the anterior abdominal wall through the umbilicus. The arteries may be cannulated percutaneously or, more commonly, by an open surgical technique as for umbilical vein cannulation. When feeding the cannula along the artery, care must be taken to optimise the final position in order not to compromise the mesenteric or renal arterial flow. Because the cannulae used are long and thin, particular care must be taken if accurate measurement of blood pressure is required.[69]

Superficial temporal artery

The superficial temporal artery has been cannulated for blood pressure measurement and arterial blood sampling. The artery is regarded as totally expendable, and is usually cannulated under direct vision following a small surgical incision anterior to the tragus of the ear.[30] Attempted cannulation below the tragus risks damage to both the parotid gland and the facial nerve. Unfortunately, the use of this artery for monitoring and blood sampling in neonates has been associated with a high incidence of contralateral hemiplegia secondary to cerebral infarction,[70–72] so it is no longer recommended for use.

KEY POINTS

- Radial artery cannulation is now a common procedure that is supported by a large body of research and a wealth of clinical experience.
- A large variety of arteries have been cannulated for blood pressure monitoring and arterial gas sampling in critical care.
- Cannulation of the umbilical artery and superficial temporal arteries is associated with a high incidence of complications, and is no longer recommended.
- Allen's test is not useful as a sole means of accurately assessing collateral blood supply when cannulation of the radial artery is planned.
- The dorsalis pedis artery is absent in 5–12% of normal individuals. Absent posterior tibial pulses are almost always pathological.

References

1. Bryan-Brown CW, Kwun KB, Lumb PD, Pia RL, Azer S. The axillary artery catheter. Heart and Lung 1983; **12**:492.
2. De Angelis J. Axillary arterial monitoring. Critical Care Medicine 1976; **4**:205.
3. Bryan-Brown CW, Lumb PD, Kathirithambi KS, Shapiro B, Azer S. Axillary artery catheterization. Anesthesiology 1979; **51**:S157.
4. Yacoub OF, Bacaling JH, Kelly M. Monitoring of axillary arterial pressure in a patient with Buerger's disease requiring clipping of an intracranial aneurysm. British Journal of Anaesthesia 1987; **59**:1056.
5. Adler DC, Bryan-Brown CW. Use of the axillary artery for intravascular monitoring. Critical Care Medicine 1973; **1**:148.
6. Gurman GM, Kriemerman S. Cannulation of big arteries in critically ill patients. Critical Care Medicine 1985; **13**:217.
7. Brown M, Gordon LH, Brown OW, Brown EM. Intravascular monitoring via the axillary artery. Anaesthesia and Intensive Care 1984; **13**:38.
8. Hanafee W. Axillary approach to carotid, vertebral, abdominal aorta and coronary angiography. Radiology 1963; **81**:559.
9. Newton TH. Axillary artery aproach to arteriography of aorta and its branches. American Journal of Roentgenology, Radium Therapy and Nuclear Medicine 1963; **89**:275.
10. Roy P. Percutaneous cathteterization via the axillary artery. A new approach to some technical roadblocks in selective arteriography. American Journal of Roentgenology, Radium Therapy and Nuclear Medicine 1965; **94**:1.
11. Molnar W, Paul DJ. Complications of axillary arteriotomies. Analysis of 1,762 consecutive studies. Radiology 1972; **104**:269.
12. Sones FM, Shirley EK. Cine coronary arteriography. Modern Concepts of Cardiovascular Diseases 1962; **31**:735.
13. Gaines PA, Reidy JF. Percutaneous high brachial aortography: a safe alternative to the translumbar approach. Clinical Radiology 1986; **37**:595.
14. Barnes RW, Foster EJ, Janssen GA, Boutros AR. Safety of brachial arterial catheters as monitors in the intensive care unit – prospective evaluation with the Doppler ultrasonic velocity detector. Anesthesiology 1976; **44**:260.
15. Mortensen JD. Clinical sequelae from arterial needle puncture, cannulation and incision. Circulation 1967; **35**:1118.
16. Bazaral MG, Welch M, Golding LAR, Badhwar K. Comparison of brachial and radial arterial pressure monitoring in patients undergoing coronary artery bypass surgery. Anesthesiology 1990; **73**:38.
17. Gravlee GP, Wong AB, Adkins TG, Case LD, Pauca AL. A comparison of radial, brachial, and aortic pressures after cardiopulmonary bypass. Journal of Cardiothoracic Anesthesia 1989; **3**:20.
18. Bell JW. Treatment of post-catheterization arterial injuries: use of survey plethysmography. Annals of Surgery 1962; **155**:591.
19. Coleman SS, Anson BJ. Arterial patterns in the hand based upon a study of 650 specimens. Surgery, Gynecology and Obstetrics 1991; **113**:409.
20. Mozersky DJ, Buckley CJ, Hagood CO, Capps WF, Dannemiller FJ Jr. Ultrasonic evaluation of the palmar

circulation. A useful adjunct to radial artery cannulation. American Journal of Surgery 1973; **126**:810.

21. Ryan JF, Raines J, Dalton BC, Mathieu A. Arterial dynamics of radial artery cannulation. Anesthesia and Analgesia 1973; **52**:1017.
22. Palm T. Evaluation of peripheral arterial pressure on the |thumb following radial artery cannulation. British Journal of Anaesthesia 1977; **49**:819.
23. Hirai M, Kawai S. False positive and negative results in Allen test. Journal of Cardiovascular Surgery 1980; **21**:353.
24. Allen EV. Thromboangiitis obliterans: methods of diagnosis of chronic occlusive arterial lesions distal to the wrist with illustrative cases. American Journal of Medical Science 1929; **178**:237.
25. Barber JD, Wright DJ, Ellis RH. Radial artery puncture. A simple screening test of ulnar anastomotic circulation. Anaesthesia 1973; **28**:291.
26. Greenhow DE. Incorrect performance of Allen's test – ulnar artery flow erroneously presumed inadequate. Anesthesiology 1972; **37**:356.
27. Bedford RF, Wollman H. Complications of percutaneous radial-artery cannulation: an objective prospective study in man. Anesthesiology 1973; **38**:228.
28. Clarke W, Freund PR, Wasse L, Curtis M, Thiele BL, Ward RJ. Assessment of adequacy of ulnar arterial flow prior to radial artery catheterization. Anesthesiology 1981; **55**:A38.
29. Slogoff S, Keats AS, Arlund C. On the safety of radial artery cannulation. Anesthesiology 1983; **59**:42.
30. Baker RJ, Chunprapaph B, Nyhus LM. Severe ischemia of the hand following radial artery catheterization. Surgery 1976; **80**:449.
31. Mangano DT, Hickey RF. Ischemic injury following uncomplicated radial artery catheterization. Anesthesia and Analgesia 1979; **58**:55.
32. Gandhi SK, Reynolds AC. A modification of Allen's test to detect aberrant collateral circulation. Anesthesiology 1983; **59**:147.
33. Ramanathan S, Chalon J, Turndorf H. Determining patency of palmar arches by retrograde radial pulsation. Anesthesiology 1975; **42**:756.
34. Brodsky JB. A simple method to determine patency of the ulnar artery intraoperatively prior to radial-artery cannulation. Anesthesiology 1975; **42**:626.
35. McSwain GR, Ameriks JA. Doppler-improved Allen's test. Southern Medical Journal 1979; **72**:1620.
36. Nowak GS, Moorthy SS, McNiece WL. Use of pulse oximetry for assessment of collateral arterial flow [letter]. Anesthesiology 1986; **64**:527.
37. Barr PO. Percutaneous puncture of the radial artery with a multipurpose Teflon catheter for indwelling use. Acta Physiologica Scandinavica 1961; **51**:343.
38. Rich GF, Lubanski RE, McLoughlin TM. Differences between aortic and radial artery pressure associated with cardiopulmonary bypass. Anesthesiology 1992; **77**:63.
39. Stern DH, Gersson JI, Allen FB, Parker FB. Can we trust the direct radial artery pressure immediately following cardiopulmonary bypass? Anesthesiology 1985; **62**:557.
40. Gardner RM, Schwartz R, Wong HC, Burke JP. Percutaneous indwelling radial-artery catheters for monitoring cardiovascular function. Prospective study of the risk of thrombosis and infection. New England Journal of Medicine 1974; **290**:1227.
41. Rulf ENR, Mitchell MM, Prakash O. Measurement of arterial pressure after cardiopulmonary bypass with long radial artery catheter. Journal of Cardiothoracic Anesthesia 1990; **4**:19.
42. Kiemeneij F, Laarman GJ, de Melker E. Transradial artery coronary angioplasty. American Heart Journal 1995; **129**:1.
43. Lotan C, Hasin Y, Mosseri M, Rozenman Y, Admon D, Nassar H, Gotsman MS. Transradial approach for coronary angiography and angioplasty. American Journal of Cardiology 1995; **76**:164.
44. Friedman SA. Prevalence of palpable wrist pulses. British Heart Journal 1970; **32**:316.
45. Colvin MP, Curran JP, Jarvis D, O'Shea PJ. Femoral artery pressure monitoring. Use of the Seldinger technique. Anaesthesia 1977; **32**:451.
46. Ersoz CJ, Hedden M, Lain L. Prolonged femoral arterial catheterization for intensive care. Anesthesia and Analgesia Current Researches 1970; **49**:160.
47. Lang EK. A survey of the complications of percutaneous retrograde arteriography. Seldinger Technic. Radiology 1963; **81**:257.
48. Becker CJ, Towbin RB. Doppler flow monitoring of the dorsal artery of the foot facilitates puncture of the femoral artery in children. American Journal of Roentgenology 1990; **155**:131.
49. Schwartz RA, Kerns DB, Mitchell DG. Color Doppler ultrasound imaging in iatrogenic arterial injuries. American Journal of Surgery 1991; **162**:4.
50. McMillan I, Murie JA. Vascular injury following cardiac catheterization. British Journal of Surgery 1984; **71**:832.
51. Cole PL, Krone RJ. Approach to reduction of vascular complications of percutaneous valvuloplasty. Catheterization and Cardiovascular Diagnosis 1987; **13**:331.
52. Altin RS, Flicker S, Naidech HJ. Pseudoaneurysm and arteriovenous fistula after femoral artery catheterization: association with low femoral punctures. American Journal of Roentgenology 1989; **152**:629.
53. Grier D, Hartnell G. Percutaneous femoral artery puncture: Practice and anatomy. British Journal of Radiology 1990; **63**:602.
54. Lechner G, Jantsch H, Waneck R, Kretschmer G. The relationship between the common femoral artery, the inguinal crease and the inguinal ligament; a guide to accurate angiographic puncture. Cardiovascular and Interventional Radiology 1988; **11**:165.
55. Huber JF. The arterial network supplying the dorsum of the foot. Anatomical Record 1941; **80**:373.
56. Palm T, Husum B. Blood pressure in the great toe with simulated occlusion of the dorsalis pedis artery. Anesthesia and Analgesia 1978; **57**:453.

57. Spoerel WE, Deimling P, Aitken R. Direct arterial pressure monitoring from the dorsalis pedis artery. Canadian Anaesthetists Society Journal 1975; **22**:91.
58. Husum B, Palm T, Eriksen J. Percutaneous cannulation of the dorsalis pedis artery. A prospective study. British Journal of Anaesthesia 1979; **51**:1055.
59. Reich RS. The pulses of the foot. Annals of Surgery 1934; **99**:613.
60. Stephens GL. Palpable dorsalis pedis and posterior tibial pulses. Archives of Surgery 1962; **84**:662.
61. Barnhorst DA, Barner HB. Prevalence of congenitally absent pedal pulses. New England Journal of Medicine 1968; **278**:264.
62. Keen JA. A study of the arterial variations in the limbs, with special reference to symmetry of vascular patterns. New England Journal of Medicine 1961; **285**:1414.
63. Johnstone RE, Greenhow DE. Catheterization of the dorsalis pedis artery. Anesthesiology 1973; **39**:654.
64. Youngberg JA, Miller ED. Evaluation of percutaneous cannulations of the dorsalis pedis artery. Anesthesiology 1976; **44**:80.
65. Spahr RC, MacDonald HM, Holzman IR. Catheterization of the posterior tibial artery in the neonate. American Journal of Diseases of Children 1979; **133**:945.
66. Egan EA, Eitzman DV. Umbilical vessel catheterization. American Journal of Diseases of Children 1971; **121**:213.
67. Cochran WD, Davis HT, Smith CA. Advantages and complications of umbilical artery catheterization in the newborn. Pediatrics 1968; **42**:769.
68. Krauss AN, Albert RF, Kannan MM. Contamination of umbilical catheters in the newborn infant. Journal of Pediatrics 1970; **77**:965.
69. Goodwin SR, Graves SA, van der Aa J. Umbilical catheters and arterial blood pressure monitoring. Journal of Clinical Monitoring 1985; **1**:227.
70. Simmons MA, Levine RL, Lubchenco LO, Guggenheim MA. Warning: serious sequelae of temporal artery catheterization. Journal of Pediatrics 1978; **92**:284.
71. Bull MJ, Schreiner RL, Garg BP, Hutton NM, Lemons JA, Gresham EL. Neurologic complications following temporal artery catheterization. Journal of Pediatrics 1980; **96**:1071.
72. Prian GW, Wright GB, Rumach CM, O'Meara OP. Apparent cerebral embolization after temporal artery catheterization. Journal of Pediatrics 1978; **93**:115.

18 • Complications

BRIAN JENKINS

Introduction

The incidence of complications associated with arterial cannulation depends upon many factors which include the site of puncture, size and shape of cannula (tapered or non-tapered), size of artery, duration of cannulation and techniques of flushing. Leaving a cannula in the artery for longer than is strictly necessary is a cause of avoidable complications. The cannula should be removed when the benefits derived from maintaining the cannula are outweighed by the risks involved.

Paediatric cannulation

Cannulation of arteries in children may carry significant risks of complications owing to the small size of the arteries in relation to the size of the cannula used. The incidence of failure is also likely to be higher than in adults, again because of the small size of the vessels. Cannulation aids such as fibreoptic light sources[1,2] and Doppler probes[3] have been used to reduce the incidence of failed cannulation.

When cannulation is possible, a significant proportion of the arterial lumen will be completely occluded by the cannula, so that the presence of an adequate collateral circulation may be even more important than in adults. Arteries that are commonly used for cannulation in adults are also used in children. In addition, some arteries such as the superficial temporal artery and the umbilical artery have been used, although their use has declined in recent years because of concern about an associated high incidence of serious complications (see Chapter 17).

Critical illness

It has been demonstrated that radial arterial lines have a significantly higher incidence of arterial occlusion in critically ill patients than other subjects.[4] This may be related to a number of factors including prolonged cannulation, the presence of systemic infection and shocked states where reduced peripheral arterial blood flow may predispose to thrombosis.[5,6] The infusion of vasoconstrictor drugs may also have a role.[7]

Cannulation for radiographic procedures

When arterial cannulation is carried out for radiological purposes, the large sizes of cannula generally used in relation to the arterial wall diameter may be a predisposing factor for subsequent thrombosis, although the short duration of most radiological procedures helps to keep the incidence within acceptable levels.

The femoral and brachial arteries have been most extensively used because of their large size. As microtechnology advances, it is likely that smaller cannulae will be developed so that the same procedures may be more commonly performed using smaller, more distal vessels such as the radial artery. Coronary arteriography is now possible using the radial artery as well as the larger vessels such as the axillary and brachial arteries.

Complications arising from damage to the arterial wall such as pseudoaneurysm and haematoma are also more common when large cannulae are used, and are more likely to be clinically significant than similar complications with smaller cannulae.

Complications

Spasm

Arterial spasm commonly occurs when a cannula is initially introduced into an artery, and may result in complete occlusion in a high percentage of cases.[8] This is due to contraction of arterial smooth muscle as a result of direct mechanical trauma. If complete occlusion occurs, perfusion to distal tissues will then depend upon the presence of patent collateral vessels until the arterial spasm is relieved. If the collateral circulation is inadequate, there may be temporary blancing of the area of skin supplied by the artery. The underperfused area should be kept warm and undisturbed. The spasm usually resolves over a period ranging from a few minutes to several hours, but if blancing is prolonged beyond 2 hours, it would seem wise to remove the cannula as a precautionary measure. The subject should be referred to a vascular surgeon, and other methods of reducing vasospasm such as an axillary sympathetic block should also be considered.[9]

Vasospasm may also occur following intermittent flushing of the cannula, and may by itself affect cannula patency.[10] This presumably occurs as a result of an arterial smooth muscle response to the cold flush solution, and is another reason to avoid intermittent flushing as much as possible.

If blanching persists following cannula removal, embolisation of clot or an arteriosclerotic plaque may have occurred, and an urgent referral to a vascular surgeon may again be necessary. Persistent spasm following cannula removal has been implicated in irreversible tissue necrosis in a neonate,[11] but it is difficult to distinguish from thrombosis unless surgical exploration is carried out. Keeping the blanched area warm may help, and artificial warming of the hand has been used to distinguish between spasm and thrombosis in studies of post-cannulation occlusion.[12]

Spasm is less common in the elderly, probably because of an associated increased incidence of arterial fibrosis and arteriosclerotic plaques, physically preventing arterial contraction. If cannulation has been attempted and has failed, spasm of the artery due to mechanical trauma may make palpation of the pulse and identification of the artery difficult. Repeated attempts at cannulation are unlikely to succeed until spasm has been reduced.

Thrombosis and ischaemia

The incidence of thromboembolism has been more extensively investigated than any other complication associated with arterial cannulation. Blood flow to distal tissues following cannulation may be assessed by a number of techniques including a modified Allen's test, Doppler techniques,[13] thermography[14] and plethysmography.[15]

Thrombosis may occur both proximally and distally from the point of cannula insertion. In the former, extension of thrombus from the site of cannula insertion is likely to be the cause, and involvement of the cutaneous branches of the radial artery has led to skin necrosis over the forearm following radial artery cannulation.[16,17] If reduced perfusion is seen distal to the site of cannula insertion, this may be due to direct extension or embolism of thrombus from the cannulation site.

Risk factors for thrombosis that have been identified are long and large-gauge cannulae,[18] prolonged cannulation,[13,19–21] multiple attempts, previous cannulation of a collateral vessel, hyperlipoproteinaemia,[22] Reye's syndrome[23] and surgical cut-down.[24]

Continuous irrigation of arterial lines with heparinised solutions has been shown to prolong the duration of catheter patency,[25] but the minimal effective concentration of heparin has yet to be established. In one study, a significant prolongation of cannula patency was demonstrated when 5 U/ml of heparin was compared with 1 U/ml,[26] but in another study no difference was apparent when 1 U/ml was compared with 0.25 U/ml.[27] Other agents such as papaverine[28] and sodium citrate 1.4%[29] have also been demonstrated to have useful antithrombotic effects. The carrier solution used may also be important, with heparinised isotonic saline reported as being significantly more effective in preventing arterial occlusion than heparinised 5% dextrose.[30]

Pretreatment with aspirin has been reported to significantly reduce the incidence of arterial occlusion,[31] presumably owing to its effect of inhibiting platelet aggregation following arterial puncture. However, other studies have failed to demonstrate a reduction.[24,32]

Excessive pressure on the artery following cannula withdrawal may result in vessel occlusion, blood stasis and subsequent thrombosis. Five minutes of gentle pressure is usually all that is required to stop haematoma formation at the puncture site, although this may need to be longer in patients with prolonged bleeding times. Removal of the catheter may result in stripping of adherent thrombus from the outside of the catheter during withdrawal, leaving thrombus in the vessel.[33] This could act as a focus for further local thrombosis and/or infection.

Infection

Infection may occur around the site of skin puncture, and embolisation of septic thrombi to tissues perfused by the artery may result in lesions such as Osler's nodes, splinter haemorrhages and Janeway lesions in distal tissues.[34,35]

Local infections may result from the use of nonsterile techniques during cannula placement, or may arise over a period of time by spread of bacteria into the arterial wound, with the incidence of infection related to the time that the cannula is *in situ*.[36] Antiseptic ointment has been shown to reduce the incidence of local infection by 3.6% and polyantibiotic ointments by 2.2%.[37] Their routine use is recommended where long-term cannulation is planned. The effect of antibiotic bonding to cannulae has also been examined. Although in studies a trend to lower infection rates was seen, this was not thought to be clinically significant.[38] In addition to being infected as a result of skin contamination, cannulae may also be infected during septicaemic episodes on intensive care.[39] The thrombus that collects on the outside of most intravascular cannulae provides an ideal culture medium for many bacteria.

Infection may also occur as a result of contamination of infusion equipment, probably due to the introduction of bacteria through three-way taps and multiple infusion devices. There has been a reported contamination rate of 46% associated with the use of three-way taps,[40] and it is suggested that covers should always be used in order to reduce the risk. An 11% rate of bacterial infection of transducer domes has been reported in patients with long-term cannulation.[41] Replacement of the infusion and transducer system every 24–48 hours is advised.

Cannulation of arteries using a cut-down approach is known to be associated with a higher incidence of infection than a percutaneous approach.[42] Umbilical artery cannulae are known to be associated with a high risk of both local and systemic infections.[43] Femoral arterial cannulation is reputed to be associated with a high risk of infection in comparison with cannulation of other arteries, presumably because of the difficulty of keeping the surrounding skin clean, especially in obese subjects.

Ensuring that the cannula is only kept *in situ* during the time of clinical need, and the use of an aseptic technique in both the initial placement of the cannula and the changes of dressings, would seem the best way to prevent serious complications due to infection.

Haemorrhage and haematoma

External haemorrhage may occur in a number of ways, the most obvious being a disconnection that allows arterial blood to leak from the site of cannulation, or if the cannula itself is removed and inadequate pressure is applied to the site of puncture. The degree of hazard will depend on the size of the artery and the size of the cannula. A moderate-sized artery may leak blood at a rate that would cause hypovolaemia within a few minutes, but a large leak from a major vessel such as the femoral artery may cause immediate life-threatening exsanguination unless the problem is rapidly identified and corrected. The incidence of accidental disconnection may be minimized by the use of Luer-Lok connections in all apparatus used.

Deranged clotting mechanisms and systemic hypertension are associated with increased risk of haemorrhage. Coarctation of the aorta may result in increased perfusion pressure to the arms and an increased risk of haemorrhagic complications during arterial puncture, particularly where large cannula are used, as in aortography via the brachial artery.[44]

When haemorrhage occurs into the tissues, it usually results in localised swelling and bruising. However, pressure effects from the haematoma may sometimes cause skin necrosis of the overlying tissue, and if nervous tissue is involved, neurological lesions may also occur (see below). When the haematoma remains in communication with the arterial lumen, transmitted arterial pressure may be felt in the haematoma, resulting in a pseudo-aneurysm. This is most frequently reported as a complication of arterial puncture in large arteries such as the femoral following radiological procedures,[45] but has also been described in smaller vessels such as the radial artery.[46,47] Colour Doppler sonography has been used to investigate persistent injuries to the femoral arterial wall,[48,49] and has a sensitivity and specificity approaching 100%.[50]

Nerve injury

Damage to neural tissue may occur following direct trauma during cannulation attempts.[51] It may also occur as a secondary complication of haematoma formation owing to pressure on adjacent neural structures, particularly in subjects with deranged clotting mechanisms. It follows that nerve damage from either mechanism is most likely to occur when a nerve is immediately adjacent to the site of arterial puncture. In practice, most of the common arterial puncture sites may be associated with this risk.

Multiple attempts at arterial cannulation are likely to result in an increased likelihood of direct damage to nerve tissue by the needle. Also, if the artery is punctured many times, haematoma formation will be more likely. Multiple cannulation attempts involving the radial artery have been cited as a contributory factor towards haematoma formation and median nerve palsy at the wrist.[52]

Enclosing structures that allow a rapid rise in tissue pressure will increase the risk of nerve damage following haematoma formation. Examples of these are the neurovascular sheath surrounding the axillary artery[53,54] and the flexor retinaculum at the wrist. Haematoma formation following radial artery cannulation has resulted in compression of the median nerve at the wrist, resulting in carpal tunnel syndrome.[52,55]

Damage to the brachial plexus following attempts at axillary artery cannulation is particularly common during radiological procedures, probably because of a combination of factors. The axillary artery is a popular site; large needles and cannulae are used which increase the chances of trauma both to surrounding nerves and the arterial wall; also, many of the patients undergoing these procedures are on anticoagulant therapy. If there is a small, persistent leak through the arterial wall and haematoma formation occurs slowly, neurological symptoms may not appear until 1–3 weeks after the procedure.[45]

Median nerve palsy has been reported following attempted brachial artery cannulation.[56,57] Damage has resulted from direct trauma to the nerve with the needle during cannulation attempts, and also secondary to haematoma formation in subjects with deranged clotting mechanisms.

Aneurysm

Aneurysm formation can occur after repeated puncture of the vessel wall,[58] but may also occur after a single traumatic episode of cannulation. It tends to be more common when large cannulae are introduced, as when angiography is performed via the femoral artery. Dissecting aneurysms have also been extensively reported following radiological procedures.[59–61] Extracorporeal aneurysms have also been reported.[62]

Arteriovenous fistula

Arteriovenous fistula has been reported following radial artery cannulation,[63] and also in other arteries such as the femoral. It is most commonly due to simultaneous puncture of an artery and an adjacent vein during cannulation attempts. The potential for this complication exists wherever an artery and a vein lie in close proximity. It has been most commonly reported following radiological procedures such as cardiac catheterisation through the femoral artery. In some cases intentional puncture of both the femoral artery and vein in the same leg is performed for right and left heart studies, and this may also be a cause.[64] Most fistulae will present with symptoms of distal ischaemia, or if the flow is large, congestive heart failure may result. Surgical repair is almost always necessary.

Accidental injection of drugs

The hazards associated with accidental injection of drugs into arteries are well known. Antibiotics[65,66] and anaesthetic drugs such as thiopentone[67] and ketamine[68] have been reported to cause skin necrosis following accidental injection. A large variety of drugs and infusions used in medical practice, such as high-concentration dextrose solutions[69,70] and sodium bicarbonate,[71] may cause similar reactions. Taking precautions to make accidental injection less likely is far easier than treating the complications that result, so prominent labelling of the arterial line and all access sites is necessary, especially when the patient is being cared for by inexperienced staff. The use of arterial cannulae without injection ports may also help to prevent this serious complication.

Embolism

Immediate loss of peripheral pulses following cannulation may result from the embolisation of atherosclerotic plaques. Severe atheroma or calcification of the arteries may be a relative contraindication to arterial cannulation because of the risk of this complication.

Retrograde flushing of thrombotic plaques through a radial artery cannula has resulted in cerebral embolisation and ischaemia,[72] but distal embolisation of thrombus[19] is more likely. Air bubbles may also be inadvertently flushed retrogradely through arterial lines, and are known to be a significant hazard. The likelihood of cerebral air embolism depends on the volume of air introduced and the distance from the cannulation site to the carotid or vertebral arteries. In the case of peripheral arteries, this may inversely correlate with the height of the subject.[72] The volume of flush solution required to produce retrograde flow from the radial artery has been reported as 5–6.3 ml in children[73] and 3–12 ml in adults.[72,74] The use of continuous flush systems is probably the best way of reducing the risk of retrograde embolism, but other methods using intermittent volume-limited flushing methods have been proposed.[75] Although these systems may help to prevent retrograde embolism they do not remove the hazard of infection potentially introduced during each flushing episode.

Placement of a cannula with the tip in close proximity to the cerebral circulation is likely to increase the risk of significant embolism. Superficial temporal artery cannulation has been reported to be associated with a high incidence of cerebral infarction in neonates.[76–78] Axillary cannulation, because of the close proximity of the cannulation site and the carotid arteries, also seems likely to pose a significant risk of this complication. The risk of retrograde embolism from the dorsalis pedis artery is vanishingly small, and this fact has been used as another argument for the routine use of this artery.[79]

If the tip of the arterial cannula becomes damaged and dislodged, this can result in embolisation to a peripheral site and necessitate surgical removal. This difficulty is most likely to occur as a result of faulty technique, such as when placement of a needle through a cannula is attempted. Long catheters and wires introduced through an arterial cannula during radiological procedures may also become damaged and dislodged.[44]

- Radiological procedures in which large cannulae are used are associated with a high incidence of complications related to arterial wall damage, such as haematoma and aneurysm formation.

Insertion failure

The Seldinger technique has been demonstrated to be associated with a lower insertion failure rate than a direct puncture technique.[80] Apart from the technique used, the failure rate will depend on many factors including the experience and skill of the operator, the depth and diameter of the artery in relation to the skin, and the blood flow through the artery. It is difficult to consider these factors in isolation from one another, but attention to the points discussed in the preceding chapters should result in an improved success rate.

Cannulation in small children is associated with a high incidence of insertion failure. As previously discussed, failure rates may be reduced with good technique and the use of localisation aids such as Doppler probes.

KEY POINTS

- Arterial cannulation is a procedure that is associated with a large variety of complications, most of which are well known and preventable.
- The incidence of complications is related to the size and type of cannula, the size of the artery cannulated and the duration of cannulation.
- Certain diseases and conditions associated with reduced peripheral perfusion such as shock and critical illness may be associated with a high incidence of ischaemic complications.
- Paediatric cannulation is associated with particular problems because of the small size of the cannulated arteries. This may result in a high incidence of ischaemic problems and a high insertion failure rate.

References

1. Cole FS, Todres ID, Shannon DC. Technique for percutaneous cannulation of the radial artery in the newborn infant. Journal of Pediatrics 1978; **92**:105.
2. Pearse RG. Percutaneous catheterization of the radial artery in newborn babies using transillumination. Archives of Disease in Childhood 1978; **53**:549.
3. Morray JP, Brandford HG, Barnes LF, Oh SM, Furman EB. Doppler-assisted radial artery cannulation in infants and children. Anesthesia and Analgesia 1984; **63**:346.
4. Davis FM, Stewart JM. Radial artery cannulation: a prospective study in patients undergoing cardiothoracic surgery. British Journal of Anaesthesia 1980; **52**:41.
5. Hall R. Vascular injuries resulting from radial artery catheterization. British Journal of Surgery 1971; **58**:513.
6. Arthurs GJ. Case report: digital ischaemia following radial artery cannulation. Anaesthesia and Intensive Care 1978; **6**:54.
7. Golbranson FL, Lurie L, Vance RM, Vandell RF. Multiple extremity amputations in hypotensive patients treated with dopamine. Journal of the American Medical Association 1980; **243**:1145.
8. Lindbom A. Arterial spasm caused by puncture and catheterization. Acta Radiologica 1957; **47**:449.
9. Dalton B, Laver MB. Vasospasm with an indwelling radial artery cannula. Anesthesiology 1971; **34**:194.
10. Sanderson RG, Schock RH. A simple technic of monitoring patency of arterial monitoring cannulas. American Journal of Surgery 1970; **120**:559.
11. Cartwright GW, Schreiner RL. Major complication secondary to percutaneous radial artery catheterization in the neonate. Pediatrics 1980; **65**:139.
12. Ryan JF, Raines J, Dalton BC, Mathieu A. Arterial dynamics of radial artery cannulation. Anesthesia and Analgesia 1973; **52**:1017.
13. Bedford RF, Wollman H. Complications of percutaneous radial-artery cannulation: an objective prospective study in man. Anesthesiology 1973; **38**:228.
14. Evans PJD, Kerr JH. Complications of arterial cannulation and thermographic assessment of sequelae. British Journal of Anesthesia 1974; **46**:318.
15. Spoerel WE, Deimling P, Aitken R. Direct arterial pressure monitoring from the dorsalis pedis artery. Canadian Anaesthetists Society Journal 1975; **22**:91.

16. Goldstein RD, Gordon MJV. Volar proximal skin necrosis after radial artery cannulation. New York State Journal of Medicine 1990; **90**:375.
17. Wyatt R, Glaves I, Cooper DJ. Proximal skin necrosis after radial-artery cannulation. Lancet 1974; **1**:1135.
18. Baker RJ, Chunprapaph B, Nyhus LM. Severe ischemia of the hand following radial artery catheterization. Surgery 1976; **80**:449.
19. Downs JB, Chapman RL, Hawkins IF Jr. Prolonged radial-artery catheterization. An evaluation of heparinized catheters and continuous irrigation. Archives of Surgery 1974; **108**:671.
20. Bedford RF. Long-term radial artery cannulation: effects on subsequent vessel function. Critical Care Medicine 1978; **6**:64.
21. Palm T. Evaluation of peripheral arterial pressure on the thumb following radial artery cannulation. British Journal of Anaesthesia 1977; **49**:819.
22. Cannon BW, Meshier TW. Extremity amputation following radial artery cannulation in a patient with hyperlipoproteinaemia. Anesthesiology 1983; **56**:220.
23. Mayer T, Matlak ME, Thompson JA. Necrosis of the forearm following radial artery catheterization in a patient with Reye's syndrome. Pediatrics 1980; **65**:141.
24. Freed MD, Rosenthal A, Fyler D. Attempts to reduce arterial thrombosis after cardiac catheterization in children: use of percutaneous technique and aspirin. American Heart Journal 1974; **87**:283.
25. Randolph AG, Cook DJ, Gonzales CA, Andrew M. Benefit of heparin in peripheral venous and arterial catheters: systematic review and meta-analysis of randomised controlled trials. British Medical Journal 1998; **316**:969.
26. Butt W, Shann F, McDonnell G, Hudson I. Effect of heparin concentration and infusion rate on the patency of arterial catheters. Critical Care Medicine 1987; **15**:230.
27. Bolgiano CS, Subramaniam PT, Montanari JM, Minick L. The effect of two concentrations of heparin on arterial catheter patency. Critical Care Nurse 1990; **10**:47.
28. Heulitt MJ, Farrington EA, O'Shea TM, Stolzman SM, Srubar NB, Levin DL. Double-blind, randomized, controlled trial of papaverine-containing infusions to prevent failure of arterial catheters in pediatric patients. Critical Care Medicine 1993; **21**:825.
29. Branson PK, McCoy RA, Phillips BA, Clifton GD. Efficacy of 1.4 percent sodium citrate in maintaining arterial catheter patency in patients in a medical ICU. Chest 1993; **103**:882.
30. Rais-Bahrami K, Karna P, Dolanski EA. Effect of fluids on the life span of peripheral arterial lines. American Journal of Perinatology 1990; **7**:122.
31. Bedford RF, Ashford TP. Aspirin pretreatment prevents post-cannulation radial-artery thrombosis. Anesthesiology 1979; **51**:176.
32. Hynes KM, Gau GT, Rutherford BD, Kazmier FJ, Fyre RL. Effect of aspirin on brachial artery occlusion following brachial arteriotomy for coronary angiography. Circulation 1973; **47**:554.
33. Formanek G, Frech RS, Amplatz K. Arterial thrombus formation during clinical percutaneous catheterization. Circulation 1970; **41**:833.
34. Fanning WL, Aronson M. Osler node, Janeway lesions and splinter haemorrhages: occurrence with an infected arterial catheter. Archives of Dermatology 1977; **113**:648.
35. Cohen A, Reyes R, Kirk M, Fulks RM. Osler's nodes, pseudoaneurysm formation, and sepsis complicating percutaneous radial artery cannulation. Critical Care Medicine 1984; **12**:1078.
36. Norwood SH, Cormier B, McMahon NG, Moss A, Moore V. Prospective study of catheter-related infection during prolonged arterial catheterization. Critical Care Medicine 1988; **16**:836.
37. Maki DG, Band JD. A comparative study of polyantibiotic and iodophor ointments in prevention of vascular catheter-related infections. American Journal of Medicine 1981; **70**:739.
38. Kamal GD, Pfaller MA, Rempe LE, Jebson PJR. Reduced intravascular catheter infection by antibiotic bonding: a prospective, randomized, controlled trial. Journal of the American Medical Association 1991; **265**:2364.
39. Band JD, Maki DG. Infections caused by arterial catheters used for hemodynamic monitoring. American Journal of Medicine 1979; **67**:735.
40. Dryden GE, Brickler J. Stopcock contamination. Anesthesia and Analgesia 1979; **58**:141.
41. Maki DG, Hassemer CA. Endemic rate of fluid contamination and related septicaemia in arterial pressure monitoring. American Journal of Medicine 1981; **70**:733.
42. Hayes MF, Morello DC, Rosenbaum RW, Matsumoto T. Radial artery cannulation by cutdown technique. Critical Care Medicine 1973; **1**:151.
43. Tooley WH. What is the risk of an umbilical artery catheter? Pediatrics 1972; **50**:1.
44. Aagard P, Davidsen HG, Andreassen M. Complications in percutaneous arteriography. Acta Chirurgica Scandinavica 1960; **119**:186.
45. Eriksson I, Jorulf H. Surgical complications associated with arterial catheterization. Scandinavian Journal of Thoracic and Cardiovascular Surgery 1970; **4**:69.
46. Wolf S, Mangano DT. Pseudoaneurysm, a late complication of radial-artery catheterization. Anesthesiology 1980; **52**:80.
47. Russell RC, Steichen JB, Zook EG. Radial-arteries pseudoaneurysms – their diagnosis, treatment and prevention. Orthopaedic Review 1979; **8**:49.
48. O'Malley CM Jr, Paulson EK, Kliewer MA, Tcheng JE, Hertzberg BS, Carroll BA. Color Doppler sonographic appearance of patent needle tracts after femoral arterial catheterization. Radiology 1995; **197**:163.
49. Sacks D, Robinson ML, Perlmutter GS. Femoral artery injury following catheterization: duplex evaluation. Journal of Ultrasound in Medicine 1989; **8**:241.
50. Schwartz RA, Kerns DB, Mitchell DG. Color Doppler ultrasound imaging in iatrogenic arterial injuries. American Journal of Surgery 1991; **162**:4.

51. Littler WA. Median nerve palsy: a complication of brachial artery cannulation. Postgraduate Medical Journal 1974; **52**:110.
52. Marshall G, Edelstein G, Hirshman CA. Median nerve compression following radial artery puncture. Anesthesia and Analgesia 1980; **59**:953.
53. Adler DC, Bryan-Brown CW. Use of the axillary artery for intravascular monitoring. Critical Care Medicine 1973; **1**:148.
54. De Angelis J. Axillary arterial monitoring. Critical Care Medicine 1976; **4**:205.
55. Koenigsberger MR, Moessinger AC. Iatrogenic carpal tunnel syndrome in the newborn infant. Journal of Pediatrics 1977; **91**:443.
56. Luce EA, Futrell JW, Wilgris EFS. Compression neuropathy following brachial artery puncture in anticoagulated patients. Journal of Trauma 1976; **16**:717.
57. Macon WL, Futrell JW. Median-nerve neuropathy after percutaneous puncture of the brachial artery in patient receiving anticoagulants. New England Journal of Medicine 1973; **228**:1396.
58. Mathieu A, Dalton B, Fischer JE, Kumar A. Expanding aneurysm of the radial artery after frequent puncture. Anesthesiology 1973; **38**:401.
59. Herman B. Complication of retrograde femoral artery catheterization. Archives of Surgery 1964; **88**:374.
60. Wolfman EF, Boblitt DE. Intramural aortic dissection as a complication of translumbar aortography. Archives of Surgery 1959; **78**:629.
61. Movitz D. Dissecting aneurysm of the femoral and popliteal artery. Surgery 1959; **45**:834.
62. Arrowsmith JJ. Extracorporeal pseudoaneurysm: an unusual complication of radial artery cannulation. Anaesthesia 1991; **46**:894.
63. Sladen A. Complications of radial artery catheterization. Current Problems in Surgery 1988; **25**:82.
64. Glaser RL, McKellar D, Scher KS. Arteriovenous fistulas after cardiac catheterization. Archives of Surgery 1989; **124**:1313.
65. Knowles JA. Accidental intra-arterial injection of penicillin. American Journal of Diseases of Children 1966; **111**:552.
66. McGrath P. Accidental intra-arterial flucloxacillin: management using guanethidine. Anaesthesia and Intensive Care 1983; **20**:517.
67. Kinmonth JB, Shepherd RC. Accidental injection of thiopentone into arteries: study of pathology and treatment. British Medical Journal 1959; **2**:918.
68. Aweibel FR, Monies-Chas I. Accidental intraarterial injection of ketamine. Anaesthesia 1976; **31**:1084.
69. Topazian RG. Accidental intra-arterial injection: a hazard of intravenous medication. Journal of the American Dental Association 1970; **81**:410.
70. Cohen SM. Accidental intra-arterial injection of drugs. Lancet 1948; **2**:361.
71. Evans JM, Latto IP, Ng WS. Accidental intra-arterial injection of drugs: a hazard of arterial cannulation. British Journal of Anaesthesia 1974; **46**:463.
72. Lowenstein E, Little JW, Lo HH. Prevention of cerebral embolization from flushing radial artery cannulae. New England Journal of Medicine 1971; **285**:1414.
73. Edmonds JF, Barker GA, Conn AW. Current concepts in cardiovascular monitoring in children. Critical Care Medicine 1980; **8**:548.
74. Chang C, Dughi J, Shitabata P, Johnson G, Coel M, McNamara JJ. Air embolism and the radial arterial line. Critical Care Medicine 1988; **16**:141.
75. Meguid M, Bevilacqua R. Management of arterial cannulas. New England Journal of Medicine 1972; **286**:376.
76. Prian GW. Complications and sequelae of temporal artery catheterisation in the high risk newborn. Journal of Pediatric Surgery 1977; **12**:829.
77. Prian GW, Wright GB, Rumach CM, O'Meara OP. Apparent cerebral embolization after temporal artery catheterization. Journal of Pediatrics 1978; **93**:115.
78. Bull MJ, Schreiner RL, Garg BP, Hutton NM, Lemons JA, Gresham EL. Neurologic complications following temporal artery catheterization. Journal of Pediatrics 1980; **96**:1071.
79. Johnstone RE, Greenhow DE. Catheterization of the dorsalis pedis artery. Anesthesiology 1973; **39**:654.
80. Beards SC, Doedens L, Jackson A, Lipman J. A comparison of arterial lines and insertion techniques in critically ill patients. Anaesthesia 1994; **49**:968.

Part 4

Arterial Catheterisation: Paediatric and neonatal procedures

19 • General Considerations

PETER JONES

Reasons for Seeking Arterial Access

The major indications for introducing cannulae into arteries are (a) continuous measurement of arterial pressure,[1] and (b) intermittent arterial blood sampling.

An arterial cannula offers convenience and reliability for patient monitoring in infants and children but is not without complications and should therefore be reserved for cases in which the risks are justified. Indications include major surgery and the management of patients experiencing rapid and substantial variations in their haemodynamic state. The percutaneous route to arterial cannulation is generally appropriate unless the vessel cannot be identified by its pulsation, when surgical cut-down may be indicated. Alternative, non-invasive methods for monitoring blood pressure have been shown to correlate well with direct measurements.[2–5] Transcutaneous monitors for oxygen and carbon dioxide tensions are well established and give continuous estimation of arterial blood tension. However, they are afflicted by practical difficulties which compromise their accuracy and continuity of service, suggesting the restriction of their use to neonatal intensive care units.[6] The use of these devices in conjunction with heel prick capillary samples for intermittent acid–base analysis should be carefully considered before arterial cannulation is undertaken in infants and children. Additional information can be obtained from invasive pressure waveforms. They can be filtered to reveal the respiratory component and have been used to monitor for apnoeic episodes.[7]

Less frequent indications for cannulation include exchange transfusions in infants of very low birthweight (approximately 1 kg);[8] haemofiltration;[9–13] and continuous monitoring of biochemical parameters. A number of catheter tip devices have been developed for continuous monitoring of oxygen tension,[14–16] arterial oxygen saturation,[17,18] haematocrit[18] and blood biochemical status in infants. These devices are introduced through cannulae and may require larger sizes than those normally recommended (see below).

Extracorporeal membrane oxygenation (ECMO) in infants requires flow rates in the range 80–120 ml/kg per hour.[19] The venous cannulae required to achieve this rate of drainage by gravity are too large for introduction percutaneously. It is therefore the general practice that both cannulae for arteriovenous ECMO and venovenous ECMO are introduced surgically.

Choosing the Artery

Anatomical considerations

Cannulation of arteries in infants and children poses extra risks when compared with the adult because the vessels are more delicately constructed, have a smaller bore and their routes follow tighter contours. In the long term, they are also more likely to be associated with structures in the event of intimal or mural trauma since any scar tissue that forms will restrict the rate of growth of the vessel. The impairment of blood flow and tissue oxygenation that would ensue from a significant stricture might be expected to affect the performance and the rate of growth of the affected limb.[20,21] The incidence of vessel occlusion and flow impairment correlates inversely with the size of cannula used.[22]

Axillary artery

The axillary artery has been recommended for cannulation when more peripheral vessels are impalpable because of shock or trauma[23] and is reasonably safe for cannulation in the critical care environment despite its being an end-artery.[24] A recent series of 62 neonates encountered no complications arising from a mean period of cannulation of 4.1 days.[25]

Brachial artery

The brachial artery has been used for both direct and percutaneous access. Being an end-artery, the consequences of its damage and occlusion are catastrophic[26] and the site can therefore no longer be recommended. The axillary artery is preferable for cannulation because it is larger and more easily palpable in a shocked child or infant.

Radial and ulnar arteries

It is considered relatively safe for either the radial or the ulnar artery (Figure 19.1) to be punctured or cannulated at the level of the wrist because the superficial and deep palmar arches provide an alternative pathway for delivery of oxygenated blood to the distal tissues in the event of either vessel becoming occluded. This logic does not support the practice of attempting to cannulate either vessel when the other is known to be damaged or occluded. Various tests, mostly based on Allen's test,[27] have been described to establish the patency of the palmar arterial arch and are considered to enhance the safety of radial artery cannulation.[28] The importance of a collateral circulation is

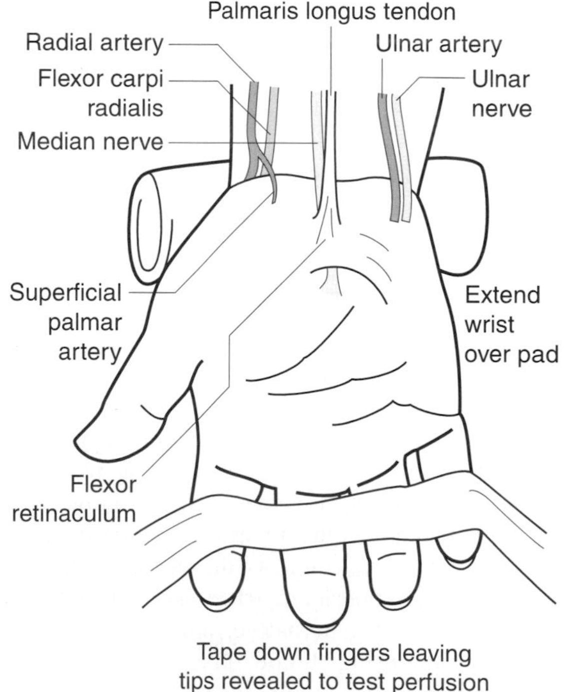

Figure 19.1 Radial and ulnar artery relations at the wrist.

highlighted in infants where the incidence of total radial artery occlusion after removal of the cannula has been recorded as more than 60%.[29] In one series including children and adults, nearly 30% had impaired flow and 10% had absent pulses after radial artery cannulation, though none had symptoms of hand ischaemia.[30] An investigation of adults and children, in which Allen's test was enhanced by strain gauge estimation of thumb blood pressure, revealed inadequate collateral circulation in 27 (adults) of 259 investigated (10%),[31] leading the authors to recommend the use of Allen's test as an exclusion test prior to cannulation. This use of Allen's test for predicting ischaemic sequelae of cannulation is contested.[22,32] The unmodified and modified (timed)[33] Allen tests are difficult to perform adequately on the neonatal wrist because of the comparatively enormous size of the operator's and assistant's fingers. Consequently, a number of alternative procedures have been recommended. Some involve the employment of specialist equipment including strain gauge plethysmography of the thumb[31,34] and ultrasonic flow probes.[22]

The radial artery is preferred for routine cannulation because it is the larger vessel and is less likely to be occluded by the cannula. It is accessible for palpation and cannulation as it runs alongside and lateral to the flexor pollicis longus tendon on the flexor surface of the wrist. A branch of the radial artery, arising at the wrist, passes through the origin of the abductor pollicis brevis to form the superficial palmar arch, together with a branch of the ulnar artery. It has been shown that the main blood supply to the fingers is via the superficial palmar arch, and that in most adults (88%) the arch is predominantly supplied by the ulnar artery, in 10% it is predominantly supplied by the radial artery, and in less than 2% the supply is exclusively from the radial artery.[35] Access for cannulation of the ulnar artery is compromised because it is closely accompanied along its medial margin at the wrist by the ulnar nerve.

As with other arteries, it is generally recommended that the cannula is inserted in a direction retrograde to that of flow within the vessel. Normally, this implies that the cannula tip points towards the axilla. Nevertheless, because an already obstructed vessel may receive blood in a retrograde direction through the palmar arches, there is a certain logic to introducing the catheter at the wrist in a downward direction in this particular circumstance.[36]

The radial artery has been successfully used for indwelling catheters and cannulae in neonates with a low incidence of complications,[37,38] avoiding the sinister problems associated with umbilical artery catheterisation.[39] It is therefore the preferred choice for arterial cannulation in infants and children even though the consequence of thrombus and embolus formation is likely to be more severe in these groups than in adults because of the greater effect of a given embolus on a small arterial tree.

Carotid artery

The carotid artery is not recommended for cannulation because of the serious consequences attending the liberation of emboli. The degree of protection afforded by the circle of Willis against the ischaemic consequence to the brain following occlusion of the carotid artery is variable and does not justify carotid artery interference. Radiological procedures are more safely undertaken by catheterisation of the femoral artery and retrograde advancement of a catheter through the aortic arch than by direct carotid puncture.

Superficial temporal artery

Cannulation of the superficial temporal artery requires its localisation by a Doppler ultrasound probe followed by percutaneous vessel puncture using a cannula-over-needle technique through a 3 mm skin incision.[40] This is claimed to offer greater reliability than radial artery cannulation with comparable thrombotic complications including a 5% incidence of retrograde thrombosis of the posterior auricular artery.[41] An alternative, surgical approach has been claimed to offer long-term effectiveness with no complications.[42] Other authors endorse the safety of the vessel for arterial cannulation, though their experience is limited.[43–45]

Internal mammary artery

The internal mammary artery is unsuitable for percutaneous access, although it can be readily cannulated during thoracic surgery.[46] It may be unwise to compromise this vessel for use as a graft in later life. Decannulation carries the risk of uncontrollable bleeding.

Umbilical artery

Each umbilical artery arises from the ipsilateral internal iliac artery (Figure 19.2). The abdominal aorta terminates by bifurcating into the left and right common iliac arteries, each of which then divides at the pelvic brim into the internal and external iliac arteries. The umbilical arteries are accessible to catheterisation at birth and, with decreasing success, for up to 4 days thereafter. In normal infants the umbilical arteries constrict within a few minutes of birth but this process is delayed in infants suffering hypoxia and acidosis.[47] Umbilical artery catheterisation was first described by Nelson in 1962.[48] A catheter is advanced into the aorta until its tip comes to rest at one of several identified sites,[49–51] though two are preferred.[52] The procedure of catheterisation is easily learned and is generally successful when it is attempted close to the moment of birth.

Severe developmental abnormalities of the abdominal wall do not preclude umbilical artery cannulation. Filston has described a technique for transposing the vessels to the lower abdomen.[53]

There have been a number of serious complications, mostly thrombotic events, which have accounted for the diminishing popularity of the technique.

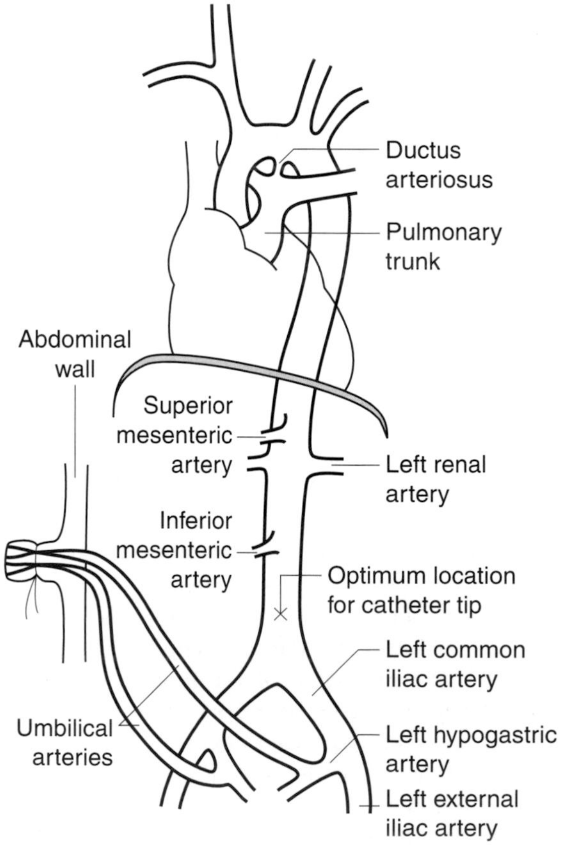

Figure 19.2 Umbilical arteries – origins and course.

Femoral artery

The femoral artery (Figure 19.3) emerges from under the midpoint of the inguinal ligament and descends medially to provide almost the entire blood supply to the leg. It is a large vessel, flanked in the groin by the femoral vein medially and the femoral nerve laterally. It overlies the hip joint, a structure that is vulnerable to damage and contamination by pathogens during attempts to access or cannulate the femoral vessels. Catheterisation of the femoral artery for monitoring purposes is readily achievable in a high proportion of at-risk children. However, it carries a 10% risk of severe catheter spasm which necessitates immediate catheter removal.[54] Nevertheless, for long-term access, it is considered to be a valuable alternative to small vessel catheterisation when the latter is not achievable, for example in children with extensive burns.[55] Femoral artery cannulation for radiological purposes carries a 5% incidence of short-term severe spasm whilst femoral artery thrombosis occurs in a further 5%, largely as a result of intimal damage.[56–58] Whilst resting blood flow appears unaffected, maximal blood flow has been shown to be significantly reduced in the catheterised leg for several years after femoral arterial catheterisation

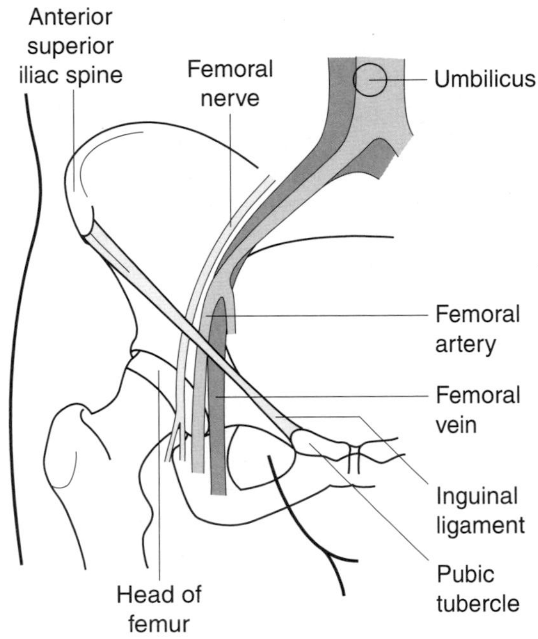

Figure 19.3 Femoral artery relations in the groin.

for radiological purposes.[59] Therapeutic (non-radiological) catheterisation in the neonatal period has been associated with ipsilateral leg growth impairment.[60] Streptokinase infusion is generally effective in treating arterial thrombosis when it occurs as a complication of femoral arterial catheterisation.[60] Compartment syndrome has been reported in association with femoral artery cannulation in an 11-month-old child.[61]

Posterior tibial artery

The posterior tibial artery (Figure 19.4) can be palpated as it terminates between the medial malleolus and the medial tubercle of the calcaneum. It lies in a groove with the tendons of tibialis posterior and flexor digitorum longus anterior to it and the tibial nerve lies posteriorly. It is at this point that the artery is accessible to cannulation. In premature neonates it can be visualised by transillumination[62] whilst in older children it is readily palpable. It is best cannulated after cutting down upon it in term infants.[63] The artery supplies the sole of the foot via the medial and lateral plantar arteries. The lateral

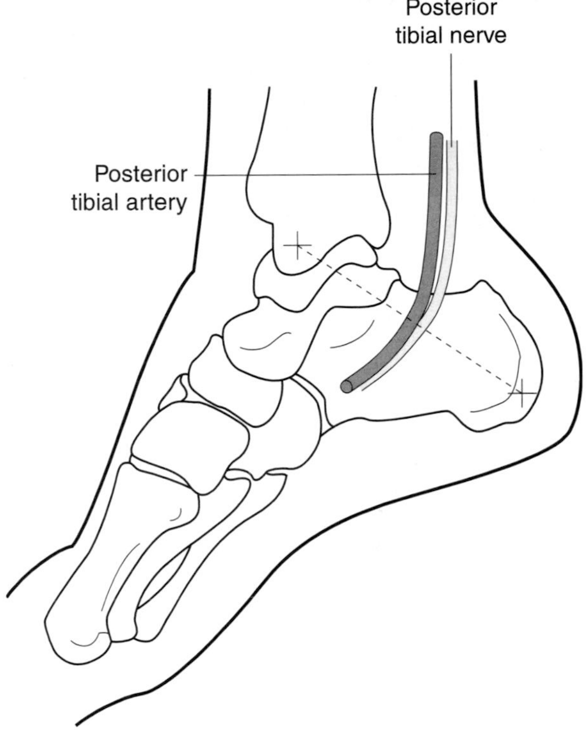

Figure 19.4 Posterior tibial artery location at the ankle.

plantar artery provides the major contribution to the plantar arch, which also receives some supply from the dorsalis pedis artery. The dependency of the foot upon blood supplied by the posterior tibial artery, combined with its close medial relation to the posterior tibial nerve, renders this vessel a somewhat contentious point for arterial access. The vessel has been used successfully in neonates.[43,63]

Dorsalis pedis artery

The dorsalis pedis is the continuation of the anterior tibial artery. It can be palpated on its course down the dorsum of the foot, lying parallel with and lateral to the extensor pollicis longus tendon. In the first intermetatarsal space, it penetrates to the sole to join the lateral plantar artery, completing the plantar arch. It is this collateral circulation that renders the vessel safe to cannulate. The vessel supplies blood to the toes. It is of small calibre but is otherwise readily accessible for cannulation. The vessel has been used clinically in adults[64] and neonates.[43] The dorsalis pedis artery is subject to significant variation in the population and has been found to be bilaterally impalpable in 5.3% of children.[65]

Choosing the Equipment

Dimensional considerations

In attempting to predict the dimensions of a vessel in an infant or child, it is reasonable to apply

Table 19.1 Dimensions of Stubs needle gauge and French gauge

Gauge number (G, g, gauge, gage)	Birmingham or Stubs needle gauge diameter (mm)	French Gauge (FG, Fg, Fr or F)
10	3.404	10.7
11	3.048	9.6
12	2.769	8.7
13	2.413	7.6
14	2.108	6.6
15	1.829	5.7
16	1.651	5.2
17	1.473	4.6
18	1.245	3.9
19	1.067	3.3
20	0.889	2.8
21	0.813	2.6
22	0.711	2.2
23	0.635	2.0
24	0.559	1.8
25	0.508	1.6
26	0.457	1.4
27	0.406	1.3
28	0.356	1.1
29	0.330	1.0
30	0.305	1.0
31	0.254	0.8
32	0.229	0.7
33	0.203	0.6
34	0.178	0.6
35	0.127	0.4
36	0.102	0.3

French Gauge (F, Fr, FG, Fg) and Charriere (Ch.) are numerically identical and are used for measuring flexible catheters where the diameter may not be constant because of dyormation. They are numerically equal to the circumference of the catheter, measured in millimeters. The abbreviations shown have appeared in iteraure or catalogues and are not necessarily 'approved'.

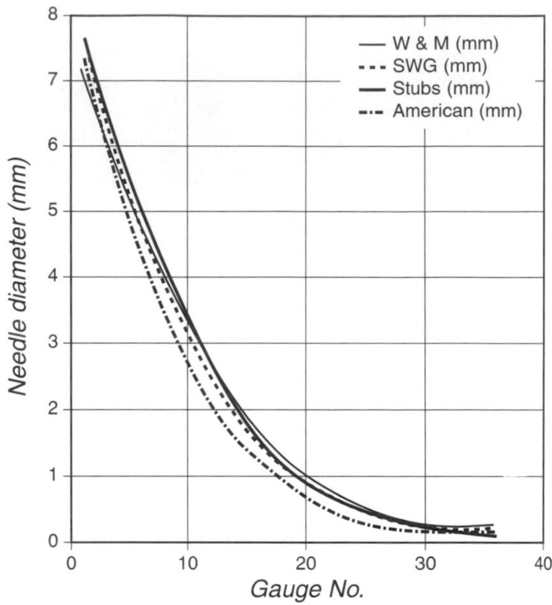

Figure 19.5 Dimensions of various wire gauges. The figure illustrates the similarities of four standard wire gauges. Stubs needle gauge (also known as Birmingham gauge), Washburn and Moen (W&M) and Imperial Standard Wire Gauge (SWG) are very similar throughout the range. Only American wire gauge is significantly different. It appears not to be used for clinical needles.

conventional scaling factors. For example, the infant is approximately a third of the length of the adult. All linear dimensions are likely to be similarly miniaturised even though there is substantial variation from this generalisation because the infant is not simply a miniature adult. On average, however, it is reasonable to reduce the dimensions of catheters and cannulae proportionally. Since the French (F) or Charrière scale represents the circumference of a catheter in millimetres, selecting a suitably miniaturised instrument for a neonate is simply a matter of dividing the size that is appropriate for adults by 3 (or, more accurately, by 3.14; see Chapter 12). Thus, a 6F catheter for an adult (2 mm diameter) would be reduced to a 2 F catheter (0.67 mm diameter) for an infant and its length would also be reduced to one third. It must be remembered that the Luer-Lok hub of the device has not been scaled and so the extracutaneous portion of the catheter cannot be so reduced. Consequently, a 5 cm catheter may not be an entirely suitable neonatal equivalent for a 15 cm adult catheter intended for femoral artery cannulation. These considerations are not assisted by the obscure nature of the most widely used size criterion in needle and catheter manufacture – the Stubs needle gauge (Table 19.1). The Stubs gauge is similar to the Standard Wire Gauge (Figure 19.5).

Catheter and cannula materials

Historically, cannulae were made of metal and therefore rigid (e.g. the Guest cannula) whilst catheters have always been manufactured from flexible material. Modern vascular cannulae are made of flexible material but achieve rigidity during insertion by being introduced over needles. They are generally relatively short. Catheters, in contrast, are much longer and are introduced through needles or cannulae or, increasingly, over a flexible wire guide such as a Seldinger wire. The ideal arterial cannula would be capable of insertion as a catheter-over-needle device, exhibiting low friction, thereby avoiding intimal damage, offering no surface upon which platelets or bacteria could become attached, becoming soft enough to be compliant with the vessel contour and totally resistant to kinking. No such material exists. In one review of 1000 radial artery cannulations, the use of polytetrafluoroethylene (PTFE, Teflon) as the catheter material significantly reduced the incidence of complications.[28] This material is now used by many manufacturers because of its slippery surface and its relative resistance to platelet adhesion. The Medicut cannula (Aloe Medical, St Louis, Mo, USA), a tapering cannula manufactured from relatively stiff polypropylene, has been criticised both for its contour and its material characteristics[66] though these claims are refuted as clinically insignificant by Marshall *et al.*[67] Flexibility is less important in arterial cannulae than in venous cannulae because they are shorter and follow a fairly straight course. Kink resistance, a quality encouraged by the use of thicker-walled tubing, is desirable because of the location of so many arterial cannulation sites over joints. Polyethylene and PTFE exhibit elastic memory. This endows cannulae made from these materials with an irritating tendency to repeatedly kink at the same place once kinking has occurred. Polyurethane, a synthetic rubber copolymer, can be formulated to possess extended physical characteristics, but its rubber-like behaviour means that it possesses very little elastic memory. It is therefore not weakened by being kinked and recovers its original contour immediately the deforming force is removed. This material has another useful quality for the manufacture of cannulae – that of temperature-dependent stiffness. It is therefore possible to fashion a cannula that at room temperature can be readily inserted as a catheter-over-needle device, but then softens at body temperature to approach the pliability of silicone elastomer, becoming sufficiently flexible to minimise the risk of intimal damage. An increasing number of cannulae and catheters are being manufactured from this copolymer.

Surface characteristics

As with venous catheters and cannulae, the surface of an arterial cannula should not permit ready adhesion by platelets. Nevertheless, the high flow velocity in an artery reduces the likelihood of thrombus formation, rendering unnecessary the use of Hydromer, anticoagulant or antimicrobial coatings, provided that the cannula does not significantly block the vessel.

Practical Aspects of Techniques

Sedation and anaesthesia

Arterial cannulation is rendered much more uncertain if the child is struggling. Some form of sedation or anaesthesia is therefore necessary in most small children if they are not seriously debilitated. Midazolam, initially 0.5 mg/kg given orally or slowly intravenously under continuous medical supervision, is a convenient sedative, but light general anaesthesia is more reliable and therefore to be preferred whenever feasible.

Positioning the child for arterial catheterisation

Unlike central venous cannulation, where the position of the vein may be somewhat obscure, localisation of the artery and its subsequent cannulation are almost always facilitated by a palpable pulsation. The approach to cannulation is usually in a retrograde direction. Consequently the point of puncture, the direction of the needle and the position of the operator become a matter of common sense. Only the angle of inclination of the introducer device to the skin needs guidance.

The posture of the patient is generally one that renders the vessel most obvious and, by placing it under slight stretch, less able to escape the advancing needle. Some form of restraining technique or device may be necessary.

Finding the vessel

In critically ill infants and children, particularly if they are obese, localisation of an artery can be difficult. A number of techniques have been developed to assist in this task.

Palpation

The first approach to localising an artery is to palpate it. With the solitary exception of the umbilical artery, only arteries that can be localised by palpable pulsation should be cannulated percutaneously. A child who is so hypotensive that no arteries are palpable should be resuscitated with fluid and inotropic drugs before an attempt is made to cannulate an artery. Impalpable arteries are better cannulated surgically. In infants and small children, in whom blood pressure is substantially lower than in fit adults, palpation requires a gentle and sensitive touch. This can be aided if the operator changes surgical gloves for the thinner latex 'procedure' gloves. It may be necessary to discard gloves altogether. Care must then be taken to avoid touching the point of needle insertion on the prepared skin, and intermittent respraying of the hands and the puncture area with alcoholic chlorhexidine is required after the fashion of Lister's 'antiseptic surgery'.

Pulse oximetry

When confronted with a femoral artery that is difficult to localise, this author exploits the pulse display of a pulse oximeter. The oximeter probe is attached to a toe of the ipsilateral foot and adjusted until a good waveform is obtained. The femoral artery may then be located as it emerges from beneath the inguinal ligament by exploring the area with a pointed but blunt object to which firm downward pressure is applied in an effort to compress the vessel. The vessel is identified by marked diminution or disappearance of the pulse waveform. A simple bleeping pulse meter would suffice but such devices are no longer readily available. A similar technique has been advocated for identifying the dorsalis pedis artery[68] in which a pulse oximeter probe is placed on the second toe, the posterior tibial artery is compressed and the front of the foot is explored with a finger or a probe until loss of pulse amplitude reveals the location of the dorsalis pedis artery. Pulse oximetry has also been used to confirm the integrity of the palmar arch as part of a modified Allen's test.[69,70]

Transillumination

The availability of intense cold light sources with fibreoptic light guides has led to the discovery that transillumination of extremities in infants can assist in revealing both arteries[62,63,71] and veins[72] for puncture. Not all light sources are suitable since some deliver substantial heat and can readily cause burns. For radial artery cannulation, the wrist is simply dorsiflexed over the probe tip. The technique can be used for displaying the radial, ulnar, posterior tibial and dorsalis pedis arteries[62] and is particularly suitable for premature infants where the vessels may be difficult to palpate. It is helpful to attach a short length of black rubber tubing over the tip of the light probe. This can then be pressed against the skin in order to eliminate the dazzle of stray light whilst minimising the possibility of contact burns.

Doppler ultrasound

In a fluid medium, the angulation of a flow-sensitive piezoelectric Doppler ultrasound probe over a vessel containing moving liquid provides an electrical signal which can be transformed into an audible sound or visual display. The characteristic sounds of blood moving in an artery and a vein are easily distinguished. The arterial signal consists of discrete bursts of relatively high-pitched noise, while the venous signal is a modulated, continuous rumble. By suitably designing the probe and maintaining a fluid sound path (usually with specially formulated gel), this principle can be exploited for localising arteries as an aid to cannulation.[73] More recently, the principle has been extended to permit a Doppler ultrasound signal to be transmitted and received down the obturator of a catheter-over-needle device (PD Access percutaneous Doppler device, Cardiovascular Dynamics Inc., Irvine, Calif, USA). Single-use transducers equipped with needles, cannulae or peel-apart introducer cannulae are available in sizes down to 22 gauge (needle size) (includes the cannula). In use, the needle is introduced through a blob of ultrasound gel or thoroughly wetted skin, preferably through a small puncture wound which can be made with a blood sampling stylet. The needle must approach the artery at an angle for the Doppler signal to be generated. The hand-held console offers both audible and visual indicators of signal strength, thereby assisting in guiding the needle to the vessel.

Ultrasound imaging

The majority of diagnostic ultrasound imaging machines are unsuited for routine use as an aid to obtaining vascular access because their probes are designed to scan too deeply into the body and the machines are too large (and expensive) for them to be routinely available in operating theatres and intensive care units to assist venous access. The Dymax Site-Rite (Dymax Corporation, Pittsburgh, Pa, USA) is a real-time ultrasound imager which is small, portable and battery-powered (Figure 19.6). It can be fitted with two specialist probes: the 7.5 megahertz probe images structures 1–4 cm beneath the skin and the 9 MHz probe views structures 0–2 cm deep. This latter probe, combined with the facility to magnify the image to twice its real size on the incorporated monochrome cathode-ray tube screen, is well suited to visualising small vessels in infants and for guiding needles and cannulae into them. The 7.5 MHz probe is better suited to visualising deeper structures, in adults. The probe can be introduced into a sterile field by encasing it in a gel-filled latex sheath. The tip of the probe is equipped with a grooved needle-guide which directs an applied needle at a steep angle towards the target area under the probe when the sheath is used. Although manufacturers encourage the use of specialist ultrasound conductive gel to achieve the link between the tissues and the probe face, an adequate image can be obtained using normal liquid skin preparation fluids as the interface. This expedient permits the probe to be applied to the prepared skin surface without the need for an isolating sheath but precludes the employment of the needle-guide. Although the Site-Rite has no colour-flow Doppler facility, adjacent arteries and veins can be easily distinguished by gently raising and lowering the probe while retaining contact with the skin surface. The vein can be seen to be readily deformed and compressed, whilst the artery retains its circular cross-sectional contour. The acute angle of the needle guide renders it

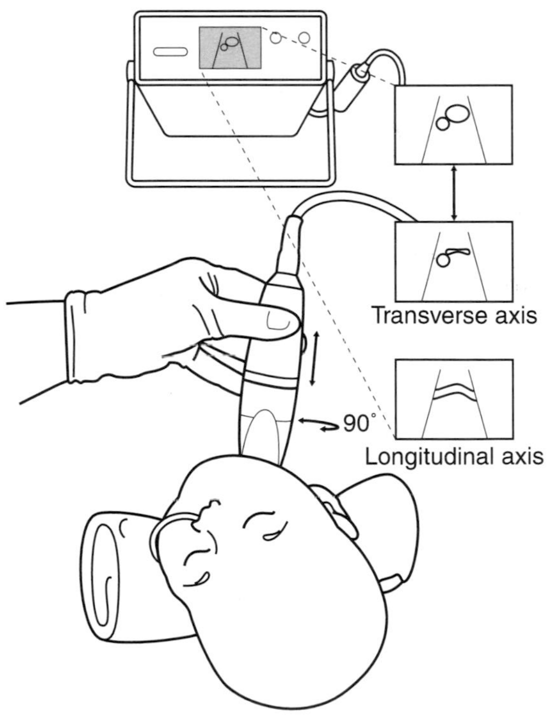

Figure 19.6 Identifying arteries and veins using the Site-Rite (Dymax, Pittsburgh, Pa, USA).

relatively unsuitable for arterial cannulation although the image is of great assistance in monitoring the progress of an exploring needle. Even when the needle is too fine to be resolved on screen, its influence in deforming the structures ahead of it defines its progress. The device enhances both the success of cannulation and the avoidance of damage to other structures.

The Site-Rite device can be used with benefit to identify and guide cannulation of several arteries, particularly the femoral and axillary arteries in children. It is sometimes helpful to rotate the face of the probe through 90° so that the artery is identified by seeing its long axis pulsating on the screen before returning to the original transverse attitude. By this means, relatively inconspicuous vessels can be more readily identified. The 9 MHz probe, combined with the ability to double the linear displayed magnification on the Mark II Site-Rite, greatly facilitates identification of superficial small vessels such as the radial artery in children.

Preparation of the insertion site

In infants and children, arteries are usually cannulated using the smallest sizes of venous cannulae. These are not particularly flexible. Although arterial cannulation sites have a gratifyingly low incidence of infectious complications, careful skin preparation remains important. Children who require vascular cannulation are often also immunocompromised, and in these patients normal skin contaminants can induce lethal septicaemia if introduced by skin puncture.[74] Surgical spirit (ethanol, degraded with methanol, methyl salicylate, diethyl phthalate and castor oil) is an effective bacteriostatic agent. Its combination with chlorhexidine provides satisfactory skin preparation when applied using a mildly abrasive cotton swab since the degreasing effect removes the loose layers of skin and oils. The process provides a better key for the adhesive dressings and tapes used to secure the cannula. Iodine, either ionic or organic, is generally unnecessary, and risks a skin eruption or worse in sensitised individuals. In its powder formulations, the residue prevents adhesive dressings from adhering properly. Excess skin preparation fluids should be carefully wiped from the skin and care should be taken to avoid spillage. Serious skin damage[75] and necrosis have been reported in neonates who were left to lie in a pool of spilt alcohol; blood alcohol estimations have revealed toxic levels of both ethanol and methanol caused by transdermal absorption in such circumstances.[76]

Securing the arterial cannula

It is an unfortunate reality that arteries are most accessible to cannulation as they pass over joints. This requires that, in children at least, some form of splint or restraining device is necessary as a part of the cannula fixation (Figure 19.7). The effect must be to restrict flexion of the joint without causing tissue damage by compression or circumferential constriction of the limb. It is preferable that purpose-designed splints are employed since improvisation with cotton wool, swabs and tongue depressors may be less than satisfactory. Tongue

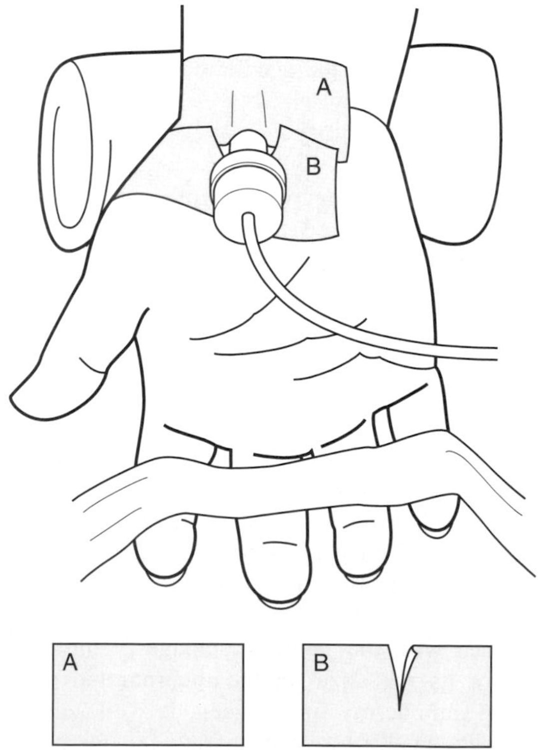

Figure 19.7 Securing the arterial cannula.

depressors have been identified as a vector for infection among debilitated neonates.[77]

The venous cannulae which are so frequently used for peripheral arterial access are less flexible than catheters. Consequently any unwarranted movement at the point of skin insertion is transmitted to the tip of the cannula which is likely to damage the adjacent vessel wall. The current vogue for fixing cannulae with self-adhesive, microporous, vapour-permeable, hypoallergenic transparent dressings is driven by the need to find a material that does not become detached when the patient sweats and is unlikely to transmit pathogens to the puncture site. Unfortunately, these materials are, of necessity, gossamer thin, and therefore unable to offer the support necessary to prevent excessive movement in an active child. The fixation offered by two strips of 2.5 cm wide zinc oxide woven stretch tape (e.g. Elastoplast, Smith & Nephew Healthcare Ltd, Hull, UK), one of which has been cut half across, is very much more secure and generally more satisfactory for fixing arterial lines to the extremities of children (Figure 19.7). This is particularly so if the cannula hub is equipped with wings. The hub itself must have Luer-Lok lugs to provide a secure locking seal with the Luer-Lok flushing/sampling line. Non-locking connectors MUST NEVER BE USED in arterial tubing systems. The line itself should be looped loosely and attached to the skin, separately from the cannula dressing. Finally, where appropriate, the limb should be gently bandaged. Some children will need to be discouraged from interfering with this assembly by having their hands swathed with cotton wool or similar padding to minimise their natural destructive dexterity, while permitting the finger or toe tips distal to the arterial cannulation site to be visible for inspection. The increased risk of ischaemic necrosis following intimal damage or the need to resite a cannula should be sufficient incentive for this practice to become more widespread.

Care of the infusion systems

Continuous arterial line flush systems have been shown to reduce occlusion incidents.[28] Intermittent flushing, even with high heparin concentrations, fails to protect arterial catheters from blockage.[37] Single-use monitoring kits designed for connection to arterial catheters provide a continuous flush by restricting the flow from a pressurised reservoir to approximately 3 ml per hour. This may be insignificant when calculating the fluid balance of adults, but in neonates and small children, particularly those with renal compromise, both the flow and composition of the flush fluid need to be considered. It may be possible to reduce the flush rate sufficiently simply by reducing the pressure in the bag of flushing fluid.

In neonates and small children, the pressurised bag infusion set provided with arterial flush kits should be replaced by a syringe pump which can be adjusted to deliver 0.5–1 ml per hour of flush. This is connected to the retained restrictor and rapid flush assembly of the monitoring kit. It is then only necessary to operate this flush while transiently actuating the purge mechanism of the pump to clear the cannula and manometer line after taking a sample of blood. The syringe drive mechanism should not be disengaged during the rapid flushing sequence because backlash in the mechanism will allow blood to re-enter the catheter where it may clot. Generally, the flush needs to be isotonic and should contain no more than 1 IU/ml of heparin.[78] This has been shown to reduce catheter occlusion but not intravascular thrombus formation.[79] It has been claimed that sodium heparin with chlorobutol should be used as the anticoagulant because chlorobutol is believed to be responsible for the improved tissue Po_2 encountered distal to a cannulated radial artery compared with the non-cannulated one.[80] Whereas saline is the preferred flush solution for adults because it does not support bacterial growth, the sodium intolerance of infants may dictate the use of 5% dextrose solution. When taking a sample of blood for analysis, it is necessary to interrupt the flush flow, then withdraw a quantity of fluid through the sampling port before taking the sample in order to minimise contamination with the flush solution. The volume of fluid to be aspirated needs to be six times the volume of the sampling path in order to ensure that there is effectively no contamination of the sample. This fluid will need to be reintroduced after the sample is taken if progressive anaemia is not to be a consequence of repeat sampling. Several manufacturers of arterial monitoring kits now offer a system which simplifies this process while minimising the risks of bacterial contamination of the patient or blood contamination of attending personnel.

Guide-wire techniques

Seldinger technique

The technique for using a Seldinger wire introducer has been dealt with elsewhere and is not be repeated here. In children, J wires are totally unsuitable for use as introducers as the arteries are insufficiently large to accommodate the curling tip as it emerges from the introducer. There will be inevitable intimal damage and possible rupture of the vessel wall if such a device is used.

Arrow Quick Flash

The disadvantage of the Seldinger wire technique is that it involves at least four separate actions. First the vessel must be cannulated, then the wire is introduced, and finally the introducing cannula or needle is removed and replaced by the chosen catheter. The technique is inherently messy and time-consuming. The QuickFlash arterial catheter (Arrow International Inc., Reading, Pa, USA) provides several features that are designed to improve the certainty of arterial cannulation (Figure 19.8). The lubricated polyurethane cannula (described by its manufacturer as a 'catheter') is transparent and the introducer needle has several holes along its shaft. Consequently, the moment the needle punctures the artery, blood can be seen in the cannula itself. This gives a more immediate indication of vessel puncture than the conventional flashback chamber in the hub of the introducer needle. The assembly includes a fine, flexible inner wire which is already located inside the lumen of the introducer needle and can be manually advanced from its split sheath into the vessel lumen. The cannula is then advanced over this wire, into the vessel. This minimises the tendency to transfix the artery while increasing the likelihood of successfully threading the cannula. The device is currently available only as a 20 gauge × 1·5 inch (3·75 cm) cannula. The spring–wire guide assembly is available in a kit which includes a polyurethane cannula (minimum size 22 gauge) in which the two components are not pre-assembled. Finally, the spring–wire guide is available without a cannula. The minimum wire diameter in this form is 0.018 inch (0.45 mm), equivalent to 26 gauge. It can be used to thread much smaller cannulae if the introducer needle is first removed. In this instance, the cannula tip must be already in the lumen of the artery before the wire is introduced.

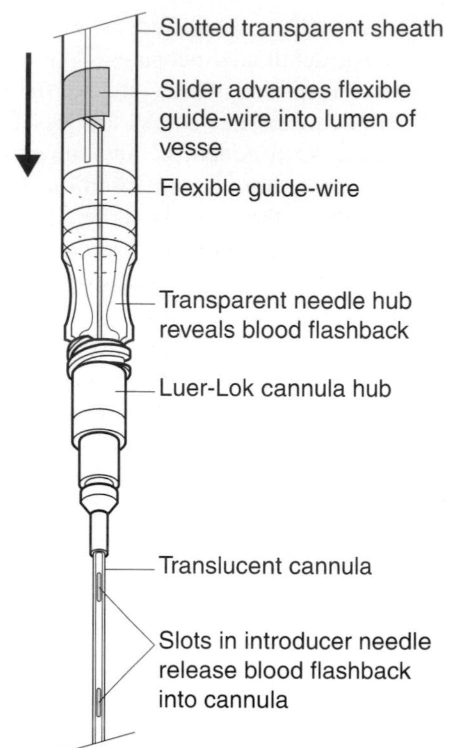

Figure 19.8 QuickFlash arterial cannula (Arrow, Reading, Pa, USA).

KEY POINTS

- Arterial cannulation in small children risks permanent damage to the vessel which may impair tissue perfusion and growth. It should be undertaken only when non-invasive measures are inappropriate.
- Selection of an appropriate artery should take into consideration the availability of alternative blood supply to the compromised tissues.
- The superficial temporal artery and the posterior tibial artery, uncommon access in adults, have both been advocated in infants.
- The umbilical arteries offer relatively easy aortic access in neonates and have been used for delivery of medication and alimentation. Users must be aware that the route has been associated with a significant incidence of severe complications and death.
- The dimensions of cannulae and catheters for use in infants and children must be suitably scaled dwon. For an infant, radial artery cannulae should be 26 gauge or smaller.
- Identification of the artery, often difficult by palpation alone, may be enhanced by trans-illumination, pulse oximetry, and by Doppler and imaging ultrasound.
- Meticulous care of the cannula, once located, is essential if it is to survive early blockage. Conventional continuous infusion techniques risk over-hydration and systemic anticoagulation and must be carefully controlled.

References

1. Modanlou H, Yeh SY, Siassi B, Hon EH. Direct monitoring of arterial blood pressure in depressed and normal newborn infants during the first hour of life. Journal of Pediatrics 1974; **85**(4):553.
2. Thick MG, Thick GC. Monitoring low blood pressure. A non-invasive technique. Anaesthesia 1978; **33**(8):726.
3. Dellagrammaticas HD, Wilson AJ. Clinical evaluation of the Dinamap non-invasive blood pressure monitor in pre-term neonates. Clinical Physics and Physiological Measurement 1981; **2**(4):271.
4. Pasch T. Measurement of blood pressure during the intraoperative period. Annales Francaises d'Anesthesie et de Reanimation 1989; **8**(5):572–5, 32.
5. Talke P. Nichols RJ, Traber DL. Does measurement of systolic blood pressure with a pulse oximeter correlate with conventional methods? [see comments] Journal of Clinical Monitoring 1990; **6**(1):5.
6. Dangel P. [Continuous monitoring of blood gases in newborn infants.] Schweizerische Medizinische Wochenschrift 1982; **112**(27–8):990.
7. Belgaumkar TK, Scott KE. Apnea in premature infants: recording by arterial catheter. European Journal of Pediatrics 1976; **123**(4):301.
8. Gortner L, Pohlandt F. [Exchange transfusion via a peripheral arteriovenous vascular access in premature infants.] Monatsschrift Kinderheilkunde 1986; **134**(4):205.
9. Paret G, Cohen AJ, Bohn DJ, Edwards H, Taylor R, Geary D, Williams WG. Continuous arteriovenous hemofiltration after cardiac operations in infants and children. Journal of Thoracic and Cardiovascular Surgery 1992; **104**(5):1225.
10. Zobel G, Trop M, Muntean W, Ring E, Gleispach H. Anticoagulation for continuous arteriovenous hemofiltration in children. Blood Purification 1988; **6**(2):90.
11. Zobel G, Haim M, Ritschl E, Muller W. Continuous arteriovenous hemofiltration as emergency procedure in severe hyperkalemia. Child Nephrology and Urology 1988; **9**(4):236.
12. Zobel G, Trop M, Beitzke A, Ring E. Vascular access for continuous arteriovenous hemofiltration in infants and young children. Artificial Organs 1988; **12**(1):16.
13. Zobel G, Ring E, Trop M, Grubbauer HM. Suction-supported continuous arteriovenous hemofiltration in children. Blood Purification 1988; **6**(1):37.
14. Soutter LP, Conway MJ, Parker D. A system for monitoring arterial oxygen tension in sick newborn babies. Bio-Medical Engineering 1975; **10**(7):257.
15. Conway M, Durbin GM, Ingram D, McIntosh N, Parker D, Reynolds EO, Soutter LP. Continuous monitoring of arterial oxygen tension using a catheter-tip polarographic electrode in infants. Pediatrics 1976; **57**(2):244.
16. Buttner W. Practical experiences with the routine application of the intravascular PO2 probe. Biotelemetry and Patient Monitoring 1979; **6**(1–2):44.
17. Wilkinson AR, Phibbs RH, Gregory GA. Continuous in vivo oxygen saturation in newborn infants with pulmonary disease: a new fiberoptic catheter oximeter. Critical Care Medicine 1979; **7**(5):232.
18. Sekelj P, Retfalvi S, Lavoie A. Measurement of blood oxygen saturation using a multichannel fiberoptic oximeter-densitometer. Canadian Journal of Physiology and Pharmacology 1977; **55**(3):585.
19. Arnold D, Kachel W, Rettwitz W, Lasch P, Brands W. [Clinical application of extracorporeal membrane oxygenation (ECMO) in neonatal respiratory failure.]

Thoracic and Cardiovascular Surgeon 1987; **35**(5):321.

20. Smith C, Green RM. Pediatric vascular injuries. Surgery 1981; **90**(1):20.
21. Guy RL, Holland JP, Shaw DG, Fixsen JA. Limb shortening secondary to complications of vascular cannulaein the neonatal period. Skeletal Radiology 1990; **19**:423.
22. Davis FM, Stewart JM. Radial artery cannulation. A prospective study in patients undergoing cardiothoracic surgery. British Journal of Anaesthesia 1980; **52**(1):41.
23. Abel M, Pringsheim W. [Intravascular monitoring by axillary artery cannulation in infants.] Anasthesie, Intensivtherapie, Notfallmedizin 1986; **21**(4):223.
24. Lawless S, Orr R. Axillary arterial monitoring of pediatric patients. Pediatric 1989; **84**(2):273.
25. Piotrowski A, Kawczynski P. Cannulation of the axillary artery in critically ill newborn infants. European Journal of Pediatrics 1995; **154**(1):57.
26. McFadden PM, Ochsner JL, Mills N. Management of thrombotic complications of invasive arterial monitoring of the upper extremity. Journal of Cardiovascular Surgery 1983; **24**(1):35.
27. Allen EV. Thromboangiitis obliterans: methods of diagnosis of chronic obstructive arterial lesions distal to the wrist with illustrative cases. American Journal of Medical Science 1929; **178**:237.
28. Mandel MA, Dauchot PJ. Radial artery cannulation in 1,000 patients: precautions and complications. Journal of Hand Surgery – American Volume 1977; **2**(6):482.
29. Hack WW, Vos A, van der Lei J, Okken A. Incidence and duration of total occlusion of the radial artery in newborn infants after catheter removal. European Journal of Pediatrics 1990; **149**(4):275.
30. Sfeir R, Khoury S, Khoury G, Rustum J, Ghabash M. Ischaemia of the hand after radial artery monitoring. Cardiovascular Surgery 1996; **4**(4):456.
31. Husum B, Palm T. Before cannulation of the radial artery: collateral arterial supply evaluated by strain-gauge plethysmography. Acta Anaesthesiologica Scandinavica 1980; **24**(5):412.
32. Wilkins RG. Radial artery cannulation and ischaemic damage: a review. Anaesthesia 1985; **40**:896.
33. Furman EF, Hairabet JK, Roman DG. The use of indwelling radial artery needles in paediatric anaesthesia. British Journal of Anaesthesia 1972; **44**:531.
34. Husum B, Berthelsen P. Allen's test and systolic arterial pressure in the thumb. British Journal of Anaesthesia 1981; **53**(6):635.
35. Mozersky DJ, Buckley CJ, Hagood COJ, Capps WFJ, Dannemiller FJJ. Ultrasound evaluation of the palmar circulation: a useful adjunct to radial artery cannulation. American Journal of Surgery 1973; **126**:810.
36. Rhee KH, Berg RA. Antegrade cannulation of radial artery in infants and children. Chest 1995; **107**(1):182.
37. Adams JM, Rudolph AJ. The use of indwelling radial artery catheters in neonates. Pediatrics 1975; **55**(2):261.
38. Schober PH. [Percutaneous cannulation of the radial artery in severely ill premature and newborn infants.] Wiener Klinische Wochenschrift 1990; **102**(16):476.
39. Todres ID, Rogers M, Shannon DC, Moylan FM, Ryan JF. Percutaneous catheterization of the radial artery in the critically ill neonate. Journal of Pediatrics 1975; **87**(2):273.
40. Prian GW. Temporal artery catheterization for arterial access in the high risk newborn. Surgery 1977; **82**(5):734.
41. Prian GW. Complications and sequelae of temporal artery catheterization in the high-risk newborn. Journal of Pediatric Surgery 1977; **12**(6):829.
42. Bause HW, Doehn M, Grossner D. [Long-term measurement of arterial blood pressure via the superficial temporal artery (author's translation)]. Praktische Anaesthesie, Wiederbelebung und Intensivtherapie 1978; **13**(3):181.
43. Aldridge SA, Gupta JM. Peripheral artery cannulation in newborns. Journal of the Singapore Paediatric Society 1992; **34**(1–2):11.
44. Galvis AG, Donahoo JS, White JJ. An improved technique for prolonged arterial catheterization in infants and children. Critical Care Medicine 1976; **4**(3):166.
45. Randel SN, Tsang BH, Wung JT, Driscoll JM, James LS. Experience with percutaneous indwelling peripheral arterial catheterization in neonates. American Journal of Diseases of Children 1987; **141**(8):848.
46. Laks H, Rongey K, Schweiss J, Willman VL. Internal mammary artery cannulation. Annals of Thoracic Surgery 1977; **24**(5):488.
47. Kitterman JA, Phibbs RH, Tooley WH. Catheterization of umbilical vessels in newborn infants. Pediatric Clinics of North America 1970; **17**(4):895–912.
48. Nelson LM, Prod'hom LS, Cherry RB. Pulmonary function in the newborn infant. Pediatrics 1962; **30**:975.
49. Baker DH, Berdon WE, James LS. Proper localization of umbilical arterial and venous catheters in newborns [abstract]. Pediatrics 1969; **43**:34.
50. Valls Soler A. [Umbilical artery catheterization. A simplified method to predict the catheter localization (author's translation)]. Anales Espanoles de Pediatria 1975; **8**(6):621.
51. Rubin BK, McRobert E, O'Neill MB. An alternate technique to determine umbilical arterial catheter length. Clinical Pediatrics 1986; **25**(8):407.
52. James LS. Complications arising from catheterization of the umbilical vessels. Report of the 59th Ross Conference on Pediatric Research, Stowe, Vermont, 1969.
53. Filston HC, Izant RJ. Translocation of the umbilical artery to the lower abdomen: an adjunct to the postoperative monitoring of arterial blood gases in major abdominal wall defects. Journal of Pediatric Surgery 1975; **10**(2):225.
54. Graves PW, Davis AL, Maggi JC, Nussbaum E. Femoral artery cannulation for monitoring in critically ill children: prospective study. Critical Care Medicine 1990; **18**(12):1363.
55. Sheridan RL, Weber JM, Tompkins RG. Femoral arterial catheterization in paediatric burn patients. Burns 1994; **20**(5):451.

56. Mortensson W, Hallbook T, Lundstrom NR. Percutaneous catheterization of the femoral vessels in children. II. Thrombotic occlusion of the catheterized artery: frequency and causes. Pediatric Radiology 1975; **4**(1):1.
57. Mortensson W, Hallbook T, Lundstrom NR Percutaneous catheterization of the femoral vessels in children. I. Influence on arterial peak flow and venous emptying rate in the calves. Pediatric Radiology 1975; **3**(4):195.
58. Mortensson W. Angiography of the femoral artery following percutaneous catheterization in infants and children. Acta Radiologica Diagnosis 1976; **17**(5A):581.
59. Skovranek J, Samenek M. Chronic impairment of leg muscle blood flow following cardiac catheterization in childhood. American Journal of Roentgenology 1979; **132**(1):71.
60. Seibert JJ, McCarthy RE, Alexander JE, Taylor BJ, Seibert RW. Acquired bone dysplasia secondary to catheter-related complications in the neonate. Pediatric Radiology 1986; **16**(1):43.
61. Selby IR, Darowski MJ. Compartment syndrome in a child occurring after femoral artery cannulation. Paediatric Anaesthesia 1995; **5**(6):393.
62. Wall PM, Kuhns LR. Percutaneous arterial sampling using transillumination. Pediatrics 1977; **59**(suppl. 6 Pt 2):1032.
63. Spahr RC, MacDonald HM, Holzman IR. Catheterization of the posterior tibial artery in the neonate. American Journal of Diseases of Children 1979; **133**(9):945.
64. Johnstone RE, Greenhow DE. Catheterization of the dorsalis pedis artery. Anesthesiology 1973; **39**(6):654.
65. Barnhorst DA, Barner HB. Prevalence of congenitally absent pedal pulses. New England Journal of Medicine 1968; **278**:264.
66. Downs JB, Rackstein AD, Klein EF, Hawkins IF. Hazards of radial artery catheterization. Anesthesiology 1973; **38**:283.
67. Marshall AG, Erwin DC, Wyse RK, Hatch DJ. Percutaneous arterial cannulation in children. Concurrent and subsequent adequacy of blood flow at the wrist. Anaesthesia 1984; **39**(1):27.
68. Katz Y, Lee ME. Pulse oximetry for localisation of the dorsalis pedis artery [letter]. Anaesthesia and Intensive Care 1989; **17**(1):114.
69. Nowak GS, Moothy SS, McNiece WL. Use of pulse oximetry to assess collateral arterial flow. Anesthesiology 1986; **64**:527.
70. Lauer KK, Cheng EY, Stommel KA, Guenther NR, Kay J. Pulse oximetry evaluation of the palmar circulation. Anesthesia and Analgesia 1988; **67**:S129.
71. Cole FS, Todres ID, Shannon DC. Technique for percutaneous cannulation of the radial artery in the newborn infant. Journal of Pediatrics 1978; **92**(1):105.
72. Kuhns LR, Martin AJ, Gildersleeve S, Poznanski AK. Intense transillumination for infant venepuncture. Radiology 1975; **116**:734.
73. Chinyanga HM, Smith JM. A modified doppler flow detector probe – an aid to percutaneous radial arterial cannulation in infants and small children. Anesthesiology 1979; **50**(3):256.
74. Ponce de Leon S, Wenzel RP. Hospital-acquired bloodstream infections with *Staphylococcus epidermidis*. Review of 100 cases. American Journal of Medicine 1984; **77**(4):639.
75. Mann NP. Gluteal skin necrosis after umbilical artery catheterisation. Archives of Disease in Childhood 1980; **55**(10):815.
76. Harpin V, Rutter N. Percutaneous alcohol absorption and skin necrosis in a preterm infant. Archives of Disease in Childhood 1982; **57**(6):477.
77. Mitchell SJ, Gray J, Morgan ME, Hocking MD, Durbin GM. Nosocomial infection with *Rhizopus microsporus* in preterm infants: association with wooden tongue depressors [see comments]. Lancet 1996; **348**(9025):441.
78. Rajani K, Goetzman BW, Wennberg RP, Turner E, Abildgaard C. Effect of heparinization of fluids infused through an umbilical artery catheter on catheter patency and frequency of complications. Pediatrics 1979; **63**(4):552.
79. Horgan MJ, Bartoletti A, Polansky S, Peters JC, Manning TJ, Lamont BM. Effect of heparin infusates in umbilical arterial catheters on frequency of thrombotic complications. Journal of Pediatrics 1987; **111**(5):774.
80. Murray JM, Mowbray A. Local tissue oxygenation following radial artery cannulation. Anaesthesia 1987; **42**(10):1070.

20 • Techniques

PETER JONES

General technical considerations

Preferred side

The peripheral arterial architecture is essentially symmetrical about the midline and therefore there is no technical reason for selecting one particular side other than accessibility during surgery or significant deformity. The aortic arch, however, is asymmetrical and may be malformed to the extent that the pressures or oxygen tensions in the two arms are different. Coarctation of the aorta may justify two separate arterial cannulation sites – one above and one below the lesion, the latter being particularly useful as a guide to the effect of circulatory interruption during surgery. Generally, the left arm is preferred for routine peripheral artery cannulation since most patients are right-handed, though in infants the possibility of a range of arterial malformations may indicate right-sided or dual cannulation.

Position of operator

The position of the operator will be indicated by individual circumstances. Preferably the operator should be in a relaxed position that does not entail excessive bending, as the procedure may take some time.

Skin preparation

The skin should be prepared in accordance with the hospital policy for percutaneous procedures using appropriate contemporary skin cleansing methods. It is generally not considered necessary to drape around the area to be punctured when a non-touch technique is used for insertion of an arterial cannula or catheter-over-needle device.

Securing the catheter or cannula

Secure the cannula with a transparent microporous dressing (e.g. Tegaderm, 3M Health Care Ltd., Loughborough, UK) and arrange for secondary strain relief of the manometer tubing with tape. The tape should not be applied to the dressing as it may cause the cannula to become dislodged. Where there is a substantial likelihood of the catheter becoming dislodged, as in the radial artery, consider using a more robust fixing method (see Figure 19.7).

TECHNIQUES FOR SPECIFIC ARTERIES

AXILLARY ARTERY

Lawless and Orr (1989)[1]

Patient category

Infants[2] and children, particularly those in whom attempts to cannulate the radial, posterior tibial, dorsalis pedis and femoral arteries have failed.

Advantages and disadvantages

Useful when other vessels are inaccessible or reduced systemic pressures make alternative cannulation sites difficult to palpate. There is some risk of thrombus occlusion of this end-artery.[3]

Position of patient

The patient lies supine and the arm is externally rotated, abducted to approximately 90°. The elbow is then bent and the patient's head laid to rest on the upturned palm.[4]

Equipment used in original description

Polyethylene catheter, 2.5 F, 2.5 cm long (Cook Inc., Bloomington, Ind, USA); polyethylene catheter, 3.0 F, 8.0 cm long (Cook Inc., Bloomington, Ind, USA); polyethylene catheter, 4.0 F, 12 cm long (Cook Inc., Bloomington, Ind, USA); Teflon catheter, 22 gauge, 2.5 cm long (Quick Cath, Travenol Laboratories, Deerfield, Ill, USA); Teflon catheter, 20 gauge, 2.0 cm long (Quick Cath, Travenol Laboratories, Deerfield, Ill, USA). All were introduced either as catheter-over-needle devices or with the aid of a Seldinger wire.

Advice on current equipment

Any narrow-gauge venous cannula or catheter[5] of appropriate length.

Anatomical landmarks

Palpate the artery high in the axilla.

Precautions and recommendations

Neurological and vascular function of the arm is checked before cannulation and 24 hours and 48 hours afterwards.

Procedure

The vessel is punctured at a point dictated by palpation of the arterial pulsation and the catheter/cannula is advanced into position. The catheter is checked radiologically and if the tip is discovered to be in the arch of the aorta it is repositioned more distally.

Success rate

All of 16 attempted cannulations were successful (100%). The average duration of use was 9 days. One cannula was removed because of possible infection risk.

Complications

There was one haematoma at the puncture site and no neurological or vascular complications.

RADIAL ARTERY

Radial artery cannulation techniques are essentially similar. Only the methods for identifying the vessel distinguish them.

RADIAL ARTERY CANNULATION USING THE PALPATION METHOD

Marshall et al. (1984)6

Patient category

Age range 1 day to 14.8 years.

Advantages and disadvantages

Convenient and accessible; an indwelling cannula spares trauma and discomfort.

Ischaemic damage may occur if post-cannulation occlusion of the vessel occurs in the absence of an adequate collateral circulation.

Position of patient

The wrist is fully supinated and extended to 45° over a sandbag and secured with an elasticated cloth tape with zinc oxide adhesive, e.g. Elastoplast.

Equipment used in original description

A 22 gauge Medicut cannula (Aloe Medical, St Louis, Mo, USA).

Advice on current equipment

Any 22 gauge or smaller venous or arterial cannula.

Anatomical landmarks

The radial artery is palpated at the wrist.

Point of insertion of needle

The point for puncture is identified a few millimetres distal to the palpated vessel.

Procedure

The skin is punctured with a stylet, making an incision large enough to admit the cannula without resistance. The assembled device is then advanced at an angle of approximately 30° to the skin using a no-touch technique. The vessel is palpated as a guide to direction. A double click indicates that first the needle and then the cannula have entered or transfixed the vein. The needle is then partially withdrawn. Blood will flood, pulsating, out of the hub of the needle if the cannula is in the vessel. If no blood is seen, the assembly is slowly withdrawn until blood flows and the cannula is advanced up the lumen of the artery. Cannulation can often be achieved without transfixing the vessel and is to be preferred. The needle is withdrawn and the cannula is immediately connected to a short manometer extension tube with Luer connectors and a three-way tap, flushed and secured with adhesive conforming tape such as Elastoplast. The wrist is then splinted with the fingers exposed but secured over the interphalangeal joints. The line is flushed using a continuous infusion of heparinised 5% dextrose (1 ml/h).

Success rate

Cannulation was 100% successful with antegrade flow demonstrated in 61 of the 66 tested. There were no long-term complications.

Complications

Three of 34 vessels tested after removal of the cannulae exhibited temporary retrograde flow but they returned to antegrade flow within 24 hours.

RADIAL ARTERY CANNULATION USING AN ULTRASONIC DOPPLER FLOW DETECTOR

Chinyanga and Smith (1979).7

Fukutome *et al.* have described the use of a 1.5 mm diameter Doppler probe to identify the diameter and trace the course of the radial artery as an aid to successful cannulation.[8]

Patient category

Infants and small children.

Advantages and disadvantages

Assists in localising the radial artery.

Requires maintenance.

Position of patient

Supine with wrist extended at 50–60° over a pad.

Equipment used in original description

Parks Model 811 ultrasonic Doppler flow detector with its probe modified by glueing a small acrylic prism to its face. This concentrates the ultrasonic energy to the ridge opposite the crystal. The ridge was flattened to make a narrow face, 1.3 mm across. A 22 gauge Bardic Angiocath (Bard Ltd, Crawley, West Sussex, UK) was also used.

Anatomical landmarks

The gelled probe is placed over the artery and its position adjusted until the audio signal is maximal. It is then firmly taped in place (Figure 20.1).

Point of insertion of needle

Approximately 5 mm distal to the probe.

Procedure

The cannula is passed through the skin and advanced towards the probe at an angle of approximately 20° to the skin. The signal is diminished as the on-target cannula masks the underlying vessel. Puncture of the artery is confirmed by blood flashback.

Success rate

The success rate was 87%.

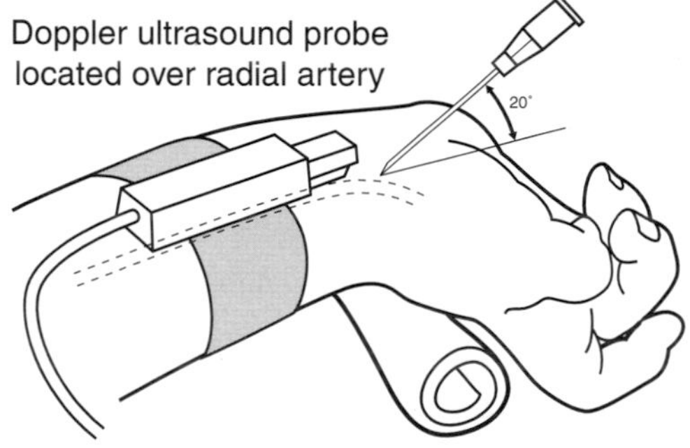

Figure 20.1 Doppler-guided radial artery cannulation (from Chinyanga and Smith, 1979).[7]

RADIAL ARTERY CANNULATION USING TRANSILLUMINATION

Wall and Kuhns (1977)[9]

Patient category

Neonates.

Advantages and disadvantages

Clear visualisation of vessels in premature infants. Ineffective in larger children.

Position of patient

For radial cannulation, the wrist is extended over the tip of the light probe.

Equipment used in original description

A 25 gauge scalp vein needle, as puncture was for sampling only. Mini-Light Portable Illuminator (Medgeneral, Minneapolis, Minn, USA) with flexible fibreoptic probe. CS2-73 Corning glass filter blank used as a heat filter. Short length of black rubber tubing applied over the end of the probe as a light seal flange.

Advice on current equipment

Any 22–26 gauge cannula would be appropriate.

Anatomical landmarks

Direct visualisation of the pulsating vessel shadow.

Precautions and recommendations

Excessive heat build-up can be a problem. The hand should be checked periodically for excessive warmth.

Procedure

The needle was introduced through the skin and the vessel was punctured under 'direct' vision.

Success rate

Twenty-four successful samples out of 25 attempts, using various arteries. Radial, ulnar, dorsalis pedis and posterior tibial artery cannulations have been performed.

Complications

None. There is a risk of burns from the infrared component of the light delivered by some sources.

UMBILICAL ARTERY

Kitterman et al (1970)10

Patient category

Neonates with poor peripheral pulses.

Advantages and disadvantages

Simple to perform, with a high initial success rate. The catheter tip can be located to provide blood samples from above or below the ductus arteriosus. Uniquely versatile – has been used for hyperalimentation.

There is a significant incidence of life-threatening complications.

The umbilical artery is the only artery to have been successfully used for total parenteral alimentation[11] though the administration of calcium gluconate by this route is contraindicated.[12] A survey in the USA (1990) revealed that 40 of 63 centres (63%) permit medications to be delivered through the umbilical artery catheter.[13]

Position of patient

Supine.

Equipment used in original description

Infants <1.5 kg: Argyle umbilical catheter 3.5 F (Aloe Medical, St Louis, Mo, USA).
Infants >1.5 kg: Argyle umbilical catheter 5 F (Aloe Medical, St Louis, Mo, USA).
Note: polyvinyl chloride, from which these catheters are manufactured, is not ideal for clot resistance.

Advice on current equipment

The author recommends a series of qualities for the optimal umbilical artery catheter:

- kink-free flexible tubing
- non-wettable surface to inhibit clot formation
- single end hole except when used for exchange transfusion
- smooth and rounded tip
- radio-opaque throughout its length
- low volume
- correct size for the vessel cannulated (8 F is too large for this application).

Polyurethane radio-opaque umbilical artery catheters, embodying the above criteria, are manufactured in 2.5 F and 3.5 F sizes by Vygon (UK) Ltd, Cirencester, UK.

Anatomical landmarks

The cut ends of the two constricted (pinhead) umbilical arteries are easily distinguishable from the umbilical vein.

Preparation

Full aseptic precautions should be taken using talc-free (and starch-free) gloves. Alcoholic chlorhexidine should be applied over the umbilical cord remnant and abdominal wall, taking care to avoid spillage pooling under the patient. The author recommends the initial application of iodine.

Precautions and recommendations

The correct location of the tip of the catheter can be monitored by ultrasonic imaging – a position 5– 10 mm above the bifurcation of the aorta is recommended as it avoids major branches of the aorta.[14]

Procedure

The catheter is shortened at its connector end by cutting and fitting it over an appropriately sized blunt needle to reduce total dead space. The area is draped using a 'circumcision drape' (small fenestrated drape). An umbilical tape is looped around the cord and tied loosely with a single knot, then tightened just enough to prevent bleeding. The cord is then cut with scissors, about 1.5 cm from the skin.

The cord is grasped in a cotton gauze swab and the cut surface is wiped. One umbilical artery is dilated using curved eye dressing forceps, permitting the opening spring to spread the tips and dilate the artery.

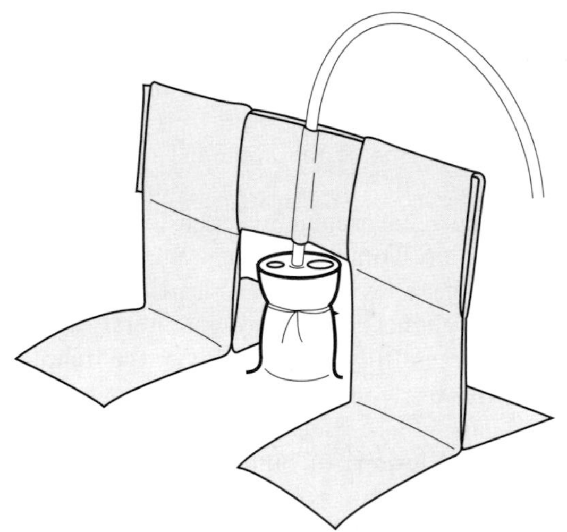

Figure 20.2 Fixing theumbilical artery catheter.

The catheter is introduced. It may encounter obstruction at the level of the anterior abdominal wall or at the level of the bladder. This is usually overcome by continued gentle force. Failing this, the catheter is withdrawn and loaded with 0.2 ml of 2% lignocaine without adrenaline (epinephrine), then reintroduced, allowing time at the obstruction for the drug to relax the spasm. If this fails, an attempt should be made to cannulate the other artery.

Gentle aspiration will withdraw blood only when the vessel has reached the internal iliac artery. The catheter should then be advanced a further 20 mm, when its tip will be at the level of the aortic bifurcation. A sample is taken and the catheter is flushed with heparinised saline.

A purse-string suture is placed in the wall of the cord, taking care not to puncture the catheter. The suture is tied and the catheter is secured by wrapping it with the ends of the suture (Figure 20.2). The stump is then dressed using a cotton swab covered with a neomycin, bacitracin and polymixin ointment and secured with tape as a non-occlusive dressing. The catheter should be firmly secured to the skin with an appropriate adhesive tape, cleaning the skin if necessary by abrasion with an alcohol-laden swab.

Alternative levels for the catheter tip may be preferred. The final position must be confirmed radiologically.

Success rate and complications

Complications of umbilical artery catheterisation

Kitterman *et al.*[10] reviewed the literature but provided no figures of their own for the technique described.

The following review highlights the substantial risk of life-threatening complications attending the use of umbilical artery catheters.

A high incidence of thrombus formation is associated with umbilical artery catheterisation. The tip of the catheter should be located below the renal arteries, it should be constantly perfused with a heparinised flush solution and should be removed as soon as possible in order to minimise serious complications.[15] Sick infants exhibit raised levels of factor VIII and reduced levels of antithrombin III (AT III), both of which encourage thrombogenesis in the presence of foreign material.[16] Aortography through the catheter has revealed incidences of thrombus formation in 24%,[17] 30%[18] and 45%[19] of catheter placements, though many are asymptomatic. More recently, ultrasonic imaging has been used to guide the placement of umbilical catheter tips[14] and to monitor the incidence and evolution of thrombotic sequelae to umbilical artery catheterisation.[20] Oppenheimer reported a 17% incidence of catheterised infants who developed echogenic lesions which resolved in 2–70 days.[21] In a series of 4000 umbilical artery catheter placements, O'Neill *et al.*[22] reported a 1% incidence of major thromboembolic problems requiring surgical intervention. These included obstruction of vessels proximal to the femoral artery involving life-threatening injury. Thromboembolic aortic occlusion induced by the use of umbilical artery catheters has been successfully treated by surgical thrombectomy.[23]

Necrotising enterocolitis (NEC) has resulted from a thrombus occluding the inferior mesenteric artery.[24] In one series of 165 infants[15] with umbilical artery catheters there were 5 deaths (3%), 12 visceral infarctions (7%) and three vascular perforations causing haemoperitoneum (2%). Haemoperitoneum has also been reported elsewhere.[25] Other studies of cases of NEC have shown a positive correlation with the use of umbilical artery (UA) catheters and their duration of use[26,27] though one study failed to confirm the relationship.[28] Umbilical artery catheterisation has been reported to adversely influence outcome in patients with NEC.[29] A study designed to establish the relationship between NEC and high or low catheter tip placement within the aorta failed to establish significance in this matter, though high catheter placement remained effective for longer, permitted more blood samples to be taken, and was less frequently the cause of emergency removal than low catheter placement.[30]

Hypertension has been reported following umbilical catheter-induced renal artery thrombosis.[31–34] Post-mortem examination of 56 infants who had UA catheters passed during life revealed a 59% incidence of thrombus in the aorta or its major branches. These thrombi rapidly developed atheromatous degeneration that extended into the underlying vessel wall and included calcification. The study stated that 'there is a need for less hazardous methods of monitoring arterial oxygen tension'.[35]

There has been one report of a case of sciatic nerve palsy following catheter-induced ischaemic gluteal necrosis.[36] Cumming and Burchfield have reported a further three cases which they attribute to accidental cannulation and obstruction of branches of the internal iliac artery, the superior and inferior gluteal arteries and the internal pudendal artery.[37]

False aneurysms of the aorta and related vessels, some mycotic,[38,39] have been reported including one causing renovascular hypertension.[33] A review of 35 mycotic thoracoabdominal aneurysms of the aorta have been reviewed by Cribari *et al.*[40]

Despite claims that total parenteral nutrition can be successfully delivered via the umbilical artery, infusions containing 10% calcium gluconate infused by this route resulted in intestinal bleeding and lesions of buttocks, anus, groins and thighs.[12]

No list of the problems would be complete without including one report of herniation of the appendix through the umbilical ring after the umbilical remnant had been cut short for the purpose of UA catheterisation.[41]

In contrast to the above catalogue of disasters, Powers and Swyer[42] found no evidence of flow reduction in the leg supplied by the catheterised common iliac artery. A study designed to investigate the relationship between intraventricular haemorrhage and high placement of UA catheter tip failed to show a significant correlation.[43]

FEMORAL ARTERY

Glenski et al. *(1987)*[44] *See Figure 19.3.*

Patient category

Neonates and children up to 4 years old.

Advantages and disadvantages

The procedure is convenient and simple.

The cannulation site is close to the perineum.

Position of patient

Supine, with an optional pad under the ipsilateral buttock.

Equipment used in original description

An 18 or 20 gauge 4 inch (10 cm) Teflon catheter-over-needle (Becton Dickinson, Rutherford, NJ, USA); 20 gauge 2 inch (5 cm) catheter for neonates and infants.

Advice on current equipment

Any small-gauge venous catheter or cannula of suitable length would be suitable, whether introduced over a needle or over Seldinger wire.

Dressings should be of the microporous transparent self-adhesive film variety and need not be changed daily.

Anatomical landmarks

Inguinal ligament, palpable femoral artery.

Point of insertion of needle

The needle is inserted at a point over the artery and at least 2 cm below the inguinal ligament.

Procedure

After taking sterile precautions, the catheter-over-needle device was introduced percutaneously and directed by palpation of the arterial pulsation to puncture the femoral artery. The catheter was advanced over the needle and then sutured in place after withdrawing the needle. A sterile dressing was applied which was changed daily.

Success rate

The success rate was 100% in 165 procedures.

Complications

Out of 165 procedures, there were 5 cases of catheter malfunction (3.0%), 4 perfusion-related complications (2.4%), and 6 cases of postoperative sepsis (3.6%).

DORSALIS PEDIS ARTERY

Modified from Johnstone and Greenhow (1973)[45]

Patient category

All.

Advantages and disadvantages

There is a collateral circulation.

The artery may be impalpable.

Advice on current equipment

A 24–26 gauge cannula-over-needle device is suitable.

Anatomical landmarks

The artery lies lateral to and parallel with the tendon of extensor pollicis longus on the dorsum of the foot.

Precautions and recommendations

Because of variation in the anatomy, the presence of an adequate collateral circulation should be confirmed by a modified Allen's test before cannulation is attempted: compress the dorsalis pedis artery by digital force, squeeze the great or second toe and confirm flushing when it is released. Alternatively, confirm that a pulse oximeter probe applied to the second toe continues to register pulsation and adequate oxygen saturation while the dorsalis pedis artery is compressed.

Point of insertion of needle

The needle is inserted slightly distal to the most obvious pulsation.

Procedure

Introduce the cannula, withdraw the introducer needle and connect immediately to a continuously flushed manometer kit.

Success rate

There were 21 successful cannulations out of 26 attempts.

Complications

Tissue necrosis has been reported.

POSTERIOR TIBIAL ARTERY

Spahr et al. *(1979)*[46]

Patient category

Neonates and older children.

Advantages and disadvantages

The posterior tibial artery is a robust vessel, which can be identified by transillumination in premature infants or cut-down in older infants. It is readily palpable and capable of percutaneous cannulation in older children.

Collateral blood supply is through the dorsalis pedis artery – a smaller vessel unlikely to provide satisfactory perfusion to the sole of the foot in the event of occlusion of the posterior tibial artery.

The posterior tibial nerve is a close posterior relation in the ankle and vulnerable to damage.

Position of patient

Transillumination

The ankle is extended over the tip of the fibreoptic light guide by grasping both in one hand.

Palpation and cut-down

With the child supine, the leg is slightly elevated on a pad and laterally rotated to bring the medial aspect of the calcaneum into view. The position may be secured by taping the leg and foot to a padded splint. The toes should remain uncovered.

Equipment used in original description

A 22 gauge needle to puncture the skin. *Note*: the text refers to a 22 gauge 'catheter' from which a 'stylet' is withdrawn. This probably is meant to indicate the use of a cannula-over-needle device. The text gives instructions that are only appropriate to such a device.

Advice on current equipment

Cannula-over-needle, PTFE or polyurethane, 24 or 22 gauge cannula, preferably with a winged hub for more secure fixing.

Anatomical landmarks

Midpoint between the posterior edge of the medial malleolus and the medial tubercle of the calcaneum. In the premature infant, the vessel can be seen to pulsate under transillumination.

Point of insertion of needle and procedure

Transillumination

The pulsation of the vessel is identified posterior and inferior to the medial malleolus. The skin is punctured over the course of the artery by the tip of a 22 gauge needle. The cannula-over-needle device is introduced at an angle of 45° to the skin surface and advanced to transfix the vessel. The introducer needle is then withdrawn to within 1 cm of the hub of the catheter. The catheter is placed flush with the skin and slowly withdrawn until flashback is seen. The cannula is then advanced carefully within the lumen of the artery, the introducer needle is removed completely and the cannula is attached to a continuous flushing device.

Cut-down

After securing the foot to a splint with tape, a 1 cm incision is made transversely, immediately below and behind the medial malleolus. The vessel is identified by blunt dissection and raised in the wound using a loop of suture material. It is cannulated by direct puncture using the 22 gauge cannula-over-needle device. No ligature is allowed to remain around the artery. The wound is closed using 5.0 silk and the cannula is connected and secured as above.

Palpation (author's technique)

With the operator's finger palpating the vessel, the 22 gauge cannula-over-needle is inserted into the skin immediately distal to the finger and advanced at an angle of 25–30° to the surface of the skin in a proximal direction (Figure 20.3). In an effort to avoid transfixing the artery, the needle assembly is slowly advanced at a much-reduced angle once flashback has been seen. The assembly is advanced into the artery for a distance sufficient to ensure that the tip of the cannula has entered the artery. The needle is then held still by one hand and the cannula is advanced with the other to its maximum extent. The needle is removed and the cannula is attached to a continuous flushing system. It is currently fashionable to secure cannulae with vapour-permeable adhesive membrane. This affords a barely adequate security for the cannula. This author recommends the use of two pieces of 2.5 cm wide brown Elastoplast or alternative zinc oxide adhesive flexible woven bandage as this provides far superior security (see Figure 19.7). The manometer line is brought back up the leg and taped in several places before the whole foot and lower limb are lightly bound in a bandage, taking care to leave the toes visible. Whilst this process precludes frequent inspection of the cannulation site, it effectively minimises incidents. All connections must be Luer-Lok and must be firmly tightened.

Success rate

Spahr quotes 17 successful cannulations on 15 infants, of which all but 4 were by percutaneous puncture. The remainder were by cut-down technique. The mean duration of use was 96 hours with the maximum being 12 days.

Complications

Two cases developed cyanotic toes – both had previously demonstrated the same phenomenon when catheterised in the umbilical artery. The patients weighed 800–3000 g.

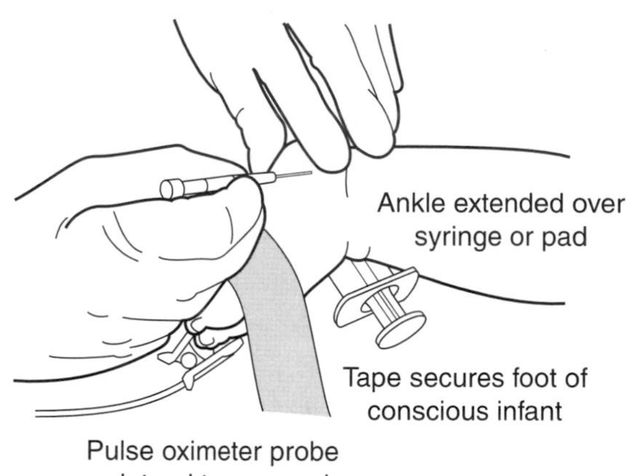

Figure 20.3 Palpation approach to the posterior tibial artery.

References

1. Lawless S, Orr R. Axillary arterial monitoring of pediatric patients. Pediatrics 1989; **84**(2):273.
2. Piotrowski A, Kawczynski P. Cannulation of the axillary artery in critically ill newborn infants. European Journal of Pediatrics 1995; **154**(1):57.
3. Chaikof EL, Dodson TF, Salam AA, Lumsden AB, Smith RB. Acute arterial thrombosis in the very young. Journal of Vascular Surgery 1992; **16**(3):428.
4. Adler D, Bryan-Brown C. Use of the axillary artery for intravascular monitoring. Critical Care Medicine 1973; **1**:148.
5. Abel M, Pringsheim W. [Intravascular monitoring by axillary artery cannulation in infants.] Anasthesie, Intensivtherapie, Notfallmedizin 1986; **21**(4):223.
6. Marshall AG, Erwin DC, Wyse RK, Hatch DJ. Percutaneous arterial cannulation in children. Concurrent and subsequent adequacy of blood flow at the wrist. Anaesthesia 1984; **39**(1):27.
7. Chinyanga HM, Smith JM. A modified doppler flow detector probe – an aid to percutaneous radial arterial cannulation in infants and small children. Anesthesiology 1979; **50**(3):256.
8. Fukutome T, Jimi N, Uehara J, Kohjiro M. [Pathway of the radial artery located with a small-caliber Doppler probe for arterial cannulation in pediatric patients.] Masui – Japanese Journal of Anesthesiology 1995; **44**(3):414.
9. Wall PM, Kuhns LR. Percutaneous arterial sampling using transillumination. Pediatrics 1977; **59** Suppl. (6 Pt 2):1032.
10. Kitterman JA, Phibbs RH, Tooley WH. Catheterization of umbilical vessels in newborn infants. Pediatric Clinics of North America 1970; **17**(4):895.
11. Hall RT, Rhodes PG. Total parenteral alimentation via indwelling umbilical catheters in the newborn period. Archives of Disease in Childhood 1976; **51**(12):929.
12. Book LS, Herbst JJ, Stewart D. Hazards of calcium gluconate therapy in the newborn infant: intra-arterial injection producing intestinal necrosis in rabbit ileum. Journal of Pediatrics 1978; **92**(5):793.
13. Hodding JH. Medication administration via the umbilical arterial catheter: a survey of standard practices and review of the literature. American Journal of Perinatology 1990; **7**(4):329.
14. Garg AK, Houston AB, Laing JM, MacKenzie JR. Positioning of umbilical arterial catheters with ultrasound. Archives of Disease in Childhood 1983; **58**(12):1017.
15. Marsh JL, King W, Barrett C, Fonkalsrud EW. Serious complications after umbilical artery catheterization for neonatal monitoring. Archives of Surgery 1975; **110**(10):1203.
16. Henriksson P, Wesstrom G, Hedner U. Umbilical artery catheterization in newborns. III. Thrombosis – a study of some predisposing factors. Acta Paediatrica Scandinavica 1979; **68**(5):719.
17. Goetzman BW, Stadalnik RC, Bogren HG, Blankenship WJ, Ikeda RM, Thayer J. Thrombotic complications of umbilical artery catheters: a clinical and radiographic study. Pediatrics 1975; **56**(3):374.
18. Olinsky A, Aitken FG, Isdale JM. Thrombus formation after umbilical arterial catheterisation. An angiographic study. South African Medical Journal 1975; **49**(36): 1467.
19. Saia OS, Rubaltelli FF, D'Elia RD et al. Clinical and aortographic assessment of the complications of arterial catheterization. European Journal of Pediatrics 1978; **128**(3):169.
20. Berger C, Durand C, Francoise M, Gouyon JB. [Ultrasonographic survey of the effect of umbilical arterial catheterization in newborn infants.] Archives de Pediatrie 1994; **1**(11):998.
21. Oppenheimer DA, Carroll BA, Garth KE. Ultrasonic detection of complications following umbilical arterial catheterization in the neonate. Radiology 1982; **145**(3):667.
22. O'Neill JA, Neblett WW, Born ML. Management of major thromboembolic complications of umbilical artery catheters. Journal of Pediatric Surgery 1981; **16**(6):972.
23. Flanigan DP, Stolar CJ, Pringle KC, Schuler JJ, Fisher E, Vidyasager D. Aortic thrombosis after umbilical artery catheterization. Archives of Surgery 1982; **117**(3):371.
24. Joshi VV, Draper DA, Bates RD. Neonatal necrotizing enterocolitis. Occurrence secondary to thrombosis of abdominal aorta following umbilical arterial catheterization. Archives of Pathology 1975; **99**(10):540.
25. Johnson JF, Basilio FS, Pettett PG, Reddick EJ. Hemoperitoneum secondary to umbilical artery catheterization in the newborn. Radiology 1980; **134**(1):60.
26. Bunton GL, Durbin GM, McIntosh N et al. Necrotizing enterocolitis. Controlled study of 3 years' experience in a neonatal intensive care unit. Archives of Disease in Childhood 1977; **52**(10):772.
27. Lehmiller DJ, Kanto WP. Relationships of mesenteric thromboembolism, oral feeding, and necrotizing enterocolitis. Journal of Pediatrics 1978; **92**(1):96.
28. Roulet M, Prod'hom LS. [Necrotizing enterocolitis in the neonatal period. Review of 19 cases proved by anatomopathologic examination.] Helvetica Paediatrica Acta 1979; **34**(5):405.
29. Cikrit D, Mastandrea J, West KW, Schreiner RL, Grosfeld JL. Necrotizing enterocolitis: factors affecting mortality in 101 surgical cases. Surgery 1984; **96**(4):648.
30. Kempley ST, Bennett S, Loftus BG, Cooper D, Gamsu HR. Randomized trial of umbilical arterial catheter position: clinical outcome. Acta Paediatrica 1993; **82**(2):173.
31. Plumer LB, Kaplan GW, Mendoza SA. Hypertension in infants – a complication of umbilical arterial catheterization. Journal of Pediatrics 1976; **89**(5):802.
32. Merten DF, Vogel JM, Adelman RD, Goetzman BW, Bogren HG. Renovascular hypertension as a complication of umbilical arterial catheterization. Radiology 1978; **126**(3):751.

33. Stevens PS, Mandell J. Urologic complications of neonatal umbilical arterial catheterization. Journal of Urology 1978; **120**(5):605.
34. Norero C, Oto MA, Morales B et al. [Renal artery thrombosis in newborn infants undergoing umbilical artery catheterization.] Revista Chilena de Pediatria 1989; **60**(6):346.
35. Tyson JE, deSa DJ, Moore S. Thromboatheromatous complications of umbilical arterial catheterization in the newborn period. Clinicopathological study. Archives of Disease in Childhood 1976; **51**(10):744.
36. Fok TF, Ha MH, Leung KW, Wong W. Sciatic nerve palsy complicating umbilical arterial catheterization. European Journal of Pediatrics 1986; **145**(4):308.
37. Cumming WA, Burchfield DJ. Accidental catheterization of internal iliac artery branches: a serious complication of umbilical artery catheterization. Journal of Perinatology 1994; **14**(4):304.
38. Fays J, Bretagne MC. Unusual evolution of a mycotic hypogastric arterial aneurysm after arterial umbilical catheterization. Pediatric Radiology 1980; **9**(1):50.
39. Dubos JP, Bouchez MC, Kacet N, Lemaitre L, Leclerc F, Lequien P, Ribet M. [Mycotic aneurysm after catheterization of the umbilical artery.] Presse Medicale 1986; **15**(19):876.
40. Cribari C, Meadors FA, Crawford ES, Coselli JS, Safi HJ, Svensson LG. Thoracoabdominal aortic aneurysm associated with umbilical artery catheterisation: case report and review of the literature. Journal of Vascular Surgery 1992; **16**:75.
41. Biagtan J, Rosenfeld W, Salazar D, Velcek F. Herniation of the appendix through the umbilical ring following umbilical artery catheterization. Journal of Pediatric Surgery 1980; **15**(5):672.
42. Powers WF, Swyer PR. Limb blood flow following umbilical arterial catheterization. Pediatrics 1975; **55**(2):248.
43. Anonymous. Relationship of intraventricular hemorrhage or death with the level of umbilical artery catheter placement: a multicenter randomized clinical trial. Umbilical Artery Catheter Trial Study Group. Pediatrics 1992; **90**(6):881.
44. Glenski JA, Beynen FM, Brady J. A prospective evaluation of femoral artery monitoring in pediatric patients. Anesthesiology 1987; **66**(2):227.
45. Johnstone RE, Greenhow DE. Catheterization of the dorsalis pedis artery. Anesthesiology 1973; **39**(6):654.
46. Spahr RC, MacDonald HM, Holzman IR. Catheterization of the posterior tibial artery in the neonate. American Journal of Diseases of Children 1979; **133**(9):945.

21 • Results and Complications

PETER JONES

See also Complications of umbilical artery catheterisation (Chapter 20).

The risks of paediatric arterial cannulation

Table 21.1 summarises the results and complications of published reports concerning arterial cannulation in infants and children. Umbilical artery cannulation is associated with an incidence of life-threatening complications that suggests that the approach should be used only when no other access route is available. Peripheral arterial cannulation is generally successful but is subject to risk of vessel damage. This may be manifested by loss of function of the cannula leading to its early removal, or to signs of tissue ischaemia which may be mild and transient or more severe, resulting occasionally in tissue necrosis. The presence of a collateral circulation permits symptoms of perfusion inadequacy to be absent in patients who are suffering long-term vessel damage or even complete blockage.[1] It is difficult to justify proceeding with cannulation of a peripheral artery without first testing for – and demonstrating the presence of – a collateral circulation, even though Allen's test may not be entirely reliable for this purpose.

The incidence of clinical infection from arterial catheters and cannulae is small. Catheter tip contamination has been reported in 3.9% of arterial catheters,[2] mostly involving *Staphylococcus epidermidis*. Though there were no instances of overt infection in that series, in which the patients were given a prophylactic antibiotic, *S. epidermidis* can be lethal in seriously ill patients.[3] Contamination of the catheter appears to occur as it passes through the skin. In the same series, catheters inserted transthoracically had a zero contamination rate. The authors recommend 3 days as the safe dwell period for arterial catheters in infants under 1 year old and 4–6 days in older children.

Recommendations for safe arterial cannulation

The general principles for safe arterial cannulation in infants and children are:

1. In neonates, avoid using the umbilical artery for arterial access except when the possibilities of peripheral arterial catheterisation have been exhausted.
2. Wherever possible, proceed with an attempt to cannulate an artery only after having confirmed that the collateral circulation is intact.
3. Use the smallest cannula practicable.
4. Consider giving the patient an appropriate antibiotic.
5. Secure the cannula properly and apply appropriate splints.
6. Ensure that all connections are made using the Luer-Lok technique.
7. Continuously flush the cannula with 1 ml/h of isotonic solution containing 1 IU/ml heparin.
8. Remove the cannula as soon as it develops any problems or is no longer required.

Table 21.1 Paediatric arterial cannulation: summary of results and complications.

Authors	Artery	Method	Age range	Successes patients (%)	Complications: Type	Complications: No. (%)	Comments	Mean duration
Abel & Pringsheim (1986)[4]	Axillary	Cannula-over-needle	9 mo	Case report of cannula in septic shock	–	–	Percutaneous using a disposable venous cannula	–
Adams & Rudolph[5]	Radial	Palpation and transfixion, intermittent flush	1 d–2.5 mo	19/20 (95%)	Blockage Ecchymoses Haematomat	13/19 (68%) 15/19 (79%) 9/20 (45%)	22 gauge Medicut, 22 gauge. Angiocath heparin 5 IU/ml	44 h
Adams *et al.* (1980)[6]	Radial	Palpation	Neonates	?	Impaired perfusion Infection	16/147 (11%) 1/147 (0.7%)		48 ± 6 h
Aldridge & Gupta (1992)[7]	Various peripheral	Percutaneous	170 newborns	Radial 138 Posterior tibial 34 Dorsalis pedis 2 Temporal 1	Transient ischaemia Blood loss Abscess Failure to aspirate	19/170 (11.2%) 4 (2.3%) 2 (1.2%) 52%	'safer than umbilical a. catheterisation'	
Bause *et al.* (1978)[8]	Superficial temporal	Arteriotomy and insertion of catheter	1–65yr	150	None	0%	Surgical cut-down	Up to 30 d
Berger *et al.* (1994)[9]	Umbilical	Cathetes	Neonates	40 cases with serial real-time ultrasound assessments	Aortic thrombosis symptomatic asymptomatic Wall-fixed catheter	 6/40 (15%) 2/40 (5%) 10/40 (25%)	Real-time ultrasound assessment must be regularly repeated	
Biagtan *et al.* (1980)[10]	Umbilical	Catheter	Neonate	Case report	Herniation of appendix through umbilical ring	–	–	–
Book *et al.* (1978)[11]	Umbilical		Neonate	5 case reports	10% calcium gluconate injected into umbilical a.	5 cases	Gut bleeding and lesions of buttock, anus, groin and thigh	–
Brush *et al.* (1990)[12]	Femoral cardiac catheter procedures	Palpation	'Children'	205/205 (29 balloon catheters)	Vascular spasm After heparin	15 (7.3%) 9 (4.4%)	Cardiac catheters responded to streptokinase	
Bunton *et al.* (1977)[13]	Umbilical	Catheter	33 wk gestation	17 infants	Necrotising enterocolitis Volvulus Abnormal blood supply	17 1/17	15/17 cases had evidence that umbilical a. catheter was implicated	
Butt *et al.* (1985)[14]	Radial (5) Post. tibial (2) Umbilical (7)	Argyl Medicut and Argyl catheters, bolus flush	Neonates	–	BP rise when arterial flush 1ml and rapid flow	–	Deliver no more than 0.5 ml slowly	–
Buttner (1979)[15]	Radial	Roche PO_2 probes	All age groups	53 probes providing continuous Po_2 measurement	–	–	Useful for controlled ventilation	<8.5 d

Chinyanga & Smith (1979)[16]	Radial	Doppler	2 mo–4 yr	20/23 (87%) 12/23 (52%) on 1st ry 19/23 (83%) on 2nd try	–		22 gauge Angiocath	–
Ciknit *et al.* (1984)[17]	Umbilical	Catheter	Neonates	Review of 101 cases of necrotising enterocolitis	Presence of Umbilical a. catheter adversely affects survivial	–	–	–
Conway *et al.* (1976)[18]	Umbilical	Po_2 electrode-tipped catheter with sampling lumen	Neonate (4 h at insertion)	36 electrodes inserted 32 functioned	–	–	–	10–190h (75h)
Cribari *et al.* (1992)[19]	Umbilical	Review of 35 cases of aortic aneurysm	Neonates	–	Mycotic aneurysm	35/?		–
Cumming & Burchfield (1994)[20]	Umbilical	Catheter	Neonates	3 case reports	Ischaemia ± infarction of iliac bone, gluteal muscles, sciatic n., perineum and skin	–	Accidental cannulation of internal illac a. branches	
Damen & Van der Tweel (1988)[2]	Intravenous, central venous, arterial and pulmonary a.	Percutaneous except for 279 transthoracic	Children	1649 catheter tips cultured, of which 58 (3.5%) positive	*Staphylococcus epidemids* cultured in 79% catheter tips	IV 0.9% Central, venous, 5.9% Arterial 3.9% PA catheter, 10.6%	0/279 positive transthoracic catheters	–
Davis & Stewart (1980)[21]	Radial, for cardiac surgery	Percutaneous, tested with US flow meter	Child – aged adult	Review of 333 cannulations	Vessel block 1 day after cannula removal 8 days after	30% 24%	Type and size of cannula matter 20 gauge Teflon best	–
Delaporte *et al.* (1987)[1]	Peripheral	Various with Doppler studies		19 cases reviewed over 1mo–2 years	Obstructed Stenosis	2/19 (10.5%) 4/19 (21%)	All vessels were symptom-free	
Dellagrammaticas & Wilson (1981)[22]	Radial (and brachial)	Percutaneous cannula and Dinamap 847 NIBP monitor	Pre-term infants (mean 30 wk)	10 infants tested	No complications	0	High degree of correlation validates NBP	
Dubos *et al.* (1986)[23]	Umbilical	Catheter	Neonate	Case report	*Staphylococcus aureus* infection leading to mycotic aneurysm of common iliac a.		Calcification around the aneurysm	–
Egan and Eitzman (1971)[24]	Umbilical (259) (mostly arterial)	–	Neonates	259/259 (100%)	Gangrene Infection Haemorrhage Extravascular catheter Complications found at necropsy	2/259 (0.8%) 5/259 (2%) 3/259 (1.2%) 2/259 (0.8%) 12/68 (17.6%)	2 catheter-related deaths	54 h
Fays & Bretagne (1980)[25]	Umbilical	Catheter	Neonate	Case report	Mycotic aneurysm	–	Surgically excised from hypogastric artery	–

Table 21.1 Continued

Authors	Artery	Method	Age range	Successes patients (%)	Complications		Comments	Mean duration
					Type	No. (%)		
Flanigan *et al.* (1982)[26]	Umbilical	Catheter	Neonates	Case Report	Acute aortic thrombosis	2 cases	Survival following successful surgical treatment	–
Fok *et al.* (1986)[27]	Umbilical	Catheter	Neonate	Case Report	Ischaemic necrosis of gluteal region and sciatic n. palsy			–
Franken *et al.* (1982)[28]	Femoral	Angiography catheters – femoral a.	Infants and children	100 unselected cases	Arterial spasm	62%	Most important factor is size of catheter relative to the artery	–
Fukutome *et al.* (1995)[29]	Radial	Mini-Doppler probe guidance	17 d–10 yr: 5–24 kg 3–5 kg < 3 kg	 11/11 (100%) 2/8 (25%) 3/4 (75%)	?	–	Mini-Doppler probe	–
Galvis *et al.* (1976)[30]	?	?	0–16 yr	57	Thromboembolic infection Blocked cannula	0% 1/57 (1.7%)	Continuous flushing technique and no stopcocks	1–31 d (mean 5.5 d)
Garg *et al.* (1983)[31]	Umbilical	Catheter and US confirmation	Neonates	56 studied using US imagin g on insertion			Recommend catheter tip 5–10mm above bifurcation	–
Glenski *et al.* (1987)[32]	Femoral	Palpation	Neonate to >4 yr	162/168 (96%) (3 went to cut-down, 3 went to radial)	Transient spasm Impaired perfusion Post-op. sepsis	6/165 (3.6%) 4/165 (2.4%) 6/165 (3.6%)	3/4 perfusion complications	72h
Goetzman *et al.* (1975)[33]	Umbilical	–	Neonates	98 surveyed	Thrombotic complication	23/98 (24%)	Revealed by aortography	–
Graves *et al.* (1990)[34]	Femoral	Percutaneous	22.3 mo	95% (60% on 1st attempt)	Impaired perfusion requiring removal	8 (11%)	Mostly in younger children	6d
Hack *et al.* (1990)[35]	Radial	Percutaneous with Dopper	26–40 wk (gestation)		Complete occulsion on removing catheter Rate proportional to duration and weight	20/32 (63%) The majority	Flow resumed after 1–29d Palmer collaterals crucial	
Hall & Rhodes (1976)[36]	Umbilical vessels and tunnelled jugular vein	5F catheters used for full TPN	Infants	80 umbilical a. 9 umbilical v. 23 IJV	No difference in infection and thrombotic phenomena		Claim umbilical artery satisfactory for TPN	11d UAC 16d UHV
Harpin & Rutter (1982)[37]	'Umbilical'	Alcoholic skin preparation	Pre-term infant	Case report	Skin necrosis of buttocks and back	Blood ethanol 259 mg/100 ml, methanol 26 mg/100 ml	Failure to remove excess skin preparation from under baby	–

Henricksson *et al.* (1979)[38]	–	–	Neonates	30 sick newborns vs. 20 healthy newborns	High factor VIII and reduced antithrombin III in sick newborn		Predispose to thrombosis around catheters	
Hodding (1990)[39]	Umbilical	Catheter		Survey of 100 institution remedication through UAC policies	Medication through UAC permitted in 40/63 (63%) of institutions			
Horgan *et al.* (1987)[40]	Umbilical	Catheter	Neonate	111 catheterisations with (59) and without (52) heparin	Thrombi detected Catheter clotting Hypertension	16/59 (27%) with heparin 18/52 (35%) without Higher in controls Higher in controls	Heparin does not reduce thromboses but minimises the sequelae	93 with heparin 101 non-heparin
Husum & Palm (1980)[41]	Radial (planned)	Strain gauge plethysmograph	11–75 yr		Thumb BP <40 mmHg when radial a. compressed	27/259 (10.4%)	Conclude Allen's test effective and mandatory	
Husum & Berthelsen (1981)[42]	Radial (planned)	strain gauge plethysmograph	11–72 yr		Thumb BP <40 mmHg when radial a. compressed	19/235 (8.1)	Conclude Allen's test effective and mandatory	
Johnson *et al.* (1976)[43]	Radial	Cut-down	5 mo	Case report, 1 child (+3 adults)	Necrosis of arm (amputated)	–	Catheter retained despite skin discolouration	–
Johnson *et al.* (1980)[44]	Umbilical	Catheter	Neonate	Case report	Haemoperitoneum	–	–	–
Johnstone & Greenhow (1973)[45]	Dorsalis pedis	Palpation	Not stated	21/26 (81%)	None stated	–	Recommend checking for collateral circulation	?
Joshi *et al.* (1975)[46]	Umbilical	–	Neonate	Case report	Necrotising enterocolitis following aortic thrombosis	–	4 similar reported cases cited	–
Kempley *et al.* (1993)[47]	Umbilical	Catheters with high and low tip placement	Neonates	308 infants 162 high tip 146 low tip	Necrotising enterocolitis Leg blanching and cyanosis Fatal aortic thrombosis	11/162 (6.7%) high 9/146 (6.2%) low more with 'low' 1 'high' group	High catheters lasted longer and were more effective	
Kessell Barker (1996)[48]	Femoral	Accidental cannulation in Down syndrome child	11 mo	–	Spasm-induced ischaemia of limb; treatment with caudal bupivacaine effective	–	Accidental drug injection – suxamethonium and atracurium	0

Table 21.1 Continued

Authors	Artery	Method	Age range	Successes patients (%)	Complications		Comments	Mean duration
					Type	No. (%)		
Kocis *et al.* (1996)[49]	Femoral	Palpation using Arrow 22 gauge polyurethane catheter	19 mo	Percutaneous 24/24 (100%) Cut-down 6/6 (100%)	Ischaemia Haemorrhage Complete obstruction Partial obstruction Clinical complication	1 (3%) 1 (3%) 6 (20%) 1 (3%) 7%	Obstruction was diagnosed by ultrasonography	6.9 days
Lawless & Orr (1989)[50]	Axillary	Palpation	1d–23 yr	16/16 (100%)	Haematoma	1 (6%)	2.5–4 F Cooke catheters and 22–20 gauge Quik Cath	9 days
Lehmiller & Kanto (1978)[51]				Autopsies on 16 cases with necrotising enterocolitis	Mesenteric thromboemboli	12/16 autopsies	UACs responsible for the emboli	
Mandel & Dauchot (1977)[52]	Radial	Cannula using Allen's test and Doppler	Infant	1000 insertions	Diminished flow Obstruction requiring embolectomy Damage requiring arterial reconstruction	24% 1 1	Critical factors: short duration, Teflon cannula, continuous flush	
Mann (1980)[53]	Umbilical	Catheter	Neonates	Case reports	3 infants developing gluteal skin necrosis	–	–	–
Marsh *et al.* (1975)[54]	Umbilical	Catheter	Infants	165 autopsies of following RDS	Visceral infarction Haemoperitoneum:	12/165 (7.3%) 3/165 (1.8%)	Umbilical a. catheters caused 5 deaths	–
Marshall *et al.* (1984)[55]	Radial (66) brachial (2) ulnar (2)	Palpation Percutaneous (62) cut-down (8)	1 d–15 yr	62/62 (100%)	Short-term retrograde flow Persistent retro-grade flow after decannulation	6/70 (8.6%) 2/70 (2.8%)	Allen's test not routine	< 3 days (elective)
McFadden *et al.* (1983)[56]	Brachial	?	10 yr	Case report	Thromboembolism	–	Saphenous vein patch	?
Merten *et al.* (1978)[57]	Umbilical	Catheters aortography and angiography	Neonates	7 case studies	Renovascular hypertension shown to have degrees of renal artery occlusion	7	Multiple lesions in other vessels found	
Mitchell *et al.* (1996)[58]	IV and radial	Tongue depressor splints	Neonates	4 case reports	Infection from *Rhizopus microsporus*	–	*Source was wooden tongue depressors*	–
Mortensson et al. (1975)[59]	Femoral (cardiac catheter)	Percutaneous	2–16 yr	98, all successful	Thrombotic occlusion Transient severe spasm	5% 5%	Conclude thrombosis due to intimal damage	0

Mortensson *et al.* (1975)[60]	Femoral (cardiac catheter)	Percutaneous	2–16 yr	49	Temporary, reduced arterial peak flow	'A few' younger children		0
Murray & Mowbray (1987)[61]	Radial	Percutaneous	Children and adults	20 with chlorbutano in heparin flush	Thumb Po_2 higher on cannulated than non-cannulated side		Chlorbutanol in heparin flush responsible	
				20 without chlorbutanol	No difference			
Norero *et al.* (1989)[62]	Umbilical	Catheter	Neonates	62 babies studied using radionuclide renal scintillography	Survived	25/62 (40.3%)		
					Renovascular hypertension	1/25		
				Iliac artery thrombosis		1/25		
				Died		37/62 (59.7%)		
				Aortoiliac thrombosis		8.8%		
O'Neill *et al.* (1981)[63]	Umbilical	Catheter	Neonate	4000 UAC inserted	Thromboembolic occlusion	41/4000 (1%)	Limbs survive when occlusion at femoral level	
Olinsky *et al.* (1975)[64]	Umbilical	Catheter	Neonate	47 catheters studied, 30 by angiography, 8 by autopsy	Arterial thrombus (angio)	9/30 (30%)	Asymptomatic	
					Arterial thrombus (autopsy)	5/8 (62.5%)		
Oppenheimer *et al.* (1982)[65]	Umbilical	Catheter	Neonate	71 infants US real-time image scanned	Clinical vascular compromise	12/71 (17%)	Images consistent with thrombus and dissection	
					US abnormal	12/71 (17%)		
Piotrowski & Kawczynski (1995)[66]	Axillary	Percutaneous, catheter-over-needle	Neonates	62	Complications	0%	All ventilated	1–10 d (mean 4.1 d)
Plumer *et al.* (1976)[67]	Umbilical	Catheter	Infants	10 case reports	Hypertension	10	5 infants died	
					Renal a. thrombosis	7/10 (all UACs)		
					Renal artery stenosis	1/10 (no UAC)		
					Idiopathic	2/10 (1 UAC)		
Ponce de Leon & Wenzel (1984)[3]	Various	Review	Neonates–adults	108 cases reviewed	*Staphylococcus epidermidis* septicaemia in A and V catheterised patients	56% of catheters cultured the organism	93% of cases had catheters or cannulae pre-infection	
Powers & Swyer (1975)[68]	Umbilical	Stimulated blood flow measured in legs	29–135 days	28 infants studied by venous occlusion plethysmography	No difference in stimulated leg blood flow (R=L)	0	Continuously flushed only with dextrose saline	4–144 h (58 h)

Table 21.1 Continued

Authors	Artery	Method	Age range	Successes patients (%)	Complications: Type	Complications: No. (%)	Comments	Mean duration
Prian (1977)[69]	Superficial temporal	Cannula by cut-down exposure then over-needle access	High-risk newborns	115 placements	Thrombosis of post. auricular a.	6/115 (5.2%)	Minor scarring	?6.5 d
					Skin slough	2/115 (1.7%)		
					Positive blood cultures	2/115 (1.7%)		
					Lost pulsatile flow	4/115 (3.4%)		
Prian (1977)[70]	Superficial temporal	Cannula by cut-down exposure then over-needle access	High-risk newborns 540–3900g	115 placements 62% functioned for >5 days			Doppler location of artery. Heparin–saline continuous infusion	6.5 d
Rajani *et al.* (1979)[71]	Umbilical	Catheter	Neonates	32 heparinised infusion flush vs. 30 non-heparinised	Catheter occlusion (heparinised)	4/32 (12%)	Heparin increases catheter patency half-life from 2 d to 7 d	2–7 d
					(non-heparinised)	19/30 (63%)		
Randel *et al.* (1987)[72]	110 radial 27 post. tibial 21 temporal	Percutaneous	Neonates	158 lines in 115 infants	Electively removed	91/158 (57.6%)	Reliable and safe compared with umbilical catheters	
					Removed for problems	67/158 (42%)		
					Infections	2/158 (1.3%)		
Rhee & Berg (1995)[73]	Radial	Percutaneous, antegrade	Paediatric	5	–	0%	Used where artery blocked proximally	–
Roulet & Prod'hom (1979)[74]	Umbilical		Neonatal	19 cases of necrotising enterocolitis reported	Emboli/thrombosis in mesenteric vessels	0	Findings suggest hypoxia and nonocclusive mesenteric arterial insufficiency	
Rubin *et al.* (1986)[75]	Umbilical	Catheter	Placement technique				Recommends a method of placing catheters tip between T6 and T10	–
Sahn *et al.* (1982)[76]	Femoral (cardiac catheters)	Percutaneous	5 d–20 yr	66	Long-term unilateral narrowing revealed by ultrasound	3/14 (21%)	These patients were symptomless	0
Saia *et al.* (1978)[77]	Umbilical	Catheterisation	Neonates	38 cases studied using aortography	Pathological change	17/38 (50%)	1 death due to catheter	
					Clinical signs	10/17 (26%)		
					Autopsy thrombus	1/8 (12%)		
Schober (1990)[78]	Radial	Percutaneous with transillumination	26–45 wk (gestation)	211/264 (80%)	Removal because aspiration ceased	53/211 (25%)	No neurological problems 1 year later	1–22 (5) d
					Removal for spasm	15/211 (7%)		
					Skin necrosis	1/211 (0.47%)		
					Infection	0%		

Seibert *et al.* (1986)[79]	Femoral indwelling catheters	?	Neonates	4 case reports	Leg shortening	–	Possible aseptic emboli to bones	–
Selby & Darowski (1995)[80]	Femoral	20 gauge cannula	?	Case report	Compartment syndrome	–	–	–
Sfeir *et al.* (1996)[81]	Radial	Cannula, Doppler ultrasound before and after	Children and adults	40 cannulae	Abnormal flow Absent pulses Ischaemia	27% 10% 0	Safe when performed 'properly'	
Shaw (1968)[82]	Radial sampling only	Palpation	Neonates 24–40 wk	122	None noted	0	23 gauge needle R better than L (preductal)	0
Sheridan *et al.* (1994)[83]	Femoral (burns patients)	Small-diameter catheters	?	81 inserted	Low incidence of infection and thrombosis	?		72 h
Skovranek & Samenek (1979)[84]	Femoral	Various	?	99 infants recatheterised after 2.7 yr	Significant reduction in maximum blood flow ipsilaterally	?	^{133}Xe clearance	?
Smith & Green (1981)[85]	Review of arterial thrombosis	Iatrogenic vascular injuries	< 2 yr		Thrombectomy Graft Rethrombosis	10/15 (67%) 1/15 (7%) 7/15 (57%)	Review of surgical treatment of arterial thromboses	–
Smith-Wright *et al.* (1984)[86]	Various arterial and venous sites	Review of 774 procedures in 467 children	–	330 arterial catheters 397 CV catheters 47 PA catheters	Bleeding Arterial obstruction: sepsis:	7/774 (1%) 3/337 (1%) 11/774 (1.4%)	'Acceptable' when set against 16% mortality in group	
Spahr *et al.* (1979)[88]	Posterior tibial	Palpation	Infants	Percutaneous 13/13 cut-down 4/4	Distal ischaemia	2/17 (12%)	Both cases previously had toe cyanosis due to umbilical catheter	96 h
Stevens & Mandell (1978)[89]	Umbilical	Catheter		2 case reports	Renovascular hypertension False aneurysm	1 1	Aortography via the UAC advocated	
Tyson & deSa (1976)[89]	Umbilical		Infants	56 autopsies	Thromboatheroma lesions	33/56 (59%)		–
UACTSG (1992)[90]	Umbilical	Catheters	Neonates	970 neonates weighing 500–1499 g	Intraventricular haemorrhage	25.8% of high catheters 23.1% of low catheters	'high' T6–8 'low' L3–5	83.4 h 74.9 h
Wall & Kuhns (1977)[91]	Radial (16) Ulnar (4) Dorsalis pedis (2) Post. tibial (2)	Transillu-mination	Neonates	24/25 (96) 17/25 (68%) 1st try 7/25 (28%) 2nd try	Transient arterial spasm Thromboembolic infection Thermal burns	25/25 (100%) 0% 0%	25 gauge scalp vein needle (blood sampling only)	0
Wessel *et al.* (1986)[92]	Femoral	Cardiac catheters	?	79 cases needing thrombectomy after catheterisation	Poor pulses Amputated extremity	15/79 (19%) 2/79 (2.5%)	Review	0

BP, blood pressure; CV, central venous; IJV, internal jugular vein; IV, intravenous; L, left; NIBP, non-invasive blood pressure; PA, pulmonary artery; R, right; RDS, respiratory distress syndrome; TPN, total parenteral nutrition; UAC, umbilical artery catheter; US, ultrasound.

References

1. Delaporte B, Didelon JL, Devaux AM, Ensel P, Samson-Dollfus D. [Peripheral arterial catheterization in neonates and infants. Remote study of the arterial permeability by the Doppler effect.] Archives Francaises de Pediatrie 1987; **44**(4):253.
2. Damen J, Van der Tweel I. Positive tip cultures and related risk factors associated with intravascular catheterization in pediatric cardiac patients. Critical Care Medicine 1988; **16**(3):221.
3. Ponce de Leon S, Wenzel RP. Hospital-acquired bloodstream infections with *Staphylococcus epidermidis*. Review of 100 cases. American Journal of Medicine 1984; **77**(4):639.
4. Abel M, Pringsheim W. [Intravascular monitoring by axillary artery cannulation in infants.] Anasthesie, Intensivtherapie, Notfallmedizin 1986; **21**(4):223.
5. Adams JM, Rudolph AJ. The use of indwelling radial artery catheters in neonates. Pediatrics 1975; **55**(2):261.
6. Adams JM, Speer ME, Rudolph AJ. Bacterial colonization of radial artery catheters. Pediatrics 1980; **65**:94.
7. Aldridge SA, Gupta JM. Peripheral artery cannulation in newborns. Journal of the Singapore Paediatric Society 1992; **34**(1–2):11.
8. Bause HW, Doehn M, Grossner D. [Long-term measurement of arterial blood pressure via the superficial temporal artery (author's trans.)] Praktische Anaesthesie, Wiederbelebung und Intensivtherapie 1978; **13**(3):181.
9. Berger C, Durand C, Francoise M, Gouyon JB. [Ultrasonographic survey of the effect of umbilical arterial catheterization in newborn infants]. Archives de Pediatrie 1994; **1**(11):998.
10. Biagtan J, Rosenfeld W, Salazar D, Velcek F. Herniation of the appendix through the umbilical ring following umbilical artery catheterization. Journal of Pediatric Surgery 1980; **15**(5):672.
11. Book LS, Herbst JJ, Stewart D. Hazards of calcium gluconate therapy in the newborn infant: intra-arterial injection producing intestinal necrosis in rabbit ileum. Journal of Pediatrics 1978; **92**(5):793.
12. Brus F, Witsenburg M, Hofhuis WJD, Hazelzet JA, Hess J. Streptokinase treatment for femoral artery thrombosis after arterial cardiac catheterisation in infants and children. British Heart Journal 1990; **63**:291.
13. Bunton GL, Durbin GM, McIntosh N *et al.* Necrotizing enterocolitis. Controlled study of 3 years' experience in a neonatal intensive care unit. Archives of Disease in Childhood 1977; **52**(10):772.
14. Butt WW, Gow R, Whyte H, Smallhorn J, Koren G. Complications resulting from use of arterial catheters: retrograde flow and rapid elevation in blood pressure. Pediatrics 1985; **76**(2):250.
15. Buttner W. Practical experiences with the routine application of the intravascular PO2 probe. Biotelemetry and Patient Monitoring 1979; **6**(1–2):44.
16. Chinyanga HM, Smith JM. A modified doppler flow detector probe – an aid to percutaneous radial arterial cannulation in infants and small children. Anesthesiology 1979; **50**(3):256.
17. Cikrit D, Mastandrea J, West KW, Schreiner RL, Grosfeld JL. Necrotizing enterocolitis: factors affecting mortality in 101 surgical cases. Surgery 1984; **96**(4):648.
18. Conway M, Durbin GM, Ingram D *et al.* Continuous monitoring of arterial oxygen tension using a catheter-tip polarographic electrode in infants. Pediatrics 1976; **57**(2):244.
19. Cribari C, Meadors FA, Crawford ES, Coselli JS, Safi HJ, Svensson LG. Thoracoabdominal aortic aneurysm associated with umbilical artery catheterisation: case report and review of the literature. Journal of Vascular Surgery 1992; **16**:75.
20. Cumming WA, Burchfield DJ. Accidental catheterization of internal iliac artery branches: a serious complication of umbilical artery catheterization. Journal of Perinatology 1994; **14**(4):304.
21. Davis FM, Stewart JM. Radial artery cannulation. A prospective study in patients undergoing cardiothoracic surgery. British Journal of Anaesthesia 1980; **52**(1):41.
22. Dellagrammaticas HD, Wilson AJ. Clinical evaluation of the Dinamap non-invasive blood pressure monitor in pre-term neonates. Clinical Physics and Physiological Measurement 1981; **2**(4):271.
23. Dubos JP, Bouchez MC, Kacet N, Lemaitre L, Leclerc F, Lequien P, Ribet M. [Mycotic aneurysm after catheterization of the umbilical artery]. Presse Medicale 1986; **15**(19):876.
24. Egan EA, Eitzman DV. Umbilical vessel catheterization. Amer. J. Dis. Child 1971;121 (March):213.
25. Fays J, Bretagne MC. Unusual evolution of a mycotic hypogastric arterial aneurysm after arterial umbilical catheterization. Pediatric Radiology 1980; **9**(1):50.
26. Flanigan DP, Stolar CJ, Pringle KC, Schuler JJ, Fisher E, Vidyasager D. Aortic thrombosis after umbilical artery catheterization. Archives of Surgery 1982; **117**(3):371.
27. Fok TF, Ha MH, Leung KW, Wong W. Sciatic nerve palsy complicating umbilical arterial catheterization. European Journal of Pediatrics 1986; **145**(4):308.
28. Franken EA, Girod D, Sequeria FW, Smith WL, Hurwitz R, Smith JA. Femoral artery spasm in children: catheter size is the principal cause. American Journal of Roentgenology 1982; **138**(2):295.
29. Fukutome T, Jimi N, Uehara J, Kohjiro M. [Pathway of theradial artery located with a small-caliber Doppler probe for arterial cannulation in pediatric patients.] Masui–Japanese Journal of Anesthesiology 1995; **44**(3):414.
30. Galvis AG, Donahoo JS, White JJ. An improved technique for prolonged arterial catheterization in infants and children. Critical Care Medicine 1976; **4**(3):166.
31. Garg AK, Houston AB, Laing JM, MacKenzie JR. Positioning of umbilical arterial catheters with ultrasound.Archives of Disease in Childhood 1983; **58**(12):1017.

32. Glenski JA, Beynen FM, Brady J. A prospective evaluation of femoral artery monitoring in pediatric patients. Anesthesiology 1987; **66**(2):227.
33. Goetzman BW, Stadalnik RC, Bogren HG, Blankenship WJ, Ikeda RM, Thayer J. Thrombotic complications of umbilical artery catheters: a clinical and radiographic study. Pediatrics 1975; **56**(3):374.
34. Graves PW, Davis AL, Maggi JC, Nussbaum E. Femoral artery cannulation for monitoring in critically ill children: prospective study. Critical Care Medicine 1990; **18**(12):1363.
35. Hack WW, Vos A, van der Lei J, Okken A. Incidence and duration of total occlusion of the radial artery in newborn infants after catheter removal. European Journal of Pediatrics 1990; **149**(4):275.
36. Hall RT, Rhodes PG. Total parenteral alimentation via indwelling umbilical catheters in the newborn period. Archives of Disease in Childhood 1976; **51**(12):929.
37. Harpin V, Rutter N. Percutaneous alcohol absorption and skin necrosis in a preterm infant. Archives of Disease in Childhood 1982; **57**(6):477.
38. Henriksson P, Wesstrom G, Hedner U. Umbilical artery catheterization in newborns. III. Thrombosis – a study of some predisposing factors. Acta Paediatrica Scandinavica 1979; **68**(5):719.
39. Hodding JH. Medication administration via the umbilical arterial catheter: a survey of standard practices and review of the literature. American Journal of Perinatology 1990; **7**(4):329.
40. Horgan MJ, Bartoletti A, Polansky S, Peters JC, Manning TJ, Lamont BM. Effect of heparin infusates in umbilical arterial catheters on frequency of thrombotic complications. Journal of Pediatrics 1987; **111**(5):774.
41. Husum B, Palm T. Before cannulation of the radial artery: collateral arterial supply evaluated by strain-gauge plethysmography. Acta Anaesthesiologica Scandinavica 1980; **24**(5):412.
42. Husum B, Berthelsen P. Allen's test and systolic arterial pressure in the thumb. British Journal of Anaesthesia 1981; **53**(6):635.
43. Johnson FE, Sumner DS, Strandness DE. Extremity necrosis caused by indwelling arterial catheters. American Journal of Surgery 1976; **131**(3):375.
44. Johnson JF, Basilio FS, Pettett PG, Reddick EJ. Hemoperitoneum secondary to umbilical artery catheterization in the newborn. Radiology 1980; **134**(1):60.
45. Johnstone RE, Greenhow DE. Catheterization of the dorsalis pedis artery. Anesthesiology 1973; **39**(6):654.
46. Joshi VV, Draper DA, Bates RD. Neonatal necrotizing enterocolitis. Occurrence secondary to thrombosis of abdominal aorta following umbilical arterial catheterization. Archives of Pathology 1975; **99**(10):540.
47. Kempley ST, Bennett S, Loftus BG, Cooper D, Gamsu HR. Randomized trial of umbilical arterial catheter position: clinical outcome. Acta Paediatrica 1993; **82**(2):173.
48. Kessell G, Barker I. Leg ischaemia in an infant following accidental intra-arterial administration of atracurium treated with caudal anaesthesia. Anaesthesia 1996; **51**(12):1154.
49. Kocis KC, Vermilion RP, Callow LB, Kulik TJ, Ludomirsky A, Bove EL. Complications of femoral artery cannulation for perioperative monitoring in children. Journal of Thoracic & Cardiovascular Surgery 1996; **112**(5):1399.
50. Lawless S, Orr R. Axillary arterial monitoring of pediatric patients. Pediatrics 1989; **84**(2):273.
51. Lehmiller DJ, Kanto WP. Relationships of mesenteric thromboembolism, oral feeding, and necrotizing enterocolitis. Journal of Pediatrics 1978; **92**(1):96.
52. Mandel MA, Dauchot PJ. Radial artery cannulation in 1,000 patients: precautions and complications. Journal of Hand Surgery – American Volume 1977; **2**(6):482.
53. Mann NP. Gluteal skin necrosis after umbilical artery catheterisation. Archives of Disease in Childhood 1980; **55**(10):815.
54. Marsh JL, King W, Barrett C, Fonkalsrud EW. Serious complications after umbilical artery catheterization for neonatal monitoring. Archives of Surgery 1975; **110**(10):1203.
55. Marshall AG, Erwin DC, Wyse RK, Hatch DJ. Percutaneous arterial cannulation in children. Concurrent and subsequent adequacy of blood flow at the wrist. Anaesthesia 1984; **39**(1):27.
56. McFadden PM, Ochsner JL, Mills N. Management of thrombotic complications of invasive arterial monitoring of the upper extremity. Journal of Cardiovascular Surgery 1983; **24**(1):35.
57. Merten DF, Vogel JM, Adelman RD, Goetzman BW, Bogren HG. Renovascular hypertension as a complication of umbilical arterial catheterization. Radiology 1978; **126**(3):751.
58. Mitchell SJ, Gray J, Morgan ME, Hocking MD, Durbin GM. Nosocomial infection with *Rhizopus microsporus* in preterm infants: association with wooden tongue depressors [see comments]. Lancet 1996; **348**(9025):441.
59. Mortensson W, Hallbook T, Lundstrom NR. Percutaneous catheterization of the femoral vessels in children. II. Thrombotic occlusion of the catheterized artery: frequency and causes. Pediatric Radiology 1975; **4**(1):1.
60. Mortensson W, Hallbook T, Lundstrom NR. Percutaneous catheterization of the femoral vessels in children. I. Influence on arterial peak flow and venous emptying rate in the calves. Pediatric Radiology 1975; **3**(4):195.
61. Murray JM, Mowbray A. Local tissue oxygenation following radial artery cannulation. Anaesthesia 1987; **42**(10):1070.
62. Norero C, Oto MA, Morales B *et al.* [Renal artery thrombosis in newborn infants undergoing umbilical artery catheterization.] Revista Chilena de Pediatria 1989; **60**(6):346.
63. O'Neill JA, Neblett WWd, Born ML. Management of major thromboembolic complications of umbilical artery catheters. Journal of Pediatric Surgery 1981; **16**(6):972.
64. Olinsky A, Aitken FG, Isdale JM. Thrombus formation after umbilical arterial catheterisation. An angiographic study. South African Medical Journal 1975; **49**(36):1467.

65. Oppenheimer DA, Carroll BA, Garth KE. Ultrasonic detection of complications following umbilical arterial catheterization in the neonate. Radiology 1982; **145**(3):667.
66. Piotrowski A, Kawczynski P. Cannulation of the axillary artery in critically ill newborn infants. European Journal of Pediatrics 1995; **154**(1):57.
67. Plumer LB, Kaplan GW, Mendoza SA. Hypertension in infants – a complication of umbilical arterial catheterization. Journal of Pediatrics 1976; **89**(5):802.
68. Powers WF, Swyer PR. Limb blood flow following umbilical arterial catheterization. Pediatrics 1975; **55**(2):248.
69. Prian GW. Complications and sequelae of temporal artery catheterization in the high-risk newborn. Journal of Pediatric Surgery 1977; **12**(6):829.
70. Prian GW. Temporal artery catheterization for arterial access in the high risk newborn. Surgery 1977; **82**(5):734.
71. Rajani K, Goetzman BW, Wennberg RP, Turner E, Abildgaard C. Effect of heparinization of fluids infused through an umbilical artery catheter on catheter patency and frequency of complications. Pediatrics 1979; **63**(4):552.
72. Randel SN, Tsang BH, Wung JT, Driscoll JM, James LS. Experience with percutaneous indwelling peripheral arterial catheterization in neonates. American Journal of Diseases of Children 1987; **141**(8):848.
73. Rhee KH, Berg RA. Antegrade cannulation of radial artery in infants and children. Chest 1995; **107**(1):182.
74. Roulet M, Prod'hom LS. [Necrotizing enterocolitis in the neonatal period. Revue of 19 cases proved by anatomopathologic examination.] Helvetica Paediatrica Acta 1979; **34**(5):405.
75. Rubin BK, McRobert E, O'Neill MB. An alternate technique to determine umbilical arterial catheter length. Clinical Pediatrics 1986; **25**(8):407.
76. Sahn DJ, Goldberg SJ, Allen HD *et al.* A new technique for noninvasive evaluation of femoral arterial and venous anatomy before and after percutaneous cardiac catheterization in children and infants. American Journal of Cardiology 1982; **49**(2):349.
77. Saia OS, Rubaltelli FF, D'Elia RD *et al.* Clinical and aortographic assessment of the complications of arterial catheterization. European Journal of Pediatrics 1978; **128**(3):169.
78. Schober PH. [Percutaneous cannulation of the radial artery in severely ill premature and newborn infants.] Wiener Klinische Wochenschrift 1990; **102**(16):476.
79. Seibert JJ, McCarthy RE, Alexander JE, Taylor BJ, Seibert RW. Acquired bone dysplasia secondary to catheter-related complications in the neonate. Pediatric Radiology 1986; **16**(1):43.
80. Selby IR, Darowski MJ. Compartment syndrome in a child occurring after femoral artery cannulation. Paediatric Anaesthesia 1995; **5**(6):393.
81. Sfeir R, Khoury S, Khoury G, Rustum J, Ghabash M. Ischaemia of the hand after radial artery monitoring. Cardiovascular Surgery 1996; **4**(4):456.
82. Shaw JCL. Arterial sampling from the radial artery in premature and full-term infants. Lancet 1968; **2**(7564):389.
83. Sheridan RL, Weber JM, Tompkins RG. Femoral arterial catheterization in paediatric burn patients. Burns 1994; **20**(5):451.
84. Skovranek J, Samenek M. Chronic impairment of leg muscle blood flow following cardiac catheterization in childhood. American Journal of Roentgenology 1979; **132**(1):71.
85. Smith C, Green RM. Pediatric vascular injuries. Surgery 1981; **90**(1):20.
86. Smith-Wright DL, Green TP, Lock JE, Egar MI, Fuhrman BP. Complications of vascular catheterization in critically ill children. Critical Care Medicine 1984; **12**(12):1015.
87. Spahr RC, MacDonald HM, Holzman IR. Catheterization of the posterior tibial artery in the neonate. American Journal of Diseases of Children 1979; **133**(9):945.
88. Stevens PS, Mandell J. Urologic complications of neonatal umbilical arterial catheterization. Journal of Urology 1978; **120**(5):605.
89. Tyson JE, deSa DJ, Moore S. Thromboatheromatous complications of umbilical arterial catheterization in the newborn period. Clinicopathological study. Archives of Disease in Childhood 1976; **51**(10):744.
90. [UACTSG] Umbilical Artery Catheter Trial Study Group. Relationship of intraventricular hemorrhage or death with the level of umbilical artery catheter placement: a multicenter randomized clinical trial. Pediatrics 1992; **90**(6):881.
91. Wall PM, Kuhns LR. Percutaneous arterial sampling using transillumination. Pediatrics 1977; **59**(Suppl 6 Pt 2):1032.
92. Wessel DL, Keane JF, Fellows KE, Robichaud H, Lock JE. Fibrinolytic therapy for femoral arterial thrombosis after cardiac catheterization in infants and children. American Journal of Cardiology 1986; **58**(3):347.

Index